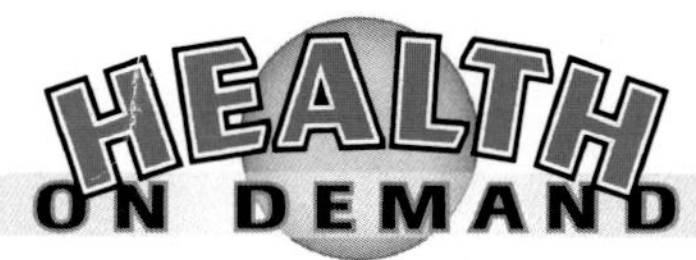

DYNAMIC HEALTH AND HUMAN MOVEMENT

Human Kinetics

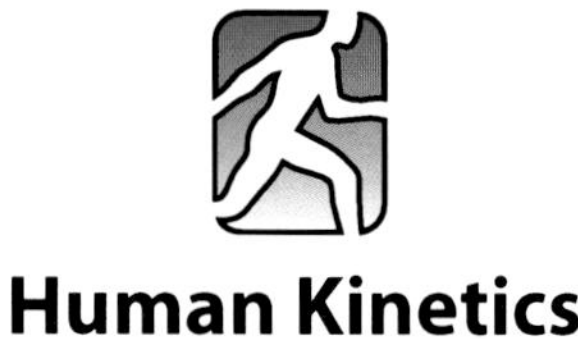

ISBN-13: 978-0-7360-9019-3

Copyright © 2010 by Human Kinetics, Inc.

All rights reserved. Except for use in a review, the reproduction or utilization of this work in any form or by any electronic, mechanical, or other means, now known or hereafter invented, including xerography, photocopying, and recording, and in any information storage and retrieval system, is forbidden without the written permission of the publisher.

The Web addresses cited in this text were current as of February 2009, unless otherwise noted.

Acquisitions Editors: Scott Wikgren, Cheri Scott, and Anna Rinaldi
Developmental Editor: Ray Vallese
Assistant Editor: Derek Campbell
Special Projects Editor: Coree Clark
Copyeditor: Alisha Jeddeloh
Proofreader: Red Inc.
Indexer: Nancy Ball
Permission Manager: Dalene Reeder
Graphic Designer: Fred Starbird
Graphic Artist: Angela K. Snyder
Cover Designer: Keith Blomberg
Photographer (interior): Neil Bernstein, unless otherwise noted
Photo Asset Manager: Laura Fitch
Visual Production Assistant: Joyce Brumfield
Photo Production Manager: Jason Allen
Art Manager: Kelly Hendren
Associate Art Manager: Alan L. Wilborn
Illustrators: Katherine Auble, Joanne Brummett, Tim Brummett, Mike Meyers, Gisela Kraus, Rachel Rogge, Becky Oles, and Heidi Richter
Printer: Mercury

Printed in the United States of America

10 9 8 7 6 5 4 3

The paper in this book is certified under a sustainable forestry program.

Human Kinetics
Web site: www.HumanKinetics.com

United States: Human Kinetics
P.O. Box 5076
Champaign, IL 61825-5076
800-747-4457
e-mail: humank@hkusa.com

Canada: Human Kinetics
475 Devonshire Road Unit 100
Windsor, ON N8Y 2L5
800-465-7301 (in Canada only)
e-mail: info@hkcanada.com

Europe: Human Kinetics
107 Bradford Road
Stanningley
Leeds LS28 6AT, United Kingdom
+44 (0) 113 255 5665
e-mail: hk@hkeurope.com

Australia: Human Kinetics
57A Price Avenue
Lower Mitcham, South Australia 5062
08 8372 0999
e-mail: info@hkaustralia.com

New Zealand: Human Kinetics
P.O. Box 80
Torrens Park, South Australia 5062
0800 222 062
e-mail: info@hknewzealand.com

E5061

CONTENTS

PREFACE

If I knew I was going to live this long, I would have taken better care of myself.

—*attributed to Mickey Mantle (and others)*

If you're like many college students, you're enjoying independence, self-exploration, meeting new friends, and experiencing new things. You might be on your own for the first time in your life, making your own lifestyle choices. It is now, during these years of growth and maturation, that your health habits, whether good or bad, are established and sometimes carried well into adulthood. And, like Mickey Mantle, you're probably not thinking about the long-term effects of the decisions you're making. This book will help you make informed decisions regarding your health and wellness. The decisions are yours, but we provide you with the best information available to help you.

People are living longer and healthier than ever before in history. Increases in life span and quality of life are due to many medical breakthroughs, countless research studies, and an increase in health literacy. In an article that received considerable attention from federal, state, and local public health officials, McGinnis and Foege (1993) argued that the real causes of death are related to behavior or the environment. The shift in public health from prevention of infectious disease to prevention of chronic disease eventually funneled down to the health education curriculum being taught in schools. State and federal government mandates the prevention-based education that is in schools today.

In Healthy People 2010, the U.S. Department of Health and Human Services defines health literacy as "the degree to which individuals have the capacity to obtain, process, and understand basic health information and services needed to make appropriate health decisions" (National Network of Libraries of Medicine 2008). Health literacy is important so that you can learn how to communicate with your doctors, read and interpret health literature, and have the skills to manage your health and prevent disease.

The importance of *Dynamic Health and Human Movement* establishes the relationship between learning and doing. Scenarios, examples, tips, and recommendations apply to your world and bridge the gap between learning about health and applying it to your everyday life. The textbook features a conversational tone and includes questions for assessment, review, and discussion; learning objectives; activities; and sidebars on topics in the news and culture to help you understand what you read and retain what you learn. Special focus is given to timely and controversial issues, encouraging you to think critically about media and advertising. Special elements on steps for behavioral change and the mind–body connection also show you how to take action to address health issues to improve mental and physical health.

As the scientific links between environment and health become stronger, awareness of how lifestyle choices affect health is more important than ever before. *Dynamic Health and Human Movement* provides you with the tools to increase your health literacy and make educated decisions about your health now and in the future.

WHAT YOU'LL FIND IN THIS BOOK

The 12 chapters in *Dynamic Health and Human Movement* cover a broad range of topics to help you make informed choices about your health and wellness.

Chapter 1, Health Promotion, explains the difference between health and wellness, the six dimensions of wellness, and the many components of fitness. It also looks at the promotion of health, wellness, and fitness in the United States. It shows you how to set goals to establish or improve healthy behaviors and helps you understand how and why we might make (or don't make) changes in our lifestyles.

Chapter 2, Fitness Basics, explores health-related fitness—the ability of your body to carry out everyday activities—and its five components: cardiorespiratory fitness, muscular strength, muscular endurance, flexibility, and body composition. It also delivers the practical information you need to stay physically active in college and throughout your adult life.

In chapter 3, Nutrition, you'll learn about the macronutrients (protein, fat, carbohydrate, and water) and micronutrients (vitamins and minerals) in the human diet and how to determine the dietary guidelines you need for maintenance, growth, and activity. The chapter also covers the safe handling of food to prevent foodborne illnesses and the specific dietary needs of vegetarians, pregnant women, and other populations.

Chapter 4, Weight Management, explains the nature and ramifications of the current obesity epidemic in the United States. It can be challenging to maintain a healthy body weight, but understanding the energy equation and applying it to your own behaviors is a great place to start. This chapter shows you how to develop and implement solutions for weight management that are effective, healthy, and long lasting.

When considering your health, don't focus solely on the physical. As explained in chapter 5, Mental Health, good mental health is important for your overall sense of well-being and your ability to adapt, maintain balance, and manage difficult situations. No one should let the stigma of mental illness prevent him or her from seeking treatment when necessary. This chapter helps you learn to recognize and deal with the signs and symptoms of mental illness in yourself or in others.

Chapter 6, Stress Management, teaches you how to handle the various kinds of stress that come from work, school, family, and major life changes. Health risks associated with stress can affect how well your body's systems function, and stress can be a factor in cancer, hypertension, and other diseases. Not everyone finds the same things to be stressful or deals with stress the same way, but you can learn some simple, positive management techniques such as meditation, muscle relaxation, and exercise.

Sometimes it can be difficult to stay healthy when everyone around you seems sick. Chapter 7, Infectious Diseases, shows you that while germs might be everywhere, you can take control of your behaviors and lifestyle choices to reduce your chance of developing an infectious disease. You'll learn about the major methods of transmission and causes of infectious diseases; the management of risk factors; the components of your immune system; and the causes, symptoms, and treatments of common infectious diseases.

Chapter 8, Chronic Diseases, explains how long-term diseases—such as cardiovascular disease, lung disease, cancer, arthritis, diabetes, and Alzheimer's disease—place burdens not only on the patients but also on society as a whole. Genetics plays a role in your risk of developing a chronic disease, but the good news is that maintaining a healthy lifestyle can be the best prevention strategy.

Do you know an HMO from a PPO? Have you thought much about your health care? For many people, college is the time when they begin to make decisions about choosing doctors, obtaining health insurance, paying for health care costs, and making choices about prescriptions and over-the-counter medications. Chapter 9, Health Care Consumerism, helps you learn how to make informed decisions about your health care. It also covers common alternative care options, including acupuncture, chiropractic medicine, massage, and herbal medicine.

Chapter 10, Environmental Health, looks at how our interactions with nature affect our own health—how environmental factors may have an adverse effect on human health or on the ecological balances that are essential to our long-term health and to the quality of the environment. You'll learn about ecosystems, climate change, and the impact of toxins, pollution, and waste. You'll get tips on going green and reducing your personal waste, and you'll learn about other ways to improve your environmental health behaviors.

How old is *old*? The answer depends on whom you ask. Chapter 11, Healthy Aging, describes how organs and body systems age, how people become more susceptible to chronic diseases, and how everyone must make decisions about treatment and care options in later years. Genetics plays a part in how you age and whether you'll be more susceptible to disease, but your lifestyle choices—such as exercising, healthy eating, and social relationships—have an even greater impact.

Chapter 12, Wellness Throughout Life, shows you how maintaining your wellness (not simply your health) is an essential part of living a healthy, happy, and productive life. Health and wellness aren't just goals to achieve but the results of a lifelong process. In this chapter, you'll learn the dimensions of wellness, the factors that influence health and wellness, and how you can change your behaviors if necessary.

WHAT YOU'LL FIND ONLINE

Dynamic Health and Human Movement is part of the Health on Demand series, and you can learn more about the series at www.HumanKinetics.com/HealthOnDemand. That Web site also provides an online student resource (OSR) that complements the textbook. For each chapter in the book, the OSR offers several extended discussions of relevant topics to help you expand your knowledge, as well as links to other pertinent sites for further exploration. In the OSR, you'll also find glossaries of terms and definitions from the book, along with answers to the review questions at the end of each chapter so that you can check your understanding of key points.

Your teacher might ask you to visit the OSR and explore its topics in conjunction with activities or assignments for chapters, but you can also check out the site on your own whenever you want to learn more about what you're reading.

REFERENCES

McGinnis, J.M., and W.H. Foege. 1993. Actual causes of death in the United States. *Journal of the American Medical Association* 270 (18): 2207-2212.

National Network of Libraries of Medicine. 2008. Health literacy. http://nnlm.gov/outreach/consumer/hlthlit.html.

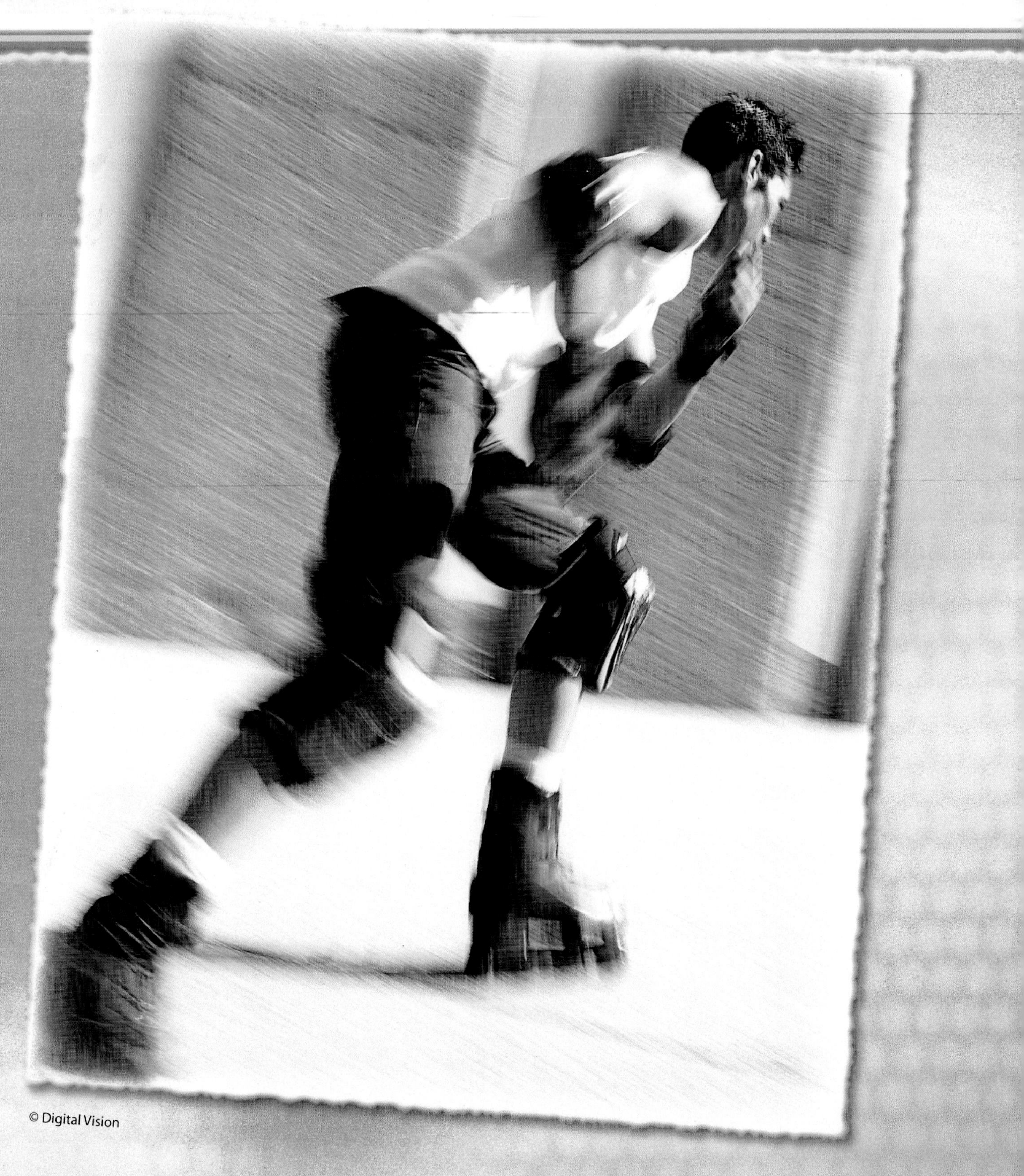

© Digital Vision

CHAPTER 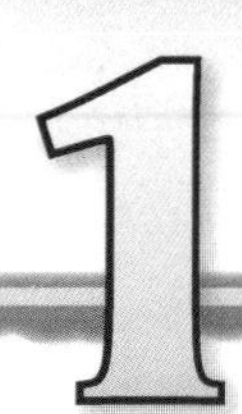

HEALTH PROMOTION

KELLI O'NEIL, MA, CSCS
University of Iowa

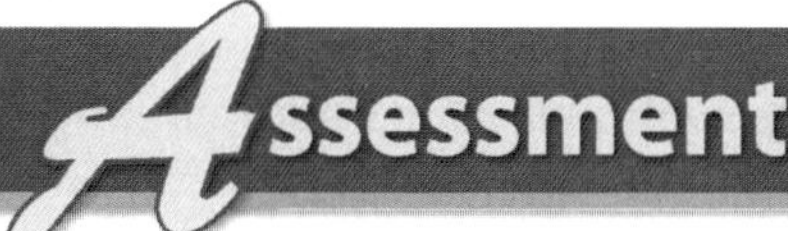

Assessment

- What are the six dimensions of wellness, and how can you attain them?
- Certain strategies can enhance the success of your behavior changes to promote your health. What are some strategies you use when you want to change a behavior?
- How much moderate-intensity physical activity should adults engage in on most days of the week?
- What can you do to improve your fitness? How is this different from enhancing health or wellness? Why is it important to know the difference?
- What is involved with setting SMART goals?
- What might motivate you to change your health behavior? Is it just fear of illness or something more?

Objectives

- Define *health*, *wellness*, and *fitness*.
- Analyze and synthesize factors influencing behavior change.
- Apply SMART goals and motivation strategies to a variety of scenarios.
- Discuss theories and models of behavior change.

Scott has not missed a day of work in 3 years. He does not eat many fatty foods. But if he wants something that is more than a block away, he drives. How would you describe Scott? Would you call him healthy, or fit, or well? What's the difference, anyway? There *is* a difference, and this chapter will teach you what it is. It'll also teach you how to set effective goals so that you can begin the process of reaching all three.

HEALTH AND WELLNESS

On a simplistic level, **health** can be defined as the absence of illness, or as the state when body and mind are absent of abnormality. René Dubos, advisor to the 1972 United Nations Conference on the Human Environment, coined the phrase, "Think globally, act locally." He expanded the Western view of health to include interaction with physical surroundings, defining health as the result of complex interactions between a person and the environment in five dimensions: physical, mental, emotional, spiritual, and social (Moore 2005). Today's definition of health often includes environmental health as a sixth dimension.

Wellness builds on this definition to acknowledge that there are varying degrees of health within each dimension. A state of wellness exists on a continuum, from premature death on one end to optimal potential in one or more dimensions of health on the other (Corbin and Lindsey 2007; Donatelle 2006). The key to wellness is balance among the dimensions of health and their interaction with the environment.

The *six* dimensions of wellness model was developed by Dr. Bill Hettler, cofounder and president of the board of directors of the National Wellness Institute (2007). The model demonstrates that all six types of wellness—physical, intellectual, emotional, social, spiritual, and occupational—must be present for a person to attain overall wellness (see figure 1.1). Your efforts to attain wellness now will become a foundation for the rest of your life.

Physical Wellness

Physical wellness refers to wellness of the physical body. It's influenced by factors such as body weight, physical fitness, and ability to perform day-to-day functions (lifting groceries or climbing stairs). You maintain physical wellness by exercising regularly, eating a healthy and well-balanced diet, making educated decisions about your health, avoiding unhealthy habits such as drug and tobacco use, and receiving adequate medical care. Remember these two tenets of physical wellness:

1. It is better to consume foods and beverages that enhance good health than those that impair it.
2. It is better to be physically fit than out of shape.

Intellectual Wellness

Intellectual wellness addresses creative and mental activities and your openness to new ideas and schools of thought. It also refers to your ability to analyze, synthesize, and act on new information. If you're intellectually well, you'll welcome lifelong intellectual growth and stimulation and you'll look for interaction with the world around you. Here are some tenets of intellectual wellness:

1. It is better to stretch and challenge your mind with intellectual and creative pursuits than to become self-satisfied and unproductive.
2. It is better to identify potential problems and choose appropriate courses of action based on available information than to wait, worry, and contend with major concerns later.

Emotional Wellness

Emotional wellness gives you the ability to get through the rigors of life. Aspects of emotional wellness include self-acceptance, self-confidence, self-control, and trust. Emotional wellness refers to the ability to deal with stress, your ability to be flexible, and your attitude toward yourself and life in general. Emotional wellness also helps you cope and become comfortable with your emotions. If you constantly strive to improve and understand your emotional wellness, you'll likely have a better outlook on life and be able to enjoy life to its fullest. You may also find you have healthier relationships because of this outlook. Remember these tenets of emotional wellness:

1. It is better to be aware of and accept your feelings than to deny them.
2. It is better to be optimistic in your approach to life than pessimistic.

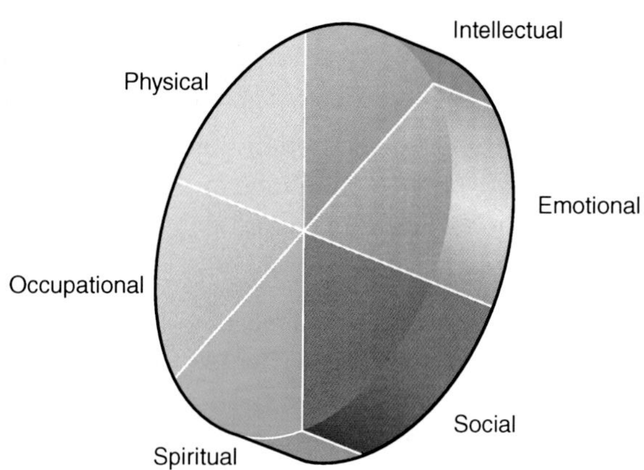

Figure 1.1 To attain overall wellness, you must have all six types of wellness.

Social Wellness

The emphasis behind **social wellness** is being a contributing member of your community and society. You should take an active role in your community and encourage effective communication among community members. The tenets of social wellness are these:

1. It is better to contribute to the common welfare of your community than to think only of yourself.
2. It is better to live in harmony with others and your environment than to live in conflict with them.

Spiritual Wellness

The dimension of **spiritual wellness** focuses on meaning and purpose in life. Aspects of spiritual wellness include the ability to forgive, to show compassion, and to love. Traditional religious beliefs and practices are part of spiritual wellness, but it also encompasses your relationships with other living things and your perception and appreciation of nature, the universe, and the meaning of life. The spiritual dimension also equips you with the ethics, values, and morals that help guide your decisions. These are the tenets of the spiritual dimension:

1. It is better to ponder the meaning of life for yourself and to be tolerant of the beliefs of others than to close your mind and become intolerant.
2. It is better to live each day in a way that is consistent with your values and beliefs than to do otherwise and feel untrue to yourself.

Occupational Wellness

Occupational wellness applies to the personal satisfaction you get from your career. As you strive for occupational wellness, you will see that you contribute your skills and talents to work that is meaningful and rewarding. Occupational wellness includes these tenets:

1. It is better to choose a career that is consistent with your personal values, interests, and beliefs than to select one that is unrewarding for you.
2. It is better to develop functional, transferable skills through structured involvement opportunities than to remain inactive and uninvolved.

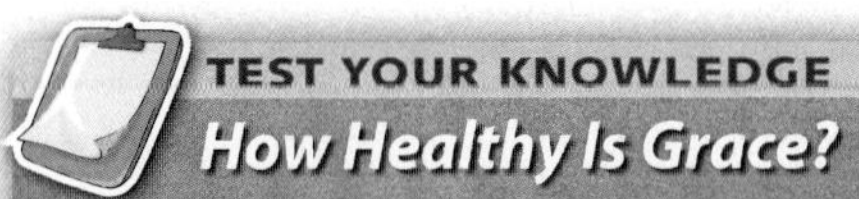

Read the following description of Grace and indicate how you think she fares for each dimension of health. Would you consider her to be well?

At age 23, Grace is a recent university graduate. She completed her English degree with honors, and she still does a lot of creative writing because she loves it. Since she graduated, she's been applying for jobs. She'd like to find something in magazine publishing, but so far she hasn't had any luck, so she's working as a substitute teacher to earn money. She's worried that she's going to need to move in with her parents soon if a better-paying job doesn't turn up, and she's starting to feel discouraged.

Grace's friends are great, though. She and her old roommate see each other several times a week and hang out on most weekends. She stays in touch with old friends from the university literary magazine through phone and e-mail, and they have a great time whenever they get together. Even with their support, though, Grace doesn't feel confident about her career situation. She prays about it a lot, and she can't help but believe there's a plan for her and her life, if she can just be patient as it unfolds.

Another thing Grace prays about is her mom's health. Her mom had a breast cancer scare recently. It turned out to be nothing, but it made Grace think about some of her own health habits. She knows she should exercise more, but her asthma seems to act up when she exerts herself, which makes it hard for her to get motivated.

Grace likes to garden; planting and weeding help take her mind off her job and money troubles. The food she grows gives her a double bonus: It saves money, and it also makes her feel connected to the earth. She did some research for a feature article on global warming, and the things she learned had an influence on her. She tries to be as easy on the environment as she can.

Where do you think Grace falls on each of the following continuums?

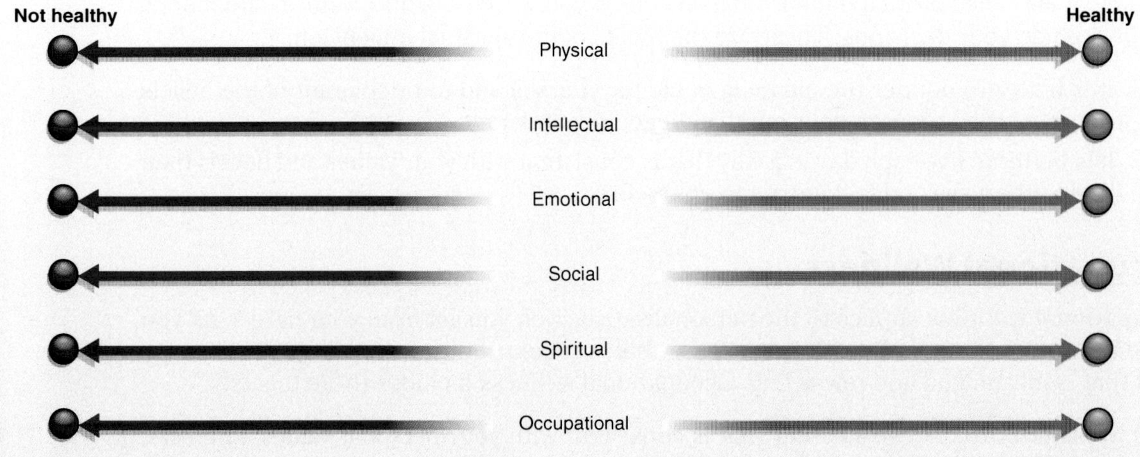

Look at Grace's overall wellness picture. What level of wellness do you think Grace has right now? What are some things she can do to improve her health and wellness?

FITNESS

The term **fitness** is sometimes used interchangeably with health or wellness. That's not the correct use of the term, though. The scope of fitness includes health-related, skill-related, and physiological components (U.S. Department of Health and Human Services [USDHHS] 2000a).

Health-Related Components

- Cardiorespiratory fitness
- Muscular strength
- Muscular endurance
- Flexibility
- Body composition

Skill-Related Components

- Agility
- Balance
- Coordination
- Speed
- Power
- Reaction time

Physiological Components

- Metabolic
- Morphologic
- Bone integrity

Health-Related Components of Fitness

There are five health-related components of fitness: cardiorespiratory fitness, muscular strength, muscular endurance, flexibility, and body composition.

Cardiorespiratory fitness refers to the ability of the cardiovascular and respiratory systems to deliver oxygenated blood to the body. As workload increases, the demand for oxygen increases. **Muscular strength** refers to the intensity of muscular contractions. **Muscular endurance** shares one main quality with cardiorespiratory fitness: stamina. It refers to the ability of the muscles to sustain a contraction or to contract repeatedly over time. **Flexibility** is the ability to move a joint through its complete range of motion (ROM). Good flexibility helps reduce risk of injury, but it's sometimes ignored or forgotten in fitness programs. The final health-related component of fitness is **body composition**. The two main elements of body composition are fat mass and fat-free mass. The proportion of fat mass to total body weight is the percent body fat. Bone, muscle, connective tissue, blood, and organs make up the bulk of its fat-free mass. You can change your body composition by increasing muscle mass while at the same time decreasing fat mass.

Skill-Related Components of Fitness

We just covered the five health-related components of fitness. Now, let's look at the six skill-related factors: agility, balance, coordination, speed, power, and reaction time. These components of fitness relate directly to performance. They relate indirectly to health in that researchers believe that highly skilled people are more likely to participate in regular physical activity (USDHHS 2000a).

- **Agility** is the ability of the body to change direction with precision and speed, which is important in sport-specific skills such as dribbling in soccer or basketball or running pass patterns in football.
- **Balance** helps the body keep a stable position both when it's stationary and when it's moving. Balance is often related to graceful movement.
- **Coordination** is the ability of the body to synchronize sensory reception with movement, such as the eye–hand coordination used in catching a ball.
- **Speed** refers to the ability to perform a task in a short time. Many sports combine speed with the performance of other skills.
- **Power** is the combination of strength (a health-related component) and speed (a skill-related component) and can be expressed as the following: force × distance / time.
- **Reaction time** is the time between a stimulus and when the body first reacts to it. The importance of reaction time is seen as a sprinter leaves the starting blocks at the start of a race or as a softball player swings at a fastball.

The development of these six skill-related components of fitness is thought to enhance athletic performance and promote physical activity (USDHHS 2000a).

What Do You Do?

Pick one of the sports in the list that follows and write a short description of how the skill-related components of fitness would be used by a player in that sport. Here's an example:

Ice Hockey

Agility—Skating around other players to maintain control of the puck
Balance—Staying stable on skates
Coordination—Puck control with the stick while skating and watching opponents
Speed—Moving down the ice to get a puck before the opponent reaches it
Power—Pushing off from a stop to accelerate quickly
Reaction time—A goalie stopping a puck with the glove

When you write the descriptions, you'll realize that each sport differs in which of the skill-related components is most important to success. Here's the list of sports to choose from:

- Lacrosse
- Volleyball
- Basketball
- Field hockey
- Soccer
- Football
- Baseball
- Golf
- Wrestling
- Gymnastics

Physiological Components of Fitness

The last aspect of fitness is physiological. There are three physiologic components: the metabolic component, the morphologic component, and bone integrity (USDHHS 2000a). Physiological components of fitness are linked to how the body adapts to habitual physical activity and are mostly unrelated to performance. In other words, people who exercise regularly tend to score higher on measures of physiologic fitness than people who don't exercise. However, having high levels of physiological fitness doesn't necessarily mean they'll be good athletes.

Metabolic fitness refers to the ability of the body to maintain balance between blood glucose and insulin levels. When this balance is not achieved, abnormalities such as diabetes and hypertension may persist. Regular physical activity promotes healthy body weight, blood pressure, cholesterol, and blood glucose, which are markers of metabolic fitness. Similar to the health-related components of fitness, metabolic fitness is generally not related to athletic performance. Regular physical activity promotes healthy body weight, blood pressure, cholesterol, and blood glucose, which are connected to heart health. Cardiorespiratory exercise contributes to heart health and to improvements in the ability to transport and utilize oxygen during exercise ($\dot{V}O_2max$). However, metabolic fitness is classified independently of $\dot{V}O_2max$.

Morphologic fitness consists of a healthy body composition, including size and mass. This physiological component of fitness is closely linked to metabolic fitness, along with the health-related body composition component. Morphological fitness measurements may include body composition, waist-to-hip circumferences, and body mass index (BMI).

Bone integrity refers to the strength and resilience of bone in regard to preventing fractures. It is typically measured through bone mineral density screenings; however, studies are also examining bone geometry as it relates to bone strength (Lloyd, Petit, Lin, and Beck 2004). Bone integrity is linked to the ability to sustain many of the health- and skill-related components of fitness.

BENEFITS AND GUIDELINES

The U.S. government has funded some important population-based measures of health, wellness, and fitness. The U.S. Surgeon General published a report on physical activity in 1996 that increased public awareness of the benefits of physical activity (USDHHS 1996).

Key benefits include the following:

- Reduced risk of dying prematurely from heart disease, and reduced risk of developing diabetes, high blood pressure, and colon cancer
- Lower blood pressure in people with hypertension
- Reduced feelings of depression and anxiety
- Improved weight management
- Improved strength and agility in older adults
- Greater sense of psychological well-being
- Enhanced building and maintaining of healthy bones, muscles, and joints

More recent studies have examined the relationship between the amount of physical activity (dose) and the resulting degree of health benefits (response) (Brown et al. 2004;

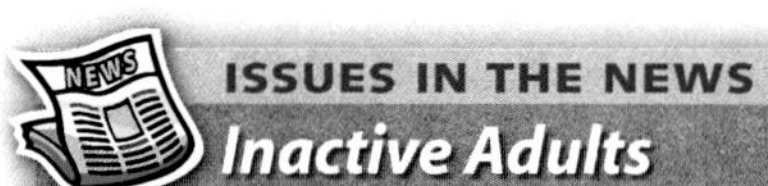

ISSUES IN THE NEWS
Inactive Adults

In spite of all the public health programs to publicize the benefits of physical activity and the risks of not getting enough activity, most adults in the United States aren't meeting the national guidelines for physical activity. Records show that some groups are more likely to be inactive than others (Ainsworth, Sternfeld, Richardson, and Jackson 2000). Identify each group in the following pairs that you think is less likely to be active. Why do you think this is the case?

- Men or women
- Younger or older
- Rich or poor
- White or nonwhite minority groups

(The second group in each pair is less likely to be active.)

Next, research effective ways to design a health promotion program for a health issue of your choice, and target that program to reach out to at least one of the groups above that is less likely to be active. What are some special program features you could include to help underrepresented groups have greater access to physical activity? Would any features work for more than one group?

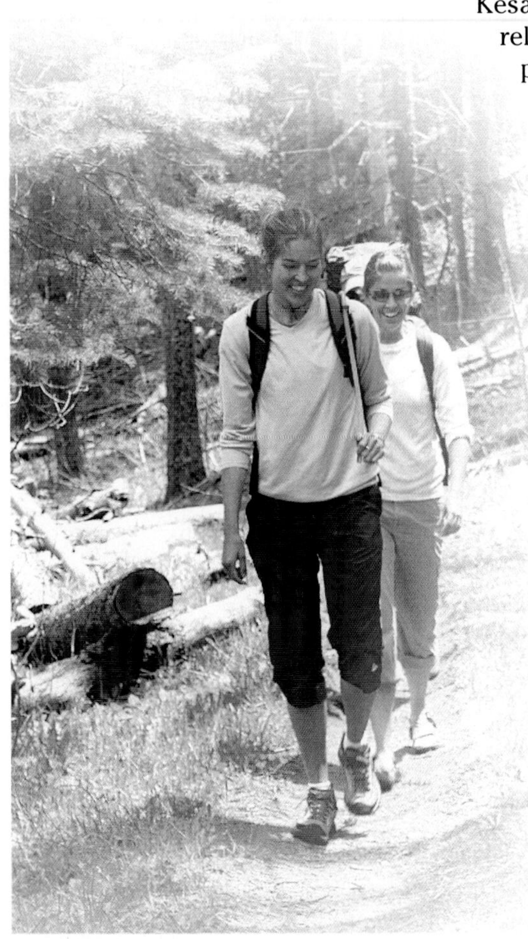

Find physical activities that you enjoy so that you will continue to participate in them.

© Human Kinetics/Luminous World Photography

Kesaniemi, Danforth, and Jensen, 2001). This dose–response relationship suggests that higher levels of physical activity promote greater health benefits (American College of Sports Medicine [ACSM] 2006; USDHHS 1996). Based on this information, the U.S. Surgeon General published standards for the minimum dose of frequency, intensity, and duration of physical activity required for achieving health benefits, which was updated in 2007. According to the most recent report, adults should engage in at least 30 minutes of moderate-intensity physical activity on all or most days of the week, or 20 minutes of vigorous-intensity physical activity on three or more days per week (ACSM 2006; Haskell et al. 2007; USDHHS 1996). Other agencies have developed additional guidelines for physical activity.

Healthy People 2010 is another government-funded health initiative in the United States. It follows a prevention-based structure that outlines key health concerns that are the focus of many health promotion programs. Healthy People 2010 is the basis for many local, state, and national public health programs and focuses on 10 leading health indicators: physical activity, overweight and obesity, tobacco use, substance abuse, responsible sexual behavior, mental health, injury and violence, environmental quality, immunization, and access to health care (USDHHS 2000b). Based on these indicators, a series of focus areas, objectives, and goals were developed to promote successful healthy behavior change for all Americans.

EFFECTIVE GOALS

Perhaps one reason why people don't develop or maintain an activity program in spite of all the evidence that activity improves health, wellness, and fitness is that they don't know how. To create healthy behavior change, it's important to develop a system of evaluation and feedback. Success in making healthy changes requires that a person acknowledge significant issues, measure current status, establish goals, and evaluate progress. The next part of this chapter discusses how to set effective goals for developing habits that will improve your health and fitness now and over the course of your life. After you've learned about goals, apply your knowledge by identifying the characteristics of the goals in figure 1.2.

Types of Goals

What does it mean to be successful? How do you know when you've succeeded? Think of an award or honor you received, a game you won, or a task you completed as a result of working hard. What were the defining characteristics of those successes? Most likely, you set goals, worked toward each goal, and then ultimately achieved them.

Long-Term and Short-Term Goals

It's often easier to reach a big goal by breaking it down into a series of smaller accomplishments. The ultimate goal, or desired end result, is a **long-term goal**, which is the outcome of sustained actions over a significant amount of time. Quitting smoking is an example of a long-term goal for someone who can't quit cold turkey.

To be successful in meeting a long-term goal, it's helpful to have a plan that involves a series of smaller, more immediate goals. These **short-term goals** are more attainable and require small, immediate changes rather than large, sustained changes. Short-term goals for quitting smoking could include chewing gum when the urge to smoke arises or taking a walk to reduce stress.

Outcome, Performance, and Process Goals

Short-term and long-term goals relate to time. Outcome, performance, and process goals involve what you do during that time.

As you'd expect, **outcome goals** focus on the end result—a product or achievement that's attained at the end of a goal phase. **Performance goals**, on the other hand, are generally comparisons (often using statistics) that measure improvement. Performance goals sometimes lead to the achievement of an outcome goal, but they can also be achieved without any change in an outcome goal. For example, a basketball team can limit turnovers (performance) and still lose the game (outcome). Finally, **process goals** emphasize a person's actions during the goal period, such as maintaining good technique during an exercise.

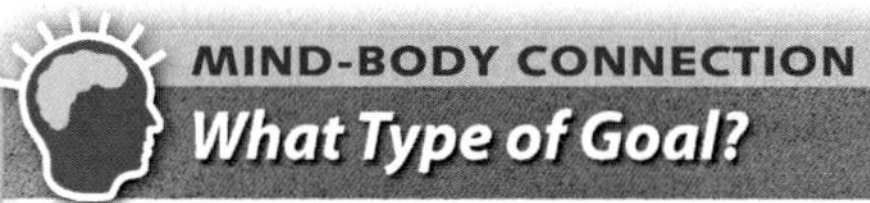

MIND-BODY CONNECTION

What Type of Goal?

Your mindset can affect the results you see physically. Following are some goal achievements related to improving health, skill, or fitness. Match the achievements with the type of goal.

1. Cut the time it takes to complete a 5K race by 12 seconds.
2. Add two poses to a yoga workout.
3. Win the state championship soccer game.
4. Point the thumb toward the pins when releasing the bowling ball.
5. Bench press 100 pounds (45 kilograms).
6. Improve free-throw shooting from 60 percent to 70 percent.
7. Turn the hips forward before swinging the baseball bat.
8. Achieve a BMI of 21.
9. Keep core tight during squats.

a. Outcome goal
b. Performance goal
c. Process goal

Answers: 1) b; 2) c; 3) a; 4) c; 5) a; 6) b; 7) c; 8) a; 9) c

Goal	Long-term or short-term?	Outcome, performance, or process?	Objective or subjective?
To finish the season with a 10–0 record			
To have a perfect passing record in tomorrow's volleyball match			
To develop lifelong friendships with my cross-country teammates			
To increase my squat 1RM by 10% in the next 6 months			
To work on team bonding during our first tournament this weekend			
To cut 12 seconds off my 1 mi (1.6 km) run time by the end of the season			
To make the cheerleading squad after tryouts tomorrow			
To increase my energy level this week by working out			

Figure 1.2 Indicate whether each goal is long term or short term; whether it focuses on outcome, performance, or process; and whether it's objective or subjective.

Objective and Subjective Goals

A final characteristic of goal types is the concept of objective versus subjective measurement of success. **Objective goals** are quantitative, and it is easy to measure success. For example, you can measure how much body fat you lose, how many push-ups you can complete, or how much you can increase your service percentage in volleyball.

Subjective goals are qualitative and represent intangible aspirations, such as "to play as a team" or "to do my best." Subjective goals usually aren't measured and reported in an empirical sense, but they can be important in developing a sense of purpose, pride, and teamwork.

Factors That Influence Behavior Change

Factors in your personal life and in your environment work together in complex ways to influence health-related behavior (see figure 1.3). The way these factors combine and overlap influences the degree to which you'll understand, sustain, and modify health-related behaviors.

Existing conditions that increase the likelihood for certain behaviors are called **predisposing factors**. For example, a person who understands the importance of dental hygiene may be more likely to practice preventive dental care than someone who lacks this type of knowledge. **Reinforcing factors** include various forms of incentives, support, and encouragement that might come from individuals, peer groups, organizations, or communities. Refer to "Setting SMART Goals" for more information on reinforcement of health-related behaviors. **Enabling factors** include features that influence the convenience and access of health-related behaviors. For example, the membership cost, location, and hours of an exercise facility influence a person's probability of joining.

Goal orientation is another noteworthy factor. It's part of personality. **Task-oriented people** tend to judge their goal performance in relation to their past performance. **Ego-oriented people**, on the other hand, prefer to compare their achievements with the achievements of others. It's good to figure out which type describes you so you can set goals that motivate you.

Predisposing factors
Race
Culture
Sex
Class
(Dis)ability
Knowledge
Access to health care
Attitude
Rewards
Support
Affordable health care
Community resources
Policy
Access to education
Encouragement
Skills
Wellness
Location
Time
Money
Government priority
Reinforcing factors
Enabling factors

Figure 1.3 The combination of predisposing factors, reinforcing factors, and enabling factors affects your approach to health-related behavior.

Setting SMART Goals

Setting effective goals helps you see clearly if you're meeting them. SMART goals have five characteristics, and each one builds on the one before it. SMART goals are **s**pecific, **m**easurable, **a**chievable, **r**ealistic, and **t**imely (adapted from Doran 1981).

A specific goal focuses less on what you want to achieve than on how you're going to achieve it. A goal to get fit, for example, is too general. A more specific goal would be, "I'm going to keep up with my sister in the 5K run we're going to do at Thanksgiving."

Specific goals are more measurable than general goals. A measurable goal makes it clear when you've achieved it. If you want to keep up with your sister, you need to figure out how fast she runs the 5K. When you can run that distance in that amount of time, you know you've met your goal.

A goal that is specific and measurable may or may not be achievable. It's important to determine whether you're willing to do what it takes to achieve the goal you've set or whether it's even possible. If you're not willing, you'll be less motivated to succeed. For example, if you don't see your sister often, you'll probably want to keep up with her during the race so you have time to talk with her. As a result, you'll think that your goal is worth attempting.

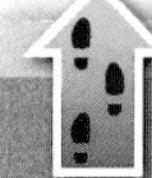

STEPS FOR BEHAVIORAL CHANGE

Matching Factors

Understanding the types of factors that affect your health-related behaviors will help you be better able to make positive changes in those behaviors. Match the following factors with each of the examples:

1. Reward system	a. Predisposing factor
2. Having physically active parents	b. Reinforcing factor
3. Recreation center close to home	c. Enabling factor

Answers: 1) b; 2) a; 3) c

When you have a goal that is specific and measurable and you're willing to do what it takes to succeed, the next step is to figure out if it's realistic. Think about predisposing, reinforcing, and enabling factors. What resources do you need to accomplish the goal you've set? Do you have the factors required for success? If your sister is a champion runner who consistently wins her age group in races, it's probably not realistic for you to think that you could keep up with her during the 5K. But if she's a casual runner, it's possible that with some training you could match her pace.

The last step in setting SMART goals is to place the goal under a time restriction. You already know that you need to be able to run a 5K at the same rate as your sister by Thanksgiving if you're going to meet your goal. That date is important because it helps you know what short-term goals you need to set to reach your long-term goal. For example, you know that you need to develop a running plan that'll gradually increase your speed and endurance over the next few months. You can set monthly goals to measure your progress so that by the time Thanksgiving rolls around, you'll be ready to have a great run with your sister.

What Do You Do?

The goals presented below are not SMART goals. Determine what parts of the SMART approach are missing and then modify each goal to meet the SMART criteria.

- Work harder in school.
- Lose 15 pounds (7 kilograms) in the next month so I can look good at my 5-year high school reunion.
- Win my fantasy football league.
- Do better at keeping my apartment clean.
- Be nicer to my family.

Motivation

Motivation is an intangible representation of desire that influences behavior. You can see behavior, but you can't see motivation. All the same, measures of motivation are often used in psychology-based research. Two broad types of motivation are intrinsic and extrinsic. **Intrinsic motivation** corresponds to feelings inside you that make you want to do something. **Extrinsic motivation**, on the other hand, refers to a system of outward rewards and punishments to influence behavior. Someone who is extrinsically motivated will do something to receive a reward or avoid punishment. Extrinsic motivation tends to work for people who are just beginning a program of behavior change. A reward system can be a successful strategy for sparking interest and helping someone begin to change behavior, but people who are intrinsically motivated tend to stick with behavior change longer.

You should know two other concepts related to motivation: reinforcement and punishment. Both are extrinsic motivators. **Reinforcement** increases the likelihood that someone will repeat a behavior, and **punishment** decreases the likelihood. There are positive and negative forms of reinforcement and punishment. Positive reinforcement provides a reward, causing the person to repeat the behavior to get rewarded again. Negative reinforcement removes a preexisting penalty or undesired activity, such as a chore, to encourage repeated behavior. A person will be motivated to repeat the behavior so as to have fewer chores to do. Positive and negative forms of punishment operate similarly. Positive punishment assigns something unwanted, such as additional chores, to discourage repeating an undesirable behavior. Negative punishment takes away something desirable, such as a privilege, with the hope of avoiding repeated unwanted behavior.

THEORIES AND MODELS OF BEHAVIOR MODIFICATION

Researchers study human behavior so they can figure out ways to help people change unhealthy behavior and maintain their new, healthier habits. Several theories and models of human behavior exist, and we'll cover four of them here. As you read about them, think about which one seems the most reasonable to you or best describes why you have changed or would change your health-related behaviors.

Self-Determination Theory

Self-determination theory says that people do things to either pursue pleasure or to avoid pain, and the degree of pleasure and pain influences motivation to move toward or away from the stimulus (National Strength and Conditioning Association [NSCA] 2004). For example, what motivates a student to study for a midterm? It may be that the student wants to gain more knowledge on the topic being studied. Or it could be that the student wants to avoid failing the test and getting a bad grade in the course. Either way the student is studying for the midterm to pursue the pleasure of learning or avoid the pain of failing an exam. This theory proposes a five-point continuum of how people determine whether they will make a choice to change behavior (see figure 1.4), and those points have varying degrees of intrinsic and extrinsic motivation associated with them (Vallerand and Losier 1999).

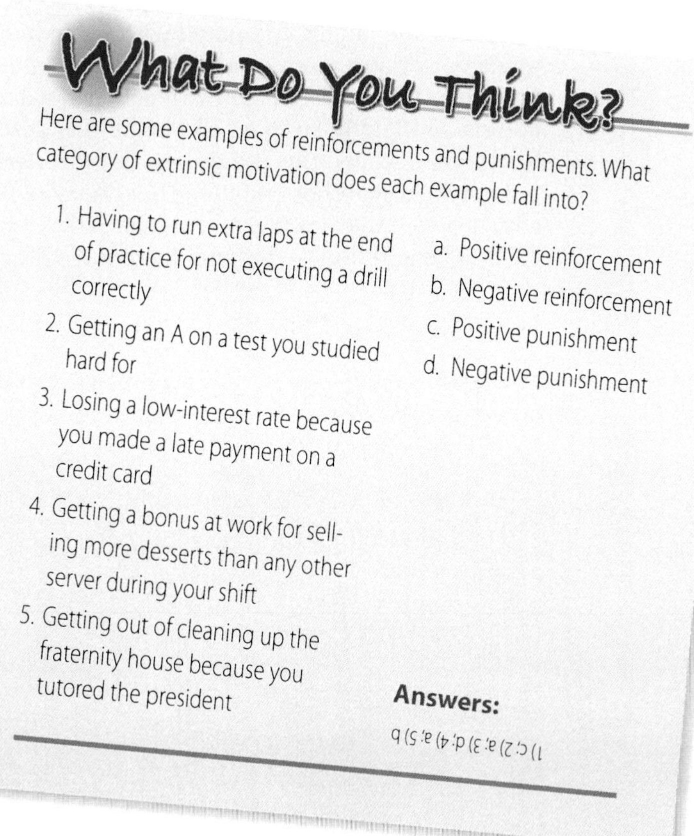

Theory of Reasoned Action and Theory of Planned Behavior

In 1967, researchers determined that people were more likely to change health behaviors when they perceived a positive outcome from the change and believed they had the support

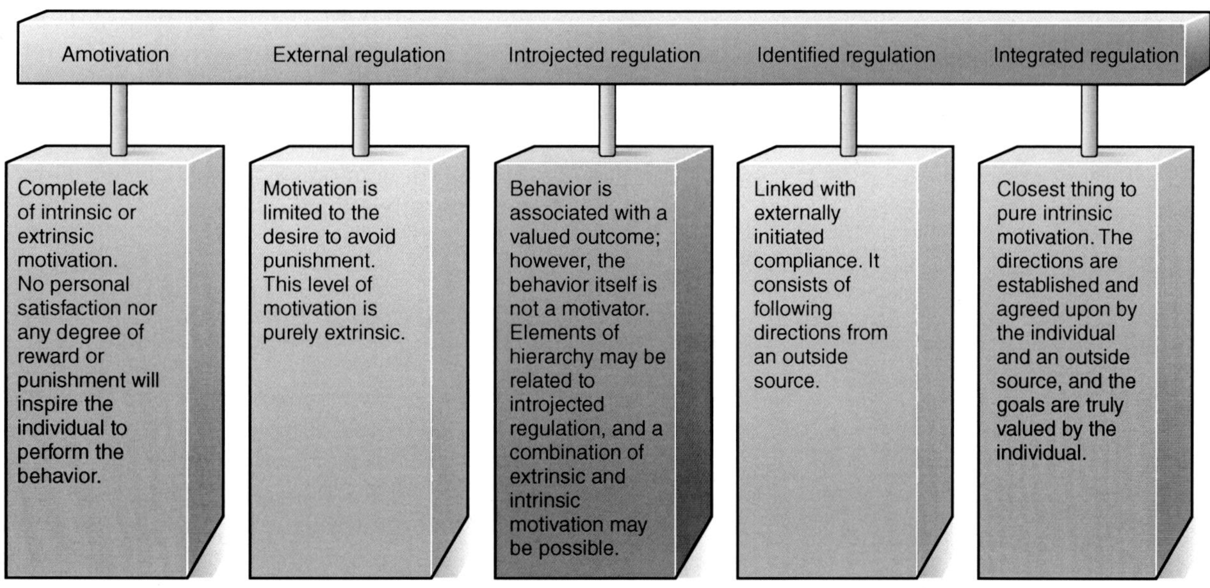

Figure 1.4 The self-determination theory of behavior modification presents a continuum that describes what motivates people to change their behaviors.

of friends and family, compared with someone who perceived a negative outcome or didn't perceive support from others. For example, under this theory, you'd likely get your blood pressure checked if you believe it is beneficial to prevent or control hypertension and if your friends and family support and value this screening effort (Glanz, Rimer, and Lewis 2002). Researchers called this the **theory of reasoned action**.

In 1986, researchers built on the theory of reasoned action when they found that people who believed they could control their behavior had stronger intentions to do so (Glanz et al. 2002). The addition of this supplement resulted in the **theory of planned behavior**.

Health Belief Model

The **health belief model** was developed in the 1950s as a method for explaining the extensive lack of preventive practices and health screenings (Glanz et al. 2002). The model incorporates four basic beliefs. People will engage in a health-related action if

1. they have an interest in health matters (health motivation),
2. they think they are susceptible to a particular illness (perceived vulnerability),
3. they think the benefits of the treatment outweigh the barriers to it (perceived barriers and benefits), and
4. they think a particular illness could be severe (perceived seriousness).

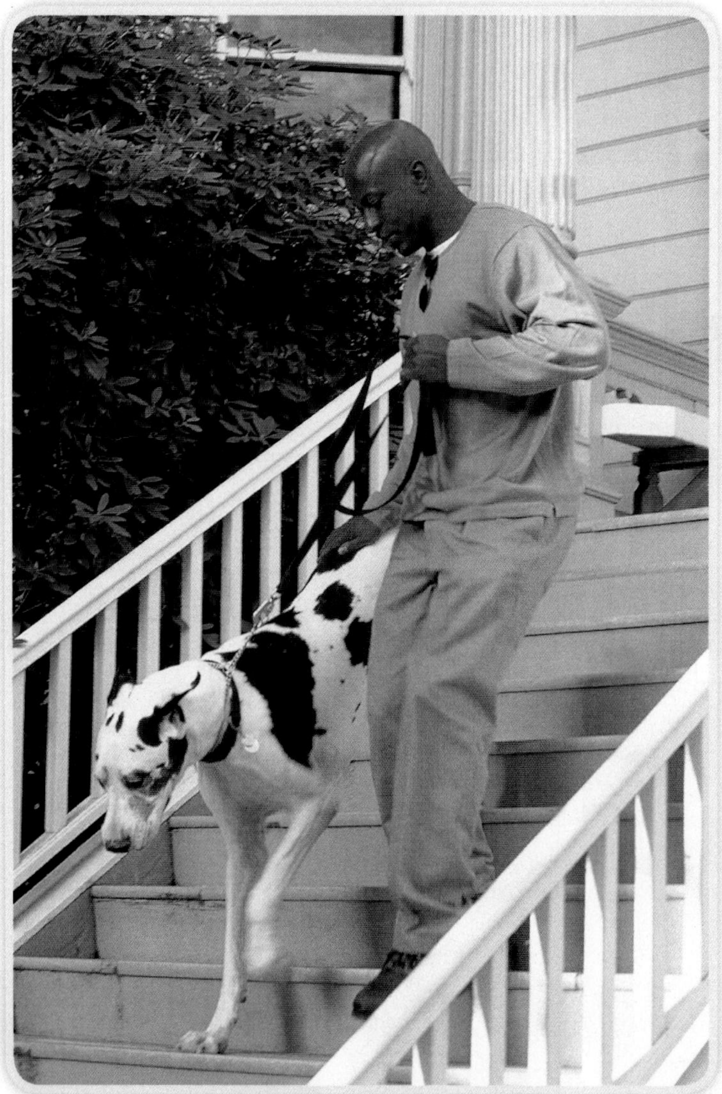

For instance, you might commit to getting daily physical activity if you 1) are interested in preventing diabetes, 2) know you're at risk for developing diabetes, 3) realize that engaging in physical activity is better than dealing with the complications of diabetes, and 4) realize that diabetes is a serious chronic disease with lifelong complications.

The health belief model is an example of a value-expectancy theory because people value the avoidance of ill health and expect to avoid ill health through a specific health-related behavior (Glanz et al. 2002). As another example, if you are motivated by the fear of HIV to start using condoms, you would expect the condoms to protect you from HIV, and you would believe that you can successfully use the condoms. The health belief model explains why people follow a recommended health action.

Transtheoretical Model

The **transtheoretical model** organizes aspects of readiness to change a behavior into five stages of change: precontemplation, contemplation, preparation, action, and maintenance (Glanz et al. 2002). Two additional stages are also sometimes included: termination and

Various factors, including the desire to prevent diabetes and other diseases, can motivate a person to engage in regular physical activity.

© Photodisc

relapse. The stages were developed in 1979 to apply to quitting smoking, but since then researchers have found that the theory can be applied more widely. The five stages in this model aren't fixed or linear. In other words, people don't progress from one stage to another in a straight line. They can cycle through some of the stages or they can jump back and forth from stage to stage.

The first stage of behavior change is the precontemplation stage. People in this stage either don't realize they have some behavior that needs to change or they deny the fact. There's no intention to change behavior within at least the next 6 months. A smoker who isn't thinking about quitting would be in the precontemplation stage.

Contemplation is typically the first stage where a person acknowledges an intention to do something, usually within the next 6 months. This is a fairly safe stage because there's little pressure to make an immediate change. A smoker who knows she should quit smoking but isn't ready to make any change right now is in the contemplation stage.

Preparation is the first active planning stage. People in this stage intend to make a change during the next month and have probably taken some steps to plan for it. A smoker who's looked into a few smoking cessation programs would be in the preparation stage.

When some behavior change has been made, a person is in the action stage. The change had to have occurred less than 6 months ago, though, for the person to still be considered in the action stage. Risk of relapse is high in this stage, and people need a lot of support and ideas about how to resist the temptation to relapse.

Maintenance is often considered the final stage in this theory. Maintenance happens when a person has sustained the new behavior for at least 6 months. There's still some risk of relapse, but it's generally lower in the maintenance stage than in the action stage.

Termination is sometimes included in the stages of change model. The risk of relapse is low and the person believes he has strong control of the situation (Glanz et al. 2002). For example, a former smoker who isn't tempted to smoke anymore, even when drinking alcohol, has reached the termination stage.

Relapse is when someone moves backward in her progress, and it can happen at any point in time, or it may never happen at all. Preparation and action are the two stages where the risk of relapse is the greatest.

HEALTH PROMOTION 101

Health, wellness, and fitness are interdependent, but they're not synonymous. Health refers to the absence of disease or abnormality in each of its dimensions. Wellness expands on that definition by including varying degrees of health within the six dimensions of wellness: physical, intellectual, emotional, social, spiritual, and occupational.

In order to enhance wellness, people often set goals. Effective goal setting provides a system of evaluation and feedback related to healthy behavior change. Goals can be classified as short-term or long-term; outcome, performance, or process; and objective or subjective. A series of complex interactions among predisposing, reinforcing, and enabling factors, along with goal orientation, influences the likelihood of beginning a program of behavior change and sticking with it. In goal setting, SMART goals (i.e., goals that are specific, measurable, achievable, realistic, and timely) ensure that goals are clear and increase the probability that they'll be successfully achieved.

Health-related behavior change is the crux of health promotion. The strategies for starting, keeping, evaluating, and understanding behavior change set the stage for the success of health-related behavior change. Ultimately, health-promotion professionals hope to minimize or eliminate a variety of diseases by enhancing health, wellness, and fitness.

REVIEW QUESTIONS

1. How are health, wellness, and fitness related? How are they different? Provide examples of each.
2. Name the six dimensions of wellness, and list one tenet of each.
3. What are the health-related components of fitness?
4. An athlete wants to increase his agility, speed, and balance. What part of fitness would be enhanced with this improvement?
5. What's the difference between metabolic fitness and morphologic fitness?
6. Name 5 of the 10 leading health indicators of the Healthy People 2010 initiative.
7. Give an example of an outcome goal, a performance goal, and a process goal.
8. Cindy finished a 1-mile (1.5-kilometer) run in 10 minutes. Her next 1-mile run is in 6 months, and she wants to finish it in under 9 minutes. She sets a goal of "run faster." Rewrite her goal so it follows the SMART goal format.
9. Describe how intrinsic motivation and extrinsic motivation work, and explain the benefit of each approach.
10. Which theory or model classifies people into categories related to their readiness to make a change?

CRITICAL THINKING

1. How would you apply strategies for behavior change differently with the subtraction of an unhealthy behavior, such as smoking, versus the addition of a healthy behavior, such as exercise? What differences may exist between people adopting each strategy in regard to motivation and goal setting?
2. Apply each of the four theories or models from this chapter to a situation where you need or want to make a change. Set goals that relate to the topic within the framework of that theory or model. How do theories and models help with the process of behavior change?

APPLICATION ACTIVITIES

1. Using yourself or a made-up example, create a profile for someone who wants to make a health-related behavior change. Include basic aspects about what changes you would like to make.
2. In class, exchange with a classmate (your "client") the behavior-change profiles that you created in the first activity. Based on what your client would like to change, set SMART goals that will lead to the change. Write several goals for the client that include short-term and long-term goals; outcome, performance, and process goals; and objective and subjective goals. Be sure to include a theory or model to support your design, and discuss ways you would use motivation in this scenario.

GLOSSARY

agility—Ability to change direction with great precision and speed.

balance—Helps the body keep a stable position both when it's stationary and when it's moving.

body composition—Components that make up the human body and the proportions of these components, specifically the relative amounts of fat and fat-free mass in the body.

CHAPTER REVIEW

bone integrity—Strength and resilience of bone in regard to preventing fractures.

cardiorespiratory fitness—Ability of the heart and lungs to deliver oxygen and nutrients to the muscles and cells during exercise.

coordination—Ability of the body to synchronize sensory reception with movement, such as the eye–hand coordination used in catching a ball.

ego-oriented people—People who prefer to compare their achievements with those of others.

emotional wellness—Ability to get through the rigors of life; aspects include self-acceptance, self-confidence, self-control, and trust.

enabling factors—Factors that influence the convenience of health-related behaviors.

extrinsic motivation—System of external rewards and punishments to influence behavior.

fitness—Marks a degree of efficiency in three categories: health-related, skill-related, and physiological fitness.

flexibility—Ability of joints to smoothly move through their full range of motion.

health—Absence of illness or abnormality; results from a series of complex interactions between a person and the environment in five dimensions: physical, mental, emotional, spiritual, and social.

health belief model—Behavior change theory that explains why people will participate in a health-related behavior.

intellectual wellness—Involves creative and mental activities and openness to new ideas and schools of thought. Also refers to the ability to analyze, synthesize, and act on new information.

intrinsic motivation—Corresponds to feelings that make you want to do something.

long-term goal—Goal that involves sustained actions over a significant length of time.

metabolic fitness—Ability of the body to maintain balance between blood glucose and insulin levels.

morphologic fitness—Healthy body composition, including size and mass.

muscular endurance—Ability to sustain a muscular contraction or to contract repeatedly.

muscular strength—Maximal force of muscle against resistance.

objective goals—Quantitative goals in which success is measured very specifically.

occupational wellness—Personal satisfaction from your career. As you strive for occupational wellness, you contribute your skills and talents to work that is meaningful and rewarding.

outcome goals—Goals that focus on the end result (a product or achievement that's attained at the end of a goal phase).

performance goals—Goals that involve comparisons (often using statistics) to measure improvement.

physical wellness—Wellness of the physical body; influenced by factors such as body weight, physical fitness, and ability to perform day-to-day functions.

power—Combination of strength and speed.

predisposing factors—Existing conditions that increase the likelihood for certain behaviors.

process goals—Goals that emphasize actions during the goal period.

punishment—Decreases the likelihood that someone will repeat a behavior.

reaction time—Length of time between a stimulus and when the body first reacts to it.

reinforcement—Increases the likelihood that someone will repeat a behavior.

reinforcing factors—Various forms of incentives, support, and encouragement that come from individuals, peer groups, organizations, or communities.

self-determination theory—Theory that people do things to either pursue pleasure or to avoid pain.

short-term goals—Goals that require small, immediate changes rather than large, sustained changes.

social wellness—Wellness that comes from being a contributing member of community and society. Relates to the depth of interpersonal relationships and how you develop and maintain associations in a variety of settings.

speed—Ability to perform a task in a short time: force × distance / time.

spiritual wellness—Meaning and purpose in life; aspects include the ability to forgive, to show compassion, and to love. Traditional religious beliefs and practices are part of spiritual wellness, but it also encompasses relationships with other living things and perception and appreciation of nature, the universe, and the meaning of life.

subjective goals—Qualitative rather than quantitative goals that represent intangible aspirations, such as "to play as a team" or "to do my best."

task-oriented people—People who tend to judge their goal performance in relation to their past performance.

theory of planned behavior—Builds on the theory of reasoned action; holds that people who believe they can control their behavior have stronger intentions to do so.

theory of reasoned action—Theory that people are more likely to change a health behavior when they perceive a positive outcome from the change and believe they have the support of friends and family.

transtheoretical model—Model of individual readiness to change a behavior that involves five stages of change: precontemplation, contemplation, preparation, action, and maintenance.

wellness—Expands upon the definition of health to acknowledge that there are varying degrees of health within each dimension: physical, intellectual, emotional, spiritual, social, and occupational.

REFERENCES AND RESOURCES

Ainsworth, B.E., B. Sternfeld, M. Richardson, and K. Jackson. 2000. Evaluation of the Kaiser Physical Activity Survey in Women. *Medicine & Science in Sports & Exercise* 32: 1327-1338.

American College of Sports Medicine (ACSM). 2006. *ACSM's guidelines for exercise testing and prescription.* 7th ed. Baltimore: Lippincott.

Brown, D.W., D.R. Brown, G.W. Heath, L. Balluz, W.H. Giles, E.S. Ford, and A.H. Mokdad. 2004. Associations between physical activity dose and health-related quality of life. *Medicine & Science in Sports & Exercise* 36: 890-896.

Corbin, C.B., and R. Lindsey. 2007. *Fitness for life.* Updated 5th ed. Champaign, IL: Human Kinetics.

Donatelle, R.J. 2006. *Access to health.* 9th ed. San Francisco: Pearson, Benjamin Cummings.

Doran, G.T. 1981. There's a S.M.A.R.T. way to write management's goals and objectives. *AMA Forum* (November): 35-36.

Glanz, K., B.K. Rimer, and F.M. Lewis. 2002. *Health behavior and health education: Theory, research, and practice.* 3rd ed. San Francisco: Jossey-Bass.

Haskell, W.L., I. Lee, R.R. Pate, K.E. Powell, S.N. Blair, B.A. Franklin, C.A. Macera, G.W. Heath, P.D. Thompson, and A. Bauman. 2007. Physical activity and public health: Updated recommendation for adults from the American College of Sports Medicine and the American Heart Association. *Medicine & Science in Sports & Exercise* 39: 1423-1434.

Kesaniemi, Y.K., E. Danforth Jr., and M.D. Jensen. 2001. Dose-response issues concerning physical activity and health: An evidence-based symposium. *Medicine & Science in Sports & Exercise* 33: S351-358.

Lloyd, T., M. Petit, H. Lin, and T. Beck. 2004. Lifestyle factors and the development of bone mass and bone strength in young women. *Journal of Pediatrics* 144: 776-782.

Moore, V. 2005. Commentary: Biological Freudianism and the quest for understanding the social origins of health. *International Journal of Epidemiology* 34: 1-2.

National Strength and Conditioning Association (NSCA). 2004. *NSCA's essentials of personal training.* Champaign, IL: Human Kinetics.

National Wellness Institute. 2007. Six dimensional wellness model. www.nationalwellness.org/index.php?id_tier=2&id_c=25.

U.S. Department of Health and Human Services (USDHHS). 1996. *Physical activity and health: A report of the Surgeon General executive committee*. Washington, DC: Author.

———. 2000a. Definitions: Health, fitness, and physical activity. www.fitness.gov/digest_mar2000.htm.

———. 2000b. Healthy People 2010. www.healthypeople.gov.

Vallerand, R.J., and G.F. Losier. 1999. An integrative analysis of intrinsic and extrinsic motivation in sport. *Journal of Applied Sport Psychology* 11: 142-169.

Other helpful resources include the following.

Centers for Disease Control and Prevention (CDC). 2008. Physical activity for everyone: How much physical activity do you need? www.cdc.gov/physicalactivity/everyone/guidelines/index.html.

University of Twente. 2004. Health belief model. www.cw.utwente.nl/theorieenoverzicht/Theory%20clusters/Health%20Communication/Health_Belief_Model.doc/.

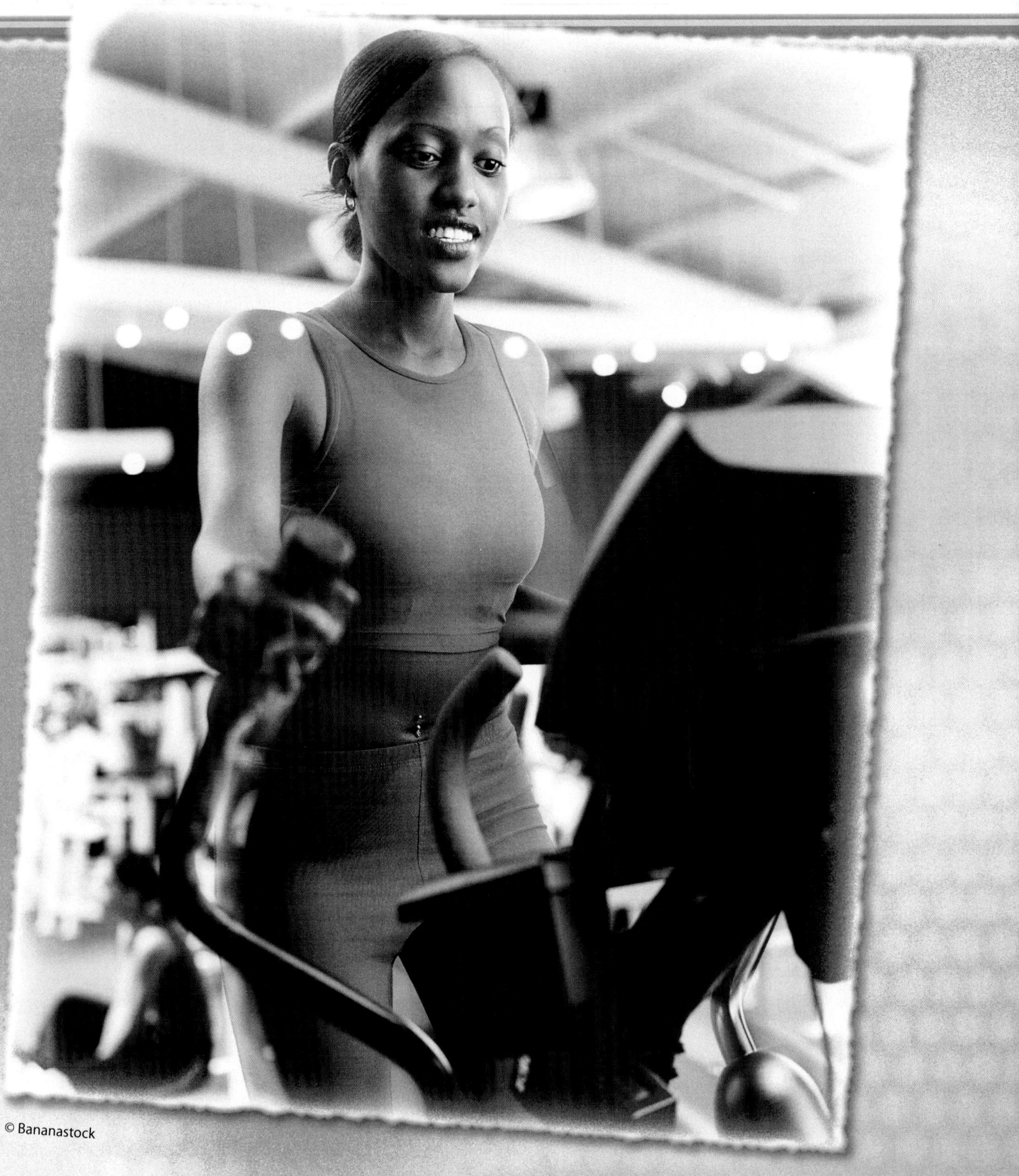

© Bananastock

CHAPTER 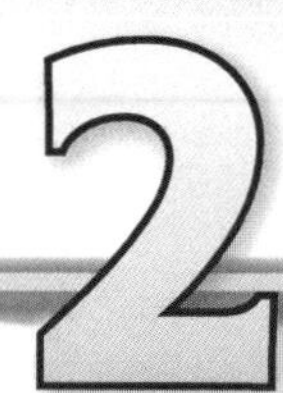

FITNESS BASICS

ANNA RINALDI, MS
University of Illinois

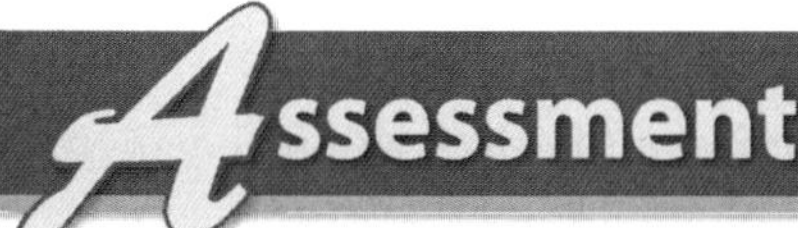

Assessment

- What's the difference between physical activity and physical fitness?
- Is "no pain, no gain" valid or just a myth?
- When doing aerobic activity, how do you know what intensity is right for you?
- How can you use the overload principle to increase your muscular strength and endurance?
- When is the best time to stretch to reduce the risk of injury?
- What are some common barriers to doing regular physical activity, and how can you overcome them?

Objectives

- Identify the five components of health-related fitness and describe the importance of each.
- Describe the benefits of cardiorespiratory fitness and how you can improve and maintain it throughout your life.
- Describe the differences between muscular endurance and muscular strength and how to incorporate both into a well-rounded resistance program.
- Identify basic types of stretches and their importance to overall health.
- Use a variety of resources to stay physically active throughout school.
- Understand how to stay physically active throughout your adult life.

If someone asked you if you were fit, how would you answer? That question would be difficult to answer unless you clarified the question by asking, "Fit for what?" For example, if you're a soccer player, you likely define fitness differently than a firefighter, a musician, an accountant, or a dancer. Regardless of what you do, though, there is a basic level of fitness, called *health-related fitness*. But before you try to answer the question, let's discuss basic fitness terminology.

PHYSICAL ACTIVITY, EXERCISE, AND PHYSICAL FITNESS

There's a difference between being physically active and being physically fit. **Physical activity** is simply moving your body. Exercise, on the other hand, is moving your body for a purpose—specifically, to improve or maintain physical fitness. **Exercise** is physical activity that is planned, structured, and repetitive and is intended to improve or maintain physical fitness.

When you carry a load of laundry to your car, you're doing physical activity. When you lift weights for half an hour to strengthen your muscles, you're exercising. Reaching to get a box of pasta from the top shelf of your cabinet is physical activity; doing a 10-minute stretching routine to improve flexibility is exercise. Going out dancing is doing physical activity; doing a workout DVD is exercising.

Physical fitness is a way of measuring how well the body can perform moderate to vigorous levels of physical activity without becoming overly tired (Insel and Roth 2007). There are three aspects of fitness: skill-related, health-related, and physiological fitness. The two aspects of fitness that can be controlled are skill-related fitness and health-related fitness. **Skill-related fitness** is what allows athletes to be good at their sports. It involves agility, balance, coordination, speed, power, and reaction time. For example, a soccer player who dribbles the ball around a defender shows agility; a softball player who keeps her foot on first base while snagging a throw from second shows coordination; and a receiver who sprints for the end zone shows speed.

This chapter is most concerned, however, about **health-related fitness**, or the ability of the body to carry out everyday activities without excessive fatigue and with enough energy left for emergencies (Donatelle 2008). There are five components of health-related fitness, each of which will be covered later in the chapter:

- Cardiorespiratory fitness
- Muscular strength
- Muscular endurance
- Flexibility
- Body composition

How Fit Are You?

It's important to know if you're fit in the five components of health-related fitness. But, as discussed at the beginning of the chapter, fitness can be relative. There are assessments that will pinpoint your level of physical fitness, however, by comparing your scores with criteria developed through scientific study that set benchmarks in each category of fitness for people of the same age and gender.

Daily activity (your lifestyle and the amount of exercise you do), genetics, nutrition, and health conditions are factors that influence fitness. Although you can't control your genetics or some health conditions, you can control most of the factors that influence your fitness and overall health and well-being.

FITT Principle

The main goal of this course is to help you develop knowledge and habits that will allow you to enjoy a long and healthy life. One foundational concept you need to know is how to gauge

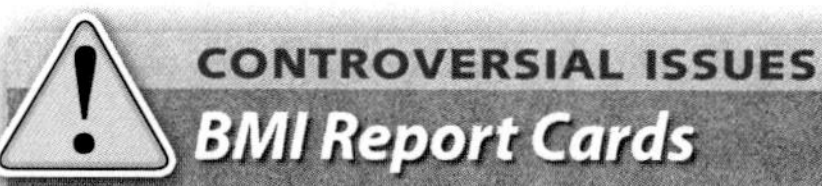

Body mass index (BMI) is a number calculated from a person's height and weight. So BMI does not directly measure body fat, and it does not factor in relative amounts of fat, muscle, and bone. Still, BMI is a valuable predictor of health risks and can be used to screen for weight categories that may lead to health problems (Centers for Disease Control and Prevention [CDC] 2007). In 2003, Arkansas became the first state in the United States to require BMI tests of all its public school students. There were complaints that the tests were embarrassing to many students and no one was offering parents any advice on how to remedy unhealthy BMIs. Do you think that BMI report cards should be sent home to parents? Or is there a better way to alert parents to their children's health status and encourage them to take a more active role in their children's health?

whether your physical activity is vigorous enough to produce fitness benefits. The acronym *FITT* makes it easy to remember the principles involved in turning physical activity into physical fitness:

- **F**requency: How often you do physical activity in a week
- **I**ntensity: How hard you're working while performing the activity
- **T**ime: How long you're doing the activity
- **T**ype: What type of activity you're doing

Later in the chapter, you'll learn how to apply the FITT principle to the various components of physical fitness (cardiorespiratory fitness, muscular strength and endurance, and flexibility).

Warm-Up and Cool-Down

Another concept to keep in mind when exercising is the importance of getting your body ready for an exercise session and letting it recover afterward. Each time you work out, you should perform a warm-up and a cool-down.

The **warm-up** prepares the body to go from rest to exercise. By warming the body up, you stretch core muscles; increase heart rate, blood flow, deep muscle temperature, respiration rate, and perspiration; and increase the viscosity of joint fluid so that the joints feel less stiff (Baechle and Earle 2000). By slowly increasing heart rate, blood flow, and body temperature, you are preparing your body for activity and reducing the risk of injury.

Do a general warm-up first that consists of 5 to 10 minutes of light movement, such as jogging or riding a bicycle, to prepare the body for exercise. Then do a specific warm-up using movements similar to those you'll be doing during the main exercise session. The specific warm-up should last for a few minutes, until you feel ready for exercise (Baechle and Earle 2000). For example, if you're going to be jumping rope, the specific warm-up might include some slow jumps. If you're going to perform biceps curls, the specific warm-up may include a set of biceps curls with little to no weight.

A **cool-down** after the workout is important, too, so that blood doesn't pool in the extremities, which could temporarily disrupt blood flow and deprive the heart and brain of oxygen. Devote 5 to 10 minutes to stretching, walking, or continuing your workout activity at a slower pace (Teague, Mackenzie, and Rosenthal 2007).

Basic Principles of Fitness

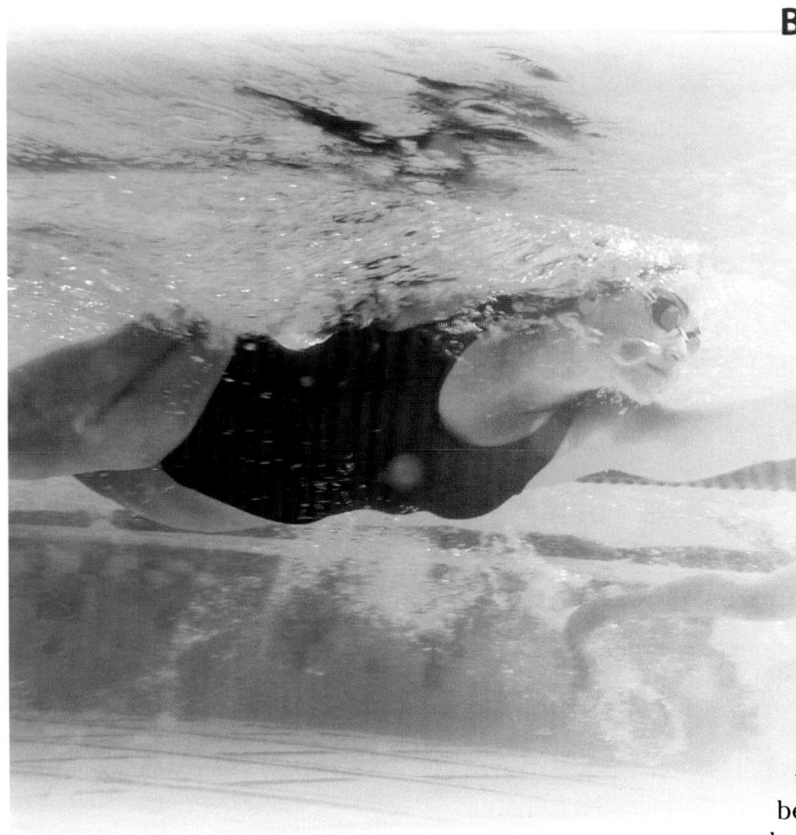

Swimming is a great aerobic exercise for improving your cardiorespiratory fitness.

© Stockbyte

To put together a good fitness program and maintain it, you'll need to remember four basic principles: overload, progression, specificity, and reversibility.

The **overload** principle is just how sounds: Muscles adapt quickly to new requirements, and if you want to make a muscle stronger, you need to make it work harder (overload it) than it's used to working (Sharkey and Gaskill 2007). Overload is relative, though. A person who isn't used to exercising needs only a little extra load to see benefits, whereas a person who is already strong needs a bigger load to see additional fitness gains.

A principle that's closely related to the overload principle is the principle of **progression**. To see consistent improvements in health-related fitness, you need to progressively increase exercise. The important thing to remember is this: If you keep doing what you've always been doing, you'll keep getting what you've always gotten.

The principle of **specificity** refers to the type of exercise you do. Exercise needs to target the training effect you want (Sharkey and Gaskill 2007). If you want to gain cardiorespiratory fitness, strength training probably won't get you far. If you want to improve flexibility, jogging isn't going to help much. Instead, if you want greater aerobic fitness, you need to do things that strengthen the heart and lungs, such as walk, swim, or bike. If you want stronger muscles, then work out with weights. If you want to be more flexible, start stretching more.

The fitness improvements you make through physical activity aren't permanent, and that's what the principle of **reversibility** refers to. When a person stops doing regular exercise (a process called *detraining*), metabolic and exercise capacity decrease significantly within as little as 1 to 2 weeks. Many training improvements are totally lost within several months (McArdle, Katch, and Katch 2001). The implications of this principle are easy to sum up: Use it or lose it. If you don't have time for your full 30 minutes of cardio or you can't fit in your usual 60 minutes of weightlifting, then do what you can. Take a brisk 10-minute walk or get in 20 minutes of weightlifting. Doing something is better than doing nothing.

People respond differently to the same training stimulus (Sharkey and Gaskill 2007). Not everyone can become a world-class bodybuilder, an elite gymnast, or a marathon runner. Heredity, maturity, nutrition, rest, sleep, fitness level, environmental factors, illness or injury, and motivation all contribute to a person's potential for improvement in health- or skill-related fitness. Although you might never be as fast, strong, or flexible as someone else, you can still maintain a level of fitness that will improve your quality of life.

All of these basic principles apply to the FITT principle discussed earlier. You don't have to constantly increase the amount of weight you are lifting to overload the muscle. You can increase the intensity by manipulating one variable while keeping all the other variables constant. Variables you can manipulate include the weight (resistance), the number of repetitions, and the speed of the movement. You could also add more exercises or increase the amount of time you spend in your workout. These principles may seem daunting, but the key is simple: Continually make minor changes to your workout program to get the best results.

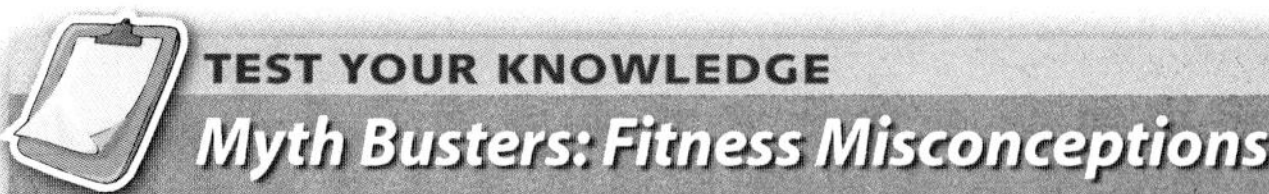

TEST YOUR KNOWLEDGE

Myth Busters: Fitness Misconceptions

Each of the following statements seems as if it could be true, but it's not. Science explains why.

Myth: If I don't eat anything before I exercise, I'll burn more calories.

Busted: You won't burn more calories by not eating; actually, the opposite is true. If you don't have enough fuel in your body to get through a workout, you won't be able to work out as long or intensely as you could if you were well fueled, so you won't be able to burn as many calories. You should consume 200 to 300 calories 1 to 2 hours before exercise.

Myth: To lose fat, you have to exercise at a low intensity in your fat-burning zone.

Busted: You do burn a higher percentage of calories from fat when your heart rate is lower. However, that's only one side of the equation. You may be burning a higher percentage of fat, but you're burning a lower number of calories overall. In weight loss, the key is burning calories, not burning fat. Given the same duration, you would burn more calories and fat working out at a higher intensity even though the percent of fat burned would be lower.

Here's an example: A 150-pound (68-kilogram) person walking for 30 minutes burns approximately 159 calories (70 percent from fat, or about 111 fat calories). The same person jogging for 30 minutes at 5.5 miles (9 kilometers) per hour burns approximately 325 calories (50 percent from fat, or about 162.5 fat calories). The higher intensity burns more calories and fat.

Myth: If I can't work out for a full 60 minutes, then I shouldn't bother working out at all.

Busted: The American College of Sports Medicine (ACSM) recommends 30 minutes of moderate activity most days of the week (ACSM 2006). It's true that more exercise is better than some, but some is better than none! You can benefit from as little as 10-minute bouts of low- to moderate-intensity activity throughout your day. It all adds up and is just as effective as 30 minutes of continuous activity. Try to incorporate more daily activity into your life to benefit from getting a little more activity here and there (Platkin 2003).

Myth: No pain, no gain.

Busted: You'll need to go to the point of discomfort to see fitness gains from exercise, but you don't have to experience pain during exercise to gain improvements. Some soreness is common for first-time exercisers. If the soreness continues, though, you're pushing too hard. Muscles can be sore for up to 48 hours after exercise. This is referred to as **delayed-onset muscle soreness (DOMS)**, which results from inflammation and microscopic tears in the tissues that surround the muscle fibers. To decrease the likelihood of DOMS or risk of injury, start off slow and ease into a new training routine. If you do too much too fast and hurt yourself, then you're back to square one or even worse off than before you started.

CARDIORESPIRATORY FITNESS

If you have a healthy cardiorespiratory fitness level for everyday living, your heart will function efficiently and won't have to work hard during daily activities. Your heart will also be able to sustain high-intensity physical activity in an emergency. The cardiorespiratory fitness level demanded by a soccer player is going to be much higher than that of a bodybuilder, construction worker, or computer technician, but anyone can benefit from a healthy cardiovascular system.

Cardiorespiratory fitness refers to the ability of the heart and lungs to efficiently deliver oxygen and nutrients to the muscles and cells by way of the bloodstream (Teague et al. 2007). The etymology of the term spells it out: *Cardio* refers to the cardiac (heart) system and *respiratory* refers to the respiratory (lungs) system. The heart and the lungs provide oxygenated blood to the body (Jackson, Morrow, Hill, and Dishman 2004).

The benefits of cardiorespiratory fitness are clear. When the heart and lungs are in good shape, the blood can carry more oxygen and the muscles can pull more oxygenated blood out of the bloodstream. The heart pumps more blood with each heartbeat and the body recovers faster from exercise. Training to improve cardiorespiratory fitness improves heart and liver function, decreases resting heart rate, decreases resting blood pressure, and decreases heart rate at any workload (Teague et al. 2007). Not only do you get benefits right away when your cardiovascular system is fit, but there are also long-term benefits, including reduced risk of heart disease, prevention of hypertension, improved blood lipids, improved overall health, and easier everyday functioning.

Guidelines

What does it take to get the benefits of cardiorespiratory fitness? A good goal is to expend 150 to 400 calories in physical activity per day or a minimum of 1,000 calories a week. Table 2.1 shows the approximate number of calories burned per hour while doing some common recreational activities. Use the column that is closest to your weight. (For every 10 pounds you weigh above the listed weight, increase the calories burned by 5 percent. For every 10 pounds you weigh below the listed weight, decrease the calories burned by 5 percent.)

Figuring out the best way to expend calories is where the FITT principle comes in. Various studies have determined the frequency, intensity, time, and type of exercise that helps develop cardiorespiratory fitness.

Frequency

To see improvements in cardiorespiratory fitness, you should do aerobic exercise 3 to 5 days a week (ACSM 2006). Most college students don't get that much exercise (Huang et al. 2003), and most other adults don't either. Figure 2.1 shows the prevalence of people across the United States who meet physical activity recommendations. Figure 2.2 shows the national average of physical activity levels in 2007. (For the figure, "recommended" physical activity is defined as doing moderate-intensity activities at least 30 minutes per day on at least 5 days per week, or doing vigorous-intensity activities for at least 20 minutes per day on at least 3 days per week. "Insufficient" physical activity is defined as doing more than 10 minutes total per week of either but doing less than the recommended level. "Inactive" is defined as doing less than 10 minutes total per week. "No leisure-time physical activity" is defined as doing no physical activities in leisure time, such as walking or gardening, in the previous month.)

Intensity

For most people, intensities within the range of 60 to 80 percent of their **heart rate reserve (HRR)** are good enough to bring improvements in cardiorespiratory fitness (ACSM 2006). People just starting a fitness program may see cardiorespiratory fitness improvements when exercising at intensity levels as low as 40 percent of HRR. As their fitness and health levels improve, they may be able to increase their intensity to produce even greater cardiorespiratory fitness benefits. People who are already in good physical condition or who are athletes need to exercise at the upper end of the HRR range to see further improvements or to maintain their cardiorespiratory fitness levels. In the next section, you'll learn how to find your HRR.

TABLE 2.1 Energy Expenditure

Activity	CALORIES USED PER HOUR				
	100 lb (45 kg)	120 lb (54.5 kg)	150 lb (68 kg)	180 lb (81.5 kg)	200 lb (91 kg)
Backpacking, hiking	307	348	410	472	513
Badminton	255	289	340	391	425
Baseball	210	238	280	322	350
Basketball (half-court)	225	240	300	345	375
Bicycling (normal speed)	157	178	210	242	263
Bowling	155	176	208	240	261
Canoeing (4 mph [6.5 kph])	276	344	414	504	558
Circuit training	247	280	330	380	413
Dance, ballet or modern	240	300	360	432	480
Dance, aerobic	300	360	450	540	600
Dance, social	174	222	264	318	348
Fitness calisthenics	232	263	310	357	388
Football	225	255	300	345	375
Golf (walking)	187	212	250	288	313
Gymnastics	232	263	310	357	388
Horseback riding	180	204	240	276	300
Interval training	487	552	650	748	833
Jogging (5.5 mph [9 kph])	487	552	650	748	833
Judo, karate	232	263	310	357	388
Racquetball, handball	450	510	600	690	750
Rope jumping (continuous)	525	595	700	805	875
Running (10 mph [16 kph])	625	765	900	1,035	1,125
Skating, ice or roller	262	297	350	403	438
Skiing, cross-country	525	595	700	805	875
Skiing, downhill	450	510	600	690	750
Soccer	405	459	540	575	621
Softball (fast pitch)	210	238	280	322	350
Swimming (slow laps)	240	272	320	368	400
Swimming (fast laps)	420	530	630	768	846
Tennis	315	357	420	483	525
Volleyball	262	297	350	403	483
Walking	204	258	318	372	426
Weight training	352	399	470	541	558

Adapted, by permission, from C.B. Corbin and R. Lindsey, 2007, *Fitness for life,* updated 5th ed. (Champaign, IL: Human Kinetics), 231.

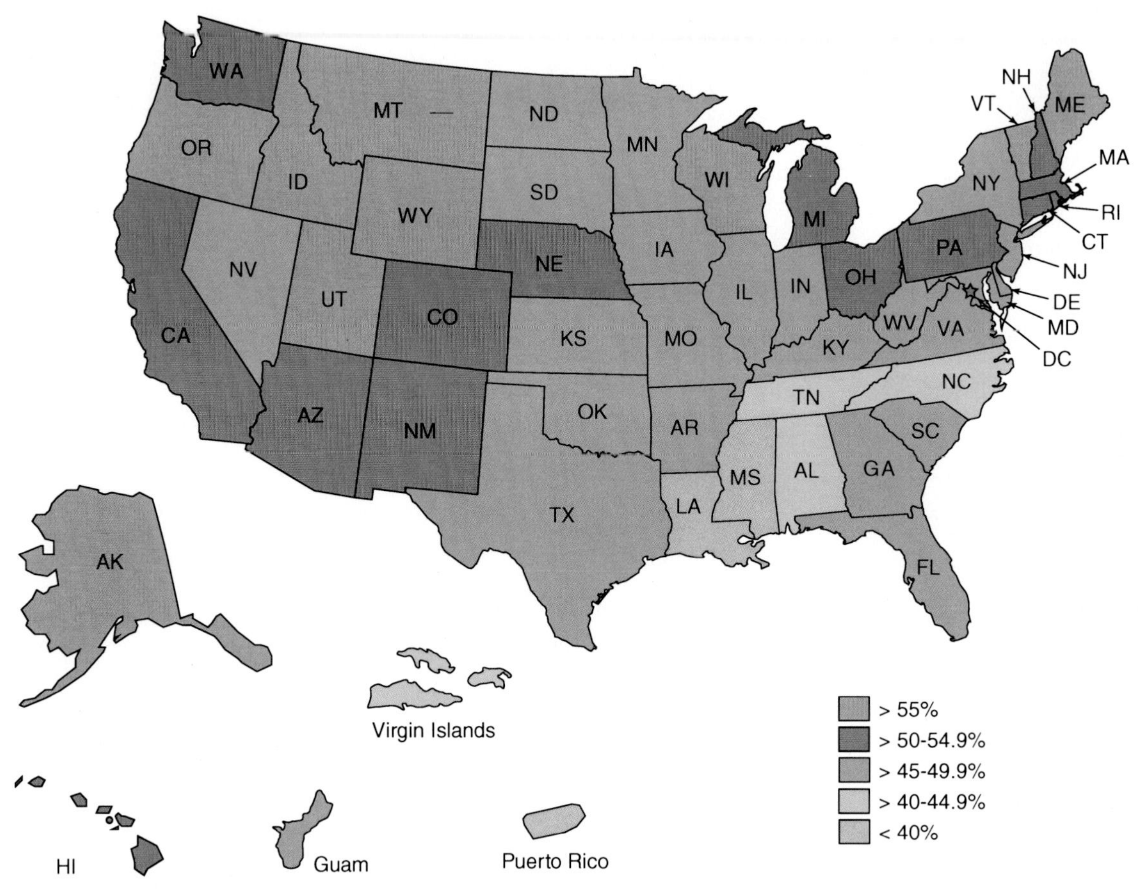

Figure 2.1 This map shows the prevalence of people by state who get the recommended amount of physical activity.

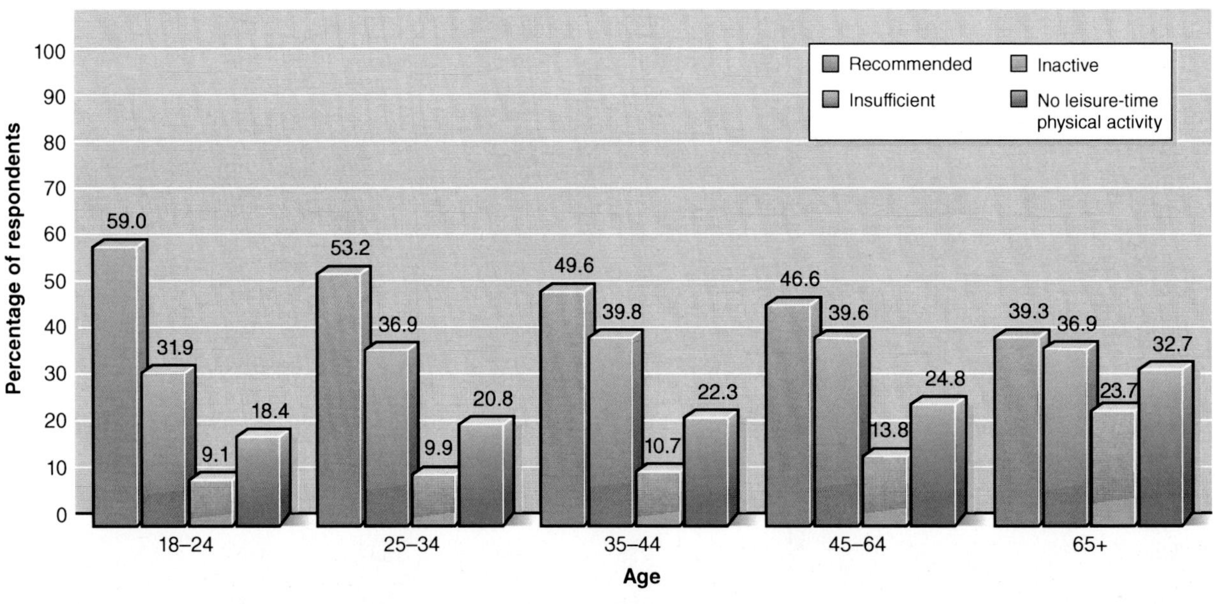

Figure 2.2 The percentage (by age) of levels of physical activity in the United States in 2007. The responses for "Recommended," "Insufficient," and "Inactive" add up to approximately 100 percent. "No leisure-time physical activity" responses represent a separate question.

Time

You need to exercise for at least 30 minutes a day (60 minutes would be even better) at moderate intensity on 3 to 5 days of the week to get the most benefit from cardiorespiratory training. It's OK, though, to do shorter bouts—10 minutes or so—several times a day to accumulate the total recommended minutes (ACSM 2006).

Type

Cardiorespiratory fitness can be achieved through two types of activity: **aerobic activity** and **anaerobic activity**. A good cardiorespiratory fitness program incorporates both types of activity to some degree. Aerobic activity is any physical activity in which you need to take in more oxygen. Any type of rhythmic activity that can be sustained for at least 20 minutes and uses large muscle groups is aerobic. Brisk walking, cycling, and swimming are common forms of aerobic activity. Anaerobic means "without oxygen," which refers to the oxygen used for metabolic demands. Anaerobic activity is high-intensity activity. Because it doesn't use oxygen, it can't be sustained for long. Examples of anaerobic activity are sprinting and weight training. The most important aspect of activity type is to do what you enjoy so you'll want to stay active.

Determining Intensity

A lot of methods exist for determining the intensity of aerobic activity, but they all measure **heart rate**. The higher the intensity, the higher the heart rate will be. The ACSM recommends exercising at a **target heart rate (THR)** zone of 60 to 80 percent of HRR to get cardiorespiratory fitness benefits (ACSM 2006). People who are just beginning a fitness program and aren't yet in good shape might want to start at 40 to 50 percent of their HRR. People who are in great shape should exercise in the higher ranges of their THR to maintain their fitness.

To determine your THR, you need to know your **maximum heart rate (HRmax)** and **resting heart rate (HRrest)**. There are physiological tests that measure HRmax very accurately, but subtracting your age from 220 is a simple method that's accurate enough. So, if you're 20, you can assume your HRmax is 200 (220 – 20 = 200). (That formula has been used as the standard for years, but more recent studies have come up with a different formula that estimates HRmax more accurately for young adults. See the Fitness Basics section of the book's online student resource for more details.)

Researchers simply took a percentage of that number and considered that to be the THR zone. They determined, for example, that exercising at 77 percent to 90 percent of HRmax is sufficient intensity to improve or maintain cardiorespiratory fitness. They simply multiplied the HRmax by 77 percent to get the lower end of the THR zone and by 90 percent to get the upper end. So, the THR for a 20-year-old would be 154 to 180 beats per minute (200 × 0.77 = 154 and 200 × 0.90 = 180).

That method of finding THR doesn't factor in current level of fitness, though. Another method, known as the **Karvonen method**, uses the HRR concept, which essentially is HRrest subtracted from HRmax. The HRrest of a fit person will be lower than that of someone who isn't fit, because a healthy heart has to beat fewer times to pump oxygen-rich blood to the muscles. For that reason, the Karvonen method tends to be a more accurate way of determining the right THR zone for exercise intensity. The equation for finding your THR range with the Karvonen method is this:

$$\text{THR range} = (\text{HRmax} - \text{HRrest}) \times \text{percent intensity} + \text{HRrest}$$

You already know your HRmax, but to use the calculation, you also need to determine your HRrest. The first thing in the morning, while you're still in bed, count your pulse for 10 seconds and multiply that number by 6 to get the number of times your heart beats in a minute. Let's say you count 10 beats during the 10 seconds you're measuring. Multiply that by 6 to get your HRrest of 60 beats per minute.

Let's work through the equation for a 20-year-old who has an HRrest of 60 and who wants to work at a THR zone of 60 percent to 80 percent.

First, we find the HRR, which again is HRmax – HRrest, or 200 – 60 = 140.

Next, we figure the low end of the THR. Multiply HRR (140) by percent intensity (60 percent) to get 84. Then add to that the HRrest (60 beats per minute) to get 144 beats per minute.

Do the same thing to find the upper end of the THR. Multiply 140 by 80 percent (112), and then add 60 to get 172 beats per minute. Our sample exerciser, then, has a THR of 144 to 172 beats per minute.

The HRrest component of the Karvonen method takes fitness into account, because without it, every person the same age would have the same THR zone. By taking HRrest into account, a fitter person will have a higher THR to aim for during exercise than if he had calculated THR without factoring in his HRrest.

What Do You Do?

Using the Karvonen method, figure out your THR for working out at 60 to 80 percent intensity.

- Your HRmax: ____________
- Your HRrest: ____________
- Your HRR: ____________
- Your THR (60 to 80 percent): ____________

Another way to determine intensity during cardiorespiratory exercise is based on perceived exertion. The Borg Rating of Perceived Exertion (RPE) scale was created to allow exercisers to rate how they're feeling during activity, taking into account personal fitness, general fatigue, and environmental factors. The scale offers an easy alternative for monitoring intensity during a workout without the use of equipment or calculations. The numbers on the scale range from 6 (meaning that you feel no exertion at all) to 20 (meaning that you feel that you're engaging in the maximum amount of exertion). Visit the Fitness Basics section of the textbook's online student resource to see the full scale.

The Borg RPE scale can be used to assess intensity for both cardiorespiratory activities and weight training. According to the ACSM, most people who are exercising at an intensity to bring about cardiorespiratory benefits have an average RPE of 12 to 16 in the range of somewhat hard to hard. (Recommendations for weight training are discussed later in the chapter.)

MUSCULAR STRENGTH AND ENDURANCE

Muscular strength is obviously beneficial in recreational activities, such as serving a tennis ball or running uphill. But strength is also important for everyday activities, such as carrying groceries, climbing stairs, or lifting boxes. Muscles provide the support necessary for good posture and keep the skeleton in proper alignment. And not only does muscular strength matter, but so does muscular endurance.

Muscular strength is the capacity of the muscle to exert force against resistance, and **muscular endurance** is the capacity of the muscle to exert force repeatedly against resistance (Teague et al. 2007). Together they allow you to perform activities of daily living with less physiologic stress, protect you from injuries, and help you maintain functional independence throughout your life.

When you increase muscle mass, you increase your metabolic rate. Muscle burns calories even at rest, so the more muscle you have, the more calories you burn throughout the day. Increased muscular strength and endurance even help build bone and prevent or postpone the bone mineral loss that comes with age (Jackson et al. 2004). On top of it all, having fit muscles improves physical appearance and self-esteem.

In the same way that cardiorespiratory training strengthens the heart, resistance training strengthens muscles and improves muscular endurance. **Resistance training** is exercise that uses free weights, bands, machines, and body weight to put resistance on the muscle through a full range of motion. There are three types of muscular contractions: isometric, concentric, and eccentric. **Isometric contractions** are the result of muscle applying force without moving,

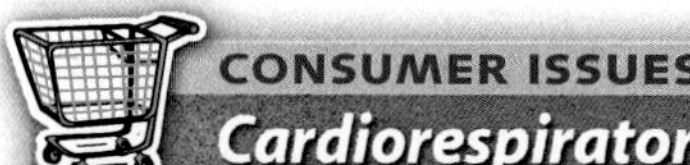

CONSUMER ISSUES

Cardiorespiratory Equipment Pros and Cons

Fitness centers have many kinds of machines for cardiorespiratory training. All can provide a good workout, and you should use whatever fits your workout style best. Be sure to try out a piece of equipment before buying it. If you belong to a gym, try a few cardio pieces to see which one works best for you. Table 2.2 shows some pros and cons of common machines (Donatelle 2008; Payne, Hahn, and Lucas 2006).

TABLE 2.2 Pros and Cons of Cardiorespiratory Workout Equipment

Equipment	Pros	Cons
Treadmill 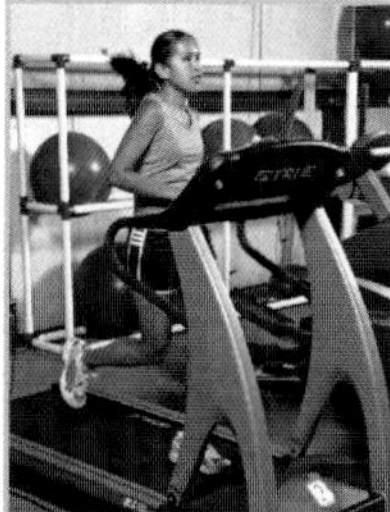	• Relatively easy to use. • Offers a wide range of intensity levels for all types of exercisers. • Improves cardiorespiratory fitness.	• Can be hard on joints and aggravate existing joint problems. • Older models may not have good shock absorption. • Using good form is critical to reducing risk of injury.
Elliptical 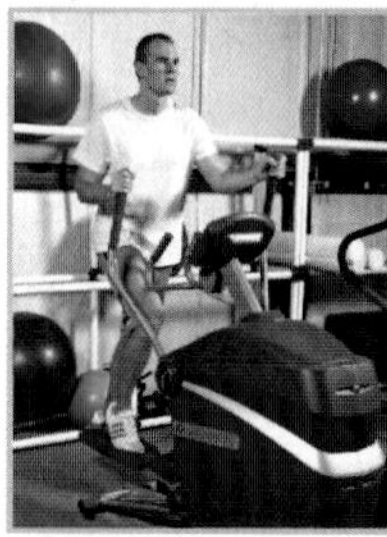	• Uses the same pattern of movement as when running or walking. • Provides less impact on joints than a treadmill.	• Requires some balance and coordination. • Need to choose a good intensity to get a good workout.
Stationary bike 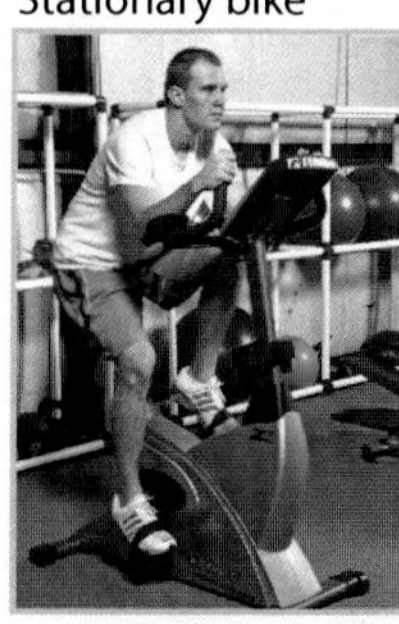	• Easy to use. • Can be used individually or in a cycling class, which offers variety. • Upright bikes are good for beginners with back problems.	• Some people find the seat to be uncomfortable for long durations. • Harder to get heart rate up; need to pay attention to resistance and cadence.
Stair stepper 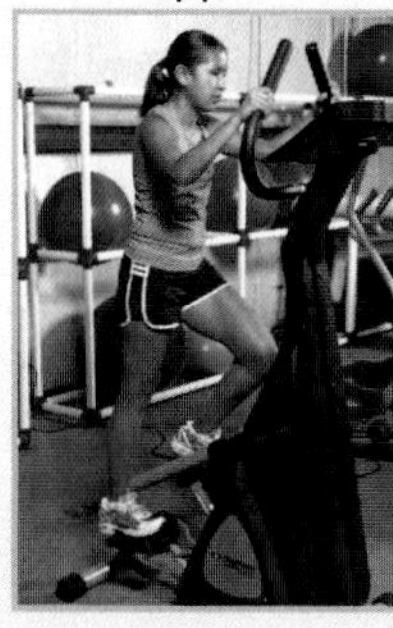	• Great for low-impact lower-body workout. • Takes a lot of energy to sustain body weight stepping up and down.	• Easy to cheat by locking arms and leaning on the machine. • May not be comfortable for those with knee pain.

such as when you flex or clench your stomach muscles. A **concentric contraction** is when a force is produced while the muscle shortens. If your arm is hanging at your side and you bend your elbow to lift your hand to your shoulder, the biceps muscle experiences a concentric contraction. An **eccentric contraction** is when a force is produced while the muscle lengthens. Lowering your hand from your shoulder to your side produces an eccentric contraction in the biceps muscle.

It's helpful to be familiar with some of the lingo related to resistance training so you can understand books or magazines you might read to help establish a resistance training routine or so you know what trainers or other exercisers in the gym mean when they talk about these things. **Weight** simply refers to the amount of resistance used during the exercise. A **repetition**, also called a *rep*, is one complete movement through a full range of motion. **Range of motion (ROM)** is the degree of movement that occurs at joint (Baechle and Earle 2000). A **set** is a series of repetitions. **Rest time** is the amount of time between sets of an exercise. Most strength training programs suggest a certain number of sets with a certain amount of weight and rest for a certain amount of time between sets. For example, you might be instructed to do 3 sets of 10 reps of a biceps curl using 5-pound (2.2-kilogram) weights, resting 30 seconds between each set.

Guidelines

It doesn't really matter if you know all the lingo, though. What matters is that you develop a program that works for you and increases your muscular strength and endurance. Your strength training exercises should focus on major muscle groups: back, shoulders, chest, arms, hips, legs, and abdominal muscles. Refer to the "Strength Training Exercises" section. As you lift, maintain normal breathing; don't hold your breath (ACSM 2006). Inhale on the easier part of the contraction and exhale on the harder part. For example, during a bench press, exhale when you push the weight up and inhale when you lower it. Holding your breath while lifting weights can make you pass out, which can be especially dangerous if you're in the middle of lifting a weight overhead.

The FITT principle can easily be used to create a well-rounded and effective muscular strength and endurance program.

Frequency

Exercise each muscle group on 2 or 3 nonconsecutive days per week (ACSM 2006). You can exercise arms, chest, and shoulders one day and legs, trunk, and back the next, but allow at least 48 hours of rest before returning to a muscle group so you don't injure the muscles from overuse. Muscles become stronger during the rest and recuperation phase. If you don't give your muscles a chance to rest, they won't recover fully, and risk of injury increases.

Intensity

According to the overload principle, muscle adapts quickly and has to be continually overloaded for progress to continue. In other words, you need to load the muscle with more than it's used to in order to coax a training effect from the body (Sharkey and Gaskill 2007). You can change the intensity of strength training exercises by varying the amount of weight you use, the number of repetitions you do, or the speed at which you move through the ROM while lifting a weight (slower speed increases intensity) (ACSM 2006). Most strength training professionals recommend a workout of 2 to 4 sets of 8 to 12 repetitions each. Depending upon your goals, you can choose from a range of 3 to 20 repetitions per set (ACSM 2006).

Your personal fitness goals will determine the intensity you'll work at. The more weight you lift, the fewer reps you'll be able to complete, and the lighter the weight you lift, the more reps you'll be able to complete.

Three training goals influence repetition number:

1. Increase muscular strength and power.
2. Increase muscle mass by enlarging muscle fibers (hypertrophy).
3. Increase muscular endurance (toning).

The number of reps influences the degree to which the goals are achieved, but you get some benefit toward all the goals in any strength program. So even though your program may be designed to accommodate your training goal to increase muscle strength and power, for example, you'll also experience some increased muscle hypertrophy and endurance.

The amount of weight you should lift depends on your training goals. You want to lift enough weight to work the muscle hard enough to get a training effect but not so much that you hurt yourself. Figuring out the right amount of weight can be tricky at first, but it'll get easier as you gain experience with resistance training.

According to the principle of **individuality**, there is no magic number for the amount of weight you should start with. The right starting weight depends on training goals and current fitness status. One way to figure out the right amount of weight for you is to base it on a percentage of **1-repetition maximum (1RM)**, which is the maximum amount of weight you can lift for no more than 1 full rep. The National Strength and Conditioning Association (NSCA) recommends lifting different percentages of your 1RM to achieve various training goals (Baechle and Earle 2000).

Your training goal determines intensity. If you want to develop strength and power, you should do 6 or fewer reps at 70 to 90 percent of your 1RM. For increasing muscle hypertrophy, do 6 to 12 reps at 67 to 85 percent 1RM. Finally, to increase muscular endurance, do more than 12 reps at less than 67 percent 1RM.

To determine your 1RM, you would have to perform a 1RM test for each exercise performed. Although this method is effective, it can be tiring and even dangerous if you don't have a spotter. An easier way to determine intensity without determining 1RM for each exercise is to use the Borg RPE scale. We already talked about how the Borg scale can help determine intensity of cardiorespiratory exercises, and it can also be used to gauge intensity of resistance training. The ACSM recommends an initial RPE rating of 12 or 13 and eventually working up to a rating of 15 or 16 for weight training for muscular endurance and hypertrophy training goals. For strength and power training goals, a target RPE of 19 or 20 would be about right for healthy populations. Again, it is important to establish a target RPE for each training exercise and environment, and the scale is just a guideline for intensity.

Time

Each repetition should take about 6 seconds total—3 seconds for the concentric phase (where the muscle shortens) and 3 seconds for the eccentric phase (where the muscle lengthens). A moderate duration is necessary to maximize both phases of the muscle contraction (ACSM 2006). Allow enough rest time between exercises to perform the next exercise with the proper form.

Type

Perform a minimum of 8 to 10 exercises to train all the major muscle groups of the body (ACSM 2006). Remember, though, to switch muscle groups so you're not training the same muscles in the same 48 hours.

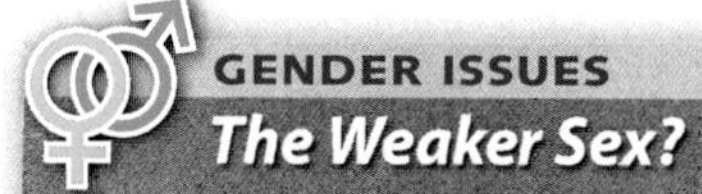

In terms of absolute strength, women are generally weaker than men because they have less muscle. When relative muscle cross-sectional area is compared, though, no difference in strength exists between the sexes, which indicates that muscle quality is not sex specific (Baechle and Earle 2000). Testosterone is the primary stimulus for initiating muscle hypertrophy, or muscle growth. The more testosterone the body produces, the greater the ability to pack on muscle. Because women do not naturally produce as much testosterone as men, their muscles generally don't get as big as men's. In other words, women don't need to worry that they'll develop big, bulky muscles from a normal strength training program (Schoenfeld 2003).

Strength Training Exercises

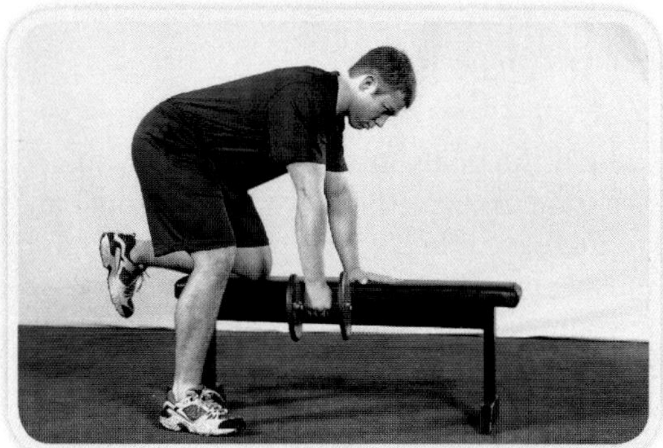
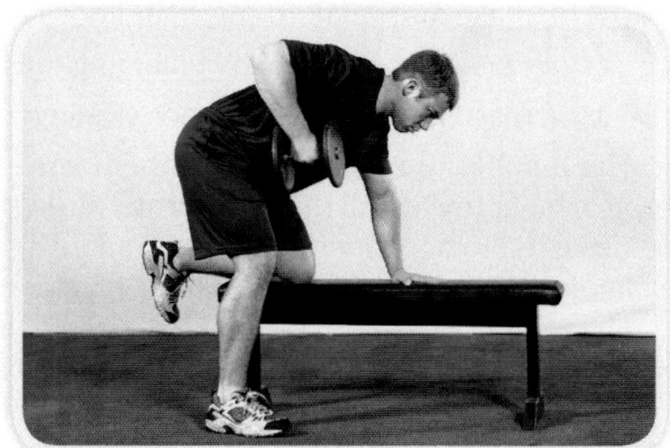

Upper back: *Dumbbell one-arm row*. Place your left knee and hand on a flat bench. Reach down with your right hand, grasp the dumbbell, and pull it up toward your torso until it touches the outside of your chest. Keep your back flat and your elbow near your side. Slowly lower the weight. Repeat with the other side.

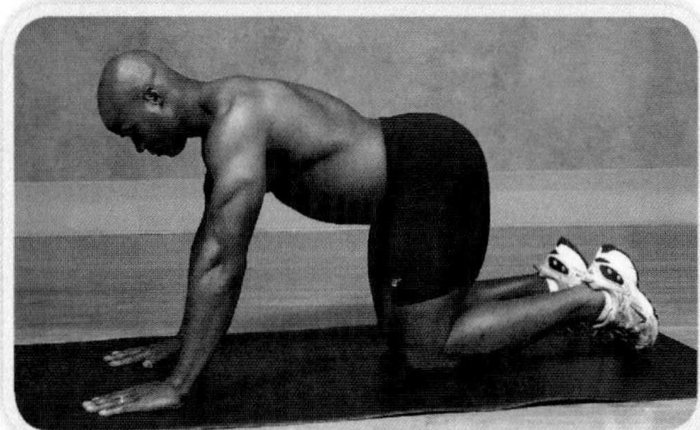
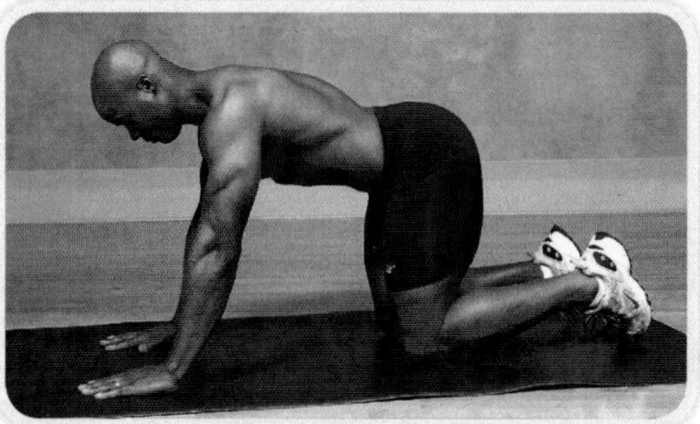

Lower back: *Four-point core activation*. Get on your hands and knees, with your hands below your shoulders and your knees below your hips. Inhale while you slowly distend the abdominal area. Then exhale while you slowly pull your belly button upward toward your spine.

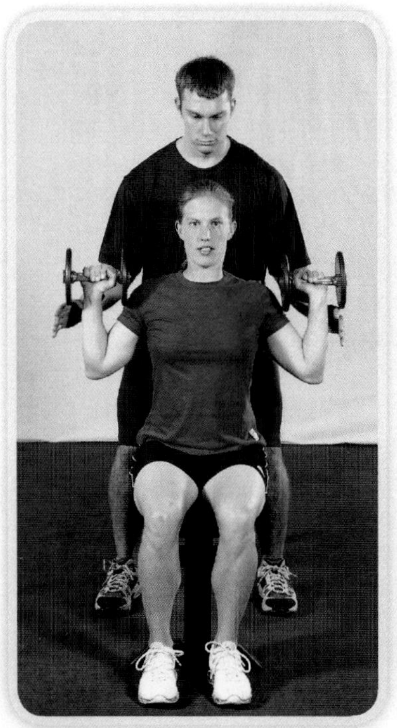
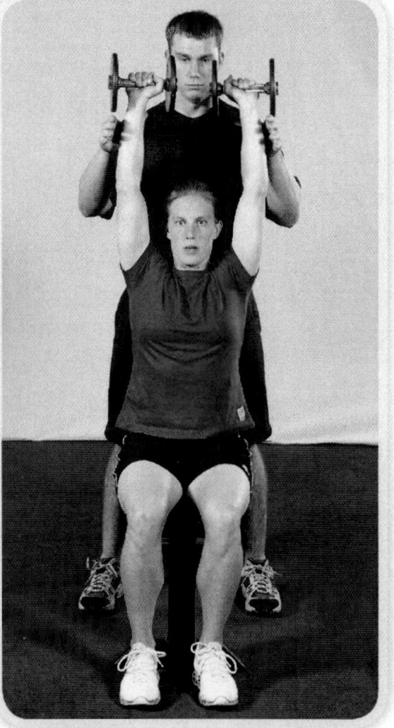

Shoulders: *Seated dumbbell shoulder press*. Sit on a bench with your thighs approximately parallel to the floor. Hold a pair of dumbbells at shoulder height with your palms facing away from you. Slowly push the dumbbells straight up to full elbow extension, but don't push so far that you lock out your elbows. Then slowly lower the weights to the starting position.

All photos on this and the next page: © Human Kinetics

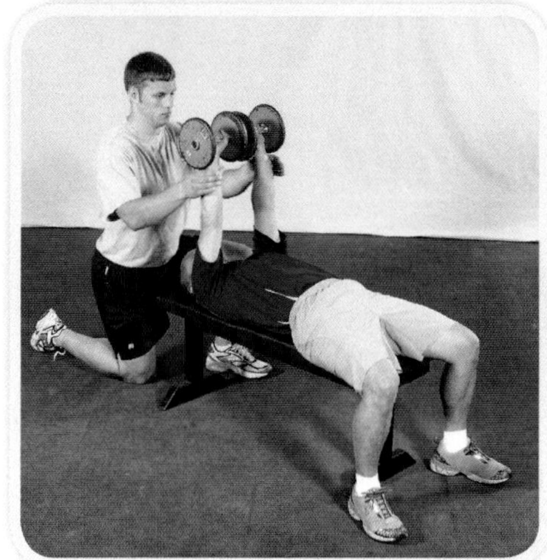

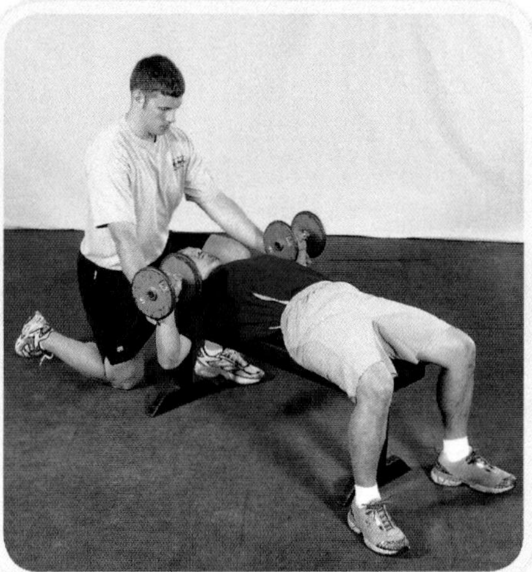

Chest: *Dumbbell bench press.* Lie on a bench with your knees bent and your feet flat on the floor. Hold a pair of dumbbells to the sides of your chest with your palms facing away from you. Slowly push the weights upward to full elbow extension, but don't lock out your elbows. Then slowly lower the weights to the starting position.

Biceps: *Dumbbell curl.* Stand with your feet about shoulder-width apart. Hold a pair of dumbbells at the sides of your thighs. While keeping your torso erect, slowly curl one dumbbell toward your shoulder, with your palm facing up. Then slowly lower the weight to the starting position and repeat with the other arm.

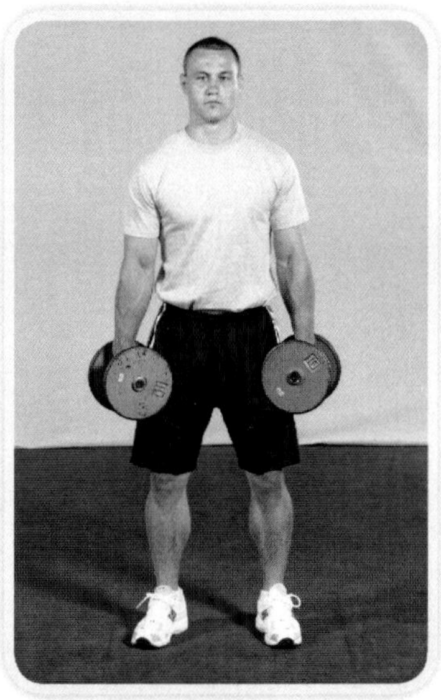

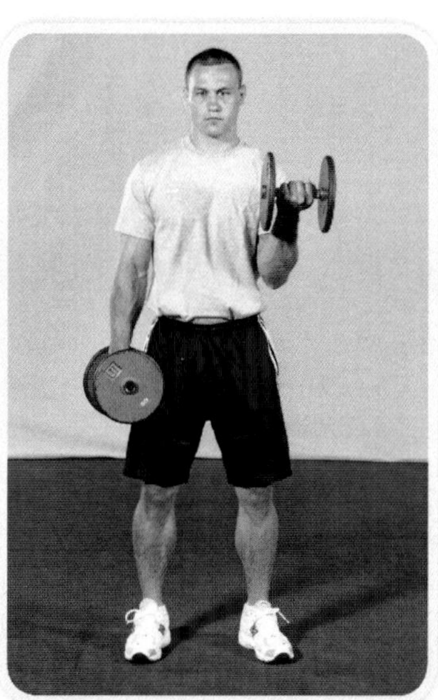

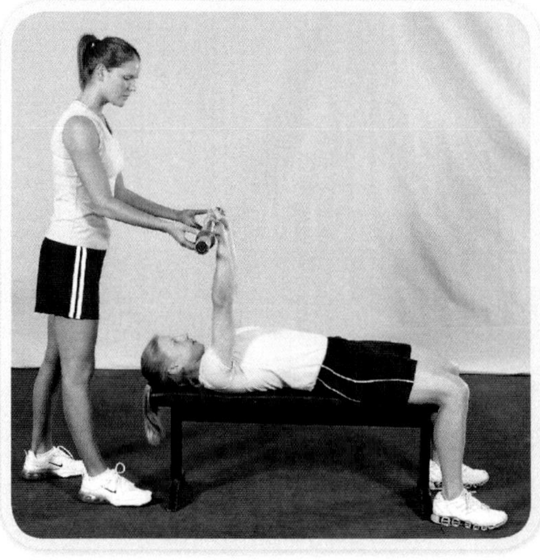

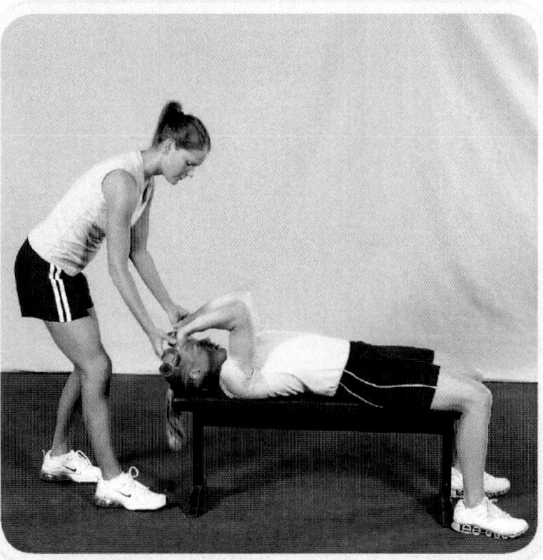

Triceps: *Barbell triceps extension.* Lie face up on a flat bench, feet flat on the floor. As the spotter hands you the bar, grasp it with your palms facing away from you, and extend your arms above your chest. Keep your upper arms and elbows stationary as you slowly lower the bar toward your head. Then slowly press it upward by extending your arms.

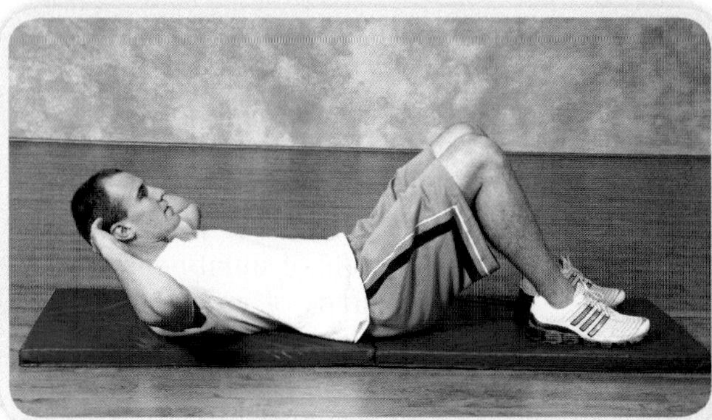
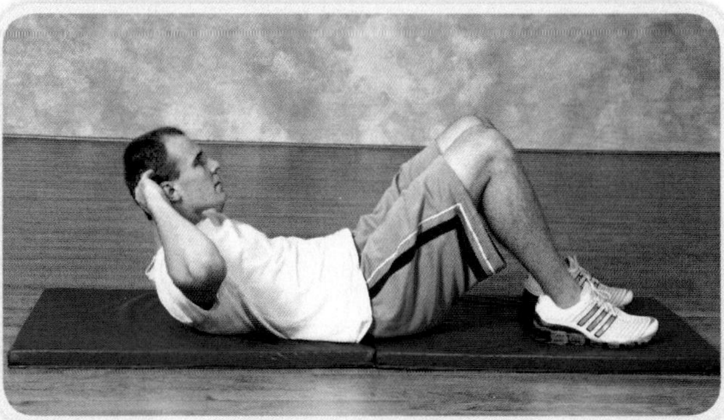

Abdominals: *Curl-up*. Lie on the floor with your knees bent and your feet flat on the floor. Lift your head off the floor, and gently touch your fingertips to the sides of your head (to prevent you from pulling up on the back of your neck). Then slowly curl your torso off the floor while keeping your feet flat on the ground.

Hips/Thighs: *Dumbbell squat*. Stand with your feet about shoulder-width apart. Hold a pair of dumbbells at the sides of your thighs. Maintain a flat or slightly arched back with your head up and eyes focused ahead and slightly above horizontal. Slowly bend at the knees and hips, as if you were sitting down, until your thighs are parallel to the floor. Do not allow your knees to move beyond your toes during the downward phase. Slowly return to your starting position.

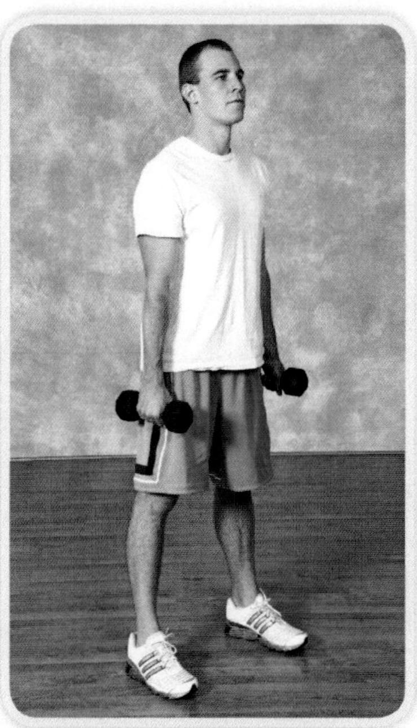
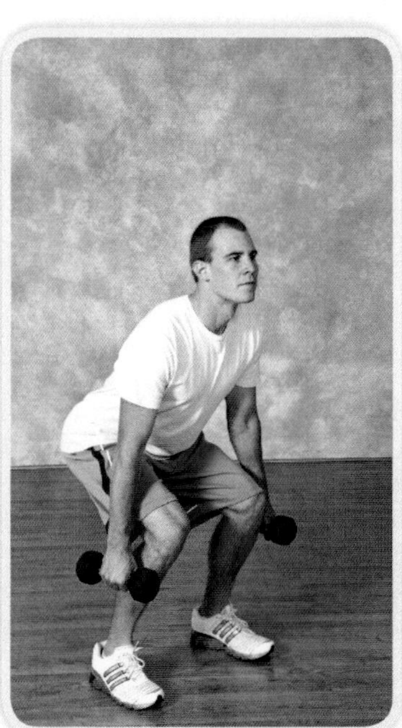

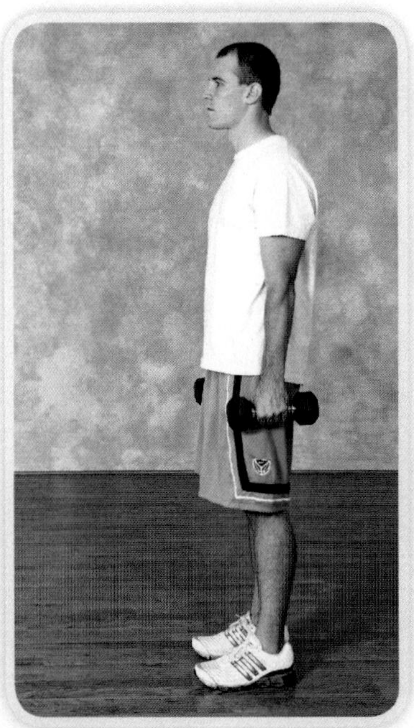
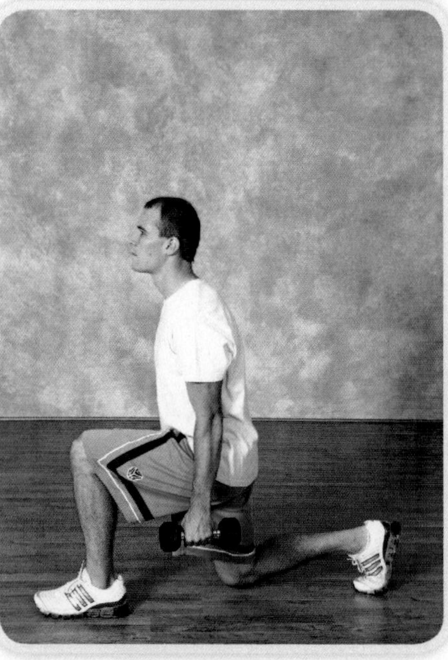

Hips/Thighs: *Dumbbell lunge*. Stand with your feet about shoulder-width apart. Hold a pair of dumbbells at the sides of your thighs. While keeping your torso erect, take a large step forward with one leg, and bend that knee until your thigh is parallel to the floor. Your front knee should not move past your front toes, and your rear knee should stop just above the floor. Push back with your front leg to return to your starting position. The torso remains erect throughout the exercise.

Hips/Thighs: *Dumbbell side lunge.* Stand with your feet about shoulder-width apart. Hold a pair of dumbbells at the sides of your thighs. While keeping your torso erect, take a large step forward at a 45-degree angle and move the dumbbells to a position in front of your torso with your palms facing each other. Bend your front knee until your thigh is parallel to the floor. Your front knee should not move past your front toes. Push back with your front leg to return to your starting position.

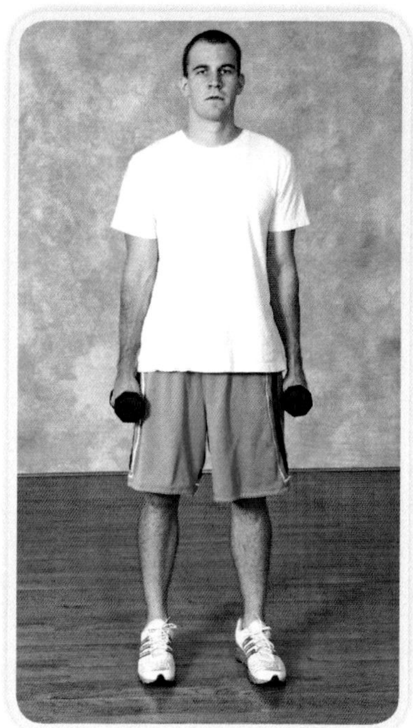

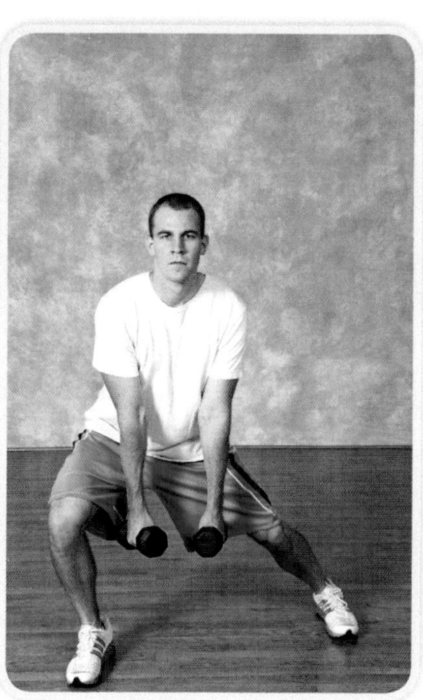

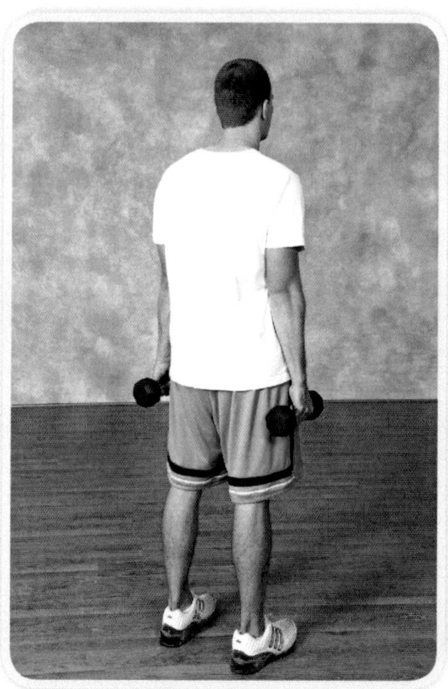

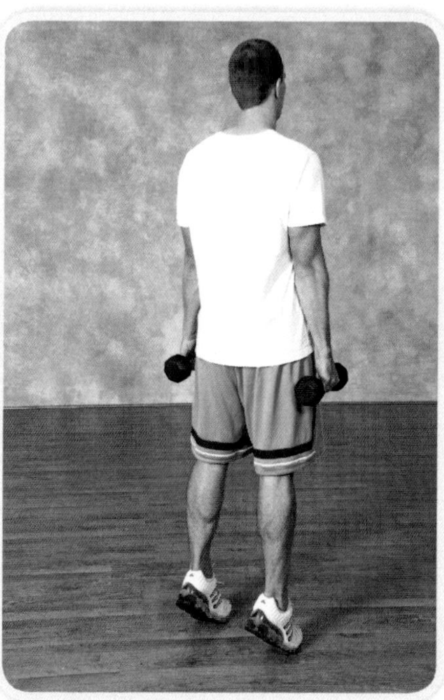

Calves: *Dumbbell heel raise.* Stand with your feet about shoulder-width apart. Hold a pair of dumbbells at the sides of your thighs. While keeping your torso erect and feet and legs parallel to each other, push your toes down and raise your heels up off the floor in a slow, controlled motion. Contract your calf muscles fully, and then lower your heels to the floor.

Building a Strength Training Program

As discussed earlier, the principle of progression says that training overload must increase as a person becomes fitter to continue to see improvements (Sharkey and Gaskill 2007). Three factors affect how quickly you will progress in your strength training. First is genetics. People have varying genetic abilities to increase strength. Second is the starting point. If you haven't been active, your initial progress will be faster than the progress of someone who has been exercising regularly. Third is commitment. Gaining and maintaining high levels of strength takes a steady commitment (Jackson et al. 2004).

Although many principles are universal in any weight training program, your goals will determine how you develop your program. The following tips can help you as you put a strength training program together.

Repetitions and weight have an inverse relationship; the higher the repetitions, the lower the amount of resistance you'll use, and vice versa. For toning and muscle endurance gains, use lighter weights but do more repetitions. For example, do 2 to 4 sets of 12 to 20 reps at no more than 67 percent of your maximum effort (Baechle and Earle 2000).

For strength gains and to build muscle, use heavier weight but do fewer repetitions and more sets. For example, do 2 to 6 sets of 3 to 12 reps at 67 percent or more of your maximum effort (Baechle and Earle 2000).

The length of time you rest between sets can also influence results. To tone your muscles and gain endurance, take shorter rests between sets (90 seconds or less) to force the muscle to respond while it's fatigued. For strength gains, use longer rest between each set (2 to 5 minutes) to move more weight during the exercise (Baechle and Earle 2000).

FLEXIBILITY

Flexibility is the ability to move a joint through its full ROM, and it's important not just for gymnastics and yoga but also for making everyday movements easier, especially with age. Stiffness can cause older people to assume unnatural body positions, which can lead to back, neck, or shoulder pain. It's especially important to pay attention to flexibility when you're doing strength training. As a muscle grows stronger, the tiny tears that were created during weight training grow back stronger. That makes the muscle tighter and starts to decrease the ROM throughout the joint.

Guidelines

The best way to improve flexibility is to do regular stretching exercises. Similar to focusing on major muscle groups for strength training, you need to stretch the muscles of the back, shoulders, chest, arms, hips, legs, and abdomen. Refer to the sample stretches on the next four pages. As with cardiorespiratory and muscular strength and conditioning programs, the FITT principle can be used to create a safe and effective stretching program (ACSM 2006).

Frequency

Stretch a minimum of 2 or 3 days per week, either at the end of your exercise session or after a warm-up. Risk of injury is lower when you stretch while your muscles are warm.

Intensity

Stretch to the end of the ROM of the joint, just until you feel discomfort or tightness, but not to the point of pain. Do 2 to 4 repetitions for each stretch.

Time

Hold each stretch for 15 to 30 seconds.

Type

Do static stretches, not ballistic stretches. That means you should hold the stretch still and not bounce as you stretch all the major muscle groups.

Flexibility Exercises

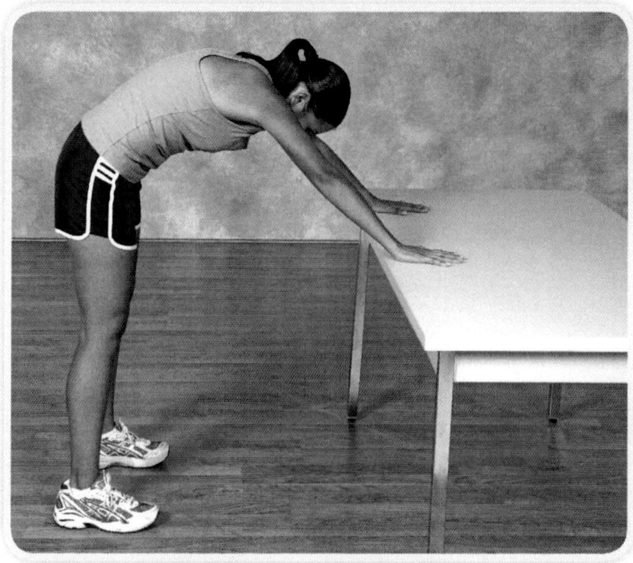

Upper back stretch. Stand a few feet away from a desk or table with your knees slightly flexed. Lean forward and push against the desk or table with both hands, bending at the waist. Press down on the surface to stretch your upper back.

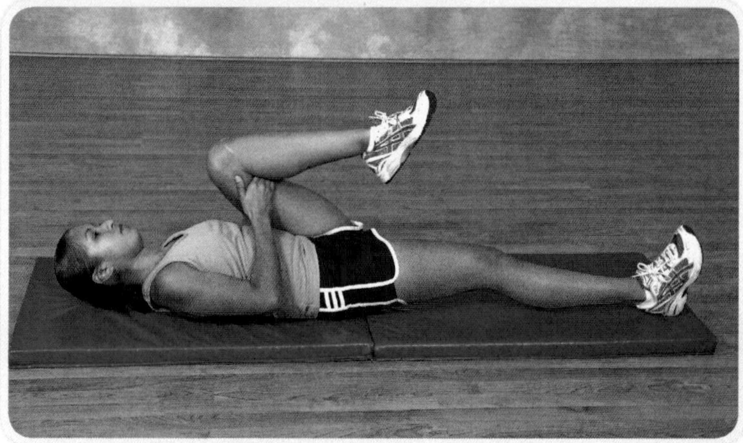

Lower back/hamstrings/gluteals stretch. Lie on the floor. Bend one knee and bring it toward your chest while keeping your other leg flat on the floor. Put both hands behind the bent knee, and pull it toward your chest to stretch your lower back. Then slowly return to the starting position.

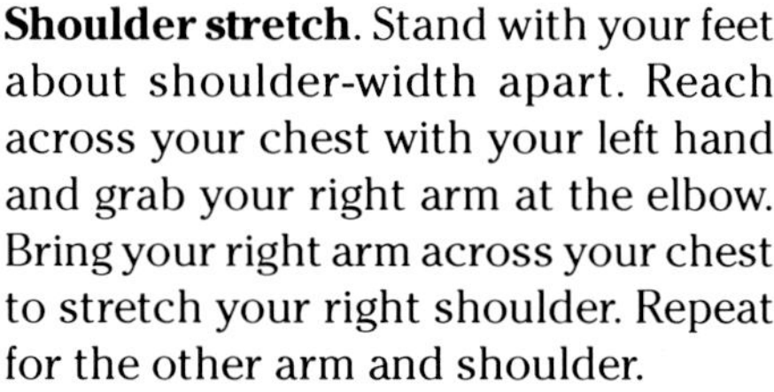

Shoulder stretch. Stand with your feet about shoulder-width apart. Reach across your chest with your left hand and grab your right arm at the elbow. Bring your right arm across your chest to stretch your right shoulder. Repeat for the other arm and shoulder.

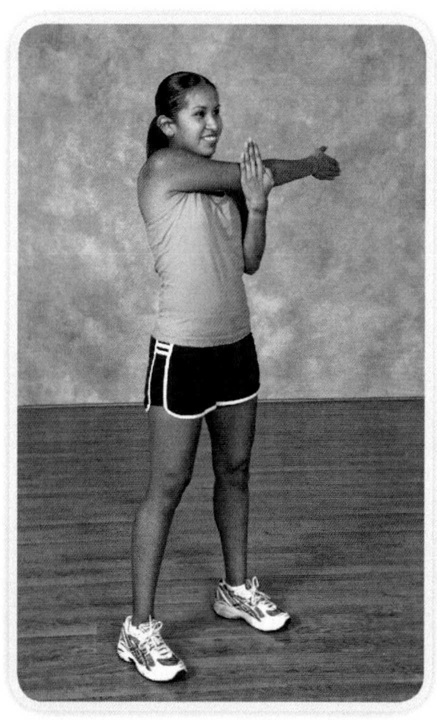

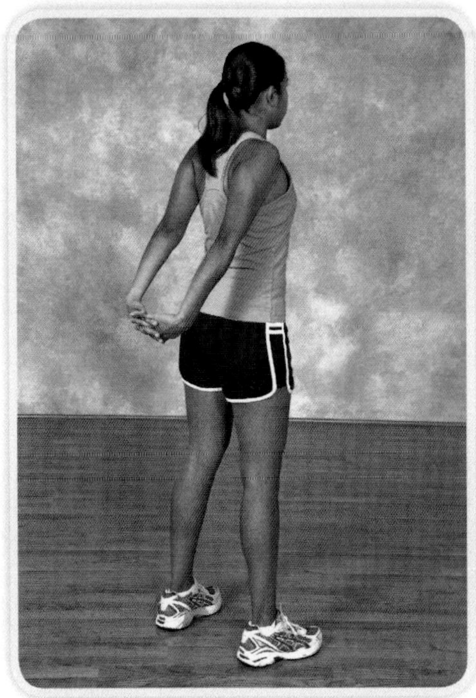

Chest stretch. Stand with your feet about shoulder-width apart. Reach both hands behind your back and lace your fingers together. Slowly lift your hands upward to stretch your chest.

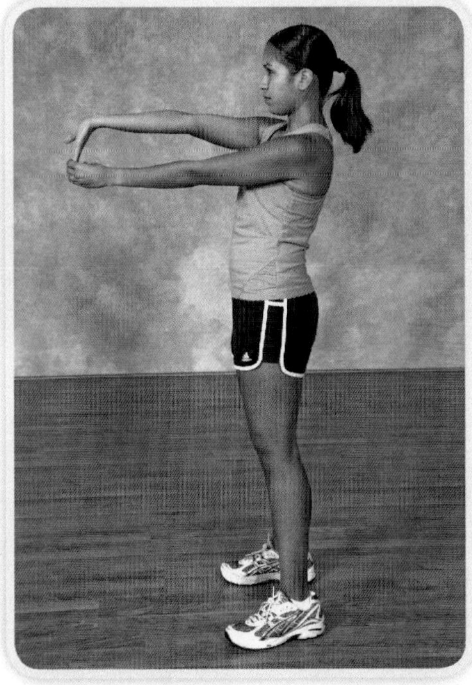

Forearm/Wrist flexor stretch. Stand with your feet about shoulder-width apart. Extend your right arm in front of you with your palm and forearm facing upward. With your left hand, grab the fingers of your right hand and slowly pull them back, stretching your biceps. Repeat for the other arm.

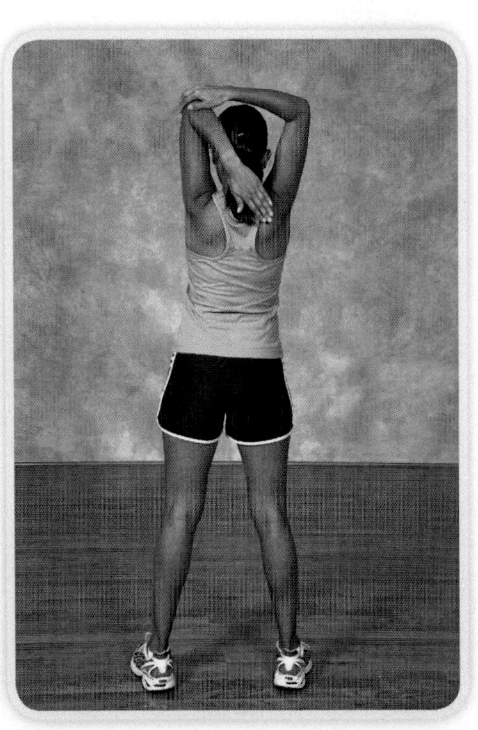

Triceps stretch. Stand with your feet about shoulder-width apart. Lift your left arm over your head, then bend your elbow and reach down your back to stretch the triceps of your left arm. Place your right hand on your left elbow, and gently apply downward pressure while reaching your left arm farther down your back. Repeat for the other arm.

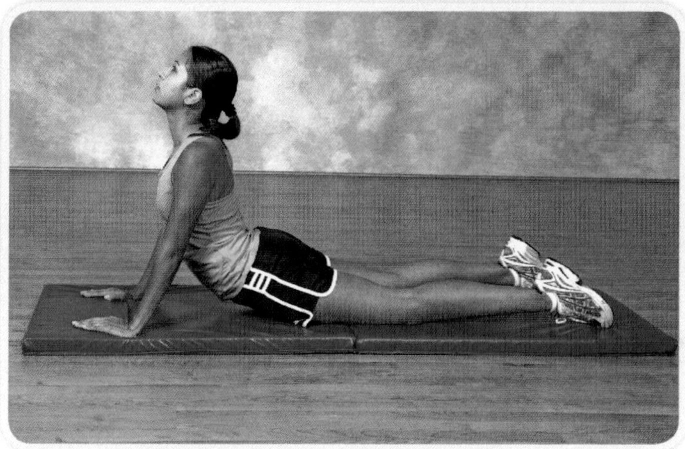

Abdominal stretch. Lie prone on the floor. Place the forearms against the floor to the sides of your chest. Slowly press down against the floor while you arch your back, lifting your head and chest off the floor. Don't arch too far, and contract your buttocks to help minimize stress on your lower back. (For an advanced stretch, as shown in the photo, place the palms of both hands on the floor to the sides of your chest.) Slowly press down against the floor while arching the back and lifting the chin.

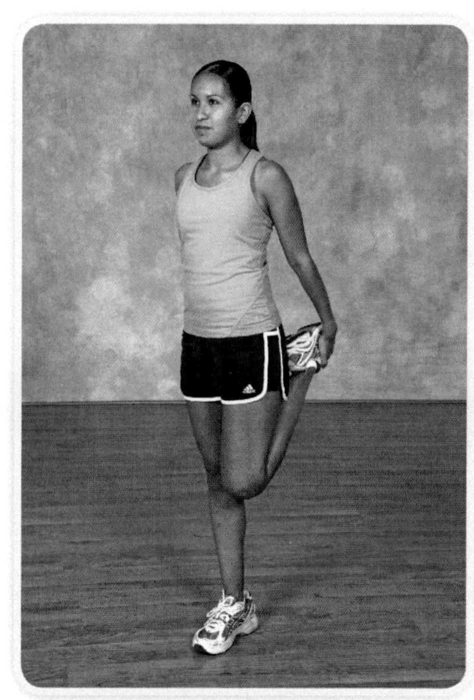

Quadriceps stretch. Stand with your feet close together. Bend your left knee. With your left hand, grab your left foot and pull it toward your buttocks to stretch your quadriceps. (You can lean against a wall with your other hand to help keep your balance.) Repeat with the other leg.

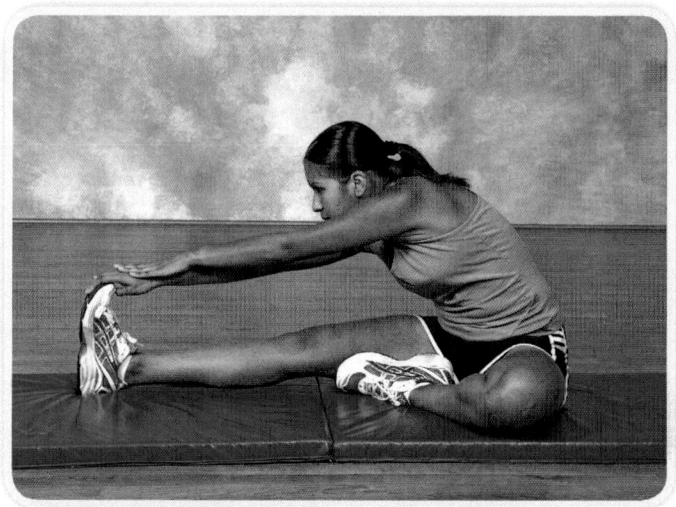

Hamstrings stretch. Sit on the floor and extend your right leg straight in front of you. Bend your left leg so the bottom of your left foot touches the knee of your right leg. Reach both hands out toward your right foot. (For an advanced stretch, as shown in the photo, grab your right toes and gently pull them back toward you.) Repeat with the other leg.

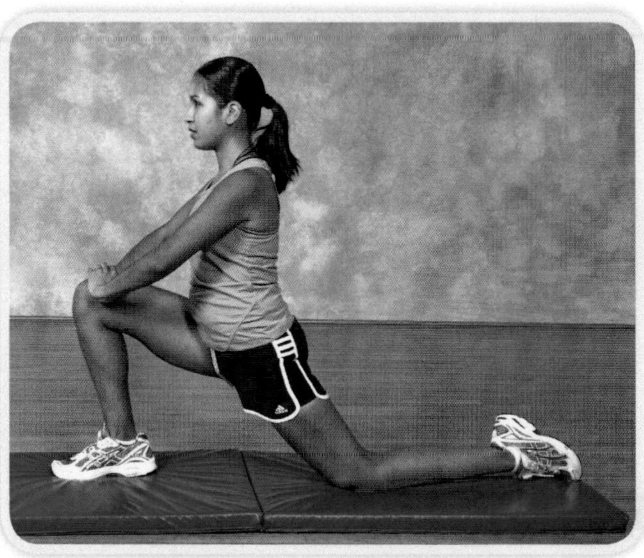

Hip stretch. Kneel on the floor with your left knee. Bend your right knee and place your right foot flat on the floor in front of you. While keeping your torso straight, lean forward toward your right leg. (For an advanced stretch, as shown in the photo, press your hands against your right knee to push your torso backward.) Repeat with the other leg.

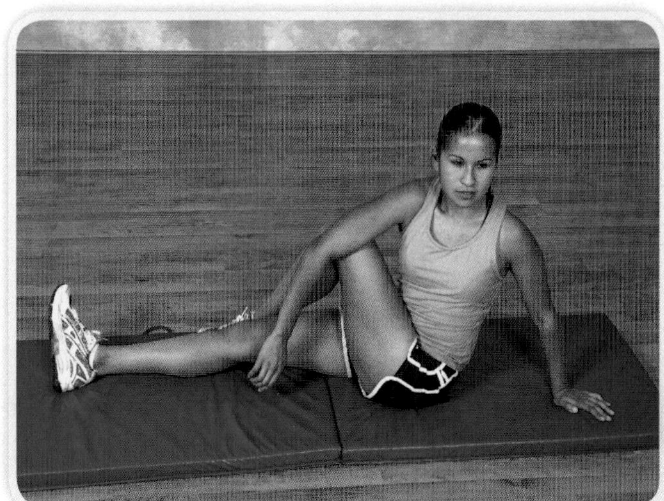

Hip stretch. Sit on the floor with your right leg extended in front of you. Bend your left knee and place your left foot flat on the ground on the outside of your right knee. Place your right elbow against the outside of your left knee, and place your left palm flat on the floor for support. Press your right elbow against your left knee while you twist your upper body to the left. Don't arch your back or bend forward at the waist. Repeat with the other leg.

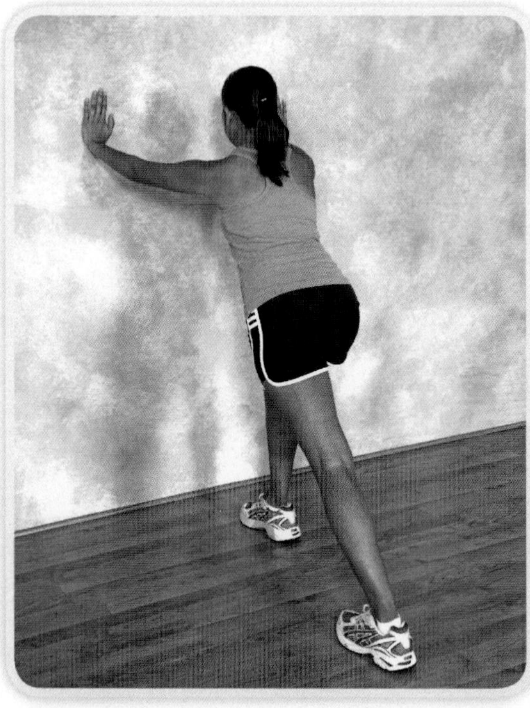

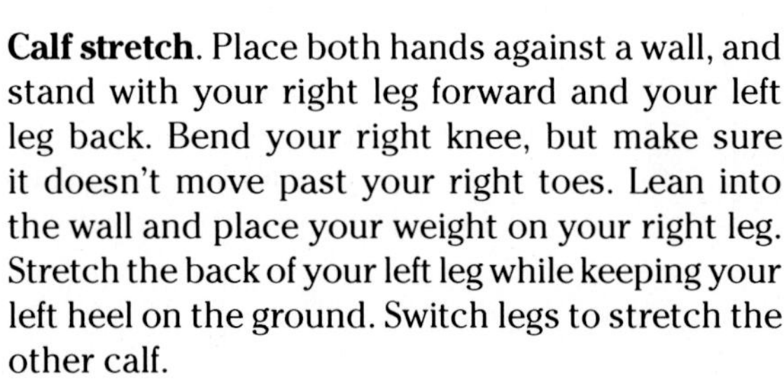

Calf stretch. Place both hands against a wall, and stand with your right leg forward and your left leg back. Bend your right knee, but make sure it doesn't move past your right toes. Lean into the wall and place your weight on your right leg. Stretch the back of your left leg while keeping your left heel on the ground. Switch legs to stretch the other calf.

Stretching to Improve Flexibility

Several types of stretches help keep muscles and joints flexible. **Passive stretching** is when a partner, stretching machine, or wall provides the force for the stretch (Baechle and Earle 2000). **Active stretching** is when you facilitate the force for the stretch. **Proprioceptive neuromuscular facilitation (PNF)** involves contracting, relaxing, and stretching opposing muscle groups.

There are three types of active stretching: static, ballistic, and dynamic. **Static stretching** is slow and controlled, and stretches are usually held for about 30 seconds (Baechle and Earle 2000). **Ballistic stretching** is when you bounce through a movement. Risk of injury is high with ballistic stretches, so it's best to avoid them. In **dynamic stretching**, you slowly move parts of the body and increase the range or speed. Dynamic stretching is particularly effective when you're getting ready for intense activity, such as sports.

PNF is usually done with a partner, but it can also be done on your own. An example of a PNF stretch is where you sit with one leg out in front of you and wrap a towel around your foot. Push against the towel with the ball of your foot to contract the calf muscle for 5 seconds. Relax for a few seconds. Then pull your toes toward you, holding the stretch for 30 seconds (Teague et al. 2007). PNF stretching takes advantage of the body's reflex response to enhance muscle relaxation and joint ROM (Jackson et al. 2004). The combination of contracting the muscle, relaxing, and then stretching enables the muscle to stretch more deeply.

BODY COMPOSITION

Body composition, the fifth component of health-related fitness, is the proportion of fat and fat-free mass (muscle, bone, and water) in the body. Healthy body composition consists of a ratio of high fat-free mass to an acceptably low fat mass. Body composition can be estimated by both laboratory and field techniques. Complexity, cost, and accuracy of the test vary depending on the type of assessment, the person being tested, the person doing the testing, and the testing situation.

A healthy body composition is influenced by gender, height, and weight. High fat levels lead to an increased risk for hypertension, type 2 diabetes, stroke, heart disease, and high cholesterol (ACSM 2006). Improving body composition will require making adjustments to the ratio of fat mass to fat-free mass. Following a sensible diet and participating in a safe and effective exercise program is the best and safest way to improve body composition.

SPECIAL CONSIDERATIONS

As important as it is to exercise to improve or maintain physical fitness, some situations require special attention. Knowing how to deal with temperature extremes, age-related concerns, and certain physical limitations will make exercise safer.

Environment and Exercise

Exercising in hot weather can be dangerous if you don't take steps to avoid overheating. Heat can cause impaired regulation of internal core temperature, loss of body fluids, and loss of electrolytes (Teague et al. 2007). Electrolytes help regulate water distribution in the body. During heat stress, the blood vessels expand and you sweat more to cool down the body. In extreme heat, the circulation system is maintaining blood pressure, and as a result it can't regulate temperature as well, which means you could be at risk for overheating. Rising core body temperatures can result in heat cramps, heat exhaustion, heatstroke, and even death. Table 2.3 describes the symptoms and treatment for heat-related disorders.

Danger from exercising in hot weather increases when humidity is high, too. The cooling effect from sweating comes from the evaporation of the sweat, not from the sweat itself, and

TABLE 2.3 Heat-Related Disorders

Heat disorder	Symptoms	Treatment
Heat cramps	Muscle cramps	Rest in cool spot, drink fluids, and avoid salty foods.
Heat exhaustion	Sweating, dizziness, nausea, fatigue, high temperature, pale skin	Rest in cool spot, cool body with water, drink cold fluids, and get medical attention if needed.
Heatstroke	Dry or sweaty hot, flushed skin; headache; vomiting; altered mental state; seizure	Cool body with ice or cold water, sip cool drinks, and get medical help.

Adapted from American Safety & Health Institute, 2007, *Complete emergency care* (Champaign, IL: Human Kinetics), 40.

when humidity is high (i.e., when there's a lot of water vapor in the air), the sweat can't evaporate (McArdle et al. 2001). The National Collegiate Athletic Association (NCAA) recommends using discretion in exercising at temperatures between 80 and 84 degrees Fahrenheit (26.6 to 28.8 degrees Celsius), especially if you're not used to exercising in the heat. When the temperature is between 85 and 87 degrees Fahrenheit (29.4 to 30.5 degrees Celsius), avoid strenuous activity in the sun. Don't exercise at all when the temperature is above 88 degrees Fahrenheit (31.1 degrees Celsius) (Murphy and Ashe 1965).

There are a couple of good strategies for keeping your body temperature from increasing too much during exercise. One is keeping the skin wet by spraying or sponging your head and body with cool water. Another strategy is **hyperhydration**, or taking in extra fluids shortly before exercising in hot environments. Drink 16 ounces (473 milliliters) when you get up, another 16 ounces an hour before activity, and 16 ounces 15 to 30 minutes before activity. Plan to consume 4 to 8 ounces (118 to 237 milliliters) every 15 minutes during activity and 24 ounces (710 milliliters) after activity (Teague et al. 2007).

Exercising in extremely cold temperatures can be dangerous, too. Excessively cold weather can cause hypothermia, or body temperature below 95 degrees Fahrenheit (35 degrees Celsius), which can be life threatening. Signs of hypothermia include shivering, feelings of euphoria, and disorientation (Teague et al. 2007). Another possible injury from exposure to the cold is frostbite, which occurs when blood vessels constrict in the extremities in an attempt to keep the core warm. The lack of blood flow can cause the temperature of the extremities to fall dangerously low, resulting in tissue damage. In extreme cases, irreversible damage requires surgical removal of the tissue.

Pay attention when exercising in windy weather, because windchill can lower external temperature (Teague et al. 2007). Air currents on a windy day increase heat loss because the insulating air layer surrounding the body that is normally warmer is continuously changed with cool air gusts. In those conditions, it's helpful to dress in layers (see "Workout Clothes" later in this chapter).

Resistance Training for Children and Adolescents

Kids can get lots of great exercise just by doing the things kids do (e.g., running around the neighborhood, riding bikes, playing pickup games). In the past, though, there's been some controversy about whether it's safe for children and adolescents to do resistance training, or lift weights. Clinicians and exercise scientists now agree that resistance exercise can be a safe and effective method of conditioning for children and adolescents, if the training is done right. A competent and caring fitness professional should supervise training sessions. The supervisor needs to carefully monitor the child's tolerance to the stress of the weights. Children should begin with light loads and then gradually increase them by 5 percent to 10 percent as strength improves. A workout should consist of 1 to 3 sets of 6 to 15 reps on 2 to 3 nonconsecutive days per week (Baechle and Earle 2000).

People With Disabilities

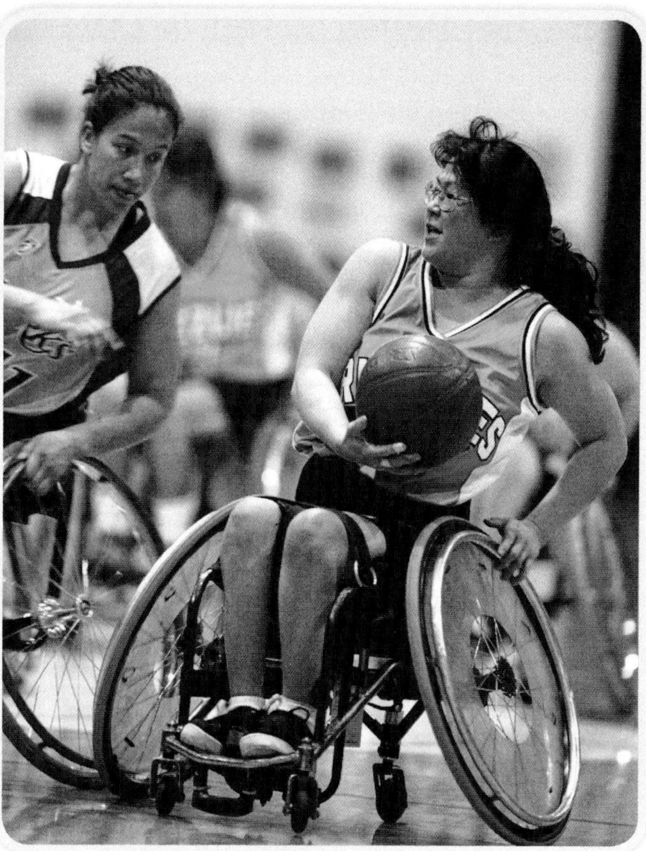

Wheelchair basketball has grown in popularity since the 1940s, when World War II veterans with disabilities began playing.

© Human Kinetics

Physical activity and exercise are especially beneficial for people with disabilities. Exercise counteracts the detrimental effects of bed rest and sedentary living patterns, and it helps maintain optimal functioning of body organs and systems (Teague et al. 2007). Laws have strengthened the rights of people with disabilities, and the U.S. government has developed programs to promote and incorporate physical activity in their lives. The best activity program for people with disabilities depends on their individual circumstances.

Pregnant Women

How active a woman was before becoming pregnant has implications for how active she can be during her pregnancy. Physical activity and exercise are usually safe for a pregnant woman, but to be sure, she should get her doctor's OK (Jackson et al. 2004). If her doctor approves, a pregnant woman should exercise comfortably, not intensely, at least three times a week and follow general safety precautions for physical activity. There are a few things that a pregnant woman should avoid during exercise, though (Jackson et al. 2004):

- She shouldn't exercise to exhaustion.
- She shouldn't overheat, keeping her body temperature under 100 degrees Fahrenheit (37.7 degrees Celsius).
- She shouldn't hold her breath.
- She shouldn't change direction or rise quickly, because she could get dizzy.
- She shouldn't do exercises that require her to lie flat on her back after the first trimester.

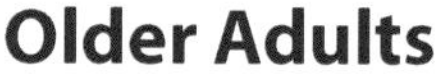

Older Adults

Functional capacity, or the physical and mental ability to perform everyday tasks, declines with age, but being fit helps maintain functional capacity during aging. The ACSM recognizes that the term *elderly* doesn't apply to a generalized age group because physiologic aging doesn't happen uniformly across populations. People who are the same chronological age can differ greatly in their physiologic age and can respond to exercise stimulus differently.

Older adults generally receive the same benefits from exercise as younger adults (Teague et al. 2007). Individual needs and physical condition influence the kind of physical activity or exercise program that is appropriate, and older adults need to use discretion when they're starting a new exercise program. Adult guidelines for cardiorespiratory fitness and general fitness programming hold true for the elderly, as long as they can meet the recommendations comfortably and safely (ACSM 2006).

Older adults should try to meet the general recommendations of 30 minutes of moderate activity daily. The first several resistance training sessions should be closely monitored by a trained professional who is sensitive to the needs of older adults. Older people who do resistance training should do 10 to 15 repetitions per set (ACSM 2006).

BEING ACTIVE IN COLLEGE

Physical inactivity reportedly contributes to more than 300,000 preventable deaths a year in the United States (U.S. Department of Health and Human Services [USDHHS] 2001). The benefits of physical activity are clear: Physical fitness usually helps people live longer and provides better quality of life. It also helps people with stress relief and weight management throughout their lives.

There are some special benefits from developing and maintaining physical fitness during college. First of all, getting involved in a physical activity program could help you meet new people and try new things. If you go to a fitness center or gym, play on an intramural team, or just walk or jog with your roommate, you can expand your social life through exercise.

What you do during your college years also helps you establish habits for the rest of your adult life. The Centers for Disease Control and Prevention (CDC) did a study in 1995, and the data indicated that patterns of weight gain start to show up in college. For example, although almost 21 percent of college students were classified as overweight, older students (25 years or older) were nearly twice as likely as those aged 18 to 24 years to be overweight (28.5 percent versus 17.2 percent in men and 29 percent versus 13.9 percent in women) (CDC 1997).

What Do You Think?

Cornell University researchers found that college freshmen gain half a pound (.2 kilogram) per week on average. That's about 11 times more weight than the average 17- and 18-year-old will gain, and nearly 20 times more than the average weight gain among adults. What makes it so easy to gain weight during college (Nichols 2007)?

The rest of this chapter will provide some practical information about how to develop a habit of being physically active, how to judge whether information you hear about exercise is reliable, and how to choose exercise apparel and equipment.

What to Believe

Fads come and go, and some sources put out incorrect or even dangerous information about health and fitness. How can you know what to believe?

Approach learning about health information in the same way you would approach research. Not all media sources are reputable, so check multiple sources that you trust, such as your family doctor, a health encyclopedia, and reputable Web sites. One good way to tell whether information is reliable and safe is if you can find the same facts in several reputable sources.

No matter what form it comes in, health information should be authored by or include quotes from certified medical professionals. You can usually trust government or public-sponsored Web sites. Be leery of anyone trying to sell you something. Above all, use common sense. If something seems too good to be true, it probably is.

What to Do

Exercise doesn't need to be a chore. To make sure you stay active, choose activities that are fun and that you enjoy. Don't pick activities that are chores just because you know they're good for you. If you don't enjoy the activity, you'll give it up. Also choose activities that are convenient. If you have a 3-hour block of time between classes, take that time to go to the recreation center or play some basketball. If you don't have a huge chunk of time, try to incorporate more activity into your daily routine. Take a 20-minute walk on your way to class or take the stairs whenever possible. Small blocks of moderate activity can add up through the day.

STEPS FOR BEHAVIORAL CHANGE

Overcoming Barriers to Activity

Here's a list of possible obstacles to regular physical activity and some ways to overcome them (Teague et al. 2007). Try to match the barrier with the strategy.

1. Going it alone
2. Not enough time
3. Not enough willpower
4. Afraid of getting hurt
5. No equipment
6. Bad weather
7. Too much traveling
8. Too many family responsibilities
9. Not a good athlete
10. Not enough energy

a. Find pockets of time where you could slip in 30 minutes of activity. Do more activity as part of your daily routine, such as using the stairs instead of the elevator to get to class, riding your bike to the store instead of driving, and so on.

b. Tell people who are important to you about your plans to become more active. Ask them to join you so you have some support. Join a running or walking club to meet other people who are interested in activity.

c. Give an activity program a chance to work. Exercise makes you more energetic over time.

d. Join some group activity classes so people are expecting you to show up. Make activity part of your weekly plan—schedule it just as you would your laundry or your homework.

e. Learn how to exercise safely. Use good warm-ups and cool-downs. Don't overdo the activity, and stay within your skill and fitness levels.

f. Choose activities such as walking or stair climbing that don't require a lot of skill. Find a friend who has your same skill level so you're not tempted to exercise beyond your abilities. Try new activities so you learn new skills.

g. Pick activities where you don't need to buy new equipment. Look in books, magazines, or online for activities that are inexpensive.

h. Have some backup activities that you can do inside if the weather is bad.

i. Exercise with your family so that you're not taking time away from them to do your activity. Find good babysitters if you need to.

j. Find accommodations that have fitness facilities on-site or nearby. Take along a jump rope or exercise band that you can use in your room.

Answers: 1) b; 2) a; 3) d; 4) e; 5) g; 6) h; 7) j; 8) i; 9) f; 10) c

Be realistic about your goals. You may not have time to be as active as you might have been in the past, but aim for 30 minutes of daily moderate activity. Try taking fitness breaks instead of food breaks. Need some energy to study? Take a quick walk instead of a trip to the vending machine; you'll find more energy in small bouts of activity than in a bag of chips. Try to find a workout buddy. A friend may provide that extra little push you'll need to be active at the end of the day.

Many students feel guilty using free time for things other than studying. Remember: sound body, sound mind. Physical activity will help you be a better student by increasing your energy and your self-confidence.

College is busy, and life is only going to get busier from here on out. Plan ahead. By using effective time management skills and planning some physical activity, you'll reduce your stress and pick up some good habits to keep your health on track for now and after college.

Where to Exercise

Budget is probably important in your consideration of where to exercise, and there are several options to fit any circumstances. Recreation centers usually cost money, and the amount varies depending on the amenities or services the facility offers. You don't have to join a fitness center, though. You can exercise right in your bedroom.

Recreation Centers

Recreation centers offer a variety of equipment for cardiorespiratory exercise, free weights, machines for strength training, and maybe even personal trainers to help you develop a program for all fitness components and to keep you on track. Recreation centers also may provide various fitness classes where you can meet new people or try new activities, such as yoga, spinning, or step aerobics.

Another way to meet new people and stay active could be to participate in intramural sport through your college. Intramural sport offers ways to play sports competitively but in a relaxed environment. Lots of sports are offered at most colleges, so you can probably find something that you'd like to play, whether it's in a coed or single-sex league.

If the usage fee for your college recreation center isn't already included in your tuition, it's probably very reasonably priced.

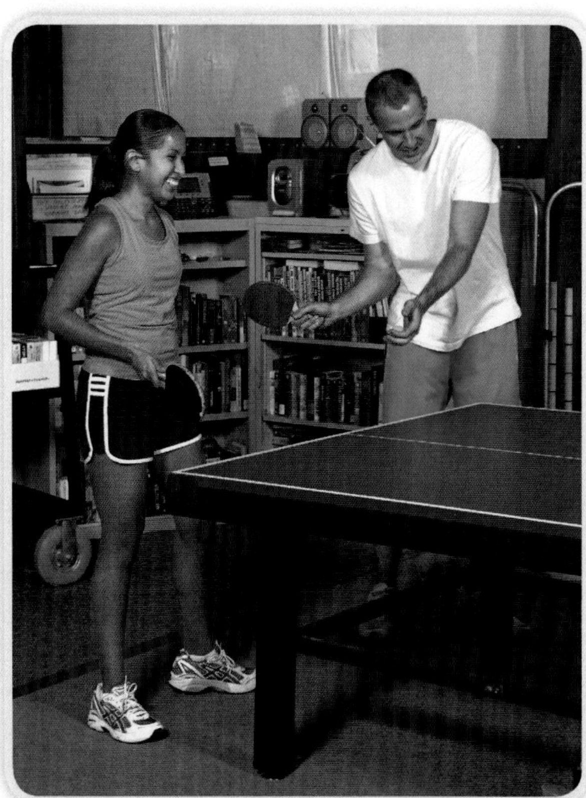

Check out the opportunities for exercise and fun at your college's recreation center.

Bedroom

If you don't feel comfortable using the rec center or if it's beyond your budget, you can do cardiorepiratory, strength, and flexibility workouts right in your bedroom for free or for just a little money. Following are some suggestions in various price ranges (Nichols 2007).

Free

- **Cardio:** Do some low-impact moves, moving the arms and legs. Stepping, jogging, or marching in place; dancing; and running the stairs are all good choices.
- **Strength:** Use body weight for resistance to work all the major muscle groups (you can find instructions for several exercises at www.abc-of-fitness.com/info/fitness-exercises.asp).
- **Flexibility:** Stretch while sitting or standing, or use furniture to help increase your ROM. You can prop your foot up on a chair, desk, or bed to stretch the hamstrings more deeply. Use the walls for stretching arms, chest, and calves.

Low Cost

- **Cardio:** Use a jump rope ($5) or just jump up and down while turning your wrists.
- **Strength:** To supplement your body weight for resistance training, you can purchase resistance bands ($15).
- **Flexibility:** A yoga DVD ($10) is a good, economical choice. It might cost a little to begin with, but you can use it over and over again.

Medium Cost

- **Cardio:** Workout DVDs ($10+) offer many options. Buy used ones online or check them out from the library.
- **Strength:** A good set of dumbbells ($20) and a stability ball ($20) are economical strength training accessories.
- **Flexibility:** Although they're not essential equipment, a yoga mat ($20) or padded exercise mat ($25+) make stretching more comfortable.

What to Wear

You don't need to buy your favorite superstar athlete's top-of-the-line sneakers or have a head-to-toe matching exercise ensemble to have a great workout. However, proper equipment and well-fitting clothes are key to an enjoyable and safe workout. The important thing is to remember that comfort and fit come before fashion.

Athletic Shoes

Shoes are made to support feet differently depending on the type of activity, so the first step in buying a good pair of shoes for your exercise program is to determine the type of athletic shoe you need to purchase (American Academy of Podiatric Sports Medicine [AAPSM] 2007). Will you be running? Playing tennis? Playing soccer? Doing a variety of activities? Find a reputable shoe store that offers a wide variety of sport-specific shoes and has knowledgeable staff to help you find exactly what you need.

No matter what activity you do, it's important to have shoes that fit correctly. When trying on shoes, wear the type of socks you normally wear when active and bring shoe inserts if you wear them. Your feet are bigger at the end of the day, so don't do your shoe shopping first thing in the morning. Have a measurement taken of both feet. If your feet are two different sizes, go with the size of the larger foot. You need between 3/8 to 1/2 inch (1 to 1.3 centimeters) between your longest toe and the end of the shoe, and the heel should fit snugly. The ball of your foot should match the widest part of the shoe, with the bend of the toe matching the toe break of the shoe. Your new shoes should fit properly when you buy them; they shouldn't need to be broken in. Test the shoes thoroughly by wearing them in the store to ensure fit and a balanced, comfortable gait (AAPSM 2007).

Replace athletic shoes often, even if they look new. It only takes 3 to 5 months of regular use before shoes lose their support and cushion (AAPSM 2007). Replacing good athletic shoes after that amount of time may seem extravagant, especially if they still look good, but you don't need to spend a fortune on athletic shoes. You can often find good deals. One option is to purchase shoes from the previous season so you can get top-of-the-line products at a lower price (Payne et al. 2006).

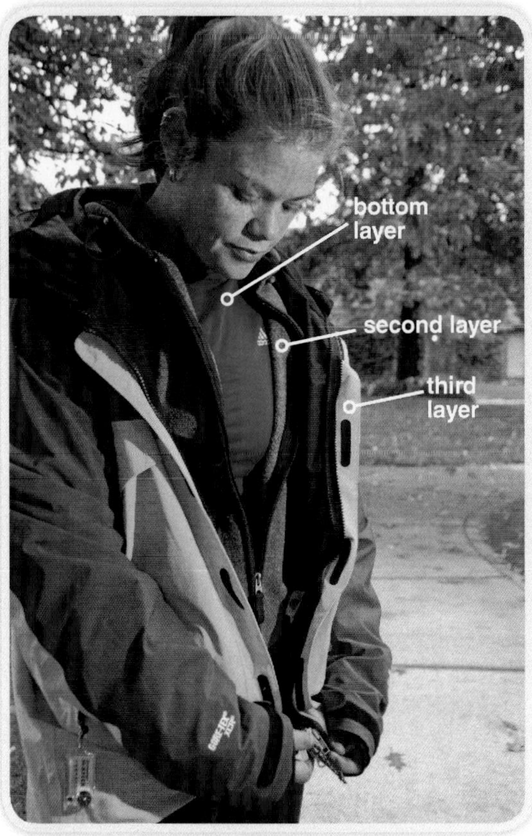

Figure 2.3 Each layer of clothing in the three-layer system has a specific function designed to keep you warm and dry in bad weather.

Workout Clothes

You don't need to buy specialized workout clothes when you start exercising, but wear comfortable clothing that allows to you move easily and maintain a steady body temperature. Choosing the right training clothes is not about fashion as much as it is about function.

If you're training outside in bad weather, use a three-layer system to stay warm and dry (see figure 2.3). The bottom layer, closest to your skin, should be the thinnest, to wick moisture away to the upper layers so that it can be dispersed to the air. Cotton isn't a good choice for the first layer, because although it can hold in heat, it absorbs and retains moisture. A lightweight microfiber channels perspiration away from the body, so it's a good first layer. The second layer is for insulation. It should retain heat and also allow excess heat to escape. Fleece is one of the most popular materials for this layer. The third, outermost layer should be made of a waterproof and windproof yet breathable material to protect you from the elements, mainly rain and wind. It needs to be light and breathable to keep you warm and dry, but it also should allow moisture to pass through.

You might also need winter accessories such as gloves, a scarf, earmuffs, a hat, or a pair of thick socks. Again, use materials made from a synthetic fiber to wick away moisture.

Safety Equipment

If you're exercising alone, especially at night, take safety precautions. Be aware of your surroundings when you're out so you can see the car up ahead or the stranger approaching you. Headphones make the workout time pass quicker, but if you wear them, make sure you can still hear what's going on around you. Stay on sidewalks when possible. If there are no sidewalks and you have to move to the street, go against traffic so that you can see vehicles approaching. Try to avoid heavily trafficked areas and construction. Certain gear can help keep you safe even on your longest workouts:

- Reflectors or lights worn on shoes or clothing. Exercise with precaution at night. Understand that you can see motorists, but they might not see you.
- Phone holders. Strap a cell phone to your arm, especially if you're going out on a path you've never taken or you're in a town you're not familiar with. Always tell someone your planned exercise route and an expected finishing time in case something happens.
- Helmet or protective padding. Depending on the activity, you might need a helmet or other protection. Even professional cyclists wear helmets in case of an accident. Don't assume you're experienced enough not to need a helmet or pads. Plan for the unexpected.
- Water bottle. Take water to ensure adequate hydration during your workout. Water is crucial for maintaining body temperature. If you'll be exercising in hot weather and dehydration is a concern, follow steps for hyperhydration previously mentioned.
- Sunscreen. Anytime you'll be outside for more than 20 minutes, you should apply sunscreen. Waterproof types will protect you even during your toughest workouts.
- Sunglasses or goggles. Protective eyewear is important for protecting your eyes from the elements. In addition, risk of injury increases when you can't see clearly.

FITNESS BASICS 101

What Do You Do?

Experts advise that people with chronic diseases, such as a heart condition, arthritis, diabetes, or high blood pressure, should talk to their doctor about what types and amounts of physical activity are appropriate. If you have a chronic disease, talk to your doctor before beginning a new physical activity program (CDC 2008).

The five components of health-related fitness are cardiorespiratory fitness, muscular strength, muscular endurance, flexibility, and body composition. Good cardiorespiratory fitness improves heart and lung function, decreases HRrest, decreases resting blood pressure, and decreases heart rate at any workload. Long-term benefits include reduced risk of heart disease, prevention of hypertension, improved blood lipids, improved overall health, and easier everyday functioning. Doing 30 minutes of moderate-intensity aerobic exercise on most, if not all, days of the week will develop or maintain the cardiorespiratory fitness levels necessary to see those benefits.

Muscular strength is the capacity of the muscle to exert force against a resistance. Muscular endurance refers to the capacity of the muscle to exert a force repeatedly against a resistance. The FITT guidelines for muscular strength and endurance provide the information you need to incorporate both into a well-rounded resistance program.

Three types of stretching—passive, active, and PNF—help improve flexibility, which is important in maintaining activities of daily living as you age. Stretching all the major muscle groups 2 or 3 days a week will keep your joints and muscles in good working condition.

Developing habits now will help you stay physically active throughout your adult life. Choose activities that are fun, make plans to fit activity into your daily or weekly schedule, and find the right equipment and clothes to make exercise as comfortable and safe as possible. Your college rec center is a good resource to take advantage of while you're in school, and your bedroom itself can function just fine as a workout facility.

Table 2.4 summarizes recommendations for general health improvements.

TABLE 2.4 Recommendations for Health Improvements

	Cardiorespiratory	Muscular strength and endurance	Flexibility
Frequency	3-5 days/week	2-3 days/week	2-3 days/week
Intensity	Moderate: 60%-80% HRR	Moderate: 2-4 sets, 8-12 reps	2-4 reps for each stretch
Time	30-60 min	6 sec per rep	Hold 15-30 sec
Type	Aerobic or anaerobic	Exercises for each major muscle group	Static

REVIEW QUESTIONS

1. What's the difference between physical fitness and health-related fitness?
2. What are the five components of health-related fitness?
3. Explain the principles of overload, progression, specificity, and reversibility.
4. For most people, intensities within the range of _____ percent to _____ percent of their HRR are good enough to bring improvements in cardiorespiratory fitness.
5. Why is the Karvonen method a more accurate way of determining the right target heart rate zone for exercise intensity?
6. Name three machines for cardiorespiratory training, and give one advantage and one disadvantage of using each machine.
7. What are the differences between muscular strength and muscular endurance?
8. Name three types of stretches that help keep muscles and joints flexible, and give an example of each type.
9. You can do cardiorespiratory, strength, and flexibility workouts right in your bedroom. For each type of workout, name one free option and one low-cost option.
10. What layers should you wear when exercising outdoors in cold weather, and why?

CRITICAL THINKING

1. List three barriers to exercise that inhibit you from participating in regular physical activity. Now come up with a strategy to overcome each barrier and describe how you will incorporate these strategies into your daily life.
2. Explain two exercise myths that you have heard that were not covered in this chapter. Use the Internet to find out if they are true or not (remember to use credible and reliable sources), and present your findings to the class.

APPLICATION ACTIVITIES

Visit the textbook's online student resource. From the Fitness Basics section, print the personal fitness contract, the program plan, and the tracking logs. Use the contract to establish your fitness goals, use the plan to chart a way to achieve your goals, and use the logs to keep track of your cardiorespiratory exercise, resistance training, and stretching.

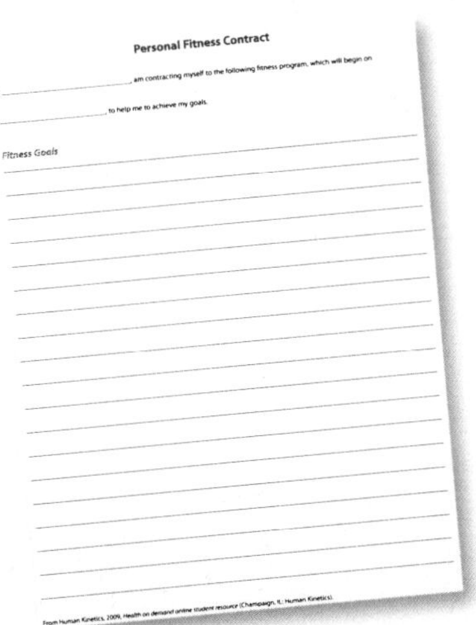
Personal Fitness Contract

Fitness Goals

Program Plan

Cardiorespiratory Exercise

Resistance Training

Tracking Log for Cardiorespiratory Exercises

GLOSSARY

active stretching—Occurs when you facilitate the force for the stretch.

aerobic activity—Any physical activity in which increased oxygen uptake is needed.

anaerobic activity—Any high-intensity activity in which oxygen is not needed.

ballistic stretching—Stretching that uses active muscular effort and bouncing instead of holding the end position.

body composition—Components that make up the human body and the proportions of these components, specifically the relative amounts of fat and fat-free mass in the body.

cardiorespiratory fitness—Ability of the heart and lungs to deliver oxygen and nutrients to the muscles and cells during exercise.

concentric contraction—Shortening phase of the muscle contraction.

cool-down—Slowing down at the end of the exercise session that reduces heart rate and prevents blood from pooling in the extremities.

delayed-onset muscle soreness (DOMS)—Soreness that occurs 24 to 48 hours following a workout as the result of the inflammation and microscopic tears in the tissues that surround the muscle fibers.

dynamic stretching—Similar to ballistic stretching except it avoids bouncing and includes movements specific to a sport or activity pattern.

eccentric contraction—Lengthening phase of the muscle contraction.

exercise—Type of planned, purposeful physical activity with the goal of improving or maintaining physical fitness.

flexibility—Ability of joints to smoothly move through full ROM.

functional capacity—Physical and mental ability to perform everyday tasks; declines with age.

health-related fitness—Level of fitness that allows the body to easily carry out everyday activities.

heart rate—Used as a guide to set exercise intensity. The higher the intensity, the higher the heart rate will be.

heart rate reserve (HRR)—Method of determining intensity that takes fitness level into account using HRrest.

hyperhydration—Strategy of taking in extra fluids shortly before exercising in a hot environment.

individuality—Everyone is unique and has individual fitness needs and adaptations to exercise.

isometric contractions—When the muscle applies force without moving.

Karvonen method—Method for calculating target heart rate ranges for training; considered more accurate than most methods because it takes HRrest into consideration.

maximum heart rate (HRmax)—The upper level of heart rate that you should be working at.

muscular endurance—Ability to sustain a muscular contraction or to contract repeatedly.

muscular strength—Maximal force of a muscle against resistance.

1-repetition maximum (1RM)—The maximum amount of weight that can be lifted through the full ROM only one time.

overload—Applying a greater load than normal to achieve a training effect.

passive stretching—Stretching that involves an external force, such as a partner or stretching machine.

physical activity—Movement produced by skeletal muscles that causes the body to work harder than normal.

physical fitness—Set of physical attributes that allows the body to perform moderate to vigorous levels of physical activity without becoming overly tired.

progression—To continue improving, the training overload must increase as you become fitter.

proprioceptive neuromuscular facilitation (PNF)—Stretching method usually performed with a partner in which passive movement and active muscle actions take advantage of the body's reflex response to enhance muscle relaxation and joint ROM.

range of motion (ROM)—Degree of movement at a joint.

repetition (rep)—One complete movement of an exercise through full ROM.

resistance training—Form of exercise that uses free weights, bands, machines, or body weight to put resistance on the muscle through full ROM.

resting heart rate (HRrest)—Heart rate while resting. The less physically fit, the higher the HRrest.

rest time—Amount of time between sets of an exercise.

reversibility—Fitness achievements are reversible if physical activity is discontinued.

set—Series of repetitions.

skill-related fitness—Ability to perform skills associated with specific sports and activities.

specificity—Type of exercise must relate to the desired results or activity.

static stretching—Slow stretch that is held without moving for about 30 seconds.

target heart rate (THR)—The range of heart rates required for exercise to result in cardiorespiratory benefits.

warm-up—Easy activity at the start of a workout to prepare the body for activity by increasing heart rate, blood flow, deep muscle temperature, respiration rate, viscosity of joint fluid, and perspiration.

weight—Amount of resistance used during an exercise.

REFERENCES AND RESOURCES

American Academy of Podiatric Sports Medicine (AAPSM). 2007. Recommended shoes. www.aapsm.org/crishoe.html.

American College of Sports Medicine (ACSM). 2006. *ACSM's guidelines for exercise testing and prescription.* 7th ed. Baltimore: Lippincott.

American Safety & Health Institute. 2007. *Complete emergency care.* Champaign, IL: Human Kinetics.

Baechle, T.R., and R.W. Earle. 2000. *National Strength and Conditioning Association's essentials of strength training and conditioning.* 2nd ed. Champaign, IL: Human Kinetics.

Centers for Disease Control and Prevention (CDC). 1997. Youth Risk Behavior Surveillance: National College Health Risk Behavior Survey—United States, 1995. *Morbidity and Mortality Weekly Report* 46 (SS-6): 1-54.

———. 2007. Body mass index. www.cdc.gov/healthyweight/assessing/bmi/index.htm.

———. 2008. Growing stronger: Strength training for older adults. www.cdc.gov/physicalactivity/growingstronger/index.html.

Corbin, C.B., and R. Lindsey. 2007. *Fitness for life.* Updated 5th ed. Champaign, IL: Human Kinetics.

Donatelle, R.J. 2008. Personal fitness. In *Access to health,* ed. R.J. Donatelle and P. Ketcham, 318-347. San Francisco: Benjamin Cummings.

Huang, T.T., K.J. Harris, R.E. Lee, N. Nazir, W. Born, and H. Kaur. 2003. Assessing overweight, obesity, diet, and physical activity in college students. *Journal of American College Health* 52 (2): 83-86.

Insel, P.M., and W.T. Roth. 2007. Exercise for health and fitness. In *Core concepts in health,* ed. P.M. Insel, W.T. Roth, and K. Price, 376-409. New York: McGraw-Hill.

Jackson, A.W., J.R. Morrow Jr., D.W. Hill, and R.K. Dishman. 2004. *Physical activity for health and fitness.* Champaign, IL: Human Kinetics.

McArdle, W.D., F.I. Katch, and V.L. Katch. 2001. *Exercise physiology: Energy, nutrition, and human performance.* 5th ed. Baltimore: Lippincott Williams & Wilkins.

Murphy, R.J., and W.F. Ashe. 1965. Prevention of heat illness in football players. *Journal of the American Medical Association* 194: 650.

Nichols, N. 2007. Dorm room workouts. SparkPeople. http://sparkpeople.com/resource/fitness_articles.asp?id=629.

Payne, W.A., D.B. Hahn, and E.B. Lucas. 2006. Becoming physically fit. In *Understanding your health,* ed. W.A. Payne, D.B. Hahn, and E. Maver, 100-126. New York: McGraw-Hill.

Platkin, C.S. 2003. Exercise facts get mixed up with fallacies. *Honolulu Advertiser,* Nov. 12. http://the.honoluluadvertiser.com/article/2003/Nov/12/il/il05a.html.

Schoenfeld, B. 2003. *Sculpting her body perfect.* Champaign, IL: Human Kinetics.

Sharkey, B.J., and S.E. Gaskill. 2007. *Fitness and health.* 6th ed. Champaign, IL: Human Kinetics.

Teague, M.L., S.L.C. Mackenzie, and D.M. Rosenthal. 2007. Fitness: Physical activity for life. In *Your health today: Choices in a changing society,* ed. M.L. Teague, S.L.C. Mackenzie, and D.M. Rosenthal, 195-224. New York: McGraw-Hill.

U.S. Department of Health and Human Services (USDHHS). 2001. *Physical activity and health: The link between physical activity and morbidity and mortality.* Atlanta: CDC.

Other helpful resources include the following.

American Council on Exercise (ACE). www.acefitness.org. ACE is a nonprofit organization committed to enriching quality of life through safe and effective exercise and physical activity.

American College of Sports Medicine (ACSM). www.acsm.org. ACSM is a professional society providing basic and applied exercise science conferences, meetings, and workshops.

National Strength and Conditioning Association (NSCA). www.nsca-lift.org. NSCA is an international nonprofit educational association that develops and presents the most advanced information regarding strength training and conditioning practices, injury prevention, and research findings.

National Weather Service (NWS). 2007a. Heat index chart. www.weather.gov/os/heat/index.shtml.

———. 2007b. Windchill index. www.weather.gov/os/windchill/index.shtml.

Racette, S., S. Deusinger, M. Strube, G. Highstein, and R. Deusinger. 2004. Weight changes, exercises, and dietary patterns during freshman and sophomore years of college. *Journal of American College Health* 53 (6): 245-251.

Silence, M. 2006. Fitness equipment: How to buy your next pair of fitness shoes. Diet Channel. www.thedietchannel.com/Fitness-Equipment-How-to-Buy-Your-Next-Pair-of-Fitness-Shoes.htm.

U.S. Department of Health and Human Services. 2008. Physical activity guidelines for Americans. www.health.gov/PAGuidelines/.

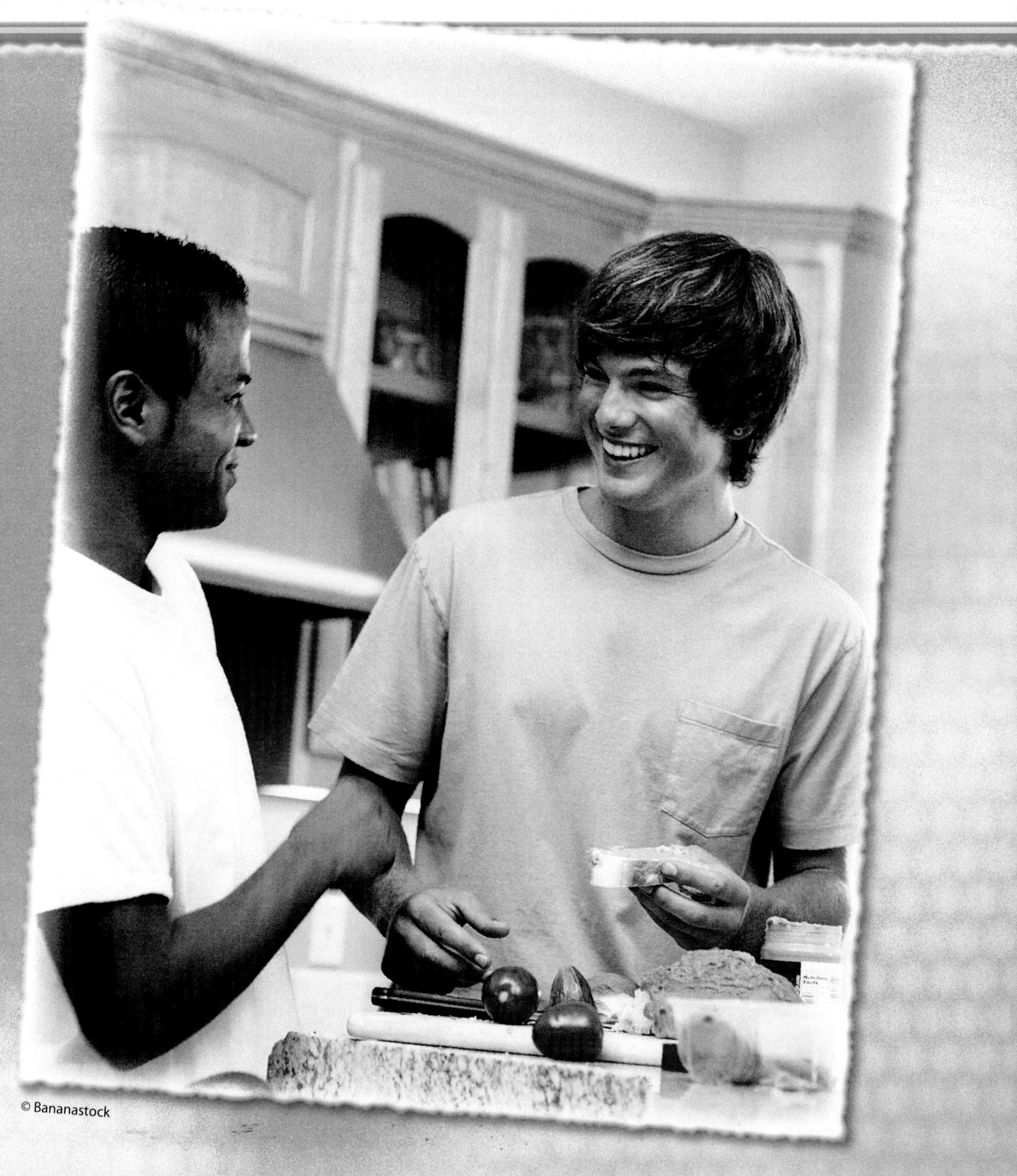

© Bananastock

CHAPTER 3

NUTRITION

STACEY L. KRAWCZYK, MS, RD, LDN
University of Illinois

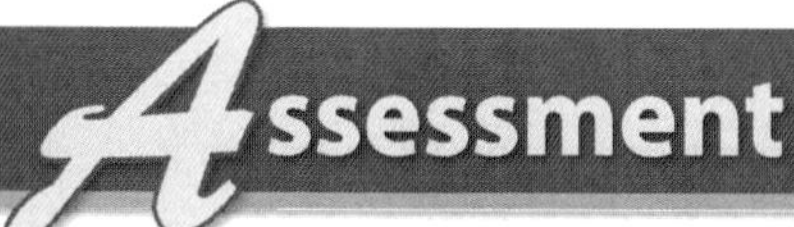

Assessment

- What foods are high in trans fat?
- What should your cholesterol levels be?
- Is it a good idea to take supplements?
- Do you drink sugar-sweetened beverages? Do you know how many calories they provide?
- What is MyPyramid, and how do you use it to make healthy food choices?
- What do all the numbers in a nutrition label really mean?
- Do you know the 10 red flags of junk science?

Objectives

- Identify the macronutrient components of the human diet and their corresponding caloric values and major functions in the body.
- Understand energy balance and how it contributes to healthy weight.
- Understand what constitutes a healthy diet according to the dietary guidelines for Americans.
- Know how to evaluate nutrition information to decipher fads and myths.
- List the best food-handling practices to prevent foodborne illness.
- Understand where to search for reliable nutrition information and resources.

Passover Seder. Labor Day cookouts. Thanksgiving turkey. Birthday cake. Food plays a huge part in most major holidays and celebrations. There's also tailgating, Sunday dinner, and chicken soup when you're sick. Food is more than just the fuel for the body. It's tied to memories, family, and culture; it's part of who you are. The aim of this chapter is to merge what you know and love about food with what's best for your body.

BODY BASICS

Nutrients are the basic components in all food. **Macronutrients** are the essential components that contribute most to the functions of the body and that supply building blocks for movement, growth, and repair. **Micronutrients** are also important to bodily functions, but they are required in only small amounts and generally need to be found in the diet.

Macronutrients

The macronutrients are protein, carbohydrate, fat, and water, and each of the first three supplies the body with energy commonly referred to as calories (water has no calories; see the later section on "Water" for more information). One gram of protein supplies 4 calories, 1 gram of carbohydrate supplies 4 calories, and 1 gram of fat supplies 9 calories. A simplified definition of **calorie** is a measure of the energy used by the body and of the energy that food supplies to the body.

Protein

Protein is a complex, nitrogen-based compound made up of amino acids in linkages called *peptide bonds*. Dietary protein is used to make the major structural protein of the body and to carry out other special functions, such as forming enzymes, hormones, and various body fluids and secretions. Protein also carries some lipids, vitamins, and minerals throughout the body. The building blocks of protein are **amino acids**, which are classified as either essential or nonessential. If the body can't make enough of an amino acid to meet its needs and has to get it through the diet, then it is essential. The body can make adequate amounts of nonessential amino acids.

Essential Amino Acids

- Leucine
- Isoleucine
- Valine
- Tryptophan
- Phenylalanine
- Methionine
- Threonine
- Lysine
- Histidine
- Arginine

Nonessential Amino Acids

- Alanine
- Aspartic acid
- Asparagine
- Glutamic acid
- Glutamine
- Glycine
- Proline
- Serine

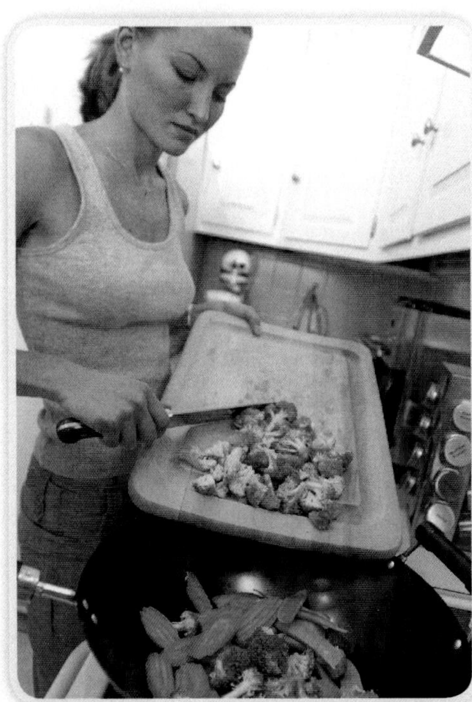

Some vegetables, such as broccoli, are high in protein.

© Human Kinetics

ISSUES IN THE NEWS

Watch Your Trans Fats

As of January 2006, the U.S. Food and Drug Administration (FDA) requires nutrition labels to list trans fat. These labeling changes are helpful, but they don't cover fast food, which often contains high levels of trans fats (TF). Fast food can even be advertised as cholesterol free and cooked in vegetable oil. Just one doughnut at breakfast (3.2 grams of TF) and a large order of French fries at lunch (6.8 grams of TF) add up to 10 grams of TF, so the lack of regulations for labeling restaurant foods can be harmful.

The Nutrition Committee of the American Heart Association (AHA) advises that healthy Americans over the age of 2 limit their intake of trans fat to less than 1 percent of total calories. Based on current data, the AHA recommends the following guidelines:

- Choose a diet rich in fruits, vegetables, whole-grain foods, high-fiber foods, and fat-free and low-fat dairy.
- Keep total fat intake between 25 and 35 percent of calories. The majority should come from fish, nuts, seeds, vegetable oils, and other sources of monounsaturated and polyunsaturated fats.
- Use naturally occurring, unhydrogenated vegetable oils, such as canola, safflower, sunflower, or olive oil.
- If you buy processed foods, choose those made with unhydrogenated oils rather than partially hydrogenated or hydrogenated vegetable oils or saturated fat.
- Use margarine instead of butter, and choose soft margarines (liquid or tub varieties) over stick forms. Some manufacturers are offering unhydrogenated margarines. Look for brands that contain less that 2 grams of trans fat per serving and list liquid vegetable oil as the first ingredient.
- French fries, doughnuts, cookies, crackers, muffins, pies, and cakes are high in trans fat; don't eat them often.
- Limit saturated fat. If you don't eat a lot of saturated fat, you won't be consuming a lot of trans fat.
- Limit commercially fried foods and baked goods made with shortening or partially hydrogenated vegetable oils. These foods are very high in fat that is likely to be hydrogenated, meaning they contain a lot of trans fat.
- Commercial shortening and deep-frying fats are made by hydrogenation and contain saturated fat and trans fat, which is just one more reason to eat fried fast food infrequently.

Reprinted, by permission, from American Heart Association. Available: www.americanheart.org/presenter.jhtml?identifier=532.

Carbohydrate

A **carbohydrate** is a chemical compound made up of carbon, hydrogen, and oxygen. Plants make and store carbohydrate as their chief source of energy. Carbohydrate is classified by its structural backbone of simple sugars, called **saccharides**.

- Monosaccharides (the simplest sugars) include glucose and fructose.
- Disaccharides (sugars formed of two monosaccharides) include sucrose, maltose, and lactose.
- Polysaccharides (sugars formed of more than two monosaccharides) include starch, dextrin, glycogen, and cellulose.

Dietary fiber is a form of cellulose that generally refers to parts of fruits, vegetables, grains, nuts, and legumes that humans can't digest. Meat and dairy products don't contain fiber. Research indicates that high-fiber diets can reduce the risks of heart disease and certain types of cancer (Pereira et al. 2004; Wakai et al. 2007). There are two types of fiber: soluble and insoluble. Soluble fiber in cereals, oatmeal, beans, and other foods has been found to lower blood cholesterol. Insoluble fiber in vegetables and fruit helps shorten transit time as foods move through the stomach and intestine. This faster transit time helps decrease the risk of cancers of the colon and rectum.

Fat

Fat includes compounds composed of the same three elements as carbohydrate (carbon, hydrogen, and oxygen), but with more carbon and hydrogen and less oxygen, which means fat can store more energy in the chemical bonds. One molecule of fat can be broken into three fatty acids and one glycerol backbone, which is why fats are chemically known as *triglycerides*. Some fats supply essential fatty acids, such as linoleic, linolenic, and arachidonic acids, which can't be synthesized in the body. Fat also maintains cell membrane integrity, regulates cholesterol metabolism, and develops prostaglandins, which help regulate body processes. The body needs dietary fat to carry fat-soluble vitamins and absorb them.

Fatty acids are classified as saturated, monounsaturated, or polyunsaturated, depending on the number of hydrogen atoms attached to the carbon atoms of the fat molecule. The greater the number of hydrogen atoms, the higher the saturated fat content. In general, the more saturated a fatty acid is, the more solid it is at room temperature, and the more unsaturated a fat is, the more liquid it is at room temperature. Liquid fat (at room temperature) is called *oil*. Saturated fat is typically more stable than unsaturated fat because it has only single bonds between the carbon and hydrogen molecules. Manufacturers of processed food value that stability because it helps increase the shelf life of food.

Trans fats are processed fats that are solid at room temperature. They naturally occur in some foods (beef, milk, butter, lamb), but the biggest source in the American diet is partially hydrogenated oils (margarine, shortening, commercial frying fats, and high-fat baked goods). Partially hydrogenated vegetable oils were developed to help take the place of highly saturated fats in food manufacturing. However, trans fats, similar to saturated fats, tend to raise blood cholesterol.

Cholesterol is a fatlike substance called a *lipid*. Cholesterol is found in all cell membranes and is necessary for the production of bile acids and steroid hormones. The body does make some cholesterol, but dietary cholesterol comes only from animal foods. Excessive cholesterol in the body can clog arteries and lead to heart disease, so it's important to monitor your blood cholesterol level. Your total cholesterol should be less than 200 milligrams per deciliter (mg/dl). Your "bad" cholesterol (low-density lipoprotein, or LDL) should be less than 160 mg/dl, and it should be less than 100 mg/dl if you have been diagnosed with heart disease. Your "good" cholesterol (high-density lipoprotein, or HDL) should be greater than 40 mg/dl if you are male and greater than 50 mg/dl if you are female. (A good way to remember which cholesterol is good and which is bad is by using a mnemonic device: **L**DL is **l**ousy and **H**DL is **h**appy.)

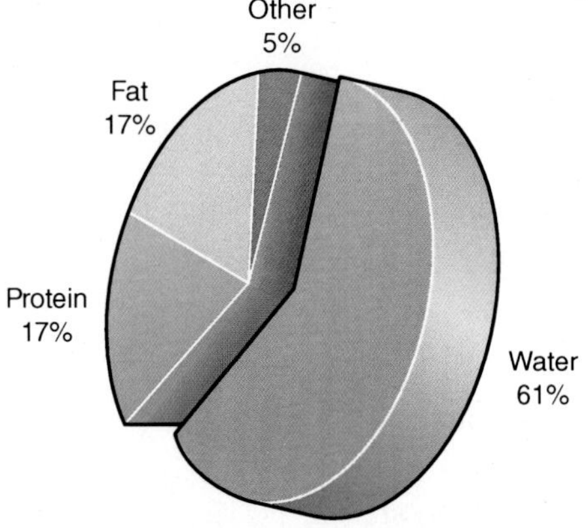

Figure 3.1 Components of a 150-pound (68-kilogram) healthy male.

Water

Water is ranked second only to oxygen as essential for life. People can survive deficiencies of energy or nutrients for months or years, but they can last only a few days without water. Water is vital to all body processes, including digestion, circulation, and lubrication of body joints. It also mediates various chemical reactions in the body.

Figure 3.1 shows how all of these components look when they're put together. An average 150-pound (68-kilogram) healthy male is composed of about 92 pounds (42 kilograms) of water, 26 pounds (12 kilograms) of fat, and another 26 pounds (12 kilograms) of protein. The rest of the weight comes from other minerals.

Micronutrients

The micronutrients are vitamins and minerals. **Vitamins** can have various forms, and different names are often used for the same vitamin. Thirteen compounds are classified as vitamins.

- Fat-soluble vitamins include vitamin A (retinol), vitamin D (cholecalciferol), vitamin E (alpha-tocopherol), and vitamin K.
- Water-soluble vitamins include vitamin C, biotin, folate, niacin (vitamin B_3), pantothenic acid, riboflavin (vitamin B_2), thiamin (vitamin B_1), vitamin B_6, and vitamin B_{12}.

Fat-soluble vitamins can be stored in the body. They're usually found with foods that contain fat and are absorbed best in the presence of a small amount of fat. Fat-soluble vitamins E and A have antioxidant properties, and in sufficient quantities they can help prevent heart disease and cancer. An **antioxidant** is a substance that reduces damage from oxidation in the body by attaching itself to free radicals. Free radicals attack tissues and remove electrons, which damages the tissue. Most water-soluble vitamins are components of enzyme systems. Many are involved in the reactions supporting energy metabolism, but vitamin C is also a strong antioxidant. Water-soluble vitamins are usually not stored in the body, unlike fat-soluble vitamins, so a daily dietary supply is necessary.

Minerals are also important nutrients found in foods, but they don't contain any carbon molecules. You need more than 100 milligrams a day of the major minerals (calcium, phosphorus, magnesium, sodium, and potassium). You need trace minerals (iron, iodine, selenium, zinc, chromium, copper, and fluoride) in smaller amounts, but their function is just as important. Sodium, chloride, and potassium are called **electrolytes**, and they work to maintain water balance and pressure between and within cells and their surrounding fluids.

You can harm your body if you take supplements that supply too many minerals because the minerals can build up and become toxic or interfere with the absorption of other nutrients. Individual mineral supplements (e.g., potassium pills) are potentially dangerous unless a doctor prescribes them for a specific purpose.

CONTROVERSIAL ISSUES

To Supplement or Not to Supplement?

From vitamins to minerals to weight-loss pills, thousands of supplements are on store shelves. Do people need dietary supplements? One thing is for sure: Selling them is big business. The total U.S. sales of dietary supplements in 2006 were estimated at more than $22 billion, with vitamins alone accounting for more than $7 billion (Zelman 2007). The rest was from sales of minerals, herbs and botanicals, sport supplements, meal supplements, and weight-loss products. The Dietary Supplement Health and Education Act, approved by the U.S. Congress in 1994, defines dietary supplements as products that

- are intended to supplement the diet,
- contain one or more ingredients (vitamins, herbs, amino acids, or their constituents),
- are intended to be taken by mouth, and
- are labeled as dietary supplements.

In August 2007, the FDA, which previously regulated dietary supplements the same way it does foods, released a new ruling to ensure that supplements

- are produced in a quality manner,
- do not contain contaminants or impurities, and
- are accurately labeled.

The FDA also provides guidelines for the use of any health claim about a manufacturer's product. The FDA must review any claims, and the manufacturer must provide evidence that the dietary supplement is both effective and safe.

As the name implies, supplements aren't supposed to replace nutritious foods in a healthy diet but to supplement them. Foods are complex and contain far more than the basic macronutrients, offering vitamins, minerals, phytochemicals, and other substances. Thus, relying on food first to supply dietary needs ensures a healthy and balanced approach.

What do the experts recommend? The American Dietetic Association (ADA) suggests that "the best nutritional strategy for promoting optimal health and reducing the risk of chronic disease is to wisely choose a wide variety of foods. Additional nutrients from fortified foods and/or supplements can help some people meet their nutritional needs as specified by science-based nutrition standards such as the Dietary Reference Intakes" (ADA 2005). Some special populations do need supplements added to their diet at the advice of a physician, including pregnant women, nursing mothers, strict vegetarians, people with certain food allergies or intolerances, senior citizens, and people with certain diseases such as cancer or kidney, cardiovascular, or bone disease.

DIGESTION, FROM BEGINNING TO END

Digestion allows the body to get the nutrients and energy it needs from the food. It helps the body break food into smaller molecules before they're absorbed by the blood and carried throughout the body to be used for energy, growth, and bodily functions. The digestive system is a series of hollow organs joined in a long tube from the mouth to the anus (see figure 3.2). The tube is lined with mucosa. In areas such as the mouth, stomach, and small intestine, the mucosa contains tiny glands that produce secretions to help digest food. Two organs outside this tube, the liver and the pancreas, also produce digestive juices that reach the intestine by way of small tubes. Many other systems (e.g., nervous, blood, hormone) also play a role in digestion.

Digestion is the mixing of food, the movement of food through the digestive tract, and the chemical breakdown of larger molecules of food into smaller molecules that the body can use. Digestion begins in the mouth when you chew and swallow, and it is completed in the small intestine. When all the digested nutrients are absorbed through the intestinal walls, fiber and waste products move to the large intestine (colon), where they remain until a bowel movement expels the feces.

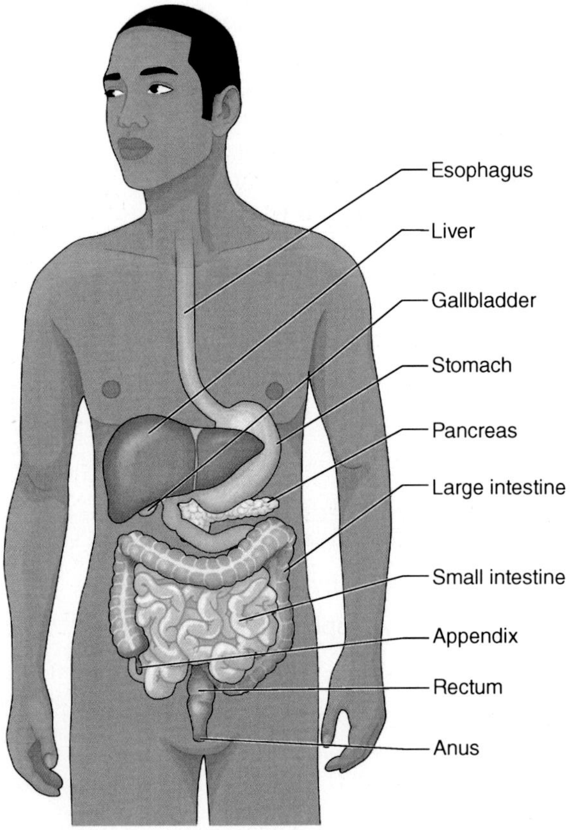

Figure 3.2 The digestive system breaks down food so it can be absorbed by the body.

EATING A BALANCED DIET

The body needs the right balance of protein, carbohydrate, fat, water, vitamins, and minerals to stay healthy, and the food you eat supplies those macro- and micronutrients. Figuring out how to get the right balance is the key. The International Food Information Council (IFIC) Foundation releases an annual report called "Food and Health Survey: Consumer Attitudes Toward Food, Nutrition and Health." Data from the 2007 report indicated that physical activity, weight, and diet are all significant factors in overall health (IFIC 2007).

Body weight seems to be one of the strongest factors that influences a decision to make a dietary change; 70 percent of people in the 2007 study said they change dietary habits to lose weight. A recent change from previous years is that more Americans (66 percent) said they're making dietary changes to improve the healthfulness of their diet. The dietary changes most often reported were changing meal and snack patterns and reducing portion sizes.

Knowing that it's important to eat a healthy diet and actually doing it are two different things, and the gap between knowing and doing is widening in the United States. A much larger percentage of adults and children are overweight and obese today than they were in the mid-1970s. Data from the National Health and Nutrition Examination Survey (NHANES) of the Centers for Disease Control and Prevention (CDC) illustrate that from the mid-1970s to 2004, the prevalence of overweight or obesity increased from 47 percent to 66 percent in adults aged 20 to 74 years (see figure 3.3). During the same time period, the prevalence of overweight children aged 2 to 5 years increased from 5 percent to 14 percent; for children aged 6 to 11 years, it increased from 7 percent to 19 percent; and for children aged 12 to 19 years, it increased from 5 percent to 17 percent (see figure 3.4) (CDC 2005).

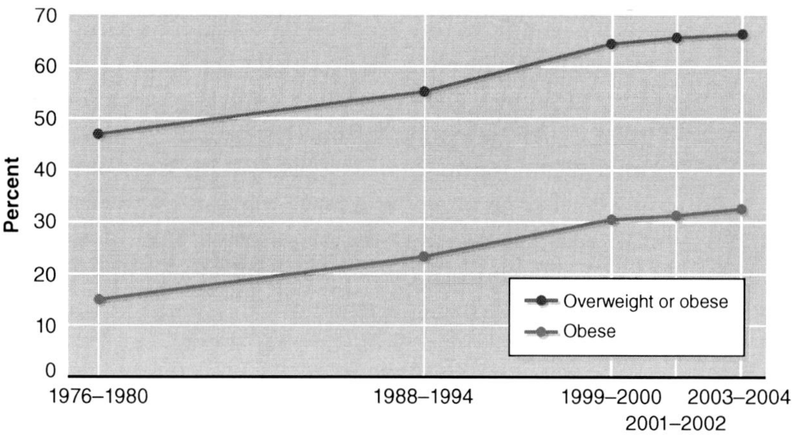

Figure 3.3 Trends in adult overweight and obesity, ages 20 years and older. (Age-adjusted by the direct method to the year 2000 U.S. Census Bureau estimates using the age groups 20 to 30, 40 to 59, and 60 years and over. Overweight defined as BMI ≥ 25; obesity defined as BMI ≥ 30.)

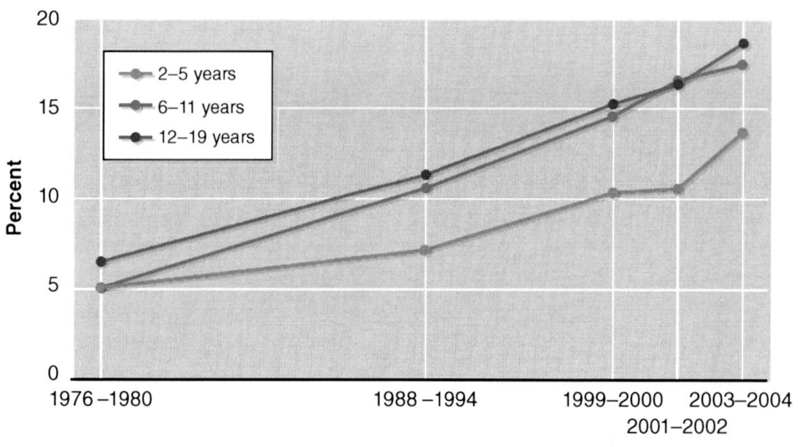

Figure 3.4 Trends in child and adolescent overweight. (Overweight is defined as BMI ≥ gender- and weight-specific 95th percentile from the 2000 CDC Growth Charts.)

People in medical and national leadership positions are concerned about the rising rate of obesity, because obesity-related chronic diseases accounted for five of the leading six causes of death in 2002 in the United States (CDC 2007). Obesity is linked to the development of many diseases and health conditions, including hypertension, dyslipidemia, type 2 diabetes, coronary heart disease, stroke, and some cancers. The estimated total cost of obesity in the United States in 2000 was about $117 billion.

Obesity and *overweight* refer to weight ranges greater than what is generally considered healthy. Health professionals refer to a screening tool called *body mass index*, or BMI, to assess people's degree of body fat. You can calculate your BMI by dividing your body weight (in kilograms) by your height (in meters) squared. A BMI between 25 and 29.9 in adults is considered overweight, and a BMI of 30 or greater is considered obese.

BMI correlates with the amount of body fat in a body, but it's not a direct measure of body fat. Some lean people, such as athletes, may have a high BMI due to high amounts of muscle, but they don't have excess body fat or corresponding health risk as a result. The BMI is simply a screening tool, and if the BMI is in the overweight or obese range, it should trigger other assessments. Two other assessments that gather further risk-factor data are waist circumference and clinical indicators for disease. Waist circumference involves the location of fat on the body. Excess body fat mainly around the waist is a risk indicator for health problems, even if the BMI falls within the normal range. Women with a waist circumference of more than 35 inches (88 centimeters) and men with a circumference of more than 40 inches (102 centimeters) are at a higher risk for certain chronic diseases.

CONSUMER ISSUES
Phytofunctional What?

Nutrition is a relatively young science. Food scientists discover new compounds and interactions of old compounds all the time. Phytochemicals, for example, are substances in plants that affect body systems and may promote health and decrease the risk of diseases such as cancer. Functional foods are food substances that may provide health benefits beyond basic nutrition. Table 3.1 describes some functional components and lists common food sources and their potential benefits.

New advances in identifying these bioactive substances and mapping the human genome have lead to an emerging field called nutrigenomics, or personalized nutrition. **Nutrigenomics** applies the human genome to nutrition and personal health to provide individual dietary recommendations. By using their unique genetic map to determine their own nutritional requirements, consumers might someday be able to reduce their risk of disease. Personalized nutrition seems promising, but research is still in the early stages. It could be many years before it's possible to have accurate and effective recommendations for personalized nutrition.

For more information, check out the Web site of the International Food Information Council Foundation (www.ific.org).

TABLE 3.1 Examples of Functional Components

Class/components	Source*	Potential benefits
CAROTENOIDS		
Beta-carotene	Carrots, pumpkin, sweet potato, cantaloupe	Neutralizes free radicals, which may damage cells; bolsters cellular antioxidant defenses; can be made into vitamin A in the body.
Lutein, xeaxanthin	Kale, collards, spinach, corn, eggs, citrus	May contribute to maintenance of healthy vision.
Lycopene	Tomatoes and processed tomato products, watermelon, red and pink grapefruit	May contribute to maintenance of prostate health.
DIETARY (FUNCTIONAL AND TOTAL) FIBER		
Insoluble fiber	Wheat bran, corn bran, fruit skins	May contribute to maintenance of a healthy digestive tract; may reduce the risk of some types of cancer.
Beta glucan**	Oat bran, oatmeal, oat flour, barley, rye	May reduce risk of coronary heart disease (CHD).
Soluble fiber**	Psyllium seed husk, peas, beans, apples, citrus fruit	May reduce risk of CHD and some types of cancer.
Whole grains**	Cereal grains, whole-wheat bread, oatmeal, brown rice	May reduce risk of CHD and some types of cancer; may contribute to maintenance of healthy blood glucose levels.
FATTY ACIDS		
Monounsaturated fatty acids (MUFAs)**	Tree nuts, olive oil, canola oil	May reduce risk of CHD.
Polyunsaturated fatty acids (PUFAs)—omega-3 fatty acids (ALA)	Walnuts, flax	May contribute to maintenance of heart health; may contribute to maintenance of mental and visual function.
PUFAs—omega-3 fatty acids (DHA/EPA)**	Salmon, tuna, marine, and other fish oils	May reduce risk of CHD; may contribute to maintenance of mental and visual function.
Conjugated linoleic acid (CLA)	Beef and lamb, some cheese	May contribute to maintenance of desirable body composition and healthy immune function.

MINERALS		
Calcium**	Sardines, spinach, yogurt, low-fat dairy products, fortified foods and beverages	May reduce the risk of osteoporosis.
Magnesium	Spinach, pumpkin seeds, whole-grain breads and cereals, halibut, brazil nuts	May contribute to maintenance of normal muscle and nerve function, healthy immune function, and bone health.
Potassium**	Potatoes, low-fat dairy products, whole-grain breads and cereals, citrus juices, beans, bananas	May reduce the risk of high blood pressure and stroke in combination with a low-sodium diet.
Selenium	Fish, red meat, grains, garlic, liver, eggs	Neutralizes free radicals, which may damage cells; may contribute to healthy immune function.
SOY PROTEIN		
Soy protein**	Soybeans and soy-based products	May reduce risk of CHD.
VITAMINS		
A***	Organ meats, milk, eggs, carrots, sweet potato, spinach	May contribute to maintenance of healthy vision, immune function, and bone health; may contribute to cell integrity.
B_1 (thiamin)	Lentils, peas, long-grain brown rice, brazil nuts	May contribute to maintenance of mental function; helps regulate metabolism.
B_2 (riboflavin)	Lean meats, eggs, green leafy vegetables	Helps support cell growth; helps regulate metabolism.
B_3 (niacin)	Dairy products, poultry, fish, nuts, eggs	Helps support cell growth; helps regulate metabolism.
B_5 (pantothenic acid)	Organ meats, lobster, soybeans, lentils	Helps regulate metabolism and hormone synthesis.
B_6 (pyridoxine)	Beans, nuts, legumes, fish, meat, whole grains	May contribute to maintenance of healthy immune function; helps regulate metabolism.
B_9 (folate)**	Beans, legumes, citrus foods, green leafy vegetables, fortified breads and cereals	May reduce a woman's risk of having a child with a brain or spinal cord defect.
B_{12} (cobalamin)	Eggs, meat, poultry, milk	May contribute to maintenance of mental function; helps regulate metabolism and supports blood cell formation.
Biotin	Liver, salmon, dairy, eggs, oysters	Helps regulate metabolism and hormone synthesis.
C	Guava, sweet red and green peppers, kiwi, citrus fruit, strawberries	Neutralizes free radicals; may contribute to maintenance of bone health and immune function.
D	Sunlight, fish, fortified milk and cereals	Helps regulate calcium and phosphorus; helps contribute to bone health; may contribute to healthy immune function; helps support cell growth.
E	Sunflower seeds, almonds, hazelnuts, turnip greens	Neutralizes free radicals, which may damage cells; may contribute to healthy immune function and maintenance of heart health.

*Examples are not an all-inclusive list.
**FDA-approved health claim established for component.
***Preformed vitamin A is found in foods that come from animals. Provitamin A carotenoids are found in many dark-colored fruits and vegetables and are a major source of vitamin A for vegetarians.
For a full list of functional components of foods, visit the International Food Information Council Web site (www.ific.org/nutrition/functional/).
Reprinted from the International Food Information Council Foundation, 2006.

What Do You Do?

Carry a small notebook with you and jot down what you drink for a day. Include the type of drink (e.g., soda, milk, water, coffee), the portion size, and the number of calories from sugar. Any surprises? This can also be a great tool for keeping track of everything you eat or drink over a couple of days. What patterns do you see? What are some easy changes that you can make to move toward a healthier diet?

Energy Equation

Simply put, overweight and obesity result from an energy imbalance over time. When you routinely take in more calories than you use for activity, body maintenance, or growth, the extra energy is deposited, generally as fat. Body weight is also influenced by genetics, metabolism, behavior, environment, culture, and socioeconomic status.

Energy In

On average, Americans spend nearly half of their food dollars on meals outside the home (Stewart, Blisard, Bhuyan, and Jayga 2004). Often, these convenience foods are high in fat, sugar, and calories and are less nutrient dense. In addition, Americans are consuming more calories in general. Food-supply data from the U.S. Department of Agriculture (USDA) estimated that daily intake of calories increased 12 percent, almost 300 calories per day, between 1985 and 2000 (Putnam, Allshouse, and Kantor 2002). Several studies have also shown that eating out more frequently is associated with obesity, higher body fatness, and higher BMI (Keystone Center 2006).

Portion sizes of restaurant meals have increased over time, too, and that means people are getting a lot more on the calories-consumed side of the equation. Table 3.2 shows how typical portion sizes increased from 1980 to 2000 and how the number of calories increased as a result (National Heart, Lung, and Blood Institute [NHLBI] 2007).

A 2007 review article from the University of Washington took a look at what could be an overarching reason for the obesity epidemic. The researcher found that refined grains, added sugars, and added fats are relatively inexpensive, good tasting, and convenient. Most energy-dense foods cost less than nutrient-dense foods, which would be attractive to people who want to keep their food costs down, such as those who have low incomes. This preference of low-cost dietary energy may be the main predictor of population weight gain (Drewnowski 2007).

Not only does what you eat have a significant impact on your calorie intake, but so does what you drink. In a 2006 report titled "What America Drinks," researchers examined beverage-consumption data from the NHANES III. They found that Americans drink sugar-sweetened beverages (soft drinks, fruit-flavored drinks, presweetened teas) to the extent that such drinks supply approximately 22 percent of total calories consumed each day (Environ International Corporation 2006). The report also found that

TABLE 3.2 Increase in Portion Size and Calories Between 1980 and 2000

Food	1980 portion size	1980 calories	2000 portion size	2000 calories
Cheeseburger	1 burger	333	1 burger	590
French fries	2.4 oz (68 g)	210	6.9 oz (196 g)	610
Regular soda	6.5 oz (192 ml)	85	20 oz (591 ml)	250
Coffee with whole milk and sugar	8 oz (237 ml)	45	Mocha latte 16 oz (473 ml)	350
Chicken Caesar salad	1.5 c	390	3.5 c	790

teenage boys drink an average of 32 ounces (946 milliliters) of sweetened beverages a day, which adds up to 387 calories, or 13 percent of total daily calories, and teenage girls drink 22 ounces (651 milliliters), or 267 calories and 12 percent of calories. That's 8,000 calories over the course of a month, just from sweetened beverages! The intake from the sugar in sweetened beverages alone is 69 to 100 pounds (31 to 45 kilograms) of sugar per teen per year (see figure 3.5).

Most Americans aren't following standard nutrition guidelines. In 2005, only 25 percent of Americans ate five or more servings of fruits and vegetables each day (CDC 2007). Though Americans don't have a problem eating the recommended number of servings of grains (10 servings per day in 2003), they don't meet the recommendations for whole grains. Instead of consuming half their servings of grains as whole grains, Americans ate only one whole-grain serving per day in 2003 (Buzby, Farah, and Vocke 2005). Foods that contain calcium don't fare any better. Soft drinks are taking the place of milk in the diets of Americans, especially for children (Environ International Corporation 2006).

What's the solution? Education is a key. Researchers found that educating college students about the dietary guidelines for Americans (which will be discussed a little later in the chapter) may lead to healthful changes in the foods they choose to eat (Kolodinsky et al. 2007). Additionally, researchers have shown that the MyPyramid recommendations in the dietary guidelines are consistent with the various recommendations suggested to control obesity and the chronic diseases associated with that condition (Krebs-Smith and Kris-Etherton 2007).

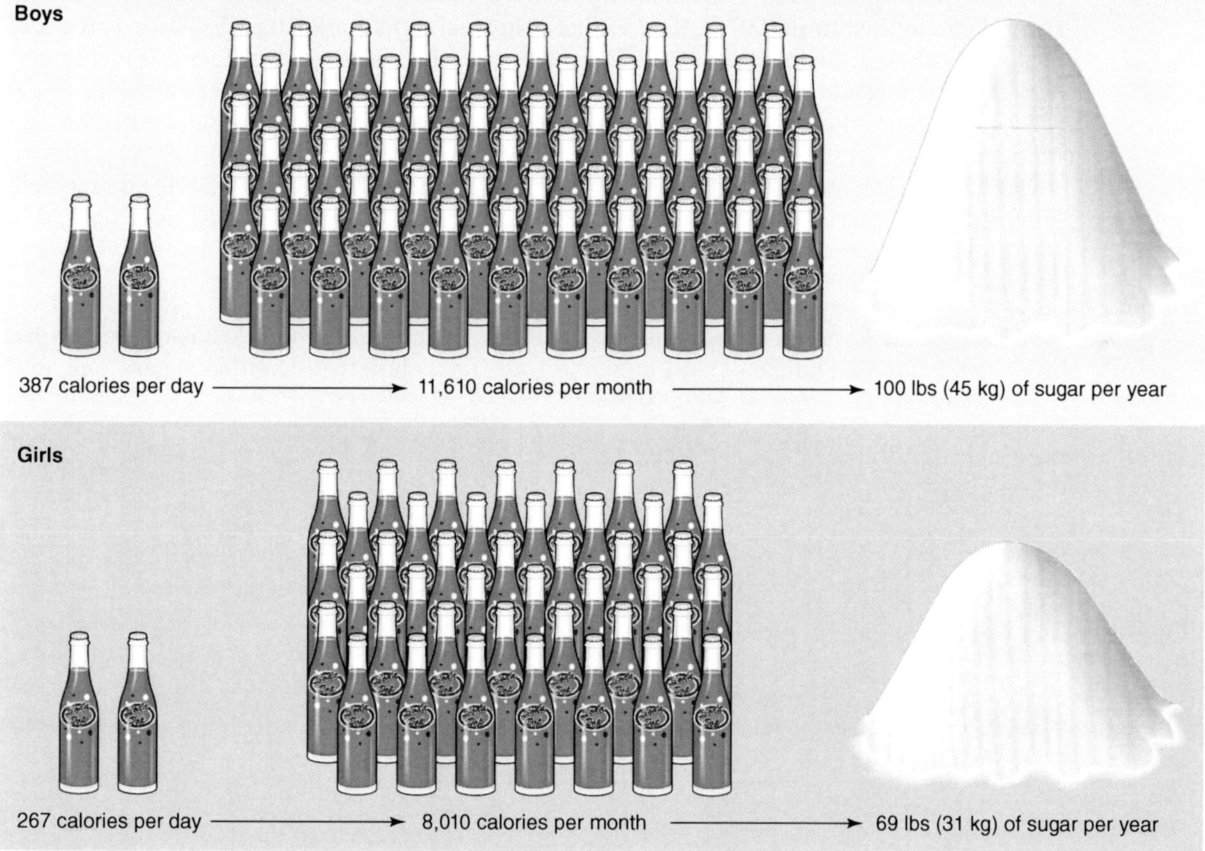

Figure 3.5 Each year, just by drinking sugar-sweetened beverages, teenage boys consume 100 pounds (45 kilograms) of sugar, and teenage girls consume 69 pounds (31 kilograms) of sugar.

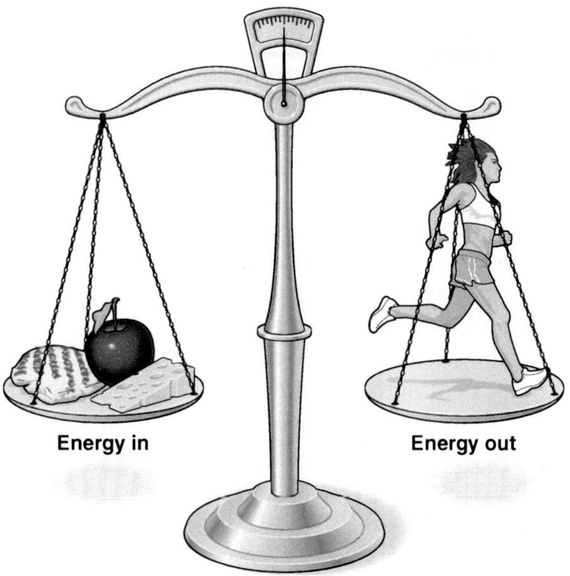

Figure 3.6 The energy equation balances energy (calories) in with energy (calories) out.

Energy Out

Figure 3.6 shows the balance between calories consumed and calories expended. As Americans are getting too much on the energy-in side of the energy equation, they're expending too little on the energy-out side. Data from the 2005 Behavioral Risk Factor Surveillance System (BRFSS) survey indicated that, on average, half of Americans don't get 30 or more minutes of moderate activity on 5 or more days during the week, nor do they get 20 or more minutes of vigorous physical activity on 3 or more days a week (CDC 2005). The current recommendation for energy expenditure to help manage body weight and prevent gradual, unhealthy body weight gain in adulthood is 60 minutes of moderate- to vigorous-intensity activity on most days of the week (U.S. Department of Health and Human Services [USDHHS] and USDA 2005). Even though the guidelines are clear, most Americans are sedentary.

Dietary Guidelines

We have already established that Americans eat out a lot, and restaurants offer many food choices that aren't healthy. Eating at home more doesn't automatically make it easier to eat a healthy diet, however. The Food Marketing Institute (2007) estimates that your local supermarket has 45,000 food products available. How can you navigate that ocean of choices to make wise decisions? As mentioned earlier, becoming educated about the USDA and USDHHS dietary guidelines can help.

The USDA and the USDHHS are required by law to jointly publish national nutrition recommendations. The first dietary guidelines for Americans were released in 1980, and they're revised every 5 years. The **dietary guidelines** are based on the latest scientific and medical knowledge and provide authoritative recommendations for Americans aged 2 years and older. The most recent recommendations can be found in *Dietary Guidelines for Americans 2005.*

The dietary guidelines have two main points (USDHHS and USDA 2005):

1. Consume a variety of nutrient-rich foods and beverages within the basic food groups, while limiting intake of saturated and trans fats, cholesterol, added sugars, salt, and alcohol.
2. Meet recommended intakes by adopting a balanced eating pattern.

What Do You Think?

Hunger does exist in the United States; 12.6 million households are food insecure. Low-income neighborhoods are underserved by full-service supermarkets and often only have access to small convenience stores where fresh produce and low-fat food items are limited. In addition, healthy foods are often more expensive, so to stretch limited food dollars many families are forced to buy cheaper, higher-calorie foods. There are fewer opportunities for physical activity in neighborhoods and schools in low-income areas, and stress due to limited access to health care and limited resources in general can also contribute to weight gain.

The focus is on how people can select healthy foods and beverages that fit into their personal habits. However, the USDA food policy and guidelines are not without their critics. Anytime the federal government releases a recommendation or guidelines, some point out the potential for influence by lobbyists. But recent studies compared the effectiveness of the MyPyramid recommendations with two other widely recommended eating plans—the Dietary Approaches to Stop Hypertension (DASH) plan and Harvard's Healthy Eating Pyramid (Reedy and Krebs-Smith 2008). Researchers found that although the guidance was slightly different in each plan, overall the emphasis on nutrient-rich foods and limited calories from added sugar and solid fat provides support for their inclusion in the evolution of optimal diets (Reedy and Krebs-Smith 2008).

MyPyramid

The dietary guidelines are illustrated by MyPyramid, which replaced the former food guide pyramid in 2005. MyPyramid highlights the personalized approach to healthy eating and physical activity in the new guidelines. MyPyramid is a simple symbol to remind you to make healthy food choices and to be active every day. Refer to figure 3.7 while reading the following description of the pyramid.

Activity is represented by the person climbing the steps on the side of the pyramid. Moderation is represented by the narrowing bands of each food group. Proportionality is represented by the widths of the food-group bands; the wider the band, the more foods in the group should make up the diet. The wider base of each group represents foods in that group with little or no solid fats or added sugars, which are the foods that should be selected more often. The narrow top area represents foods that contain more added sugars and solid fats. The person climbing the steps to the top of the pyramid also illustrates that as you become more active, you can include more of the foods at the top of the pyramid in your diet. Variety is symbolized by the six color bands that illustrate all five food groups plus the fats and oils that are needed each day for a healthy diet.

For the grains group, choose foods from whole-grain sources at least half of the time. Examples of these foods would be whole-wheat bread, brown rice, oatmeal, and whole-grain cereals. To "vary your veggies" and "focus on fruits," explore the variety of fresh, frozen, canned, and dried options that are available. The milk group includes calcium-rich foods, which should include low-fat or fat-free dairy products or other calcium sources such as fortified foods and beverages. Last, "go lean with protein." This food group includes lean meats, poultry, and fish, as well as other nonmeat protein sources.

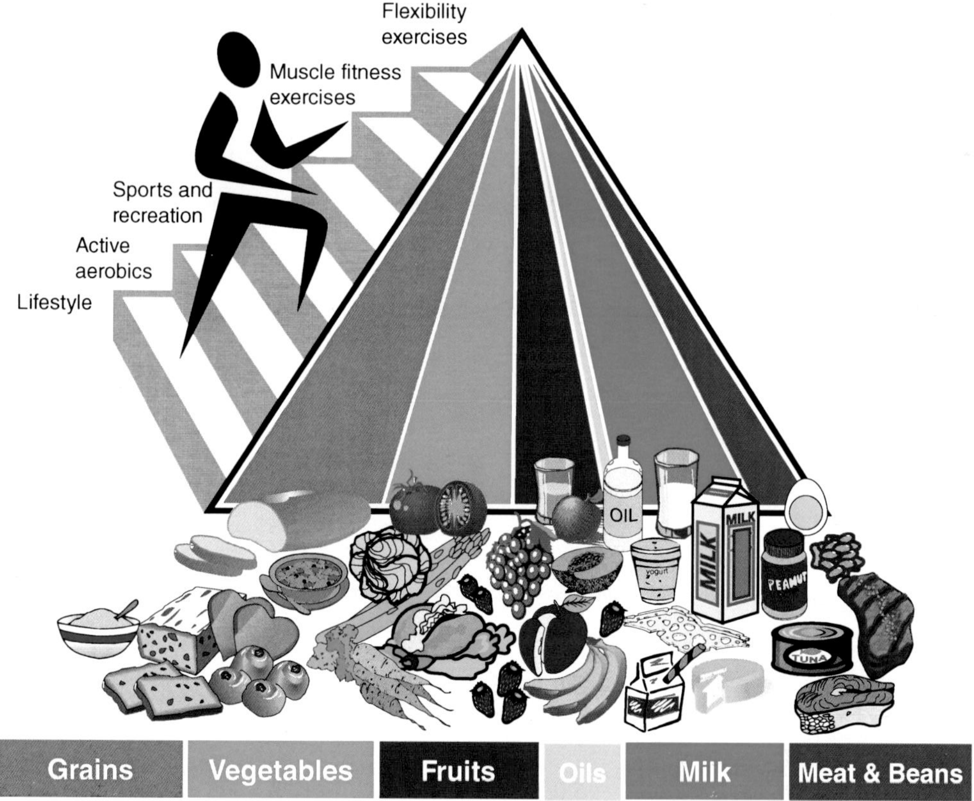

Figure 3.7 MyPyramid illustrates the dietary guidelines for Americans.

U.S. Department of Agriculture and the U.S. Department of Health and Human Services.

MyPyramid focuses on personalization. Everybody is different (age, gender, activity level), so no single recommendation would work. At www.mypyramid.gov, you can enter your personal data to generate a MyPyramid plan that fits your characteristics. The MyPyramid in figure 3.7, for example, represents a 2,000-calorie diet.

A new concept in MyPyramid is discretionary calories. Because MyPyramid is based on personal data, a certain amount of calories is built in to allow for flexibility of food choices. Physical activity increases calorie use, so when you do more activity, you gain a larger discretionary calorie allowance (see table 3.3).

What does a healthy diet for a college student look like? First, if you walk to class most of the day, you should get the recommended minimum 30 minutes of physical activity. But can you make healthy choices to meet recommendations for your diet based on your schedule and time constraints? Here is a sample menu that has 1,795 calories and some purposeful planning:

Breakfast (383 calories): Flavored fat-free, sugar-free yogurt (6-ounce [177 milliliters] cup), .5 cup dried fruit, 1 ounce (28 grams) fat-free granola, 1 small (6-ounce [177 milliliters]) latte

Lunch (242 calories): Chicken (2 ounces [57 grams]) and cheese (2 ounces [57 grams]) quesadilla (whole-wheat tortilla), .5 cup raw carrots

Dinner (775 calories): Whole-wheat pasta (1 cup) with tomato sauce and meatballs (3 ounces [85 grams] meatballs), mixed greens (1 cup) with cucumber (.5 cup), low-fat salad dressing (1 Tbsp [15 milliliters]), garlic bread (one slice)

Snacks (395 calories): Apple with 2 tablespoons (30 milliliters) peanut butter, .5 cup grapes, .5 ounce (14 grams) hard pretzels, 1 cup low-fat popcorn, 1 cup tomato juice

If you're not sure what a typical serving of food should look like, use the following guide to help visualize your food choices.

TABLE 3.3 Number of Discretionary Calories by Age and Activity Level

	NOT PHYSICALLY ACTIVE*		PHYSICALLY ACTIVE**	
Age and sex	Estimated total calorie need	Estimated discretionary calorie allowance	Estimated total calorie need	Estimated discretionary calorie allowance
Females 14-18	1,800	195	2,000-2,400	265-360
Males 14-18	2,200	290	2,400-3,200	360-650
Females 19-30	2,000	265	2,000-2,400	265-360
Males 19-30	2,400	360	2,600-3,000	410-510
Females 31-50	1,800	195	2,000-2,200	265-290
Males 31-50	2,200	290	2,400-3,000	360-510
Females 51+	1,600	130	1,800-2,200	195-290
Males 51+	2,000	265	2,200-2,800	290-425

*These amounts are appropriate for people who get less than 30 minutes of moderate physical activity most days.

**These amounts are appropriate for people who get from 30 minutes (lower calorie level) to 60 minutes (higher calorie level) of moderate physical activity most days.

One Serving of Fruits or Vegetables

- Baseball = 1 medium fruit
- 1/2 baseball = 1/2 cup fresh fruit
- Large egg = 1/4 cup raisins
- Baseball = 1 cup salad greens
- Fist = 1 baked potato

One Serving of Meat and Alternatives

- Deck of cards = 3 oz meat, fish, or poultry
- Ping-pong ball = 2 tbsp peanut butter

One Serving of Fat

- 1 die = 1 tsp margarine or spread
- Thumb tip = 1 tsp oil

One Serving of Dairy and Cheese

- 4 stacked dice = 1 1/2 oz cheese
- 1/2 baseball = 1/2 cup ice cream

One Serving of Grains

- Fist = 1 cup of cereal
- CD or DVD = 1 pancake
- 1/2 baseball = 1/2 cup cooked rice or pasta
- Cassette tape = 1 slice of bread

GENDER ISSUES

What Color Is Your Diet?

In 2005, 28.7 percent of women ate fruits or vegetables five or more times a day, compared with only 19.6 percent of men (CDC 2005). A growing body of research shows that fruits and vegetables are critical to promoting health. An easy way to assess how healthy your meal may be is to check the hue of your plate. If the food on your plate is mostly colorless, there's a good chance you're eating a lot of breaded and fried foods. If your plate resembles the colors of the rainbow, then you're probably choosing healthy fruits and veggies of different colors. Visit www.fruitsandveggiesmorematters.org for more information.

Other Key Recommendations

Other key recommendations in the dietary guidelines cover fat, sodium, potassium, sugar, alcohol, and food safety. To help prevent the development of certain chronic diseases, Americans are supposed to eat less than 10 percent of their calories from saturated fats and less than 300 milligrams a day of cholesterol. New to the 2005 version of the guidelines is a caution to eat trans fats in amounts that are as low as possible. Total fat intake should be between 20 and 35 percent of dietary calories, focusing on fat from polyunsaturated and monounsaturated fats, such as those from fish, nuts, and vegetable oils.

The dietary guidelines recommend selecting foods and beverages with little added sugar or sweetener. The largest proportion of added sugar in the American diet comes from beverages sweetened with high-fructose corn syrup.

Sodium is abundant in the U.S. food supply, mostly because there are so many processed and ready-to-eat foods. Americans are encouraged to eat a diet with less than 2,300 milligrams of sodium a day (approximately 1 teaspoon [5 milliliters] of salt). To accomplish that, try not to add salt when you're making your own food, and choose prepared foods that have less added salt. Eat potassium-rich foods, such as fruit, vegetables, and low-fat milk products. Eating more potassium and less salt can help lower blood pressure (USDHHS and USDA 2005).

What about alcohol? *Dietary Guidelines for Americans 2005* says, "Those who choose to drink alcoholic beverages should do so sensibly and in moderation—defined as the consumption of up to one drink per day for women and up to two drinks per day for men" (USDHHS and USDA 2005). Alcohol provides 7 calories per gram to the diet, but research isn't

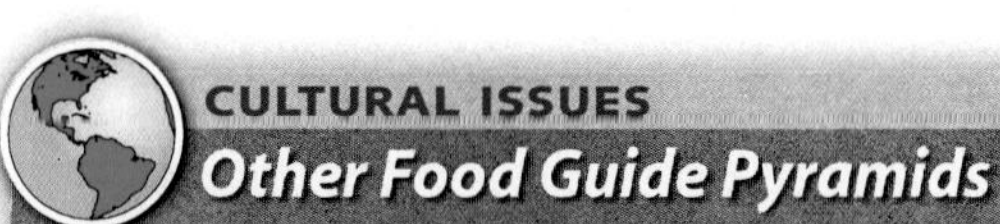

Since the introduction of the Food Guide Pyramid in 1992, which became MyPyramid in 2005, many critics have taken the lead in questioning the one-size-fits-all approach to the guidelines. Health and civil rights advocates have criticized the federal dietary guidelines as being insensitive to African Americans, Latinos, Asian Americans, and Native Americans. Oldways is a nonprofit organization that has created ethnic food guide pyramids (www.oldwayspt.org/pyramids.html). You can also find links to ethnic food pyramids on the Web site for the USDA Food and Nutrition Information Center at http://fnic.nal.usda.gov (at the site, search for "ethnic food guide pyramids").

conclusive as to whether it provides any health benefits. The guidelines caution that certain groups shouldn't consume alcohol:

- Women of childbearing age who may become pregnant
- Women who are pregnant or lactating
- Children and adolescents
- People who have trouble restricting their intake
- People with specific medical conditions
- People who are taking medications that can interact with alcohol
- People who do activities that require attention, skill, or coordination, such as driving or operating machinery

The last key recommendation added to the dietary guidelines in 2005 focuses on food safety. To avoid microbial foodborne illness, safe food-handling practices are necessary, which we'll discuss later in the chapter.

Dietary Guidelines for Vegetarians

The current interest in global sustainability, animal rights, and healthful diets has led to the increase in the availability and acceptability of vegetarian meals and food products. In 2000, an estimated 2.5 percent of the U.S. adult population consistently followed a **vegetarian** diet, never eating meat, fish, or poultry (ADA 2003). Fewer than 1 percent considered themselves to be **vegan**, or a vegetarian who eats no animal products or animal by-products (dairy, eggs) and who uses no animal products (fur, silk, wool) or skin (leather). However, 20 to 25 percent of American adults report that they eat four or more meatless meals weekly, or maintain a semivegetarian lifestyle. In 2006, the Vegetarian Resource Group commissioned a national study to estimate the percentage of the population that adheres to a vegetarian diet. That year, 2.3 percent of adults aged 18 years or older said they never eat meat, fish, or fowl (down just a bit from the 2000 estimates). Additionally, 6.7 percent of participants said they never eat meat (Stahler 2006). Nine percent of females said they don't eat meat, which makes them almost twice as likely as males (5 percent) to abstain from eating meat. However, the percentage adhering to a vegetarian diet (no meat, fish, or poultry) was almost evenly split between genders, with 3 percent of women and 2 percent of men being vegetarian.

There are differing forms of vegetarian diets. Ovo vegetarians eat eggs, lacto vegetarians consume dairy products, and pesco vegetarians eat fish. Those forms of vegetarianism can be combined, too, so there are lacto–ovo vegetarians, for example.

Vegetarian diets offer a number of health advantages. Because vegetarians don't eat animal protein, they also consume lower levels of saturated fat and cholesterol. In addition, vegetarian diets offer higher levels of carbohydrate, fiber, magnesium, folate, vitamins C and E, carotenoids, and phytochemicals. Some vegans may have lower intakes of vitamin B_{12}, vitamin D, calcium, zinc, and occasionally riboflavin, so they need to thoughtfully plan meals to ensure they get the recommended intake of those nutrients, or else they need to consider taking supplements to make up for any deficits.

In a national study, researchers looked at five studies that involved more than 76,000 people. Results showed that death from heart disease was 31 percent lower among vegetarian men compared with nonvegetarian men and 20 percent lower among vegetarian women compared to nonvegetarian women (ADA 2003).

Vegetarian diets offer many health benefits, but people who follow them still must be purposeful in their planning. Adolescents and some adults often follow a vegetarian lifestyle for ethical reasons, but they choose high-fat dairy foods, fried vegetables, and so on, which cancels out some of the health benefits of a meatless diet. Below are some quick tips for making better choices in a vegetarian diet. Your local grocery store or dorm cafeteria probably has lots of variety to choose from.

- Soy products such as tofu, soymilk, soy cheese, soy yogurt, or textured soy protein
- Dried or canned beans of all varieties including black, pinto, garbanzo, and kidney
- Veggie burgers and crumbles
- Cereals, especially iron fortified
- Whole-grain pasta, rice, and breads
- Variety of fruits and vegetables
- Nuts, including peanut butter (a great source of protein)
- Low-fat milk, cheese, and other dairy products (for nonvegans)
- Eggs and fish (for nonvegans)

For more information on a vegetarian lifestyle, check out the vegetarian starter kit at The Physicians Committee for Responsible Medicine Web site (www.pcrm.org/health/veginfo/).

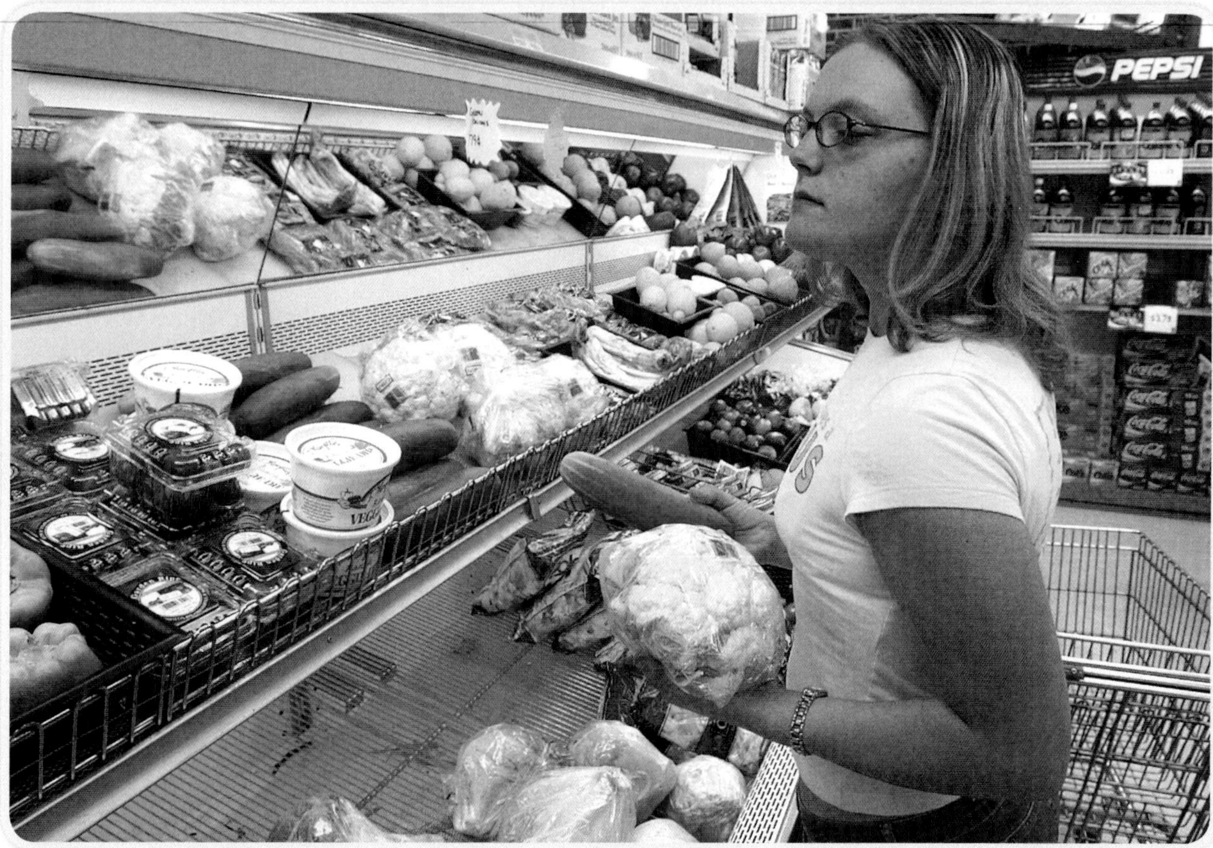

Your local grocery store offers an estimated 45,000 different products, and it can be a challenge to make healthy food choices when shopping. The fruits and vegetables available in the colorful produce section are a good place to start; try to have five or more servings of fruits and veggies per day.

© Human Kinetics/Kelly Huff

Reading Labels

The nutrition label on food products is probably familiar to you; you've seen it hundreds of times. It includes excellent information, so if you're not sure how to use it, it's worth learning how. The goal of the nutrition facts is to give enough nutrient-specific information about a product so you can compare products and make an educated selection of which one best fits into your meal planning. Figure 3.8 shows a label for a box of macaroni and cheese.

The first thing to look for is the serving size and the servings per container (number 1 in figure 3.8). The size of the serving influences the number of calories (number 2) and the nutrient amounts listed on the label (numbers 3 and 4). The percent daily value, or % DV (number 6), stands for the percentage of the nutrient that is generally recommended in a standard 2,000-calorie diet (see the footnote at number 5). Using the percent daily value helps you figure out if a particular food is a good source of the nutrients you may be concerned about, and it allows you to make comparisons between products. Here's a good rule of thumb: If a food provides 5 percent daily value or less, it is a low source of that nutrient (e.g., low fat, low sodium); if a food provides 20 percent daily value or higher, it is a high source of that nutrient (e.g., high fiber, high saturated fat).

You can use the nutrition facts label not only to limit those nutrients you typically want to cut back on (fat, saturated fat, trans fat, cholesterol, and sodium) but also to increase those nutrients you want to eat in larger amounts (dietary fiber, particular vitamins and minerals). Some nutrients on the label do not have a percent daily value (trans fat, protein, sugars). Either there is no established daily reference intake, as in the case with trans fat and sugar, or the American diet provides sufficient quantities that it is not necessary to list it unless a specific health claim is made. If you're trying to limit trans fat or sugar in your diet, compare the labels of similar products and choose the food with the lower amount of those nutrients.

Nutrition Facts
1 Serving Size 1 cup (228g)
Servings Per Container 2
Amount Per Serving
2 Calories 250 Calories from Fat 110
% Daily Value* 6
Total Fat 12g 18%
3 Saturated Fat 3g 15%
Cholesterol 30mg 10%
Sodium 470mg 20%
Total Carbohydrate 31g 10%
Dietary Fiber 0g 0%
Sugars 5g
Protein 5g
Vitamin A 4%
4 Vitamin C 2%
Calcium 20%
Iron 4%
5 * Percent Daily Values are based on a 2,000 calorie diet. Your Daily Values may be higher or lower depending on your calorie needs.
Calories: 2,000 2,500
Total Fat Less than 65g 60g
Sat Fat Less than 20g 25g
Cholesterol Less than 300mg 300mg
Sodium Less than 2,400mg 2,400mg
Total Carbohydrate 300g 375g
Dietary Fiber 25g 30g

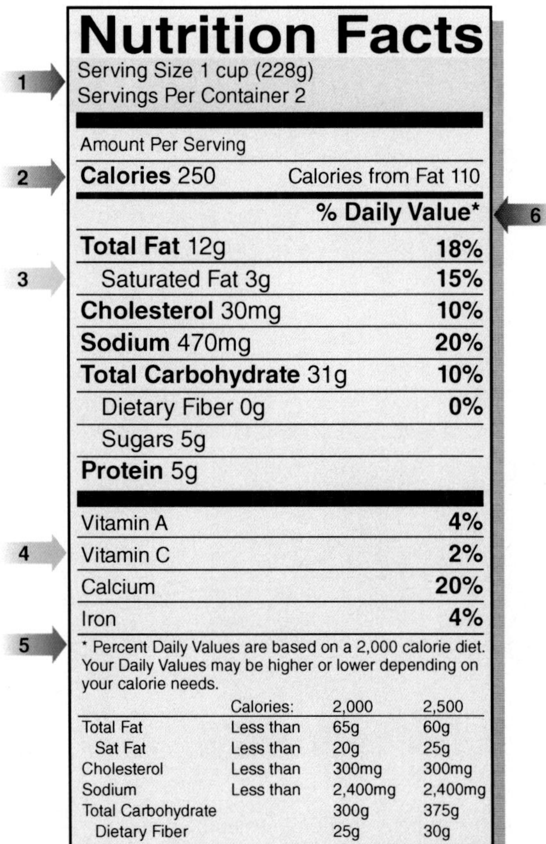

Figure 3.8 Do you know how to read nutrition labels, such as this one from a box of macaroni and cheese?

What about all those health claims listed on labels? You can't look at those alone without reading the nutrition label. Specific guidelines must be followed before a food manufacturer can apply for a health claim, and the responsibility of the claim rests with the manufacturer, FDA, or, in the case of advertising, with the Federal Trade Commission (FTC). Claims can fall into three categories: health claims (for example, "Diets high in calcium may reduce the risk of osteoporosis"), nutrient-content claims (describing the level of a nutrient in the product using terms such as *free*, *high*, and *low*, or comparing the level of a nutrient in a food to that of another food using terms such as *more*, *reduced*, and *lite*), and structure and function claims (for example, "Calcium builds strong bones").

Food trends increasingly cater to a grab-and-go, eat-on-the-run philosophy. Prepackaged, portion-controlled serving sizes are the fastest-growing market segment of the snack industry (Warner 2005). Portion-controlled packaging, such as 100-calorie cookie packs, provides built-in portion control of a tasty snack. That convenience costs more than buying the food in a regular-size package and portioning it out at home, but it does help consumers who want the portion control without buying diet versions of their favorite snacks. These snack foods are less nutrient dense than, say 100 calories of an unprocessed food, such as a piece of fruit, a handful of nuts or seeds, or a handful of baby carrots. The nutrient-dense unprocessed foods might even be more satisfying than, say, 23 thin chocolate wafer cookies or 9 potato chips.

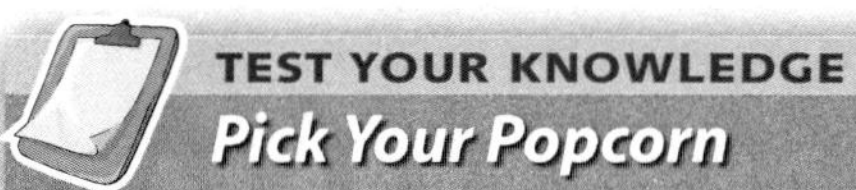

TEST YOUR KNOWLEDGE

Pick Your Popcorn

Below are food labels for two kinds of popcorn. Compare them and evaluate which appears to be the better choice. Look at serving size, total calories, calories from fat, trans fat, cholesterol, sodium, and so on. If one appears to be healthier than the other, does that mean you should never have the other one? The answer probably depends on your own health situation. Figure out your limits for those kinds of foods based on the dietary guidelines and your health.

Nutrition Facts

Serving Size: Makes 5 cups popped
Servings Per Bag: About 12.5 cups popped

Amount Per Serving	1 Cup Popped	
Calories		20
Calories from Fat		0
		%DV*
Total Fat	0g	**0%**
Saturated Fat	0g	**0%**
Trans Fat	0g	
Cholesterol	0mg	**0%**
Sodium	40mg	**2%**
Total Carbohydrate	4g	**1%**
Dietary Fiber	1g	**6%**
Sugars	0g	
Protein	<1g	
Vitamin A		**0%**
Vitamin C		**0%**
Calcium		**0%**
Iron		**0%**

Nutrition Facts

Serving Size: Makes 3.5 cups popped
Servings Per Bag: About 10.5 cups popped

Amount Per Serving	1 Cup Popped	
Calories		45
Calories from Fat		30
		%DV*
Total Fat	3g	**5%**
Saturated Fat	1g	**4%**
Trans Fat	1g	
Cholesterol	0mg	**0%**
Sodium	85mg	**4%**
Total Carbohydrate	5g	**2%**
Dietary Fiber	1g	**4%**
Sugars	0g	
Protein	1g	
Vitamin A		**0%**
Vitamin C		**0%**
Calcium		**0%**
Iron		**0%**

Organic Foods

Since October 2002, the USDA has allowed organic food manufacturers to use a designated seal for foods that are at least 95 percent organic. That year, the U.S. total retail sales of organic foods totaled $9 billion (ADA n.d.). Organic meat, poultry, eggs, and dairy products are produced without antibiotics or hormones, and organic produce is produced without the use of conventional pesticides and fertilizers. Before foods can be labeled as organic, the farm is inspected and certified to ensure that all the regulations are being followed to earn the USDA organic label. Although organic foods generally are grown with lower levels of pesticides, the jury is still out as to whether these foods are healthier or safer than conventionally grown foods.

FOOD SAFETY

Now that you know more about what to eat for a healthy diet, it's time to move on to how to prevent what you eat from unintentionally making you sick. The CDC estimates that 76 million cases of foodborne disease occur each year in the United States. Most of the cases are mild and cause symptoms for only a day or two, and most people don't seek medical help. Some infections, though, result in serious illnesses and even death. Each year, foodborne diseases result in approximately 325,000 hospitalizations and 5,000 deaths in the United States (Mead et al. 1999). The most vulnerable populations are the elderly, the very young, pregnant women, and those who already have an illness that reduces their immune system functions.

The opportunities for food to become contaminated as it is produced or prepared are many, especially as the amount of imported food increases. More than 250 foodborne diseases have been identified that result from bacteria, viruses, parasites, or poisoning from toxins produced by the organism (Mead et al. 1999). Cross-contamination of foods and the addition of harmful chemicals or unsanitary food processing leads to an increase in foodborne illnesses.

Raw foods from animals are the most likely to be contaminated, including beef, chicken, eggs, unpasteurized milk and cheese, and raw shellfish. Fresh fruits and vegetables, notably prewashed, bagged leafy greens, also bring a risk of contaminated processing practices, and they are generally not heated to sufficiently kill the organisms before being eaten. Most foodborne outbreaks are discovered only after people have suffered the typical symptoms of foodborne illness: nausea, vomiting, abdominal cramps, diarrhea, a high fever, blood in the stool, or prolonged vomiting.

It's not all bad news, though. The American food supply is among the safest in the world. The almost 300 million people living in the United States eat several meals and snacks each day and rarely get sick from their food. In addition, the USDA provides helpful guidelines for handling, cooking, and storing foods to help prevent foodborne illness.

Buying, Handling, and Preparing Food Safely

Food safety starts before you even bring your food home. Think about food safety while you're grocery shopping. Pick up the cold or frozen items last. Don't buy meat or poultry that's in a torn package. Never buy food that's past the sell-by or use-by expiration dates. If you buy meat that's marked down because it's getting close to its expiration date, use it the same day you purchase it (U.S. Department of Agriculture [USDA] 2006).

Always refrigerate perishable food within 2 hours of buying it (1 hour when the temperature is above 90 degrees Fahrenheit [32.2 degrees Celsius]). Keep your refrigerator temperature

CONTROVERSIAL ISSUES

Eating Cloned Meat

Food from healthy clones of cattle, swine, and goats is as safe as food from noncloned animals, the U.S. Food and Drug Administration (FDA) reported in January 2008. It was reported that no hazards had been identified that might indicate food consumption risks in healthy clones of cattle, swine, or goats. The report states, "We therefore conclude that food products derived from cattle, swine, and goat clones pose no more risk than food derived from sexually reproduced animals" (paragraph 2 under Summary of the Risks Assessments; FDA 2008a).

Under current law, the FDA only requires labeling if there may be health concerns or a material difference in the composition of food. Since the FDA has not identified any safety concerns or found any material difference in food, it is currently not requiring any additional labeling relating to food derived from adult clones of cattle, swine, and goats or the offspring of clones of any species traditionally consumed as food (FDA 2008b). However, food products from cloned animals or their offspring will not reach store shelves for years.

How do you feel about consuming cloned meat and dairy products? Will you eat it? Do you think it is safe? Should packages be labeled if they are derived from a cloned animal?

at or below 40 degrees Fahrenheit (4.4 degrees Celsius); your freezer should be at or below 0 degrees Fahrenheit (–17.7 degrees Celsius). Cook or freeze fresh poultry, fish, ground meats, and variety meats (the organ meats, feet, and tails of butchered animals) within 2 days; cook or freeze other beef, veal, lamb, or pork within 3 to 5 days. Perishable foods such as meat and poultry should be wrapped securely to maintain quality and to prevent meat juices from getting on other food. If you're going to freeze meat in its original packaging, put foil around the package first.

You can store canned foods with high acid content, such as tomatoes, grapefruit, and pineapple, for 18 months (no refrigeration necessary) if the can remains in good condition and has been stored in a cool, clean, and dry place. Canned meats and vegetables with low acid content will keep on the shelf for 2 to 5 years. Throw away food that's in dented, leaking, bulging, or rusted cans (USDA 2006).

When you're handling food, remember the four Cs of food safety (USDA 2006).

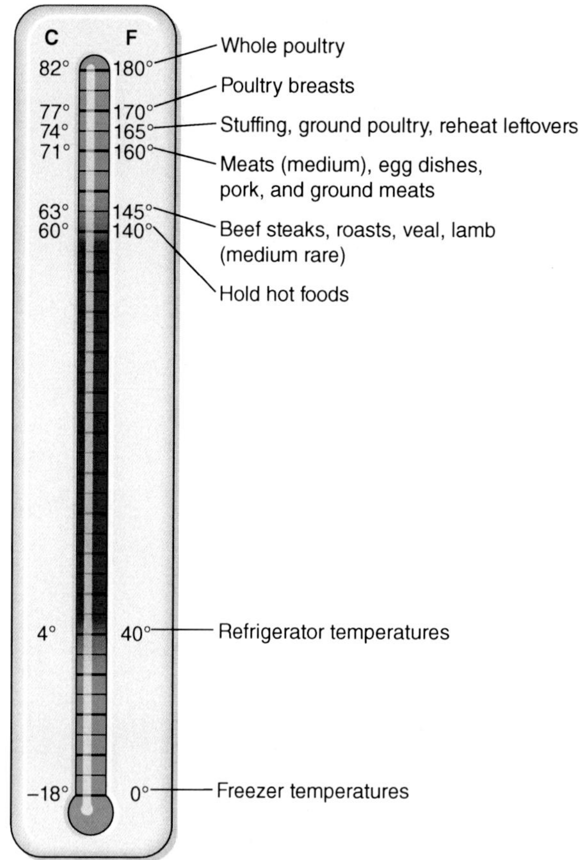

Figure 3.9 To help prevent foodborne illness, always cook, refrigerate, and freeze food items to the proper temperature.

1. **Clean:** Always wash your hands with warm soapy water for 20 seconds before and after handling food. When you're done preparing food, clean counters and cutting boards with a solution of 1 tablespoon (15 milliliters) of bleach in 1 gallon (4 liters) of water.
2. **Cook:** Cook each item to the proper temperature. Cook beef, veal, and lamb steaks, roasts, and chops to 145 degrees Fahrenheit (62.7 degrees Celsius); cook pork to 160 degrees Fahrenheit (71.1 degrees Celsius). Let ground beef, veal, and lamb reach 160 degrees Fahrenheit (71.1 degrees Celsius). All poultry should reach a minimum temperature of 165 degrees Fahrenheit (73.8 degrees Celsius). See figure 3.9.
3. **Chill:** Refrigerate food promptly. Always marinate meat and poultry in a sealed container in the refrigerator. Cold storage times are available for both refrigerating and freezing at www.fsis.usda.gov/Fact_Sheets/Basics_for_Handling_Food_Safely/index.asp.
4. Don't **Cross-contaminate:** Keep foods (especially raw meat and poultry) separated from each other on countertops and cutting boards.

Thawing food in the refrigerator allows for slow, safe thawing. Make sure juices from thawing meat and poultry do not drip onto other food. For faster thawing, place food in a leakproof plastic bag and submerge in cold tap water. Change the water every 30 minutes. Cook immediately after thawing. Cook meat and poultry immediately after microwave thawing (USDA 2006).

If you defrosted meat and poultry in the refrigerator, you may refreeze them before or after cooking. If thawed by other methods, cook before refreezing (USDA 2006).

When serving food, hot food should be held at 140 degrees Fahrenheit (60.0 degrees Celsius) or warmer. Cold food should be held at 40 degrees Fahrenheit (4.4 degrees Celsius) or colder. When serving food at a buffet, keep food hot with chafing dishes, slow cookers, and warming trays. Keep food cold by nesting dishes in bowls of ice or use small serving trays and replace them often. Perishable food should not be left out more than 2 hours at room temperature (1

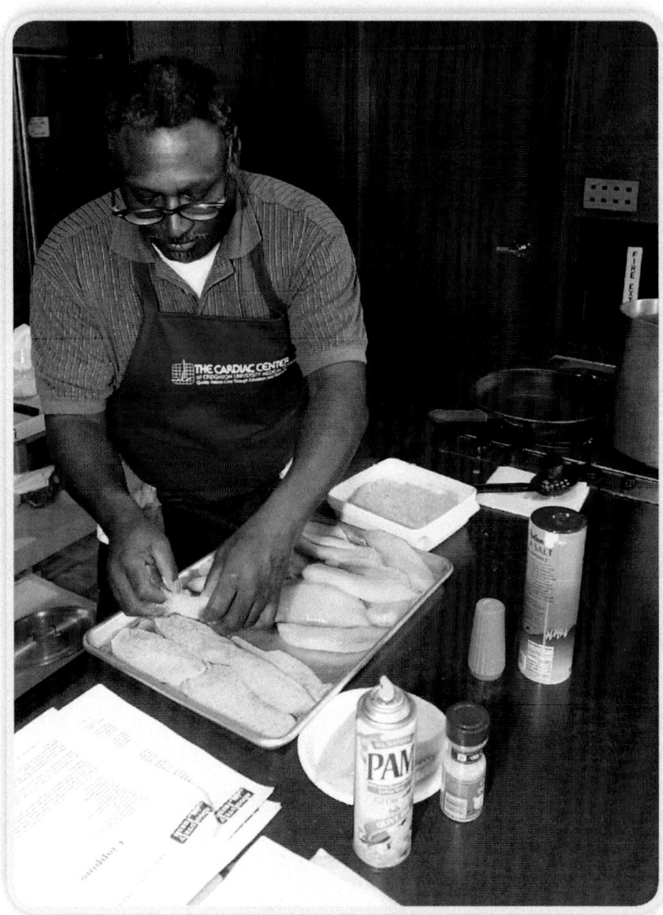

Wash your hands with soap before and after preparing food so that you don't get or pass on the bacteria that cause foodborne illness.

© Human Kinetics

hour when the temperature is above 90 degrees Fahrenheit [32.2 degrees Celsius]) (USDA 2006).

Discard any food left out at room temperature for more than 2 hours (1 hour if the temperature was above 90 degrees Fahrenheit [32.2 degrees Celsius]). Place food in shallow containers and immediately put in the refrigerator or freezer for rapid cooling. Use cooked leftovers within 4 days (USDA 2006).

Avoiding Foodborne Illnesses

Foodborne illnesses are caused when the four Cs of preparing food aren't followed properly. Some of the illnesses come from bacteria such as *E. coli*, *Salmonella*, *Listeria monocytogenes*, *Campylobacter*, and *Clostridium botulinum* (CDC 2006).

Botulism toxin is produced by *Clostridium botulinum* in an environment without oxygen and with little acidity. The botulism spores are heat resistant, and if food that contains these spores isn't properly processed at the correct temperature for the correct duration, the spores survive canning. Most cases of botulism poisoning come from home-canned vegetables, but there have been outbreaks involving commercially processed food, too (CDC 2006). Symptoms of botulism illness occur 4 to 36 hours after a person has ingested the bacteria, and they include inability to swallow, double vision, and progressive paralysis of the respiratory system. If these symptoms appear, get medical help right away. The illness can be fatal.

Campylobacter is a bacteria that comes mainly from raw poultry, cow or sheep meat, and unpasteurized milk. Symptoms of the illness caused by the bacteria include diarrhea, abdominal cramping, fever, and sometimes bloody stools. These systems occur about 2 to 5 days after the bacteria are consumed, and they last from 7 to 10 days (CDC 2006). Seek medical help if the symptoms are severe, if you become dehydrated, or if you are immunocompromised.

Eating undercooked ground beef or visiting a farm can put you at risk for getting *E. coli*. Beef can become contaminated with the bacteria during slaughter, and the bacteria can be mixed into the meat during grinding. Because the bacteria are present in the ground in some areas, they can be found on produce, such as sprouts and lettuce. You can also pick up the bacteria from swimming in or drinking contaminated water. People who don't wash their hands well after using the restroom or cleaning a baby's dirty diaper can infect others. Symptoms of illness from *E. coli* appear about 2 to 5 days after becoming infected and last 5 to 10 days. Symptoms include severe bloody diarrhea and abdominal cramps, usually with no fever (CDC 2006). Symptoms are generally severe enough that you will need to go to the hospital.

Listeriosis bacteria (*Listeria monocytogenes*) are found in soft cheese, unpasteurized milk, hot dogs and deli meats, imported seafood products, frozen cooked crab meat, cooked shrimp, and cooked surimi (imitation shellfish). Listeriosis bacteria resist heat, salt, and acidity better than many other microorganisms. They survive and grow even in the refrigerator. Symptoms of listeriosis can appear as long as 7 to 30 days after the bacteria are consumed, but most people report symptoms within 48 to 72 hours after eating the contaminated food

(CDC 2006). Symptoms include fever, headache, nausea, and vomiting. The bacteria primarily affect pregnant women and their fetuses, newborns, the elderly, people with cancer, and people with impaired immune systems. In infants, it can be fatal (CDC 2006), but the severity of symptoms can vary among other populations.

Salmonella bacteria are found in raw meats, poultry, eggs, milk and other dairy products, shrimp, frog legs, yeast, coconut, pasta, and chocolate. Symptoms occur about 8 to 12 hours after eating and include abdominal pain, diarrhea, and sometimes nausea and vomiting. The illness from salmonella lasts a day or less and is usually mild (USDA 2006).

Other bacteria that can affect food include *Clostridium perfringens*. The food poisoning happens when food isn't kept hot; the bacteria grow at the warm temperatures of 120 to 130 degrees Fahrenheit (48.8 to 54.4 degrees Celsius). To be safe, keep gravy and stuffing at 140 degrees Fahrenheit (60.0 degrees Celsius). Bacillary dysentery is caused by *Shigella* bacteria, which are found in milk and dairy products. Bacillary dysentery appears when people handle food without properly washing their hands. Staphylococcal (staph) food poisoning, caused by *Staphylococcus* bacteria, also occurs when people who haven't washed their hands well handle food (USDA 2006).

Using the guidelines for food buying, handling, and preparation described in this chapter will help you avoid getting or passing on any of the bacteria that cause foodborne illness.

JUNK SCIENCE

> "Lose 30 pounds in 30 days!"
>
> "Eat as much as you want and still lose weight!"
>
> "Try the thigh buster and lose inches fast!"

Messages like those bombard you from television ads, online pop-up ads, spam e-mail, and so on. How can you know what's true? Nutrition science is still evolving and the media often respond immediately to reports before all the facts are in. Is there some way to critically evaluate the information that comes your way?

The Internet is a wonderful tool for finding information on just about any topic you want to research, including health and medical concerns. The problem is that a lot of misinformation is published on the Web and in other media, and you have to develop a discerning eye to sift through the junk to find the truth.

There are plenty of trusted sources on the Web, including these:

- www.nutrition.gov—Clearinghouse for government nutrition guidance and Web sites
- www.eatright.org—Web site for the American Dietetic Association (ADA)
- www.mypyramid.gov—Consumer tool for applying the dietary guidelines
- www.fruitsandveggiesmorematters.org—Practical strategies to incorporate more fruits and vegetables into your diet
- www.americanheart.org—Web site for the American Heart Association (AHA)
- www.cancer.gov—National Cancer Institute Web site on cancer research
- www.cancer.org—American Cancer Society Web site on cancer research and education
- www.foodallergy.org—Web site for the Food Allergy and Anaphylaxis Network
- www.ific.org—Web site for the International Food Information Council (IFIC)
- www.nationaldairycouncil.org—Dairy nutrition education and research
- www.nof.org—Web site for the National Osteoporosis Foundation (NOF)
- www.foodsafety.gov—Gateway to government food safety information
- www.win.niddk.nih.gov—Web site for the Weight-Control Information Network
- www.webmd.com—Comprehensive health and medical news and information Web site
- www.vrg.org—Information for vegetarian diets

When you're searching for information, you'll undoubtedly come across sites that aren't on that list. When that happens, you need to critically evaluate the information you find. In 1995, the Food and Nutrition Science Alliance released the following tool to help interpret dietary information on the Web. Any combination of these signs should raise suspicion about the accuracy of the information and cause you to delve deeper into the subject (Goldberg 1995).

Ten Red Flags of Junk Science

1. Recommendations that promise a quick fix
2. Claims that sound too good to be true
3. Simple conclusions drawn from a complex study
4. Recommendation based on a single study
5. Dramatic statements that are refuted by a reputable scientific organization
6. Recommendations based upon studies without peer review
7. Recommendations based upon studies that ignore differences among individuals or groups
8. Dire warnings of danger from a single product
9. Lists of so-called good and bad foods
10. Recommendations made to help sell a product or made by the manufacturer itself

Food and nutrition misinformation can be a serious barrier to public health. A false sense of security in a miracle cure might cause someone to wait too long before getting appropriate health care. Some additional tips for evaluating the source of the information include these:

- Can you identify the sponsor or owner of the article or Web site that might indicate a potential bias?
- Can you name the contributors and their credentials and affiliation?
- Does the site link you to credible Web sites with supporting data or guidelines?

Another tool that you can use in your myth busting is www.quackwatch.com, a nonprofit organization whose purpose is to combat health-related frauds, myths, fads, fallacies, and misconduct.

Americans are obsessed with dieting and are always looking for a quick fix. Some people are willing to try the latest diet published in a popular magazine, discussed on talk shows, or displayed on the shelves of the local bookstore. A fad is a practice or interest followed for a short time with exaggerated enthusiasm, or a craze. Because the fad diet of the month constantly changes, a good resource to check the facts of the diet can be found by doing a quick search at a trusted resource such as the Weight-Control Information Network, AHA, or WebMD Web sites (see the previous list for URLs).

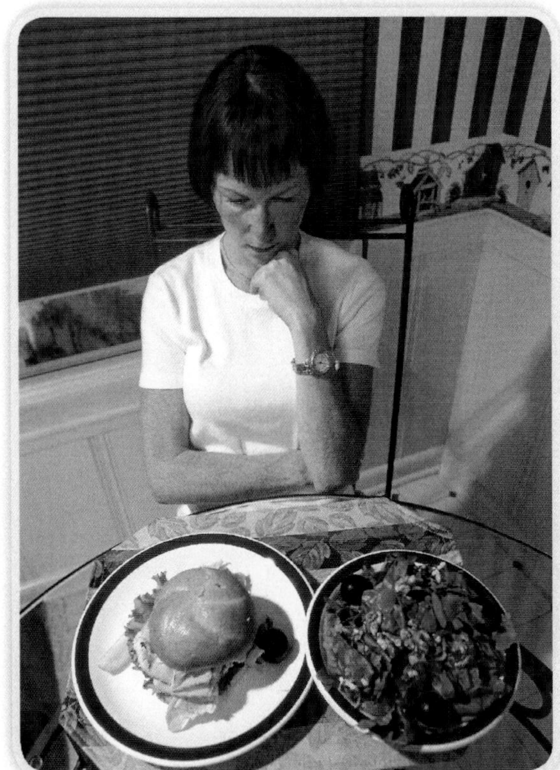

Make nutritional choices based on facts from trusted sources, not on fad diets or misinformation.

© Bill Crump/Brand X Pictures

NUTRITION FOR SPECIAL POPULATIONS

The information at MyPyramid.gov includes nutrition recommendations for almost all Americans over the age of 2. However, it's worth noting a few basic facts related to some special populations.

STEPS FOR BEHAVIORAL CHANGE

Smart Food Choices

Are you ready to make changes to your eating behavior? Here are some specific steps you can take to make smart food choices.

Question the Cooking Method

- Stay away from breaded, battered, or fried foods. Instead, eat broiled, grilled, steamed, or sautéed foods.
- Avoid foods in heavy cheese or cream sauces. Instead, stick to foods in a light broth or tomato sauce.

Protein

- Limit amount of red meat consumed.
- Choose lean cuts of meat.
- Eat a variety of fish and seafood cooked in a healthy way.

Grains

- Eat a variety of whole grains.
- Choose brown rice and whole-wheat pasta and bread.

Fruits and Veggies

- Hit the salad bar first.
- Avoid full-fat dressings and limit the amount used.
- Ask yourself, "What color is my diet right now?" Evaluate how many fruits and veggies are on your tray.
- Choose thin-crust pizza with veggies instead of meat and extra cheese.
- Explore the variety of fresh, frozen, canned, and dried options that are available.

Dairy

- Choose low-fat and fat-free dairy.

Fat and Sweets

- Eat in moderation.

Portions

- Eat proper serving sizes.
- Eat only what you need in all-you-can-eat dining.
- Eat slowly and listen to your body. Stop eating when you are full.

Smart Snacks to Keep Handy

- Fresh fruits or veggies
- Canned fruits in light syrup
- Oatmeal
- Granola bars
- Fiber-rich cereal
- Nuts
- Trail mix
- Microwave popcorn
- Canned tuna
- Peanut butter
- Low-sodium soups
- String cheese
- Low-fat milk
- Low-fat cottage cheese or yogurt
- Bottled water

Infants

Infants grow quickly during their first year. Their birth weight doubles after about 5 months and triples by the first birthday. Their length increases by half during the same time. Appropriate nutrition is essential during this time; infants who don't receive sufficient calories, vitamins, and minerals won't reach their expected growth. Calorie needs per pound (half kilogram) of body weight are higher during the first year of life than at any other time.

Breast milk can provide all the nutrients a healthy baby needs for growth during the first 4 to 6 months of life. Newborns generally feed more often than older infants (from 8 to 12 times a day). When babies are 6 months old, they are physically ready to eat semisolid food. Pediatricians advise parents not to give whole cow or soy milk to babies under a year old. Breast milk and commercially prepared infant formula are the only fluids recommended before that age to help prevent iron-deficiency anemia and to provide all the nutrients the baby needs for growing. Caregivers can introduce juice and water at around 6 months, but mostly to help with cup training.

Toddlers

Three meals and two snacks usually provide the 1,000 calories a day that toddlers (children between the ages of 1 and 2) need for growth and energy (USDA 2001). Toddlers need foods from the same food groups as adults, but the serving sizes should be two-thirds of the adult serving size. Toddlers should eat servings from these food groups every day:

- Meat, fish, poultry, eggs (two to three servings)
- Dairy products (three servings equivalent to 2 cups of milk each day)
- Fruit and vegetables (three servings each)
- Cereal, grains, potatoes, rice, breads, pasta (six servings)

As toddlers develop an awareness of their environment and start to realize that they have some control over what they eat, they have a tendency to get picky about their food. They're no longer growing as fast as they did when they were infants, and their appetites may be erratic. Food jags also start during the toddler stage. Food jags are when children demand the same food over and over and then suddenly reject it. The best way to handle a toddler at this stage is with patience and continued offerings of healthy foods and regular meals and snacks.

Pregnant Women

The demands of pregnancy require an additional 300 calories a day to gain sufficient weight to support a healthy pregnancy and baby. Half of a peanut-butter sandwich with a glass of milk, for example, is enough to fill that requirement. One of the main assessment tools that doctors use throughout the pregnancy is weight gain. The amount of weight gain depends on prepregnancy weight status. The MyPyramid daily nutrition recommendations also apply during pregnancy:

- 6 to 7 ounces (170 to 198 grams) of grains

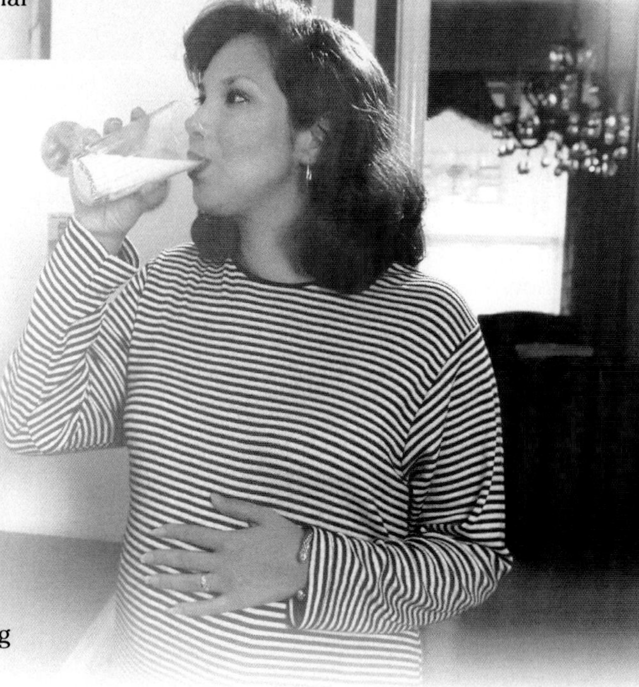

A pregnant woman might think she must "eat for two," but she needs to take in only an extra 300 calories per day.

© Bill Crump/Brand X Pictures

- 2.5 to 3 cups of vegetables
- 2 cups of fruit
- 3 cups of calcium-rich foods
- 5.5 to 6 ounces (156 to 170 grams) of lean meat and beans

Obstetricians will usually prescribe a prenatal supplement to help provide pregnant women and women who are trying to get pregnant with the extra iron and folic acid needed.

Food safety is important during pregnancy, because pregnant women and developing babies are more vulnerable to foodborne illnesses. As mentioned earlier, listeriosis is an illness caused by bacteria in unpasteurized milk; soft cheese; prepared and uncooked meats, poultry, and shellfish; and uncooked hot dogs or deli meats (USDA 2006). It's fine for pregnant women to eat up to 12 ounces (340 grams) of fish or shellfish each week, but certain fish can be dangerous. Large fish such as shark, swordfish, king mackerel, and tilefish contain high levels of mercury, a toxic heavy metal. Five of the most common types of seafood that are low in mercury are shrimp, canned light tuna, salmon, pollack, and catfish (U.S. Environmental Protection Agency [EPA] 2004).

NUTRITION 101

The human diet is composed of macronutrients and micronutrients. Protein, fat, carbohydrate, and water make up the bulk of our diets. Vitamins and minerals are micronutrients because they are important but only required in much smaller amounts in our diets. When all the components are eaten to meet but not exceed the body's needs for maintenance, growth, and activity, healthy body weight is achieved. Following the dietary guidelines for Americans in the personalized form of the MyPyramid food plan enables each person to meet those needs.

Besides eating foods that are healthy for the body, you must pay attention to how you handle the foods to prevent foodborne illnesses. Additionally, a lot of information about nutrition is available on the Internet, but for reliable information you should stick with well-trusted sources. Finally, certain populations, such as vegetarians, infants, and pregnant women, have specific dietary needs. The information in this chapter will help you develop a healthy diet that combines the foods and traditions you love with what's best for your body.

CHAPTER REVIEW

REVIEW QUESTIONS

1. How many calories are in 1 gram of protein? Carbohydrate? Fat? Alcohol?
2. What is BMI, and how is it calculated?
3. Name the food groups of MyPyramid.
4. On a nutrition facts label, what does "% DV" mean?
5. Name the four Cs of food safety.
6. What are the macronutrient components of the human diet?
7. Is a daily dietary supplement usually necessary for fat-soluble vitamins? What about water-soluble vitamins?
8. How many extra calories per day are required for the average pregnant woman?
9. To whom do the dietary guidelines for Americans apply?
10. Of the six leading causes of death, how many are accounted for by obesity-related chronic diseases?

CRITICAL THINKING

1. The Food and Nutrition Science Alliance established 10 red flags of junk science. Name 5 of the red flags, and for each, explain why the flag raises suspicion about the accuracy of the information in question.
2. Explain the energy equation, and describe what happens on each side of the equation.

APPLICATION ACTIVITIES

1. The Cultural Issues sidebar in this chapter points out that the USDA Food and Nutrition Information Center includes links to food guide pyramids that are specific to other cultures. Check out these other guides by visiting http://fnic.nal.usda.gov and typing "ethnic food guide pyramids" in the search box. Select one food guide from another culture. How does its information compare to MyPyramid? Write a 1- to 2-page paper detailing your findings.
2. Visit http://hp2010.nhlbihin.net/portion/, the National Institute of Health's Portion Distortion Web site, to learn about how much food portion sizes have changed in the last 20 years. Take the Portion Distortion I and Portion Distortion II quizzes. How do the portion sizes you choose in your daily diet compare with what is recommended? Are you active enough to burn off those extra calories? If the portions you eat are larger than what is recommended, what steps could you take to improve your habits? Write a 1- to 2-page reflection paper to report on your results.

GLOSSARY

amino acids—The building blocks of protein, classified as either essential or nonessential.

antioxidant—Any substance that reduces oxidative damage such as that caused by free radicals, or highly reactive chemicals that attack molecules by capturing electrons and thus modify chemical structures.

calorie—Measure of the energy used by the body and of the energy that food supplies to the body.

carbohydrate—Macronutrient made up of carbon, hydrogen, and oxygen.

cholesterol—A fatlike substance that is made by the body and is found naturally in animal foods such as meat, fish, poultry, eggs, and dairy.

dietary fiber—Parts of fruits, vegetables, grains, nuts, and legumes that humans can't digest. The two basic types of fiber are insoluble and soluble.

dietary guidelines—Guidelines published every 5 years since 1980 by the USDHHS and the USDA to promote health and to reduce risk for major chronic diseases through diet and physical activity.

digestion—Allows the body to get the nutrients and energy it needs from the food. It breaks food down into smaller molecules before they're absorbed by the blood and carried throughout the body to be used for energy, growth, and maintenance of body functions.

electrolytes—Sodium, chloride, and potassium work to maintain water balance and pressure between and within cells and their surrounding fluids.

fat—Macronutrient composed of the same three elements as carbohydrate (carbon, hydrogen, and oxygen) but with more carbon and hydrogen and less oxygen, which means it can store more energy in the chemical bonds.

fatty acids—May be saturated, monounsaturated, or polyunsaturated, depending on the number of hydrogen atoms attached to the carbon atoms of the fat molecule. The greater the number of hydrogen atoms, the higher the saturated fat content.

macronutrients—Substances essential in large amounts to the growth and health of the body.

micronutrients—Compounds essential in minute amounts to the growth and health of the body.

minerals—Micronutrients that don't contain any carbon molecules.

nutrients—Substances that an organism must obtain from its surroundings for growth and the sustenance of life.

nutrigenomics—Personalized nutrition that applies the human genome to nutrition and personal health to provide individual dietary recommendations.

protein—Complex, nitrogen-based macronutrient made up of amino acids in linkages called *peptide bonds*.

saccharides—Simple sugars that form the structural backbone of carbohydrate.

trans fats—Processed fats that are solid at room temperature, including partially hydrogenated or hydrogenated vegetable oils and shortening. Often used in commercial baked goods.

vegan—Vegetarian who eats no animal products or animal by-products (dairy, eggs) and who uses no animal products (fur, silk, wool) or skin (leather).

vegetarian—Person who does not eat meat, fish, or poultry.

vitamins—Micronutrients that come in various forms and may be water soluble or fat soluble.

water—Ranked second only to oxygen as essential for life. Water is vital to all body processes, including digestion, circulation, and lubrication of joints. It also mediates various chemical reactions in the body.

REFERENCES AND RESOURCES

American Dietetic Association (ADA). 2003. Position of the American Dietetic Association and Dietitians of Canada: Vegetarian diets. *Journal of the American Dietetic Association* 103 (6): 748-765.

———. 2005. ADA position statement: Fortification and nutritional supplements. *Journal of the American Dietetic Association* 105 (8): 1300-1311.

———. n.d. Organic foods versus conventional foods. http://eatright.org/cps/rde/xchg/ada/hs.xsl/home_4143_ENU_HTML.htm.

Buzby, J., H. Farah, and G. Vocke. 2005. Will 2005 be the year of the whole grain? www.ers.usda.gov/AmberWaves/June05/Features/Will2005WholeGrain.htm.

Centers for Disease Control and Prevention (CDC). 2005. CDC Behavioral Risk Factor Surveillance System 2005 data. http://apps.nccd.cdc.gov/brfss/index.asp.

———. 2006. Fight Bac! Partnership for Food Safety Education. www.fightbac.org.

———. 2007. *Physical activity and good nutrition: Essential elements to prevent chronic diseases and obesity*. Atlanta, GA: Author.

Drewnowski, A. 2007. The real contribution of added sugars and fats to obesity. *Epidemiologic Reviews* 29: 160-171.

Environ International Corporation. 2006. What America drinks: How beverages relate to nutrient intakes and body weight. www.environcorp.com.

Food Marketing Institute. 2007. Supermarket facts: Industry overview 2007. www.fmi.org/facts_figs/?fuseaction=superfact.

Goldberg, J.P. 1995. *Junk science*. Chicago: Food and Nutrition Science Alliance.

International Food Information Council Foundation (IFIC). 2007. *2007 Food and Health Survey: Consumer attitudes toward food, nutrition, and health*. Washington, DC: Author.

Keystone Center. 2006. The Keystone Forum on Away-From-Home Foods: Opportunities for prevention of weight gain and obesity. www.keystone.org/spp/documents/Forum_Report_FINAL_5-30-06.pdf.

Kolodinsky, J., J.R. Harvey-Berino, L. Berlin, R.K. Johnson, and T.W. Reynolds. 2007. Knowledge of current dietary guidelines and food choice by college students: Better eaters have higher knowledge of dietary guidance. *Journal of the American Dietetic Association* 107 (8): 1409-1413.

Krebs-Smith, S., and P. Kris-Etherton. 2007. How does MyPyramid compare to other population-based recommendations for controlling chronic disease? *Journal of the American Dietetic Association* 107: 830-837.

Mead, P.S., L. Slutsker, V. Dietz, L.F. McCaig, J.S. Bresee, C. Shapiro, P.M. Griffin, and R.V. Tauxe. 1999. Food-related illness and death in the United States. www.cdc.gov/ncidod/eid/vol5no5/mead.htm.

National Heart, Lung, and Blood Institute (NHLBI). 2007. Portion Distortion I and II Slide Set Quiz. http://hp2010.nhlbihin.net/portion/.

Pereira, M.A., E. O'Reilly, K. Augustsson, G.E. Fraser, U. Goldbourt, B.L. Heitmann, G. Hallmans, P. Knekt, S. Liu, P. Pietinen, D. Spiegelman, J. Stevens, J. Virtamo, W.C. Willett, and A. Ascherio. 2004. Dietary fiber and risk of coronary heart disease: A pooled analysis of cohort studies. *Archives of Internal Medicine* 164: 370-376.

Putnam, J., J. Allshouse, and L.S. Kantor. 2002. U.S. per capita food supply trends: More calories, refined carbohydrates, and fats. *Food Review* 25 (3).

Reedy, J., and S.M. Krebs-Smith. 2008. A comparison of food-based recommendations and nutrient values of three food guides: USDA's MyPyramid, NHLBI's Dietary Approaches to Stop Hypertension Eating Plan, and Harvard's Healthy Eating Pyramid. *Journal of the American Dietetic Association* 108: 522-528.

Stahler, C. 2006. How many adults are vegetarian? www.vrg.org/journal/vj2006issue4/vj2006issue4poll.htm.

Stewart, H., N. Blisard, S. Bhuyan, and R.M. Jayga Jr. 2004. *The demand for food away from home—full-service or fast food?* [Agricultural Economic Report Number 829]. Washington, DC: USDA Economic Research Service.

U.S. Department of Agriculture (USDA). 2001. *Feeding infants: A guide for use in the child nutrition programs*. Alexandria, VA: USDA Food and Nutrition Service.

———. 2006. Safe food handling. www.fsis.usda.gov/Fact_Sheets/Basics_for_Handling_Food_Safely/index.asp.

U.S. Department of Health and Human Services (USDHHS) and USDA. 2005. *Dietary Guidelines for Americans 2005*. www.health.gov/dietaryguidelines/dga2005/document/pdf/DGA2005.pdf.

U.S. Environmental Protection Agency (EPA). 2004. What you need to know about mercury in fish and shellfish. www.epa.gov/waterscience/fishadvice/advice.html.

U.S. Food and Drug Administration (FDA). 2008a. Animal cloning: Risk management plan for clones and their progeny. www.fda.gov/cvm/CloningRA_RiskMngt.htm.

———. 2008b. Animal cloning: FAQs about cloning for consumers. www.fda.gov/cvm/CloningRA_FAQConsumers_Final.htm.

Wakai, K., C. Date, M. Fukui, K. Tamakoshi, Y. Watanabe, N. Hayakawa, M. Kojima, M. Kawado, K. Suzuki, S. Hashimoto, S. Tokudome, K. Ozasa, S. Suzuki, H. Toyoshima, Y. Ito, and A. Tamakoshi for the JACC Study Group. 2007. Dietary fiber and risk of colorectal cancer in the Japan Collaborative Cohort Study. *Cancer Epidemiology Biomarkers and Prevention* 16: 668-675.

Warner, M. 2005. Snack makers use a calorie count to appeal to dieters. *New York Times*. www.nytimes.com/2005/05/30/business/30portion.html.

Zelman, K.M. 2007. The truth behind the top 10 dietary supplements: What you need to know about the most popular dietary and nutritional supplements on the market. www.webmd.com/diet/features/truth-behind-top-10-dietary-supplements?page=6.

Other helpful resources include the following.

American Association for Retired Persons (AARP). 2008. Size does matter: Master portion control. www.aarp.org/health/staying_healthy/eating/size_does_matter.html.

Food Resource and Action Committee. 2006. The paradox of obesity and hunger. www.frac.org/html/hunger_in_the_us/hunger&obesity.htm.

Fraser, G.E. 1999. Associations between diet and cancer, ischemic heart disease, and all-cause mortality in non-Hispanic white California Seventh-Day Adventists. *American Journal of Clinical Nutrition* 99: 595-598.

Harvard Health Publications. 2008. Artificial sweeteners: Okay in moderation. *Harvard Women's Health Watch* 11(11): 2-3.

U.S. Department of Agriculture (USDA). 2008a. USDA National Nutrient Database for Standard Reference. www.nal.usda.gov/fnic/foodcomp/search/.

———. 2008b. What are "added sugars"? www.mypyramid.gov/pyramid/discretionary_calories_sugars.html.

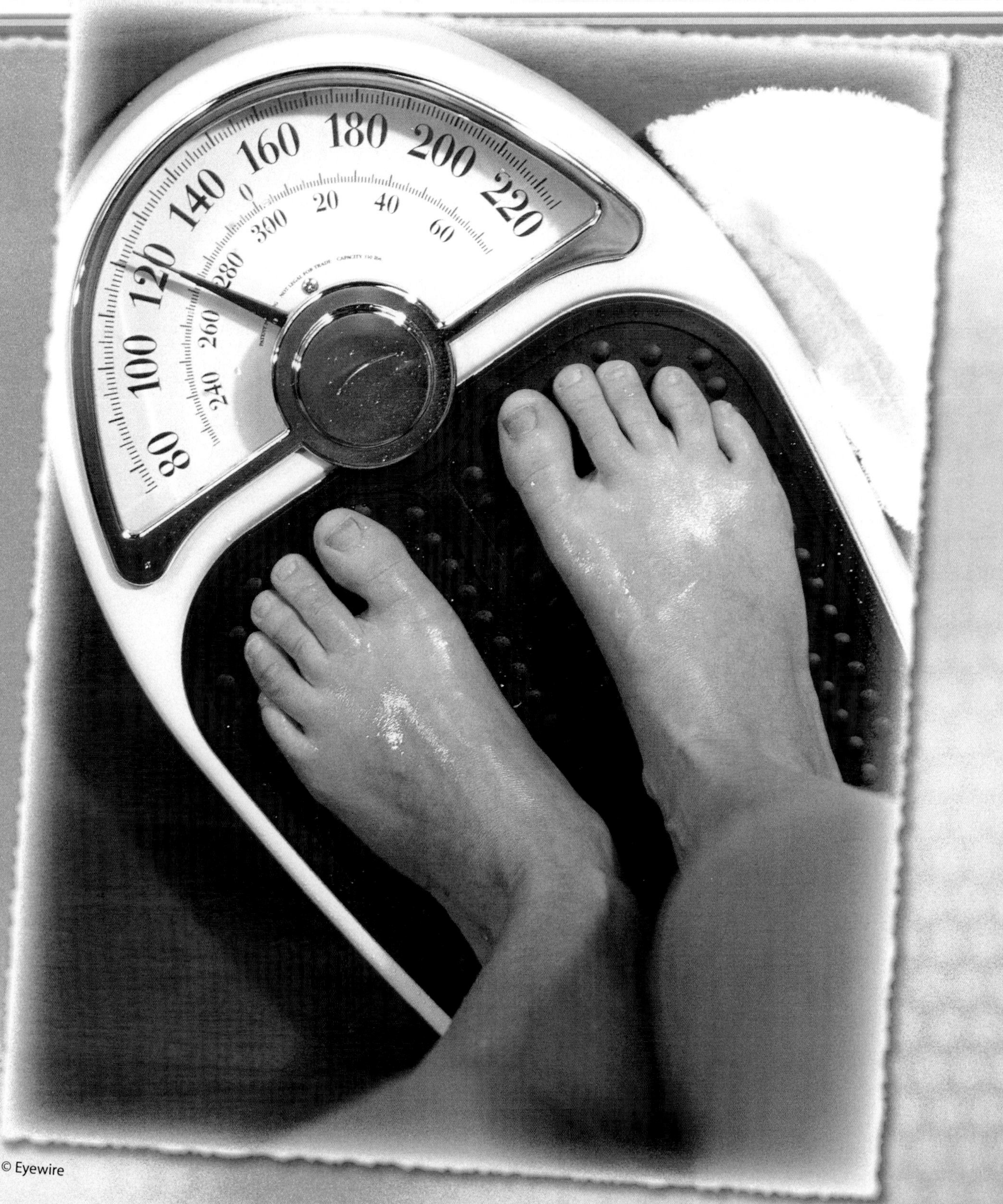

© Eyewire

CHAPTER 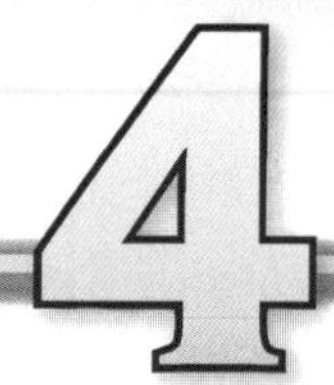

WEIGHT MANAGEMENT

LORI NEIGHBORS, PHD, RD
University of Wisconsin–Milwaukee

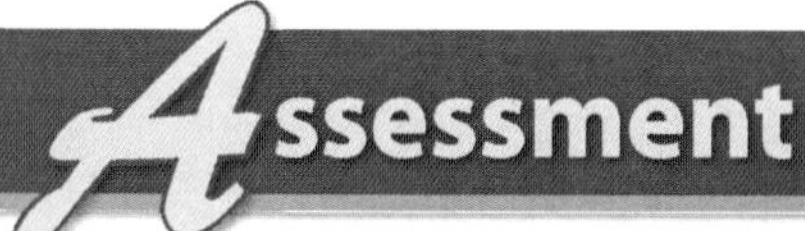

Assessment

- Did you know that the World Health Organization (WHO) classifies around 400 million people worldwide as obese, including 20 million children under the age of 5?
- What's the difference between hunger and appetite?
- Do people eat more food when dining alone or when dining with others?
- Are you an apple or a pear? What does that mean for your health?
- Is it true that some people are overweight because of their genes or heredity?
- Why should you avoid dieting if you want to lose weight?

Objectives

- Understand the concept of energy balance and how it contributes to body weight.
- Describe the state of affairs regarding body weight in the United States, including the obesity epidemic.
- Describe various methods used to evaluate body weight and to diagnose underweight, overweight, and obesity.
- Discuss body weight influences from genetic, social, and environmental perspectives.
- Describe the physical, social, and mental health ramifications associated with too little or too much body weight.
- Describe treatment options for those with too little or too much body weight.
- Critically evaluate popular weight management options for safety, efficacy, and long-term success.

Do some observing the next time you a walk down a busy street. What do you notice about the body weight of the people around you? According to national statistics, chances are that about 6 out of every 10 adults you observe are overweight or obese. What you can't see is that one out of every three men and almost one in every two women will be trying to lose weight. Despite weight-loss efforts, the United States and other industrialized nations such as Germany, the United Kingdom, and India are in the midst of an obesity epidemic. Given the myriad consequences associated with excess body weight, promoting healthy long-term weight management has moved to the forefront of public health efforts, yet a solution that works for the masses remains elusive.

The weight-loss industry has come a long way since the first popular diet book appeared in 1864. It was a 21-page pamphlet by William Banting titled "Letter on Corpulence, Addressed to the Public." Today, bookstore shelves are lined with self-help books about weight loss, each with its own formula to help people shed unwanted pounds. Infomercials promote products and services promising that, "For only three payments of $49.99, you can achieve the body you want in only 2 months!" Weight-loss treatment has even evolved into a form of entertainment; reality TV shows such as NBC's *The Biggest Loser* and VH1's *Celebrity Fit Club* publicly chronicle the weight loss struggles of overweight and obese participants.

If any of these products or programs held the magic bullet for weight loss, society would look very different than it does today. The weight-loss industry has exploded into a multibillion-dollar enterprise because when it comes to weight management, there is no magic bullet and one size does not fit all. However, there are some general approaches and techniques pertaining to food, eating, and activity that have been found to help with the causes and consequences of energy imbalance. Most of the chapter focuses on weight management from the perspective of losing weight and maintaining a healthy weight, because those are areas that many people need to learn about. We will also briefly cover the opposite situation that affects some people—underweight.

HOW DID WE GET HERE?

Body weight and body fat have been increasing in the United States for some time. Data from the National Health and Nutrition Examination Survey of the Centers for Disease Control and Prevention (CDC) illustrate that from the mid-1970s to 2004, the prevalence of overweight or obesity increased from 47 percent to 66 percent among adults aged 20 to 74 years (see figure 4.1). During the same time period, the prevalence of overweight children aged 2 to 5 years increased from 5 percent to 14 percent; for children aged 6 to 11 years, it increased from 7 percent to 19 percent; and for children aged 12 to 19 years, it increased from 5 percent to 17 percent (see figure 4.2) (CDC 2005). You can see an animated map of the United States that shows the increased prevalence of obesity over the past 20 years at www.cdc.gov/nccdphp/dnpa/obesity/trend/maps.

We are living in what the World Health Organization (WHO) has labeled an **obesogenic environment**. We are surrounded by influences, conditions, and trends that make healthy lifestyle choices more difficult and consequently promote weight gain and the maintenance of excess body weight. In

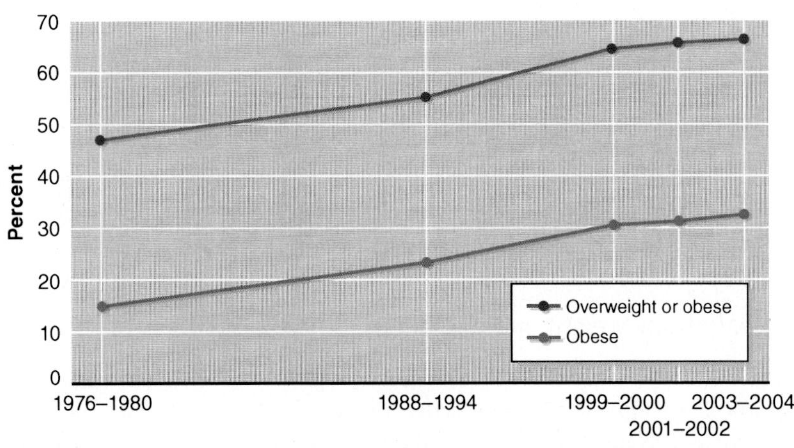

Figure 4.1 Trends in adult overweight and obesity, ages 20 years and older. (Age-adjusted by the direct method to the year 2000 U.S. Census Bureau estimates using the age groups 20 to 30, 40 to 59, and 60 years and over. Overweight defined as BMI ≥ 25; obesity defined as BMI ≥ 30.)

the United States and other Westernized nations, people are exposed to a toxic food and activity environment where energy-dense foods are widely available, inexpensive, and marketed heavily. At the same time, energy-saving devices and other changes in lifestyle have led to an increase in sedentary behavior and a decline in physical activity.

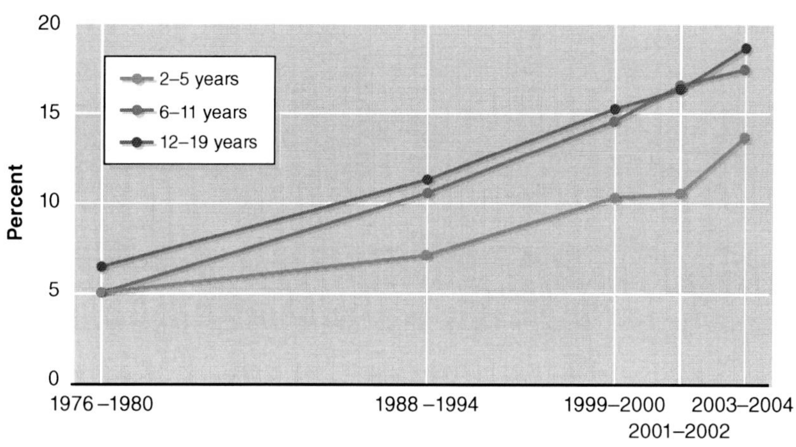

Figure 4.2 Trends in child and adolescent overweight. (Overweight is defined as BMI ≥ gender- and weight-specific 95th percentile from the 2000 CDC Growth Charts.)

Toxic Food Environment

Many environmental influences affect what foods we buy, where we eat, and how much we consume. These influences include trends in the food supply, food prices, eating out, portion size, and food-related advertising and promotion.

Simply put, there is more energy, represented as calories from food and drink, available per person per day in the United States' food supply than ever before. On average, in 1970, there were 3,300 calories available from the food supply per person compared with 3,800 calories in 1994. Given that a moderately active adult requires about 2,000 to 2,600 calories per day, the 15 percent increase in the calories from food available for consumption means that the U.S. food supply can provide the average adult almost double the amount of calories needed by the body. Between 1970 and 1996, the amount of added fat and oils in the food supply increased 22 percent. Although fruits and vegetables have become increasingly available over the years, fruit and vegetable intake remains below recommended levels.

We have more options to eat out than ever before. Between 1972 and 1995, the number of commercial eating places (e.g., restaurants, fast-food restaurants, convenience stores, delis) grew by 89 percent, and fast-food restaurants increased by an astounding 147 percent. As society becomes more and more pressed for time, people spend fewer hours preparing food and they eat out more often. That usually means they're consuming greater amounts of calories and fat.

Exposure to television commercials, especially for fast food or convenience foods, may influence consumers' food choices toward high-fat, high-energy foods. Given that about 98 percent of U.S. households own a television and spend about 2 hours a day watching it, children and adults are exposed to a great number of food-related advertisements. The amount of money food manufacturers spend on advertising may surprise you. In 1997, food manufacturers spent $7 billion on advertising, 28 percent of which was spent advertising foods from fast-food restaurants (Frazao 1999). In the same year, the U.S. Department of Agriculture (USDA) spent a fraction of that amount—about $333.3 million (about 3 percent of the amount spent by food manufacturers)—on nutrition education, evaluation, and demonstration. The foods that are most heavily advertised are those that are most often overconsumed.

What Do You Do?

The next time you sit down to watch TV, keep track of the total minutes of commercials that are shown and the minutes of commercials that are related to food or drink. What proportion of those commercials advertise or promote healthier foods (such as fruits and vegetables) versus less healthy foods (such as hamburgers, sugary drinks, or pizza)?

Portion size is another feature in the toxic food landscape. Both at restaurants and grocery stores, the portion sizes of prepared foods are exploding (Young and Nestle 2002). Large portions and so-called value meals lead many consumers to believe they got a bargain. At 7-Eleven convenience stores, the 16-ounce (473-milliliter) Gulp costs just under 5 cents an ounce, but a 32-ounce (946-milliliter) Big Gulp costs only 2.7 cents an ounce. However, the larger portions contain more calories. A growing body of research indicates that people eat and drink more when they're served more (e.g., Rolls, Morris, and Row 2002), so the bargains may be contributing to our growing waistlines.

Toxic Physical Activity Environment

Physical activity levels have declined sharply over the past half-century. Specific influences in the environment affect physical activity, including television, computers, transportation, and occupational activity. Almost every home in the United States has a television, and an increasing number have a computer. Time spent in front of a TV or computer screen has been on the rise over the past few decades and is associated with an increase in sedentary behavior (and snacking).

People are less likely to walk or bike as a means of transportation than in previous years (Committee on Physical Activity 2005). Americans are driving more and walking or cycling less than they did in the past. In 1960, roughly two-thirds of trips for all daily travel were made by car; by 2000, that figure had increased to more than four-fifths. In 1969, about half of students between the ages of 5 and 15 years walked to school. This number has dropped dramatically, to about 15 percent in 2001.

For many Americans, the work environment no longer provides the opportunity for physical activity that it once did (Brownson, Boehmer, and Luke 2005). As a whole, the proportion of the U.S. workforce employed in jobs requiring high energy expenditure has declined steadily since the 1970s, while the proportion of the workforce employed in low-activity jobs increased sharply between 1950 and 1970 and has since leveled off. In 1950, for example, approximately 30 percent more people had high-activity occupations than low-activity occupations. In 2000, twice as many people had low-activity jobs than high-activity jobs.

National Weight Management Recommendations

As you may now realize, many factors influence physical activity and eating behavior, making it challenging to maintain a healthy lifestyle and body weight. The body-weight challenges faced by American society have prompted the government to develop national recommendations pertaining to body weight. *Dietary Guidelines for Americans 2005* includes these key recommendations (U.S. Department of Health and Human Services [USDHHS] and USDA 2005):

- To maintain body weight in a healthy range, balance calories from foods and beverages with calories expended.
- To prevent gradual weight gain over time, make small decreases in food and beverage calories and increase physical activity.

The guidelines get more specific for special populations:

- *Those who need to lose weight.* Aim for a slow, steady weight loss by decreasing calorie intake while maintaining adequate nutrient intake and increasing physical activity.
- *Overweight children.* Reduce the rate of weight gain while allowing growth and development. Consult a health care provider before placing a child on a weight-reduction diet.
- *Pregnant women.* Ensure appropriate weight gain as specified by a health care provider.
- *Breastfeeding women.* Moderate weight reduction is safe and does not compromise weight gain of the nursing infant based on health care providers' specifications.
- *Overweight adults and overweight children with chronic diseases or those on medication.* Consult a health care provider about weight-loss strategies before starting a weight-reduction program to ensure appropriate management of other health conditions.

BASIC REGULATION OF EATING AND BODY WEIGHT

To better understand the weight-control concerns facing society, it is important to have a solid understanding of factors that influence the regulation of eating and body weight. These include hunger, energy balance, and theories about body weight regulation.

Hunger, Satiation, Satiety, and Appetite

What is the difference between hunger and appetite? Satiation and satiety? You might think those words mean the same thing, but when it comes to understanding the regulation of eating and body weight, they're quite different. The body receives internal cues, or sensations, that help you know when to start and stop eating (see figure 4.3). The first sensation is hunger, which prompts eating. **Hunger** is a physical sensation that signals the physiological need to find and consume food. The second sensation is **satiation**, which signals the body to stop eating. **Satiety**, the third sensation, determines how much time is spent not being hungry and not eating between meals. Research has suggested that many people are not very good at regulating the frequency and amount of food consumed based on these internal signals. One reason for this is another food-related cue: appetite.

The desire for food is often referred to as **appetite**, which is not the same as hunger. Hunger is the physiological need for food, but appetite is a subjective, psychological desire to eat food, which may or may not be the result of hunger. In contrast to hunger and satiety, appetite is generally stimulated by external cues, or cues from the environment.

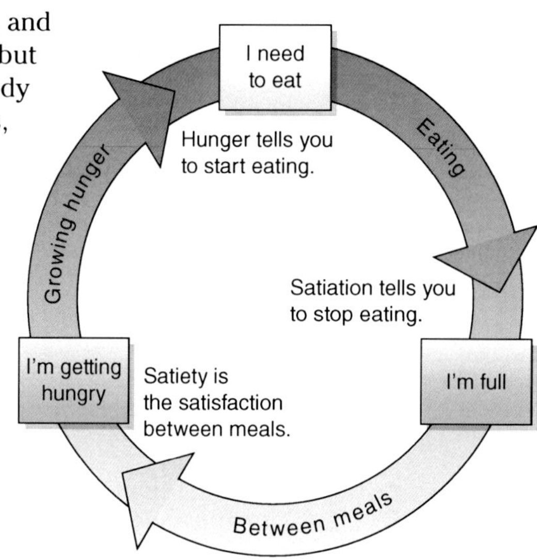

Figure 4.3 Hunger, satiation, and satiety are cues that tell you when to start and stop eating.

Think about the last time you ate a large holiday dinner. Even though you felt stuffed, did you still find room for ice cream or pie? That's appetite. The loss of appetite (e.g., from illness or medication) can prevent you from consuming food even when you might have a physiological need for it. Think about the last time you had a severe cold. Did you eat more or less than usual? Chances are, food didn't sound that good to you. If so, you didn't have an appetite for food.

Energy Balance

The balance between **energy intake** and **energy output** determines body weight in healthy people. Simply put, when you consume more calories (energy from food) than you burn off through physical activity and body processes, your body is in a state of **positive energy balance**. If you remain in that state, you'll gain weight. The reverse is also true. When your body burns off more calories than consumed, the result is **negative energy balance**, which leads to weight loss. Energy balance is defined by the following equation:

energy intake = energy output

(protein + carbohydrate + fat + alcohol) = (basal metabolism + physical activity + thermic effect of food + thermogenesis)

The terms included on the energy output side o]f the equation will be discussed in more detail later in the chapter. Briefly, the contributors to energy output are as follows:

- Basal metabolism represents the energy needed to sustain the metabolic activities of cells and tissues and to maintain vital body systems and processes.
- Thermic effect of food is the energy it takes to digest food.
- Thermogenesis is the generation of heat to maintain body temperature.

Although the concept of energy balance might seem simple, the human body is a complex machine that feeds on input from numerous internal and external forces to regulate eating behavior, energy balance, and body weight. Some of the internal forces include hormones and genetics. External forces include the sensory properties of food, portion size, and the food environment.

Energy Intake

Energy intake is critical in regulating body weight because there is greater flexibility in energy intake than there is in energy expenditure. For example, day-to-day variability in energy intake is estimated to be 25 percent, but energy expenditure varies by only about 8 percent (Jebb 2002).

> **What Do You Think?**
>
> Are there times when you eat although you're already full? Universities and some restaurants offer all-you-can-eat buffet options for meals. Do you find that you eat more at a buffet-style meal? How do you think this all-you-can-eat mentality affects your waistline?

So, how do you determine how much to eat? How do you know when you're full? Do you eat only when you're hungry, or are other factors involved? Research about the regulation of eating and body weight has revealed a complex interplay of internal and external factors that influence food consumption and energy balance. A network of internal body systems, including gastrointestinal, metabolic, and hormonal signals, stimulate or inhibit food consumption. Those systems send signals that end an eating episode, trigger the next meal, or influence energy intake over the next few days, weeks, or even months. Energy intake regulation becomes even more complex when you factor in the variety of cognitive, social, and environmental factors that can override the internal physiological control of food intake.

Diet Composition

The nutritional characteristics of the food you consume (e.g., macronutrients, fiber, energy density) influence how much you eat as well as how full or how satisfied you feel after eating. For example, foods high in dietary fiber enhance feelings of fullness and delay hunger in numerous ways, such as slowing the rate at which the stomach empties, creating a greater volume of food in the gastrointestinal tract, and promoting the release of cholecystokinin, a hormone that works with the brain to inhibit food intake (Burton-Freeman, Davis, and Schneeman 2002). Consuming foods that contain protein appears to have a stronger effect on satiation than consuming foods high in fat or carbohydrate (Paddon-Jones et al. 2008).

The **energy density** of foods (or the amount of calories in a given volume) also affects eating behavior. Foods such as candy and peanut butter that provide a lot of calories in a small amount of food have a high energy density, whereas fresh fruits and vegetables, which are high in water (volume), are generally low in calories and so have a low energy density. Studies show that people tend to eat a consistent volume of food, but when they choose foods with low energy density, they automatically decrease the amount of energy they consume without increasing hunger (Bell et al. 1998; Bell and Rolls 2001). Figure 4.4 shows three foods with different levels of energy density.

Gastrointestinal Sensations

The stomach is a large tank that can hold up to 4 cups of food for several hours, until the food is able to enter the small intestine. As food enters the stomach and small intestine, they stretch (or distend) and send signals to the brain to suppress the urge to eat.

Hormonal and Neurological Factors

Scientists continually uncover new hormonal and neurological factors that play a role in regulating energy intake. Hormones influence eating behavior through their direct or indirect

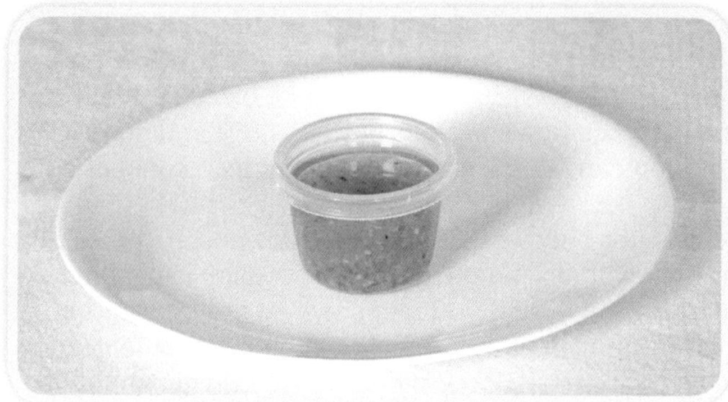

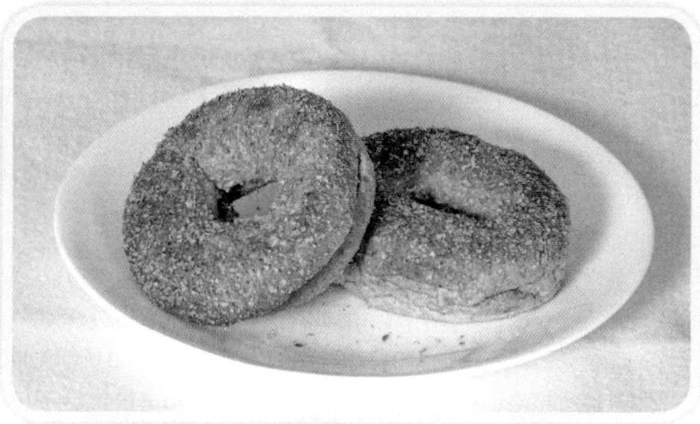

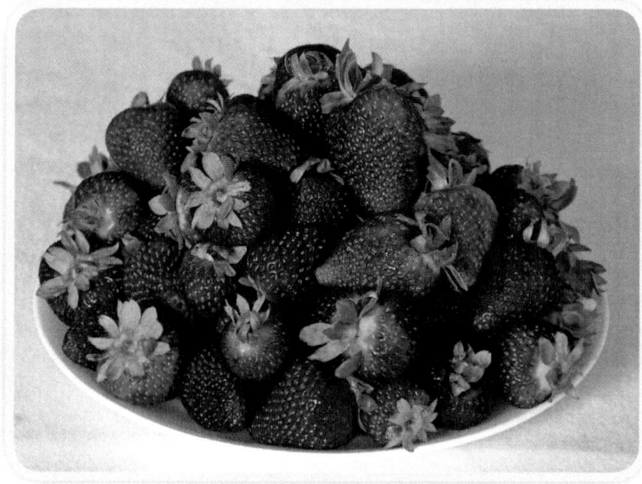

Figure 4.4 Each amount of food shown equals approximately 500 calories. But if you're going to consume that number of calories, would you rather get them from 11 tablespoons of salad dressing, 2 plain wheat bagels, or 3.4 pounds (1,542 grams) of fresh strawberries? Which plate looks like it would be more filling?

effects on the brain. For example, decreases in the neurotransmitter **serotonin** and increases in **neuropeptide Y** are associated with an increased appetite for carbohydrate. The levels of neuropeptide Y may also rise during food deprivation, which means it might be a factor that leads to an increase in appetite after dieting.

The hormone **ghrelin** is produced by the stomach and acts on the **hypothalamus** to stimulate hunger and feeding. Another hormone, **cholecystokinin (CCK)**, is released by the intestinal tract when fat, protein, and fiber reach the small intestine. At the brain level, CCK helps inhibit food intake.

A good deal of research has focused on the hormone **leptin**, a compound that is secreted by fat tissue. Leptin tells the central nervous system how much fat the body is storing. When researchers gave leptin to obese mice who lacked it, the hormone helped the mice reach a normal weight (Schwartz, Baskin, Kaiyala, and Woods 1999). But mice aren't people. Research has shown that overweight people have high concentrations of leptin in the blood, and they don't respond to leptin by reducing their food intake. Research has also found that obese patients respond poorly to leptin, which suggests they have some level of leptin resistance.

Cognitive, Social, and Environmental Factors

Humans have the capacity to eat when they're not hungry or in need of food. Food and eating have meaning beyond simple nourishment. As a result, many cognitive, social, and environmental factors influence eating behavior. For example, think about how many children are raised to be members of the clean-plate club. Many parents encourage children to eat all the food on their plates. When kids do as they're told, they might be ignoring their internal cues of fullness. The duty to eat everything served often remains even after members of the clean-plate club grow up.

A lot of people use food as a mechanism to cope with emotional or stressful situations. They use food as a reward, comfort, or solution to boredom, and food marketers often try to link food products with emotion. For instance, a Hershey's chocolate campaign had the tagline, "Find your Hershey's happiness." Associating emotion (both positive and negative), stress, and boredom with food consumption can be unhealthy and might lead some people to overeat.

The presence of other people influences not only what you eat but how much you eat. In some cases, simply watching the eating behavior of a parent, friend, or stranger can influence your own eating behavior. Think about how much food you ate, how fast you ate, and how much you paid attention to what you were eating during a recent big holiday or celebratory meal compared with a meal while you were at home alone. When we spend enjoyable time with family and friends, we can easily lose track of the quantity of food we consume. Interestingly, food consumption has been shown to increase by 47, 58, 69, 70, 72, and 96 percent when people eat with 2, 3, 4, 5, 6, and 7 or more people, respectively (de Castro and Brewer 1992). One explanation for that phenomenon is that the presence of familiar and friendly people makes meals longer, more enjoyable, and more relaxing and distracts us from monitoring what and how much food ends up in our stomachs.

Numerous other factors influence eating behavior. Distraction can initiate, obscure, or extend food consumption. If you eat while you're watching television, for example, you might activate an eating script that leads you to eat while distracted, even when you're not hungry. Cultural norms also influence what and how much you eat. In certain cultures, it's considered rude to refuse food when someone offers it. Some people are influenced by the clock, and they'll eat at mealtime even if they aren't hungry. The perceived variety of food available can also increase consumption. A simple study found that people eat 43 percent more M&M candies when they're eating from a bowl with 10 colors than they do from a bowl with only 7 colors (Kahn and Wansink 2004).

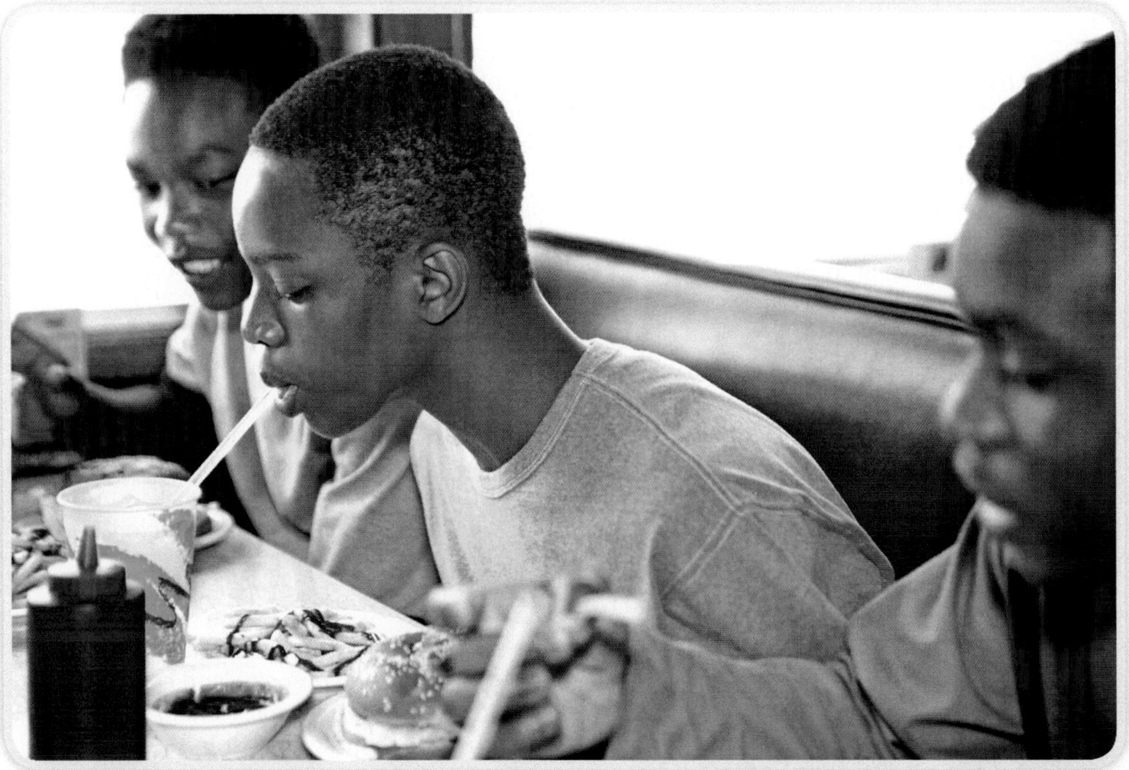

Research has shown that people consume more food when eating with friends or family than when eating alone.

© Bananastock

Scientists are continuing to uncover additional factors that influence energy intake. Package size, plate size, lighting, and other environmental factors can make you eat far more than you might realize. Did you know that cup shape influences how much you drink? If you were given a tall, skinny glass and a short, wide glass, you'd likely serve yourself more and drink 30 to 35 percent more out of the short, wide glass (Wansink and van Ittersum 2005). In another study, nutrition experts attended what they thought was an ice cream social but in reality was an experiment. They got either a 17-ounce (503-milliliter) bowl or a 34-ounce (1-liter) bowl and either a 2-ounce (59-milliliter) or 3-ounce (89-milliliter) ice cream scoop and were invited to serve themselves (Wansink, van Ittersum, and Painter 2006). After they dished up their ice cream, they completed a brief survey, and the researchers weighed the ice cream. The guests with the larger bowls served themselves 31 percent more than those with smaller bowls, and they weren't even aware of it. The people who got the larger ice cream scoop dished up 14.5 percent more ice cream than those with the smaller scoop. And guess which groups ate more ice cream?

Other research suggests that people will eat more of a particular snack food when it's visible and nearby. In one study, 40 employees were given candy in either clear or opaque dishes and had the dishes placed on their desks. Those given clear dishes had their hand in the candy 71 percent more often than those who were given candy in opaque dishes. When the candy was directly on their desks, the employees consumed 77 more calories than they did when researchers placed the dish about 2 yards (2 meters) away (Wansink, Painter, and Lee 2006).

Energy Output

All of the seen and unseen influences take a toll on the calories you consume. Trouble arises when energy output doesn't keep up with intake. The body uses energy for three main purposes: basal or resting metabolism, physical activity, and digestion, absorption, and processing of food.

Basal and Resting Metabolic Rate

Most of the energy from the food we consume is spent on the basic body functions required to sustain life. Basal metabolism (also known as **basal metabolic rate [BMR]**) represents the minimum amount of energy spent during a fasting state to keep a resting, awake body alive and performing basic bodily functions (e.g., heartbeat, lung respiration, and liver, brain, and kidney function). BMR accounts for 60 to 70 percent of the total energy used by the body. **Resting metabolic rate (RMR)** is similar to BMR (the terms are often used interchangeably even though they are not identical), except that it measures the activity required to keep the basic body functions going in a nonfasting, non-completely-rested state. Measurement of RMR is typically performed 3 to 4 hours after eating or performing significant physical activity, and because the body is not completely at rest at the time of assessment, RMR tends to be about 6 percent higher than BMR. Because the conditions required to accurately assess BMR are more difficult to meet, measurement of RMR is more common.

The energy used by the organs and resting muscles makes up the greatest portion of RMR. Other tissues, such as fat and bone, are less metabolically active and require less energy. A lean, muscular person burns more energy at rest than a person who weighs the same but has a higher percentage of body fat.

Many factors increase or decrease RMR. Factors that increase RMR include stress, caffeine, smoking, increased lean body mass, pregnancy and lactation, increased total body weight, hot and cold temperatures, fever, and hyperthyroidism (medical condition where the thyroid gland excessively produces thyroid hormones). Factors that decrease RMR include aging (lean body mass declines with age), female gender (women have generally less lean body mass than men), hypothyroidism (medical condition marked by insufficient production of thyroid hormones), and energy restriction. If you suddenly deprive your body of adequate energy from food by going on a starvation or semistarvation diet, for example, your RMR adapts to conserve energy by dropping as much as 15 percent in 2 weeks. When you start to eat normally again, your RMR goes back to normal (Ravussin and Swinburn 1992).

Energy Expenditure for Physical Activity

Physical activity has a big impact on how much energy the body burns beyond basal energy needs. How active or inactive you choose to be determines your total calorie expenditure for the day. If you're like most people, physical activity accounts for 15 to 30 percent of your total energy expenditure. That measurement will vary depending on the type, intensity, and duration of your activities. Walking for 30 minutes expends less energy than running for 30 minutes, for example.

All activity counts, even activities you might not think of as exercise. **Nonexercise activity thermogenesis (NEAT)** is the energy the body burns when doing activities of daily life such as typing, doing yard work, fidgeting, or walking up a flight of stairs. Table 4.1 includes examples of such activities; note that people of different weights burn a different amount of calories.

Energy Expenditure to Process Food

The energy you put in your body in the form of food requires energy (albeit a small amount) to process and use. The energy used by the body to digest, absorb, and metabolize food is referred to as the **thermic effect of food (TEF)**. Generally, TEF peaks about 1 hour after eating and dissipates within 5 hours. Food composition also affects TEF. For example, the TEF value of a protein-rich meal is higher than the TEF value of a meal rich in fat, because it takes more energy to metabolize amino acids than to transfer absorbed fat into adipose stores. For a typical diet, TEF accounts for about 10 percent of total energy expenditure.

TABLE 4.1 Energy Burned in Daily Activities

	CALORIES USED PER HOUR				
Activity	**100 lb (45 kg)**	**120 lb (54.5 kg)**	**150 lb (68 kg)**	**180 lb (81.5 kg)**	**200 lb (91 kg)**
Applying makeup	91	109	136	163	181
Attending class	82	98	122	147	163
Brushing teeth	91	109	136	163	181
Carrying groceries	113	136	170	204	227
Gardening	181	218	272	327	363
Homework	82	98	122	147	163
Laundry	98	117	146	176	195
Light cleaning (such as dusting)	113	136	170	204	227
Making the bed	91	109	136	163	181
Mopping	159	191	238	286	318
Packing or unpacking boxes	159	191	238	286	318
Playing board games	68	82	102	122	136
Raking the lawn	195	234	293	351	390
Sleeping	41	49	61	73	82
Walking the dog	136	163	204	245	272

To see how many calories you burn doing other select activities, visit www.caloriesperhour.com and use the activity calculator.

Thermoregulation

Birds and mammals, including humans, regulate their body temperatures within fairly narrow limits. Substantial changes in the environmental temperature result in involuntary activities to maintain the internal temperature of the body, which expends energy. This process is called **thermoregulation**. Shivering is an example of thermoregulation. The contribution of thermoregulation to overall energy needs is small.

Determining Energy Needs

Direct and indirect calorimetry are the two main ways to determine energy expenditure. **Direct calorimetry** is based on the principle that energy used is ultimately degraded into heat, and the amount of heat released from the body provides a direct measure of metabolic rate. For this method, researchers put a subject into an insulated chamber about the size of a small bedroom. The heat that the body releases raises the temperature of a layer of water surrounding the chamber. By measuring the water temperature in the direct calorimeter before and after the body releases heat, scientists can directly measure the amount of energy the body spends. As you may have guessed, measurements obtained through this method, although widely accepted, are costly, complex, and not readily available for use outside research environments.

Indirect calorimetry is a widely used method for estimating energy expenditure. This method measures oxygen consumption and carbon dioxide production rather than directly measuring heat transfer. It is based on the predictable relationship that exists between the body's use of energy and oxygen. For example, a person who consumes a typical diet of carbohydrate, fat, and protein needs 1 liter of oxygen to yield about 4.85 calories of energy. Indirect calorimetry is more feasible and participant friendly than direct calorimetry; instruments to measure oxygen consumption can be mounted on carts or carried in backpacks. New metabolic measurement devices such as the BodyGem can even fit in the palm of the hand.

Many equations have been developed to help estimate energy needs, and they have varying degrees of accuracy. The Food and Nutrition Board has published a series of equations for estimating the energy needs, called **estimated energy requirements (EER)**, throughout the life span (Food and Nutrition Board 2005). In the following equation, the EER is defined as the average dietary energy intake that is predicted to maintain energy balance in a healthy adult of a defined age, gender, weight, height, and level of activity consistent with good health. To determine a person's EER, you need to know his or her age in years, weight in kilograms, and height in meters. Use table 4.2 to estimate the person's overall physical activity level.

Women aged 19 and older:

$$\text{EER} = 354 - (6.91 \times \text{age}) + \text{physical activity} \times (9.36 \times \text{weight} + 726 \times \text{height})$$

Men aged 19 and older:

$$\text{EER} = 662 - (9.53 \times \text{age}) + \text{physical activity} \times (15.91 \times \text{weight} + 539.6 \times \text{height})$$

TABLE 4.2 Physical Activity Estimates for Estimating Energy Requirements

Activity level	Physical activity (men)	Physical activity (women)
Sedentary (e.g., no exercise)	1.00	1.00
Low activity (e.g., walks the equivalent of 2 mi [3.2 km] per day at 3-4 mph [5-6.5 kph])	1.11	1.12
Active (e.g., walks the equivalent of 7 mi [11 km] per day at 3-4 mph [5-6.5 kph])	1.25	1.27
Very active (e.g., walks the equivalent of 17 mi [27 km] per day at 3-4 mph [5-6.5 kph])	1.48	1.45

Early Theories of Body Weight Regulation

Many theories have emerged to explain why some people become overweight or obese and others do not. The more popular theories include set-point theory and fat cell theory.

Set-Point Theory

In adults, body weight is generally maintained at a stable level for long amounts of time. **Set-point theory** was originally posed to explain why repeated dieting is often unsuccessful in producing long-term changes in body weight or shape. The set-point theory proposes that humans have a genetically predetermined body weight or body-fat content that the body closely regulates. According to the theory, every person has a built-in feedback mechanism that dictates how much fat the body should carry (similar to a thermostat for fat). The body transmits information to a central control center located in the hypothalamus. The control center then sends signals to modulate food intake or energy expenditure to correct any deviations from the determined set point.

The set-point theory has not been widely accepted for several reasons. During adulthood, many people experience significant long-term weight changes. Further, most adults gain weight slowly over time. Also, if people are placed into a different social, physical, or emotional environment, they can change and maintain weight at a new level. Many researchers have challenged the set-point theory on the basis of its simplicity and on other grounds, and there is little scientific research to support it.

Fat Cell Theory

According to **fat cell theory**, people have a certain number of fat cells, and that number influences how easily body fat is gained or lost. The theory proposes that some people develop **hypertrophic obesity**, or a greater-than-average number of fat cells, during critical times in their lives, particularly during childhood. In hypertrophic obesity, fat cells are larger than normal. This is compounded by the physiological fact that fat cells have a maximum size. When fat cells are filled to capacity, they divide, generating more fat cells. When a person reaches a body weight that is about 40 percent overweight or more, fat tissue is likely to contain both bigger fat cells and more of them. That condition is called **hyperplastic obesity**.

Unfortunately, fat cells don't disappear when you lose weight. They do get smaller but, beyond a certain point, they don't shrink any further, and the body attempts to refill them with fat. The only way to permanently remove fat cells from the body is through liposuction. The fat cell theory lends some explanation for why obese people may have a difficult time losing weight and keeping it off, but it doesn't fully address the question of why they became obese in the first place.

WAYS TO ASSESS WEIGHT AND FATNESS

People can estimate and evaluate their body weight and body fat in many ways. Some methods are simple and somewhat crude indicators of body weight and body composition; other methods are more complex and precise.

Height–Weight Tables

Height–weight tables provide a gender-specific body weight range that has been calculated from a health perspective as desirable for a given height. Some tables provide different weight ranges for different body frame sizes in addition to height. Examples of height–weight tables include the Metropolitan Life Insurance Company height and weight tables. Other assessment methods tend to relate body weight status to disease risk more accurately, and as a result, the popularity of height–weight tables has decreased.

Body Mass Index

One of the most common ways to estimate body weight status is the **body mass index (BMI)**. Calculated by dividing a person's body weight (in kilograms) by height (in meters) squared, BMI is a fairly reliable indicator of body fatness in most people. Although BMI doesn't assess body fatness directly, it's an inexpensive and easy way to assess body weight.

For men and women aged 20 and older, **underweight** is defined as a BMI below 18.5, **normal weight** as 18.5 to 24.9, **overweight** as 25.0 to 29.9, and **obese** as above 30.0 (see table 4.3). Obesity is further subdivided into three classes: I (BMI of 30.0 to 34.9), II (35.0 to 39.9), and III (40.0 and above). The ranges are based on epidemiological data showing that risk of dying increases as BMI exceeds 25.0. However, until a BMI of 30, the increase in mortality risk is modest. Figure 4.5 shows the curve illustrating the link between BMI and mortality.

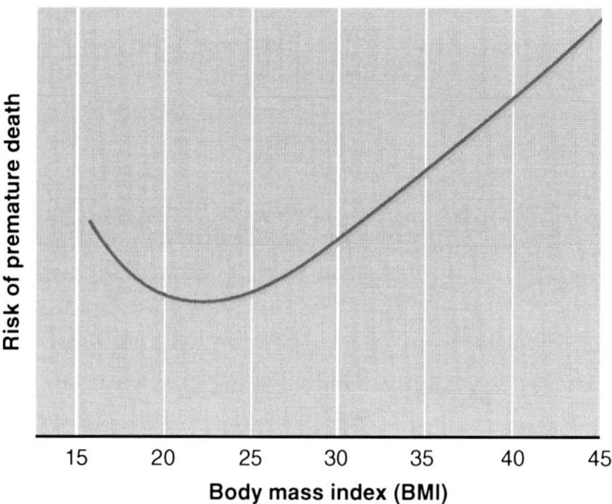

Figure 4.5 A BMI that is too low or too high increases the risk of mortality.

To lower the risk of developing diseases associated with excess body fat, the National Institutes of Health (NIH) suggests that people who are obese or overweight and have two or more risk factors (e.g., high blood pressure, triglycerides, or blood sugar; family history of heart disease; physical inactivity; smoking) should consider losing weight.

Body-Fat Ranges

Fat has numerous essential functions in the body and also serves as a storage form of energy. Some researchers suggest that body fat may be a better measure of weight-related disease risk than BMI (Gallagher et al. 2000). The American Council on Exercise suggests that an acceptable range of body fat is 18 to 25 percent for men and 25 to 31 percent for women (women have a higher acceptable range because they have a higher proportion of essential body fat required for the body to function). Body-fat ranges are lower for athletes or people attempting to attain a high level of fitness: 13 to 24 percent for women and 5 to 17 percent for men. Health problems can occur when the body stores too much or too little body fat, indicated by levels above or below the acceptable range.

Direct Measurement of Body Fat

Several measurement methods can directly estimate body fat. **Skinfold measurements** assess body fat using calipers to measure the amount of fat directly under the skin (subcutaneous fat) at various sites around the body (e.g., triceps, calf, upper thigh). When performed by a trained professional, skinfold measurements correlate well with other body-fat estimation measurements; however, estimates may be inaccurate if an inexperienced technician does the measurements.

Dual-energy X-ray absorptiometry (DXA) is an accurate method of estimating body fat, although the equipment required is expensive and not widely available. DXA measures body fat by scanning the body and passing small doses of radiation through the body. Detectors quantify the proportions of tissue as fat, lean tissue, or bone.

Hydrodensitometry, also known as *underwater weighing* or *hydrostatic weighing*, is often considered the gold standard for estimating body composition. Underwater weighing is based on the fact that body fat is less dense than water and fat-free mass is denser than water, which means that body fat increases buoyancy and fat-free mass decreases it. During hydrodensitometry, the person being weighed breathes out as much air as possible to increase buoyancy and decrease the underwater weight. Then the weighing can be done and the percent fat can be calculated based on the underwater weight. This procedure requires that the person being weighed be completely submerged in a tank of water, and a trained technician has to conduct the procedure.

Another common, quick, and inexpensive technique to estimate body composition is **bioelectrical impedance analysis (BIA)**. BIA technology sends a low-voltage, painless electric current through the body to determine the electrical impedance (a measure of the opposition offered by an electric circuit to the flow of an alternating current) of body tissues, which provides an estimate of total body water. Fatty tissue resists electrical flow more than lean tissue does because of its lower electrolyte and water content. Using values of total body water derived from BIA, fat-free mass and body-fat percentage can be estimated. The technique typically involves attaching surface electrodes to various locations on the arm and foot. Today, numerous BIA body-fat scales and handheld devices are on the market.

Body-Fat Distribution

The distance around the waist is positively correlated with abdominal fat content: The greater the distance around the waist, the more abdominal fat there is. A large **waist circumference** is a risk factor for developing type 2 diabetes, hypertension, and cardiovascular disease. Determine your waist circumference by placing a measuring tape snugly around your waist. Risk for adverse health conditions increases with a waist measurement greater than 40 inches (102 centimeters) among men and greater than 35 inches (88 centimeters) in women. An estimate of waist circumference can be used in conjunction with BMI to estimate one's risk for developing weight-related diseases (see table 4.3).

TABLE 4.3 Disease Risk Relative to BMI and Waist Circumference (WC)

Classification	BMI (kg/m²)	Men: WC ≤ 102 cm (40 in.) Women: WC ≤ 88 cm (35 in.)	Men: WC > 102 cm (40 in.) Women: WC > 88 cm (35 in.)
Underweight	<18.5	No risk	No risk
Normal	18.5-24.9	No risk	No risk
Overweight	25.0-29.9	Increased risk	High risk
Obesity (class I)	30.0-34.9	High risk	Very high risk
Obesity (class II)	35.0-39.9	Very high risk	Very high risk
Obesity (class III)	≥40.0	Extremely high risk	Extremely high risk

Are you an apple or a pear? Similar to waist circumference, extra body fat around the midsection (i.e., apple shape, which is more common among men) can increase the risk for developing diseases such as heart disease and type 2 diabetes compared with excess fat around the hips and thighs (i.e., pear shape, which is more common among women). To determine your **waist-to-hip ratio (WHR)**, use a measuring tape to measure the circumference of your hips at the widest part of the buttocks and the circumference of the smallest part of the natural waist (just above the belly button). The WHR is easily calculated by dividing waist circumference by hip circumference.

A large study of heart disease conducted in 52 countries with more than 27,000 participants found that WHRs over 0.85 in women and over 0.9 in men were strongly associated with an increased risk for myocardial infarction (heart attack), and those ratios predicted heart disease better than BMI and waist circumference (Yusuf et al. 2005). As with most of the body weight and shape assessment measures, the WHR is a guideline for evaluating body size.

Subjective Assessment

There are many ways to objectively assess body weight and body fat. However, the subjective evaluation of body weight and body fatness, often referred to as **body image**, also affects health behavior.

Body image can be defined in many ways. In the 1930s, Paul Schilder, a neurologist by training, was responsible for moving the study of body image out of the field of neuropathology (study of diseases of the nervous system) and emphasizing a biopsychosocial approach. Schilder is credited with providing one of the first multidimensional definitions of body image. He believed that conscious and unconscious processes contribute to the total image that people have of their body. That image is influenced by emotions, attitudes, wishes, and social relationships. Sociocultural trends play a role, too, including what society considers the ideal body to be, your level of exposure to the ideal, and how important the ideal body is to you. Perceptions of your physical appearance and weight status, how satisfied you are with specific aspects of your body (e.g., weight, muscularity, fatness), and body esteem factor into body image, too.

Body image is an important part of weight management because how you think and feel about your body strongly influences how you manage your weight, including what you eat and how you exercise. In a nationally representative study of American adults, 9 out of 10 said that most of their fellow Americans are overweight. But just 7 out of 10 said the same thing about people they knew. And when they were asked about themselves, fewer than 4 out of 10 adults (39 percent) said they were overweight. However, estimates suggest that almost 70 percent of American adults are overweight or obese (Taylor, Funk, and Craighill 2006).

Generally speaking, women consider themselves overweight—often incorrectly so—and try to manage their weight more often than men do. Conversely, men often don't consider themselves overweight when they actually are. People who have **eating disorders** such as **anorexia nervosa** or **bulimia nervosa** are extreme examples of those who have a harmful relationship between body image and weight management.

People should always try to engage in healthy eating and activity behaviors, but not everyone will weigh or look the same. How you view your physical appearance and your desire to lose (or gain) weight should be balanced with **self-acceptance**. Extreme attempts to achieve a potentially unattainable body weight or shape may undermine self-esteem and result in emotional or physical harm.

HEALTH EFFECTS OF OVERWEIGHT, OBESITY, AND UNDERWEIGHT

Overweight and obesity are complex public health issues. Almost every day a news story reports the latest causes and physical, psychological, and social consequences of excess body weight. Although the media tend to focus on the obesity epidemic, underweight is also a serious health concern with a myriad of physical, psychological, and social consequences.

Physical Health Consequences of Excess Weight

Excess body weight takes a toll on physical health. Typically, the more overweight a person is, the more frequent and severe the physical health consequences are. The good news for people who are overweight and obese is that weight loss doesn't have to be extreme before they see improvements in health. Losses of 5 to 10 percent of initial body weight can lead to substantial improvements in risk factors for diabetes and heart disease. If a person weighs 200 pounds (91 kilograms), he would begin reaping health benefits after losing 10 to 20 pounds (4.5 to 9 kilograms). (The following physical health consequences are from NIH. Available: http://win.niddk.nih.gov/publications/health_risks.htm.)

Type 2 Diabetes

In this disease, blood sugar (blood glucose) levels are above normal. High blood sugar is a major cause of heart disease, kidney disease, stroke, amputation, and blindness. Type 2 diabetes is the most common form of diabetes in the United States. It is most often associated with old age, obesity, family history of diabetes, previous history of gestational diabetes, and physical inactivity.

More than 85% of people with type 2 diabetes are overweight. Researchers don't know exactly why people who are overweight are more likely to develop this disease. It may be that being overweight causes cells to change, making them resistant to the hormone insulin. Insulin carries sugar from the blood to the cells, where it is used for energy. When a person is insulin resistant, cells can't take up blood sugar, resulting in high blood sugar. In addition, the cells that produce insulin must work extra hard to try to keep blood sugar normal. This may cause these cells to gradually fail.

Coronary Heart Disease and Stroke

Coronary heart disease (CHD) means that the heart and blood flow are not functioning normally. Often, the arteries have become hardened and narrowed. If you have CHD, you may suffer from a heart attack, congestive heart failure, sudden cardiac death, angina (chest pain), or abnormal heart rhythm. In a heart attack, the flow of blood and oxygen to the heart is disrupted, damaging portions of the heart muscle. During a stroke, blood and oxygen do not flow normally to the brain, possibly causing paralysis or death.

People who are overweight are more likely to develop high blood pressure, high levels of triglycerides (blood fats) and LDL cholesterol (bad cholesterol), and low levels of HDL cholesterol (good cholesterol). These are all risk factors for heart disease and stroke. In addition, excess body fat—especially abdominal fat—may produce substances that cause inflammation. Inflammation in blood vessels and throughout the body may raise the risk of heart disease.

Metabolic Syndrome

Metabolic syndrome is a group of obesity-related risk factors for CHD and diabetes. People have metabolic syndrome if they have three or more of the following risk factors:

- A large waistline. For men, this means a waist measurement of 40 inches (102 centimeters) or more. For women, it means a waist measurement of 35 inches (88 centimeters) or more.
- High triglycerides or taking medication to treat high triglycerides. A triglyceride level of 150 milligrams per deciliter (mg/dl) or higher is considered high.
- Low levels of HDL (good) cholesterol or taking medications to treat low HDL. For men, low HDL cholesterol is below 40 mg/dl. For women, it is below 50 mg/dl.
- High blood pressure or taking medications to treat high blood pressure. High blood pressure is 140 mmHg or higher for systolic blood pressure or 90 mmHg or higher for diastolic blood pressure.
- High fasting blood glucose (sugar) or taking medications to treat high blood sugar. This means a fasting blood sugar of 100 mg/dl or higher.

Metabolic syndrome is strongly linked to obesity, especially abdominal obesity. Other risk factors are physical inactivity, insulin resistance, genetics, and old age. Obesity is a risk factor for the metabolic syndrome because it raises blood pressure and triglycerides, lowers HDL (good) cholesterol, and contributes to insulin resistance. Excess fat around the abdomen carries even higher risks.

Cancer

Cancer occurs when cells in one part of the body, such as the colon, grow abnormally or out of control. The cancerous cells sometimes spread to other parts of the body, such as the liver. Being overweight may increase the risk of developing several types of cancer, including cancers of the colon, esophagus, and kidney. Overweight is also linked with uterine and postmenopausal breast cancer in women. Gaining weight during adulthood increases the risk for several of these cancers, even if the weight gain does not result in overweight or obesity.

It is not known exactly how being overweight increases cancer risk. It may be that fat cells release hormones that affect cell growth, leading to cancer. Also, eating or activity habits that lead to being overweight may contribute to cancer risk.

Sleep Apnea

Sleep apnea is a condition in which a person stops breathing for short amounts of time during the night. A person who has sleep apnea may suffer from daytime sleepiness, difficulty concentrating, and even heart failure.

The risk for sleep apnea is higher for people who are overweight. A person who is overweight may have more fat stored around the neck, which makes the airway smaller. A smaller airway can make breathing difficult, loud (snoring), or stop altogether. In addition, fat stored in the neck and throughout the body may produce substances that cause inflammation. Inflammation in the neck is a risk factor for sleep apnea.

Osteoarthritis

Osteoarthritis is a common joint disorder that causes the joint bone and cartilage (tissue that protects joints) to wear away. Osteoarthritis most often affects the joints of the knees, hips, and lower back.

Extra weight may place extra pressure on joints and cartilage, causing them to wear away. In addition, people with more body fat may have higher blood levels of substances that cause inflammation. Inflammation at the joints may increase the risk for osteoarthritis.

Gallbladder Disease

Gallbladder disease includes gallstones and inflammation or infection of the gallbladder. Gallstones are clusters of solid material that form in the gallbladder. They are made mostly of cholesterol and can cause abdominal pain, especially after consuming fatty foods. The pain may be sharp or dull.

People who are overweight have a higher risk for developing gallbladder disease. They may produce more cholesterol, a risk factor for gallstones. Also, people who are overweight may have an enlarged gallbladder, which may not work properly.

Fatty Liver Disease

Fatty liver disease occurs when fat builds up in the liver cells and causes injury and inflammation in the liver. It can sometimes lead to severe liver damage, cirrhosis (buildup of scar tissue that blocks proper blood flow in the liver), or even liver failure. Fatty liver disease is similar to alcoholic liver damage, but it is not caused by alcohol and can occur in people who drink little or no alcohol.

People who have diabetes or prediabetes (when blood sugar levels are higher than normal but not yet in the diabetic range) are more likely to have fatty liver disease than people without these conditions. People who are overweight are more likely to develop diabetes. It is not known why some people who are overweight or diabetic get fatty liver disease and others do not.

Pregnancy Complications

Overweight and obesity raise the risk of pregnancy complications for both mother and baby. Pregnant women who are overweight or obese may have an increased risk for gestational diabetes (high blood sugar during pregnancy), preeclampsia (high blood pressure during pregnancy that can cause severe problems for both mother and baby if left untreated), and Cesarean delivery or complications with Cesarean delivery. Babies of overweight or obese mothers have an increased risk of defects of the brain and spinal cord, stillbirth, prematurity, and being large for gestational age.

Pregnant women who are overweight are more likely to develop insulin resistance, high blood sugar, and high blood pressure. Overweight also increases the risks associated with surgery and anesthesia, and severe obesity increases operative time and blood loss.

Some studies have shown that gaining excess weight during pregnancy—even without becoming obese—may increase risks. It is important to consult with an obstetrician or other health care provider about how much weight to gain during pregnancy.

Social and Psychological Health Consequences of Excess Weight

Most people in the United States think being fat is a bad thing and is something people should be able to control. Americans value leanness and muscularity among men and thinness among women (it is possible to be thin without having much lean body mass if you have a high percentage of body fat and a low body weight). With the growing prevalence of overweight and obesity, fewer and fewer people have the supposedly ideal body, but many continue to strive for it. Being overweight or obese thus creates a psychological burden.

Social Stigma

Overweight or obese people who live in societies that consider fat to be a negative attribute are often socially stigmatized. Stigmatization of overweight and obese people in the United States is widespread and has been documented in employment, health care, education, and social relationships.

In 2001, leading experts in the field published a review of **weight stigmatization** in health care, education, and employment. In health care, they reported that 24 percent of nurses said they are repulsed by obese people and 39 percent of physicians said that their obese patients are lazy. In education, obese students were less likely to be accepted to college despite having equivalent application rates and academic performance as nonobese peers, and overweight students received less family financial support for college than normal-weight students. In employment, obese women between the ages of 18 and 25 earned 12 percent less than nonobese women (Puhl and Brownell 2001).

Stigmatization also occurs in interpersonal relationships. Overweight and obese people are considered less desirable for sexual relationships (Chen and Brown 2005) and for dating partners (Sobal, Nicolopoulos, and Lee 1995). A study conducted in the 1960s asked fifth- and sixth-grade students to rank six pictures of children in order of whom they would most like for a friend. Children rated the obese child last among children with crutches, in a wheelchair, with an amputated hand, and with a facial disfigurement (Richardson, Goodman, Hastorf, and Dornbusch 1961). Researchers repeated this study 40 years later and found an increase in prejudice against the obese child (Latner and Stunkard 2003).

MIND-BODY CONNECTION

Coping With Weight Stigma

Have you been a victim of weight-based discrimination, or have you observed someone who was a victim? Weight-related teasing, bullying, and other forms of weight-based discrimination are unfortunately commonplace. A four-component model that involves recognition, readiness, reaction, and repair might help those working with overweight people who have been stigmatized (Sobal 1991).

1. Recognition—awareness that obesity is stigmatized and understanding about stigma
2. Readiness—anticipation, preparation, and prevention of stigmatizing acts
3. Reaction—immediate and long-term coping with stigmatizing acts
4. Repair—recovery from problems resulting from stigmatization and reform of actions and values of others

It is clear that a pervasive bias against overweight people exists in U.S. society, resulting in stigmatization and discrimination in various settings. The implications of these findings are dire. Stigmatization of obese patients by health care professionals may affect clinical judgments and also discourage obese patients from seeking medical care. Stigmatization in the workplace can affect wages, promotions, and disciplinary actions. In the education system, overweight and obese children face serious challenges (e.g., teasing, fewer college opportunities) that can affect learning and opportunities for future employment. In interpersonal relationships, the rejection of overweight and obese people offers them fewer desirable romantic partners and fewer opportunities for social mobility through both friendship and marriage.

Psychological Health and Weight Management

Much less is known about the psychological ramifications of overweight and obesity than about the physical and social consequences. You just read about how research indicates that discrimination of overweight people is widespread. Generally, obese people are less liked and viewed less favorably than people of normal weight. Many negative characteristics are attributed to obese people; they're often seen as lazy, stupid, sloppy, and ugly. They're bombarded with messages implying that they're unacceptable. It shouldn't be surprising that, for overweight and obese people living in this kind of culture, there are psychological consequences associated with overweight and obesity, including negative body image and low self-esteem (Friedman and Brownell 2002).

Because obesity is viewed as unattractive and the result of personal misbehavior, many overweight people develop a negative body image. Negative body image is associated with psychological and eating disorder symptoms. For example, some obese people (particularly those who have experienced discrimination because of their weight) are more prone to have distorted perceptions of their body size, to be more dissatisfied and preoccupied with their physical appearance, and to be more reluctant to participate in social situations (Schwartz and Brownell 2002). Cognitive-behavioral therapy even without accompanying weight loss can help overweight and obese people with negative body image.

Excess weight is frequently associated with low self-esteem for several reasons (Johnson 2002):

- Current cultural definitions of beauty and attractiveness, particularly regarding Caucasian women, consider fatness to be unattractive.
- Overweight and obese people are often targets of antifat messages in the media, insults from others, social rejection, comedians telling fat jokes, and bullying.
- Many people assume that larger people lack self-discipline and don't care about themselves or their health.
- People regard weight control and diet failures as personal failures. A failed diet attempt is often internalized and the blame is rarely placed on the flawed process of dieting.

All of these factors take a toll on self-esteem. Some overweight people postpone life events in anticipation of getting a slimmer body. They make poor choices because they feel inferior. They may even sabotage healthy relationships.

But just as not all overweight and obese people have physical health problems, not all are afflicted with the psychological effects of being overweight. Researchers have identified some commonalities among overweight people that make them more resilient to the potential psychological distress that comes from living in a society that stigmatizes being overweight (Johnson 2002):

- They don't view other overweight people with dislike or disgust.
- They don't base their self-regard on others' approval.
- They realize that not all outcomes are deserved and not all things (including weight) are under personal control.
- They are able to blame the bias and prejudice of critics rather than themselves.

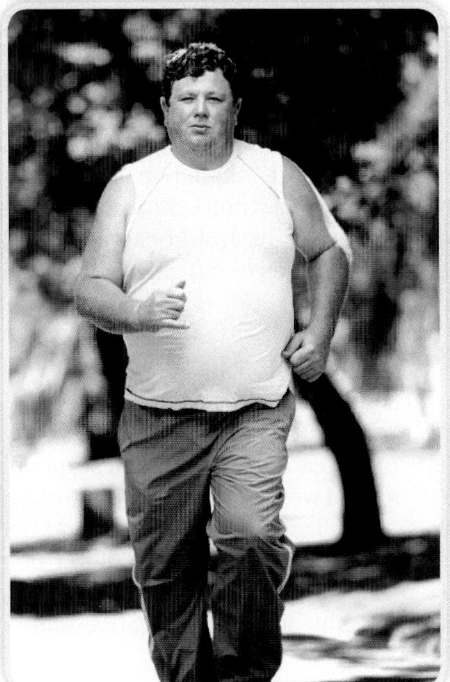

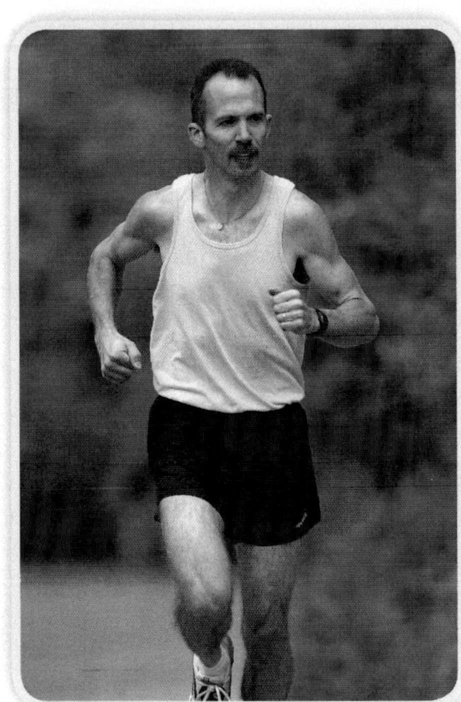

What conclusions about these two joggers might an observer draw based solely on their weight?

© Getty Images/Stockbyte

© Human Kinetics

That research provides suggestions for how other overweight people can develop that same resilience (Johnson 2002):

- Appreciate the functional nature of your body.
- Focus on your talents, accomplishments, and strengths.
- Don't put anything on hold while waiting to lose weight.
- Reject the notion of figure flaws.
- Don't use the opinions of others as the basis for your self-concept.
- Delve into the history of cultural preferences concerning the size and shape of the human body (the current thin ideal is by no means omnipresent).
- Get regular exercise (it's been found to increase self-esteem irrespective of physical health benefits).
- Use positive self-talk and avoid body-related self-criticism.
- Look for size-acceptance support groups.
- Do not become preoccupied with dieting.

Consequences of Too Little Weight

The attention focused on overweight and obesity almost eclipses the problem of underweight. However, just as excess weight can take a toll on the body, so can a lack of weight. Underweight is frequently defined as having a body weight that is 15 to 20 percent or more below the desired weight for height, or having a BMI under 18.5. Underweight in the United States receives far less attention in public health than overweight does, because a much smaller proportion of the U.S. population meets the criteria for underweight.

Being underweight may seem preferable to being overweight, but the reality is that being underweight is also associated with many health risks. People who have a low BMI have greater mortality risk than people with a normal BMI, especially with aging (see figure 4.5). The specific health risks often relate to the underlying cause of why a person is underweight (e.g., disease state, genetics, stress) but may also include reduced function of the pituitary, thyroid, gonadal, and adrenal glands; loss of energy; malnutrition; susceptibility to injury and infection; and a distorted body image.

CAUSES OF OVERWEIGHT, OBESITY, AND UNDERWEIGHT

A lot of factors influence body weight status. They include genetics, gender, race and ethnicity, age, socioeconomic status, and psychological factors.

Genetics

In recent decades, obesity has reached epidemic proportions in places where calorie-rich foods are abundant and opportunities for physical activity are declining. Even in the same environment, though, some people gain weight and others easily maintain a healthy weight. Biology and heredity may provide some clues as to why those differences exist.

Although genetic changes in populations as a whole occur too slowly to be blamed for the rapid rise in obesity in the United States, genes do appear to play a role in the development of obesity. Much is known, and even more is not, about the role of genetics in the development of obesity. For example, genes can directly cause obesity in people with certain disorders, such as **Prader-Willi syndrome**, a condition where the body does not ever feel full. However, in most people, genes do not always predict future health or weight status.

Biological relatives tend to resemble each other in many ways, including body weight. People with a family history of obesity could be predisposed to gain weight. Within the same environment, some people store more energy as fat than others do. Think about it. Do you know someone who eats a lot but stays lean? Do you know someone else who seems to gain weight readily despite efforts to prevent it? In those cases it's possible genetics are at work. Scientists haven't yet learned, though, how the genes that predispose someone to obesity affect energy regulation and metabolism, or why weight management interventions are more effective for some people than for others.

A question that has yet to be resolved is to what extent family patterns are caused by the environment rather than by heredity. Because of the interplay between genetics and the environment, the heredity component is difficult to estimate. Researchers are making progress, though, and they estimate that genes alone generally account for 50 to 90 percent of variations in body fat (Barsh, Farooqi, and O'Rahilly 2000). Researchers in the United Kingdom found that diet and lifestyle are less influential in a child's weight than genetics are. They studied more than 5,000 pairs of identical and fraternal twins and found that children's BMI and waist circumference were linked to genetic factors 77 percent of the time and to environmental factors 23 percent of the time (Wardle, Carnell, Haworth, and Plomin 2008).

There is much more to learn about nature (genes and biology) versus nurture (environment) in the development of overweight and obesity. At this point, however, there are three important conclusions:

1. For those who are genetically predisposed to obesity, prevention of obesity is the best option, although prevention may require individual interventions and support.
2. Obesity is a chronic, lifelong condition resulting from taking in too many calories and performing too little activity, modulated by a susceptible genotype. For that reason, preventing weight gain to begin with is the best option for good health.
3. Genes are not destiny. In almost all instances, obesity can be prevented or managed with the right approach.

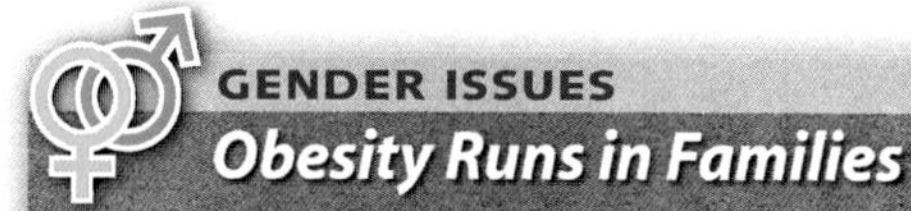

GENDER ISSUES

Obesity Runs in Families

Obesity has been shown to run in families. It is now clear that this is due in part to shared genetic characteristics. If one parent is obese, the child has twice the risk of becoming an obese adult. The risk is even greater if both parents are obese. Interestingly, maternal obesity appears to influence the child's risk of being obese to a greater extent than paternal obesity does (Mafeis, Talamini, and Tato 1998).

Gender

In general, men and women view their bodies differently. At young ages, girls are more likely than boys to label themselves overweight or too heavy and to try to lose weight. Boys, on the other hand, are typically more concerned about their height and how muscular they are. They often try to gain weight (most often as muscle mass). By early adulthood, most women want to lose weight, whether they're overweight or not.

Women face unique weight management challenges throughout their lives, such as pregnancy. During pregnancy, body weight and fat stores increase to meet the physiological needs of the growing fetus. (It's estimated that the energy requirement for an entire pregnancy is about 80,000 calories!) Many women end up gaining more than the recommended amount of weight during pregnancy and have a difficult time returning to their prepregnancy weight. In 2008, the USDA Center for Nutrition Policy and Promotion released nutrition guidance and recommendations for pregnant and breastfeeding women (e.g., MyPyramid for Pregnancy and Breastfeeding, available at www.mypyramid.gov/mypyramidmoms/) to help women manage their nutrition and body weight during this phase of the life course.

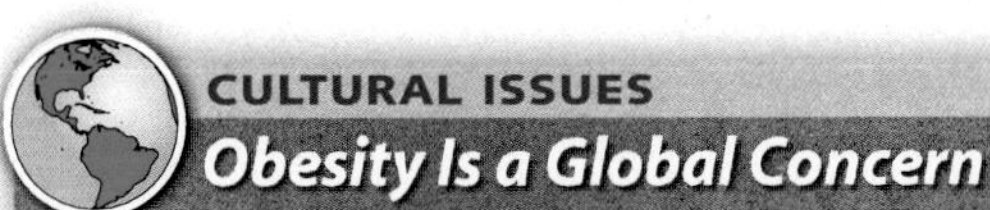

CULTURAL ISSUES
Obesity Is a Global Concern

A 2005 study examined medical records of 168,000 people aged 18 to 80 years from 63 countries across five continents who visited their primary care doctor on one of two specific half-days. The International Day for the Evaluation of Abdominal Obesity (IDEA) study looked at two measures of fatness—waist circumference and BMI. With the exception of South and East Asia, findings suggest that excess body weight is pandemic, with one-half to two-thirds of the global population overweight or obese. Additionally, researchers found that as abdominal fatness measured by waist circumference increased, so did the presence of heart disease and diabetes mellitus. This relationship was observed at all levels of BMI, even in some apparently lean people (Balkau et al. 2007).

Race and Ethnicity

Racial and ethnic groups interpret and manage body size and weight differently. For example, estimates suggest that obesity is more common among African American and Mexican American women than among Caucasian women, although racial and ethnic disparities in obesity were not observed among men (Ogden, Carroll, McDowell, and Flegal 2007). It is likely that this difference is due to metabolic, behavioral, and perceptual factors. African American men and women have a lower RMR than Caucasians. In addition, there may be sociocultural pressures that promote heavier body weights among some minority populations. For example, traditional soul food is typically high in fat, sugar, and sodium. African American women tend to eat a diet that is higher in fat and engage in less physical activity than Caucasian women.

Age

Degenerative loss of muscle mass and strength and increase in body fat are both hallmarks of the aging process. Lean body mass tends to peak when adults are in their 30s and 40s and is followed by a steady decline with age. This decline in lean body mass is associated with weakness, disability, and morbidity. In contrast to muscle mass, body weight tends to increase until about 60 years and is a major concern among people between the ages of 50 and 69. After age 60, weight tends to decline with age.

People in less technologically developed societies don't show this pattern of weight change, which suggests that reduced physical activity and changes in eating habits, rather than the process of aging itself, may be causing the change in body weight. Healthy eating and exercise programs may help prevent or reverse much of the proportional decrease in muscle mass and increase in total body fat experienced with aging.

Socioeconomic Status

Socioeconomic status has been an important factor associated with obesity, because it influences energy intake and energy expenditure and as a result affects body weight and body fat. Socioeconomic status influences access to resources, knowledge of nutrition and health, food choices, and physical activity at work and during leisure time. In general, in industrialized countries such as the United States, people with low socioeconomic status, particularly women, are more likely to be obese than their counterparts with high socioeconomic status. However, some studies suggest that this disparity may be on the decline (Zhang and Wang 2004).

ISSUES IN THE NEWS

Cost of Healthy Eating

A study published in 2007 found that healthy food may be too expensive to permit low-income families to meet certain national dietary recommendations (Cassady, Jetter, and Culp 2007). For example, a low-income family would have to devote 43 to 70 percent of its food budget to fruits and vegetables to meet the 2005 dietary guidelines, which recommend five to nine servings of fruits and vegetables a day. Reducing prices could be an effective way to help low-income families buy nutritious foods. Offering incentives for buying healthy foods and changing people's attitudes about the desirability of fruits and vegetables could also be effective strategies.

Psychological Factors

Life can be stressful. Some people cope with that stress by smoking, drinking alcohol, shopping, gambling, and eating. Food can be used for entertainment, to alleviate boredom or stress, as a pick-me-up when tired, or as a distraction from problems. Using food as a coping mechanism may be associated with binge eating and excess body weight. People with healthy lifestyles have adopted mechanisms that don't involve food, such as developing social support networks, to cope with the stresses of life.

Causes of Underweight

Few people in the United States are underweight, but the causes of underweight vary just as widely as the causes of overweight. The most common causes of underweight and unintentional weight loss include the following:

- Dietary intake insufficient to meet activity needs
- Excessive activity, such as in the case of athletes in training
- Eating disorders (e.g., anorexia nervosa) that stem from a distorted body image and result in the extreme restriction of food intake or compulsive overexercising
- Poor absorption and metabolism of food
- Metabolic and genetic factors
- Prolonged exposure to psychological and emotional stress that affects eating behavior
- Addiction to alcohol or other drugs
- An underlying disease that results in loss of appetite, increased metabolic rate, or muscle wasting (e.g., burns, cancer, acquired immunodeficiency syndrome [AIDS])

Underweight is often a symptom of an underlying disease, so it should be assessed medically.

EMBRACING A HEALTHY WEIGHT MANAGEMENT LIFESTYLE

You can quit smoking to reduce your chances of getting lung cancer, and you can quit drinking alcohol to avoid becoming dependent on it. But people struggling to lose weight can't completely quit eating to solve their problem. There are some guidelines to follow, though, that can help people reach and maintain a healthy weight. Setting health goals is the first step.

Setting goals is helpful in healthy behavior change. When it comes to weight loss, the NIH recommends an initial goal of losing 10 percent of starting weight within 6 months, or .5 to 2 pounds (.2 to .9 kilogram) per week. That can usually be done by eating about 500 to 1,000 fewer calories per day. It may seem to be a modest amount of weight loss for people who are very overweight, but even moderate weight loss can significantly reduce the severity of obesity-related risk factors. It's also important to lose weight slowly. Weight does not go on quickly, and for long-term weight loss it should not come off quickly.

Another approach to goal setting is to focus on healthy behaviors rather than just on weight loss. For example, you can set a goal to eat a certain number of fruit and vegetable servings a day, to perform physical activity on a certain number of days each week, or to take the stairs rather than the elevator every second opportunity. These are SMART goals—specific, measurable, achievable, realistic, and timely. When the focus is on the process of changing habits and not just on losing weight, people are more successful in meeting their goals.

Fewer and fewer children and adults are at a healthy body weight. Many weight problems are lifestyle problems, and long-term weight management is not something that you start and stop. When it comes to weight control, some introspection is helpful and could lead to gradual lifestyle changes. Most successful approaches require people to take on new eating and activity habits that incorporate behavior and cognitive modification.

Healthy Eating

Learning how to eat in a healthy way means looking at the nutritional components of food. This includes everything from total calories to the various nutrients provided by portions.

Total Calories

Remember, to maintain body weight, the energy you take in must equal the energy you expend. To reduce body weight, the energy you expend must exceed the calories you consume from food and beverages. To lose weight at the recommended rate of 1 to 2 pounds (.2 to .9 kilograms) per week, you must burn about 3,500 to 7,000 calories per week more than you eat (3,500 calories equal 1 pound [.2 kilogram]). It's hard to do that by only cutting down on the calories you take in, because it means you need to omit 500 to 1,000 calories each day. Instead, take advantage of that energy balance equation! You can achieve successful weight loss by reducing your calorie intake by 250 to 500 calories per day and increasing the amount of energy you burn through physical activity by 250 to 500 calories. Cutting out 500 to 1,000 calories a day can be tough, but cutting out 250 to 500 calories is easier than you might think. For example, replacing one regular soda with diet soda will save about 150 calories. Watching portion sizes will also help decrease total calorie intake, which means that reading nutrition labels is important because many foods have smaller serving sizes and are more energy dense than you might expect. For example, see the two popcorn labels in figure 4.6.

Dietary Fat

The body needs some dietary fat to function normally, but you should limit dietary fat intake to less than 30 percent of total calories. Saturated fat should make up no more than 10 percent of total calories. There are about 9 calories in each gram of fat, so if your daily calorie requirements are 2,000 calories, you should limit your total fat intake to 65 grams and saturated fat to 22 grams.

Complex Carbohydrate and Fiber

A lot of people try to lose weight by omitting carbohydrate from their diets, which is not a good idea. Complex carbohydrate should make up about half of total calorie intake. Examples of foods rich in complex carbohydrate include whole-grain breads and pastas, vegetables, fruits, and legumes. Eating those types of foods regularly can also help provide the recommended 20 to 30 grams of fiber a day, because foods with complex carbohydrate are also

Nutrition Facts
Serving Size: Makes 5 cups popped
Servings Per Bag: About 12.5 cups popped

Amount Per Serving	1 Cup Popped	
Calories		20
Calories from Fat		0
		%DV*
Total Fat	0g	**0%**
Saturated Fat	0g	**0%**
Trans Fat	0g	
Cholesterol	0mg	**0%**
Sodium	40mg	**2%**
Total Carbohydrate	4g	**1%**
Dietary Fiber	1g	**6%**
Sugars	0g	
Protein	<1g	
Vitamin A		**0%**
Vitamin C		**0%**
Calcium		**0%**
Iron		**0%**

Nutrition Facts
Serving Size: Makes 3.5 cups popped
Servings Per Bag: About 10.5 cups popped

Amount Per Serving	1 Cup Popped	
Calories		45
Calories from Fat		30
		%DV*
Total Fat	3g	**5%**
Saturated Fat	1g	**4%**
Trans Fat	1g	
Cholesterol	0mg	**0%**
Sodium	85mg	**4%**
Total Carbohydrate	5g	**2%**
Dietary Fiber	1g	**4%**
Sugars	0g	
Protein	1g	
Vitamin A		**0%**
Vitamin C		**0%**
Calcium		**0%**
Iron		**0%**

Figure 4.6 Compare the nutrition label on the left, which represents a typical "light" microwavable popcorn, to the label on the right, which represents a full-flavor popcorn.

often rich sources of fiber. Fiber helps provide feelings of satiation and fullness, which can help prevent overeating.

Sugars and Refined Carbohydrate

It's OK to eat highly processed foods and foods with added sugars occasionally, but those foods shouldn't be a core component of your diet. Foods such as candies, cakes, and brownies with high sugar content provide a lot of calories and fat but few other nutrients. Satisfy your sweet tooth with other types of foods, such as oranges, small amounts of dried fruit, and grapes. Such foods provide sweetness along with additional nutritional value.

Protein

Protein is an essential component of the diet. Proteins function as enzymes, hormones, and antibodies, as well as structural components (e.g., collagen) and transport components (e.g., protein pumps help control cell volume, nerve impulses, and drive the active transport of sugars and amino acids into cells; protein carriers transport substances in the bloodstream for delivery throughout the body). In the United States, men eat an average of 88 to 92 grams of protein a day, and women eat about 63 to 66 grams (St. Jeor et al. 2001). High-protein diets, where more than 30 percent of daily calorie intake comes from protein, have been around since the 1960s and have regained popularity. High-protein diets are probably not harmful for most healthy people for a short length of time, but no long-term scientific studies support their overall effectiveness and safety. Many foods high in protein are also high in fat and saturated fat, but moderate amounts of protein help promote a sense of fullness, so you should eat some protein at each meal. Healthy people should consume about 0.8 grams of healthy, low-fat protein per kilogram of body weight. That comes out to 10 to 15 percent of total daily calorie intake.

Energy Density

It's hard to control food portions, especially when dinner plates are so big and restaurants serve extra-large helpings. One strategy that can help people who don't feel full quickly or who like to eat a lot is to eat large servings of foods that contain few calories. We covered energy density earlier in this chapter. It refers to the amount of energy (calories) in food for a given amount of weight. Some foods, especially those with a lot of fat such as chips, cookies, nuts, and butter, are very energy dense. They provide a lot of calories in a small amount of food. In contrast, certain foods have very low energy density, such as nonstarchy vegetables, fruits, nonfat milk, and soups. Those foods often have a high water content that fills you up without adding a lot of calories. Choosing foods with low energy density may help manage hunger and body weight. You can find more information about this well-researched concept in the Volumetrics eating plan (www.volumetricseatingplan.com).

Eating Habits

You can adopt a variety of eating habits to help lose weight or prevent weight gain. If you eat four to five small meals and snacks (including a healthy breakfast) per day, you can stave off hunger and prevent overeating later. Research consistently shows that people eat more when they are served more, so keeping tabs on portion size is also an important aspect of weight control. Experiment with healthful substitutions for certain high-calorie, high-fat foods. For example, try making scrambled eggs with an egg substitute. Try using light salad dressing instead of the full-fat variety. And try chocolate-chip meringue cookies for dessert rather than regular chocolate-chip cookies.

To establish good eating habits, don't set up hard and fast food rules or label certain foods as completely off-limits. People often want what they can't have, so if you restrict yourself too much, you can set up a cycle for disinhibition and guilt. All foods in moderation can fit into a healthy eating plan. When it comes to eating, it's hard to be perfect. Making the healthier choice more often than not, learning to control portion size, and making healthy substitutions are behaviors that define moderation.

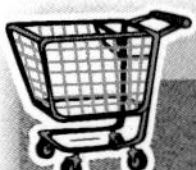

CONSUMER ISSUES

Portion Distortion

For food companies, the costs to increase the size of the food products they sell are small, but the ramifications for what and how much we eat are large. Portion sizes of many food products began to grow in the 1970s and rose sharply in the 1980s, exceeding standard serving sizes. This trend has been found to parallel the rise in overweight and obesity (Nielsen and Popkin 2003; Young and Nestle 2002). For example, in the 1950s, the family-size bottle of Coca-Cola was 26 ounces (769 milliliters), an amount that barely exceeds the single-serve bottle (20 ounces [591 milliliters]) today! In the mid-1950s, McDonald's offered only one size of French fries, equivalent to today's small order. It was about one-third the weight of the largest size available in 2001. Even today's plates hold more than they did in the past. An informal survey of the restaurant industry in 1994 found that plate size has increased from 10 inches (25 centimeters) to 12 inches (30 centimeters).

Larger portions provide more food and far exceed portion-size recommendations from the USDA and FDA, but that's not the end of it. Studies show that when people are served more food, they consume more food (Rolls, Morris, and Row 2002). And when they have larger glasses, plates, and bowls, they serve themselves and consume more food and beverage (Wansink and Cheney 2005; Wansink, Painter, and North 2005; Wansink and van Ittersum 2005).

Look at the nutrition facts label on packaged food items. It provides information about the calories, protein, fat, vitamins, and minerals in a defined serving of that food item. Be prepared to be surprised. The serving amount may be much smaller than you think it is!

Improving Physical Activity

An active lifestyle is key to maintaining a healthy weight and fitness level. Becoming and remaining physically active promotes physical health, reduces risk of disease, and improves mental health and body image. Most people lose weight by eating less, but being physically active is what will keep the weight off. Start exercising slowly to avoid soreness and injury and gradually increase the intensity.

Initially, try to do some moderate physical activity for 30 to 45 minutes on 3 to 5 days per week, but any amount of activity is better than nothing. Set a long-term goal to accumulate at least 30 minutes or more of moderate-intensity physical activity on most, and preferably all, days of the week. *Dietary Guidelines for Americans 2005* suggests that people who want to lose weight should get 60 minutes of physical activity per day. To maintain weight loss, 60 to 90 minutes per day is recommended (USDHHS and USDA 2005). The lists that follow give an idea of how long you need to do certain activities for the activities to be considered moderate. A moderate amount of physical activity is roughly equivalent to physical activity that uses 150 calories of energy per day, or 1,000 calories per week. Some activities can be performed at various intensities; the suggested durations in these lists correspond to expected intensity of effort.

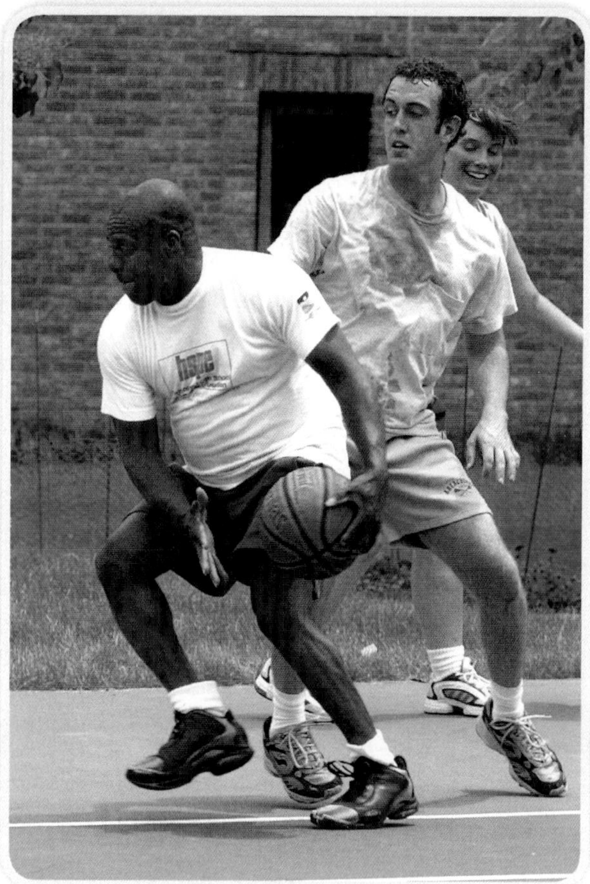

Playing basketball can be a fun way to get your recommended amount of physical activity.

© Human Kinetics

- Washing and waxing a car for 45 to 60 minutes
- Washing windows or floors for 45 to 60 minutes
- Playing volleyball for 45 minutes
- Playing touch football for 30 to 45 minutes
- Gardening for 30 to 45 minutes
- Wheeling yourself in a wheelchair for 30 to 40 minutes
- Walking 1.75 miles (2.8 kilometers) in 35 minutes (20 minutes per mile [1.6 kilometers])
- Shooting baskets for 30 minutes
- Bicycling 5 miles (8 kilometers) in 30 minutes
- Dancing fast (social dancing) for 30 minutes
- Pushing a stroller 1.5 miles (3 kilometers) in 30 minutes
- Raking leaves for 30 minutes
- Walking 2 miles (3.2 kilometers) in 30 minutes (15 minutes per mile [1.6 kilometers])
- Doing water aerobics for 30 minutes
- Swimming laps for 20 minutes
- Playing wheelchair basketball for 20 minutes
- Playing a basketball game for 15 to 20 minutes
- Bicycling 4 miles (6.4 kilometers) in 15 minutes
- Jumping rope for 15 minutes
- Running 1.5 miles (2.4 kilometers) in 15 minutes (10 minutes per mile [1.6 kilometers])
- Shoveling snow for 15 minutes
- Stair-climbing for 15 minutes

Cognitive and Behavior Modification

What events start and stop your eating? What factors influence your food choices? Early in the chapter you read about many of the individual, social, and environmental influences on eating behavior. Now that you're more aware of the influences, how do you address them to improve eating and activity habits?

Research has suggested that aspects of **behavior therapy**, or behavior modification and **cognitive-behavioral therapy**, can aid weight control. These approaches focus on examining behaviors, thought processes, and environments to reduce the likelihood of engaging in behaviors, habits, and circumstances that contribute to excessive food consumption and inhibit physical activity.

A variety of cognitive-behavioral tools can be helpful in weight control. These include self-monitoring, chain breaking, stimulus control, emotion and stress management, social support, contingency management, and cognitive restructuring.

Self-Monitoring

Self-monitoring is a tool for tracking behavior that can help with weight control. Keeping a food diary, for example, that lists when, where, and how you're feeling when you eat can raise awareness of the foods you eat and the situations that might lead to unhealthy eating patterns. The diary can encourage new habits and discourage poor ones. Other items to keep track of could include the servings of fruit and vegetables consumed each day, body weight, or information about exercise.

Chain Breaking

Chain breaking is a strategy to identify and separate behaviors that tend to occur together and encourage overeating. For example, many people snack too much when they talk on the phone or watch TV. The ABC model of behavior, which stands for antecedent, behavior, and consequences, may help break the behavior chain. First identify the antecedents, or the events that trigger the behavior. Next, examine the behavior itself. Finally, consequences (either positive or negative) discourage or reinforce the behavior.

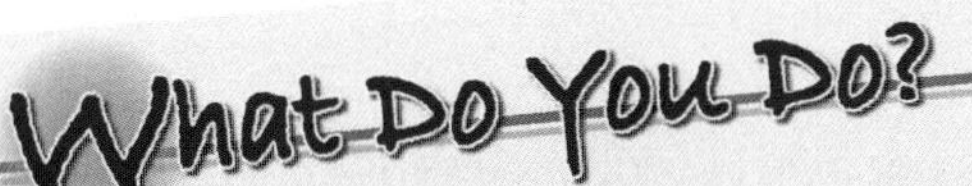

Identify the antecedent, behavior, and consequences in the following example: You feel tired and run-down after a day of classes and you want to unwind and watch TV before dinner. You grab a bag of chips and eat most of them while you watch the news. Afterward, you feel guilty for not sticking to your eating plan, so you overeat at dinner. Write down how you could turn this scenario around so that the behavior and consequences to the antecedent are different.

Stimulus Control

Stimulus control, or environmental management, means altering the environment to increase the likelihood you'll engage in healthy behaviors. For example, if there are foods that you can't stop eating if they're around, then you wouldn't buy them often. Other examples would be putting foods that are less healthy out of sight and putting fruit or other healthy foods out where they're easy to see. Consider placing comfortable walking shoes in plain sight near the door to remind you to exercise.

Managing Emotions

Managing emotions and stress is profoundly important if you turn to food before, during, or after emotional or stressful situations. A lot of people use food for comfort, but that pairing can be dangerous for weight management. If you find yourself in a similar situation, try to use reframing (finding the positive aspects within a potentially negative situation), disengagement (withdrawing from the situation), imagery, and self-soothing (comforting yourself using a method that does not involve food) to manage negative emotions. Using physical activity instead of food to cope is a great remedy for a bad mood and stress.

Social Support

Social support means getting others on board to participate in or otherwise provide healthy emotional or physical support for your efforts. Find family and friends to provide praise and encouragement. Look for a registered dietitian or other weight-control professional to help with accountability and advice. Join a support group of people who are dealing with weight control. Such groups can provide empathy because the members are probably experiencing challenges similar to yours.

Contingency Management

Contingency management means being prepared for the high-risk eating situations that are likely to occur from time to time. For example, consider rehearsing how you might respond when friends or family try to encourage you to eat too much at a party. One simple response that often works well is simply, "Thanks, but I'm not hungry."

Cognitive Restructuring

No one eats perfectly or exercises perfectly all of the time. You'll miss an exercise session from time to time, eat something high in fat, or eat too much. People who are trying to lose weight find those scenarios discouraging and start to have thoughts such as, "I'm a failure," or "Well, since I ate a cookie, it doesn't matter what I do now. I might as well eat the whole box." **Cognitive restructuring** simply means restructuring how you think about something. "I'm not perfect all the time, and one cookie is not going to ruin my day," is a good way to restructure the negative message. Labeling some foods as off-limits may encourage all-or-nothing thinking. If you eat a food that you've labeled off-limits, you could start to feel guilty and discouraged. Take a different approach, and try to manage food choices with the principles of moderation and portion size.

Self-Help Approaches for Weight Management

Hundreds of books are available to help with weight control, and some are better than others. An easy-to-follow manual or an eating and activity plan in a self-help book can help some people find success. It's important, though, to look past the glitz, glamour, and claims on the covers to find a plan that is likely to result in long-term weight control. Be on the lookout for the following red flags:

- Extravagant claims touting a scientific breakthrough, the final solution, or quick and easy weight loss. If there really were a magic solution to weight control, society would be much thinner than it is now.
- Overly restrictive eating patterns, including diets that restrict or omit entire food groups, endorse the consumption of only a few food items, or promote peculiar eating patterns (e.g., "Eat only between noon and 5 p.m."). Those methods are generally not effective, and people can't maintain them over the long term. They will probably lead to discouragement.
- The promise to cure a disease.
- Endorsing or requiring special nutrition supplements such as herbs and powders.

Self-help weight-loss support groups can be found in many communities. The groups are led by peers also struggling with weight or by someone who has previously lost weight and kept it off. These groups can be valuable, because they provide an outlet for sharing personal weight-loss struggles, empathy, motivation, information, and new ideas. They can also reduce the isolation and alienation many overweight and obese people feel in a society oriented toward leanness.

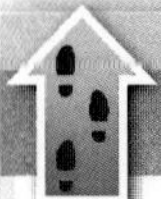

STEPS FOR BEHAVIORAL CHANGE

Seven Steps to Success

These seven steps can help you make positive behavior changes.

- **Step 1: Identify your purpose.** Ask yourself why you want to manage your weight. Is it to improve your overall health? Did a doctor tell you to? Do you have an upcoming event (such as a wedding) that you want to look good for? Think about your reasons for losing weight. For long-term weight control, the motivation should be salient and long term. You have a better chance of success when seeking to adopt a healthy lifestyle than when trying to quickly lose weight for a one-time event.
- **Step 2: Set the right goals.** Setting the right goals is an important step. Most people trying to lose weight focus just on weight loss. However, the most productive areas to focus on are the eating and exercise behaviors that will lead to long-term weight change. Try to set specific, measurable goals about increasing your activity level or the servings of fruits and vegetables that you eat.
- **Step 3: Find small successes.** Shaping is a behavioral technique in which you select a series of short-term goals that get closer and closer to the ultimate goal. An example of a short-term goal could be reducing your fat intake from 40 percent of your calories to 35 percent and then later to 30 percent. Shaping is based on the concept that nothing succeeds like success. Small wins can be extremely encouraging, and setting short-term goals is less daunting than attempting a more drastic change.
- **Step 4: Reward success (but not with food).** Rewards that you control can be used to encourage attainment of behavioral goals, especially those that have been difficult to reach. An effective reward is desirable, timely, and contingent on meeting your goal.
- **Step 5: Balance your (food) checkbook.** Self-monitoring refers to observing and recording some aspect of your behavior (e.g., calorie intake, servings of fruits and vegetables, exercise sessions) or an outcome of the behavior (e.g., weight). Self-monitoring of a behavior can be particularly helpful as a barometer to see how you are doing. It also increases your awareness of eating or activity patterns you may not otherwise notice (e.g., always eating sweets after a stressful encounter).
- **Step 6: Avoid a chain reaction.** Stimulus control involves learning what social or environmental cues seem to encourage undesired eating or sedentary behavior and then changing those cues. For example, you might realize that you're more likely to overeat while watching television, or whenever treats are on display near the office coffeepot, or when you're around a certain friend. You might then try to sever the association of eating with the cue (don't eat while watching television), avoid or eliminate the cue (leave the coffee room immediately after pouring coffee), or change the circumstances surrounding the cue (plan to meet with your friend in settings where there's no food).
- **Step 7: Get the (fullness) message.** Changing the way you go about eating can make it easier to eat less without feeling deprived. It takes 15 or more minutes for your brain to get the message that you've been fed. Slowing the rate of eating can allow you to start to feel full by the end of the meal. Eating lots of vegetables can also make you feel fuller. Another trick is to use smaller plates so that moderate portions don't appear meager. Changing your eating schedule can be helpful, especially if you tend to skip or delay meals and overeat later.

From NHLBI. Available: www.nhbli.nih.gov/health/public/heart/obesity/lose_wt/behavior.htm.

Commercial Approaches

Commercial weight-control programs provide eating and activity counseling for groups or individuals, and they often involve group support. A growing number of these programs are offered over the Internet. The food and eating plans endorsed by commercial weight-control programs vary widely. Some companies employ credible health professionals such as doctors and registered dietitians to develop and guide these programs at the corporate level; others might be run by people who are not specialists in food, nutrition, and physical activity. Be careful when choosing a commercial weight-control program, and don't be afraid to ask questions. At the minimum, be sure to examine the training and education of the staff, risks of the products or program, cost, and success and failure rates of previous participants.

Professional Counselors

People who need additional help managing body weight or improving eating and activity habits should seek out professionals for individually tailored advice. Registered dietitians, physicians, psychologists, licensed therapists, and personal trainers can all provide support, education, and advice about weight management. The underlying issue for many people who are struggling to control weight may or may not have to do with food, eating, and activity. Delving deeper into the meaning of food and eating with a mental health professional may provide insight into the reasons behind the struggles with weight management. Be sure to carefully scrutinize the credentials and training of professionals before committing to receive their services or participate in their programs.

Pharmaceutical Approaches

The pharmaceutical industry has long been on the hunt for a magic pill that will treat obesity. Nothing like that has been discovered yet, but some options are available that have varied degrees of success. Doctors consider using weight-loss drugs for people with a BMI of 30 or above or those with a BMI of 27 or higher who also have other obesity-related conditions such as hypertension, diabetes, or dyslipidemia. The U.S. Food and Drug Administration (FDA) has approved two major classes of antiobesity drugs: appetite suppressants and fat-absorption inhibitors.

Appetite suppressants promote weight loss by manipulating chemicals in the brain to make the body feel full. Phentermine (Fastin, Pro-Fast, and Zantryl) and sibutramine (Meridia) are the most commonly prescribed appetite suppressants in the United States. The main side effects of phentermine are sleeplessness and nervousness, and sibutramine is associated with increases in blood pressure and heart rate.

Fat-absorption inhibitors literally inhibit the absorption of fat. Xenical (orlistat) was approved in 1999 and is the only example of this type of treatment approved for use in the United States. Xenical works by blocking about 30 percent of dietary fat from being absorbed by the body. The unabsorbed fat is eliminated in bowel movements. Some people experience unpleasant side effects that are worsened by eating foods high in fat, including abdominal cramps, gas, leakage of oily stool, and inability to control bowel movements. Additionally, because Xenical reduces the absorption of fat-soluble vitamins (A, D, E, K), it might be necessary to take a vitamin supplement while taking Xenical. In 2007, the FDA approved an over-the-counter product, Alli, that contains orlistat.

Weight management drugs should always be taken as directed under a doctor's supervision. However, the long-term effects of these drugs are still being discovered. In some instances, the FDA may approve a drug and later discover damaging side effects. This occurred in the mid-1990s, when the appetite suppressant Redux (combination of phentermine and fenfluramine), otherwise known as **fen-phen**, was frequently prescribed to treat obesity. However, in September 1997, fenfluramine and Redux were withdrawn from the market because they caused heart valve damage. Phentermine is still available by prescription because it has not been associated with the adverse health effects of the fenfluramine–phentermine combination.

Weight-loss drugs are generally not recommended for long-term use. It's important, then, for people who are taking them to learn about and adopt healthy eating and activity habits that can be maintained over the long term to prevent regaining weight.

Surgical Options

Surgical options to treat severe obesity have become more popular over the past few years. Gastrointestinal surgery for obesity, or **bariatric surgery**, is an option of increasing popularity for people with a BMI of 40 or more or for people with a BMI between 35 and 39.9 who also have a serious obesity-related health problem. Surgery is generally viewed as a last-ditch effort, used when other legitimate, less invasive methods have been attempted with little long-term success.

The most common types of bariatric surgery work in one of two ways. Adjustable gastric banding and vertical banded gastroplasty restrict the amount of food that can be consumed, but they don't interfere with the digestive process. Roux-en-Y gastric bypass restricts the amount of food that can be consumed and also affects the amount of calories and nutrients the body can absorb. In adjustable gastric banding, for example, a doctor places a hollow band of silicone rubber around the upper end of the patient's stomach, creating a narrow passageway into the rest of the stomach (see figure 4.7*a*). This band is tightened, allowing the patient to be able to eat only 1/2 to 1 cup of food at a time without discomfort. In the Roux-en-Y gastric bypass, a small stomach pouch about the size of a walnut is surgically created, and a Y-shaped section of the small intestine is attached directly to the pouch, permitting food to bypass the lower stomach and 2 feet (61 centimeters) of the intestines (the duodenum and the first portion of the jejunum) (see figure 4.7*b*).

Many patients who have bariatric surgery lose a dramatic amount of weight in a short time. However, the long-term effectiveness of these procedures depends on how well patients learn to manage a new way of eating. Additionally, many serious side effects are associated with the procedures, including dumping syndrome (rapid emptying of stomach contents into the small intestine resulting in nausea, vomiting, dizziness, cramping, and diarrhea), vitamin and mineral deficiency, dehydration, gallstones, blood clots in the legs, intolerance to certain foods, hypoglycemia, incision hernia, and even death. Many patients require long-term follow-up care and lifelong vitamin supplementation to avoid life-threatening complications.

Finally, bariatric surgery is an expensive option. Procedures cost between $20,000 and $35,000, and that doesn't include the cost of body-contouring surgery that is often required later to remove excess skin. Insurance coverage for weight-loss surgery varies by insurance company and state. Patients must meet certain standards and must wait for completion of the approval process before they can have the surgery.

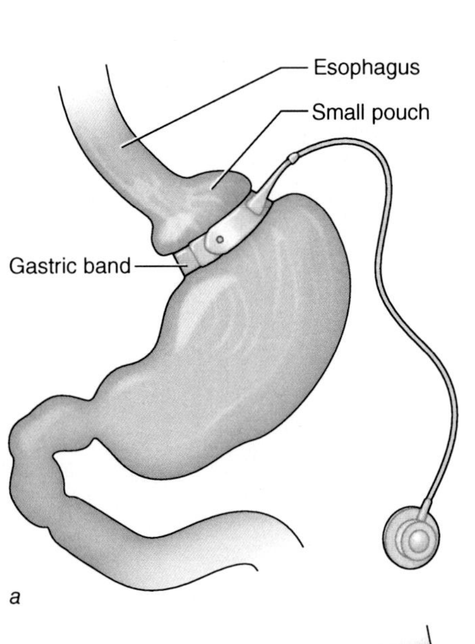

Figure 4.7 Two common types of bariatric surgery include *(a)* adjustable gastric banding and *(b)* Roux-en-Y gastric bypass.

DIETING IN THE UNITED STATES

The diet industry in the United States is lucrative. New eating plans are constantly popping up, and old ones resurface. Establishing a healthy eating plan that you can maintain for the rest of your life is the key to successful weight management.

Dieter's Cycle

The term *dieting* can mean different things to different people. For some, it's the simple desire to lose weight. For others, it's the periodic, short-term use of a weight-loss behavior. For still others, it's just trying to maintain their current weight. For many, however, dieting often leads to a dieter's cycle: Start a new diet, follow strict rules about food and eating, experience weight loss, break the diet rules, feel discouraged and guilty, abandon the diet, regain weight, and start the next new diet (see figure 4.8). This pattern of restriction, weight loss, disinhibition, and weight gain can be emotionally and possibly even physically damaging.

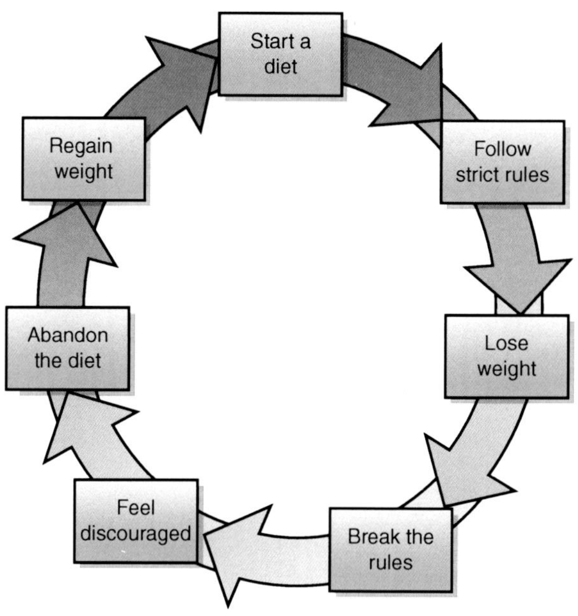

Figure 4.8 Some people get stuck in the dieter's cycle and fail to make long-term progress.

Weight cycling, or yo-yo dieting, is the repeated loss and regain of body weight. Cyclers might lose and regain 5 to 10 pounds (2 to 4.5 kilograms) or as much as 50 pounds (22.5 kilograms) or more. The jury is still out on whether weight cycling results in health problems. Some studies suggest that weight cycling may increase the risk of high blood pressure, high cholesterol, and gallbladder disease. Other studies suggest there is no link between weight loss and regain and physical health. Even less is known about the effects of weight cycling on behavior and psychological factors. People who perceive themselves as weight cyclers tend to have lower self-esteem, body image, and life satisfaction.

In general, if you need to lose weight, avoid dieting and instead prepare to make sustainable healthy lifestyle changes. A healthy eating plan and physical activity are the keys to success.

Popular Diets

Many people who want to lose weight attempt the latest diet to hit the market, and the next one, and the next one, and each tends to have short-lived success. Most popular diets lead to some initial weight loss simply because the dieters cut down on their food intake and watch what they eat. Diet fads change with time, but diet plans tend to cluster into three types: low-carbohydrate, high-protein diets; low-fat diets; and novelty diets.

Low-Carbohydrate, High-Protein Approaches

Low-carbohydrate, high-protein diets are in fashion again. Diets such as Protein Power, Dr. Atkins' New Diet Revolution, and Sugar Busters all severely restrict foods that contain starches and sugars. These diets revisit an idea that became popular in the 1970s (with historical roots going back 200 years): Carbohydrate makes us fat. The protein in these diets often comes from animal sources, meaning that fat, saturated fat, and cholesterol intake can be high. The Nutrition Committee of the American Heart Association (AHA) has issued a science advisory warning that high-protein diets have not been proven effective and pose health risks (St. Jeor et al. 2001). The report covered the Atkins, Zone, Protein Power, Sugar Busters, and Stillman

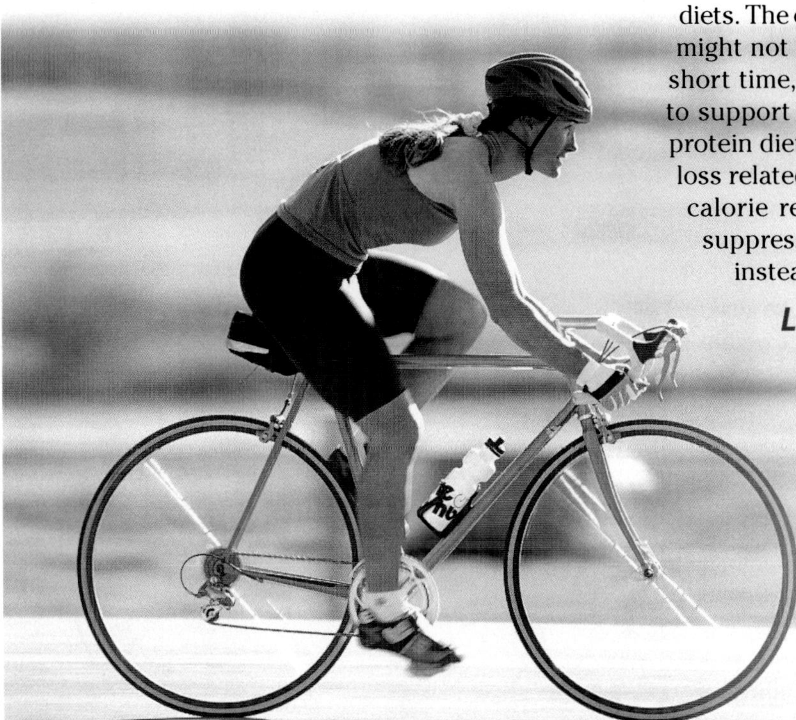

Unlike fad diets, regular physical activity can help you lose weight and keep it off.

© Eyewire

diets. The committee stated that although these diets might not be harmful for most healthy people for a short time, there are no long-term scientific studies to support their overall efficacy and safety. In high-protein diets, weight loss is initially high due to fluid loss related to reduced carbohydrate intake, overall calorie restriction, and ketosis-induced appetite suppression (ketosis is when the liver burns fat instead of glucose for energy).

Low-Fat Approaches

Dietary Guidelines for Americans 2005 recommends maintaining a healthy eating plan that has a total fat intake between 20 and 35 percent of total calories (USDHHS and USDA 2005). Very-low-fat diets (which often turn out to be high-carbohydrate diets) are even more restrictive. Generally, diets of this nature, such as the Pritikin program and Dr. Dean Ornish's program, recommend that about 5 to 10 percent of calories come from fat. This approach is generally not harmful for healthy adults. People adopting a very-low-fat eating plan consume large amounts of whole grains, fruits, and vegetables. However, this diet so different from the typical North American lifestyle that it could be hard for people to sustain over the long term.

Novelty Diets

Many diets are simply gimmicks. Most of them focus on one specific food or food group (e.g., the grapefruit diet) and exclude almost all others. For example, the rice diet was designed in the 1940s to lower blood pressure, and it has resurfaced as a weight-loss diet. The logic behind many of these diets is that you will only be able to eat so much of the select food for so long before becoming bored, so you'll reduce your calorie intake. The reality is that most people are not able to eat only one or a few foods for an extended length of time, so they get frustrated, quit the diet, and regain weight quickly.

Very-Low-Calorie Approaches

A **very-low-calorie diet (VLCD)** is used to help treat severe obesity (BMI at or above 30), particularly if a person has obesity-related diseases such as type 2 diabetes. VLCDs are usually doctor supervised and use commercially prepared formulas to promote rapid weight loss. The formulas often contain appropriate amounts of vitamins and micronutrients to help prevent nutritional deficiencies that are likely to occur at such low calorie levels (often fewer than 800 calories a day). VLCD formulas are not the same as over-the-counter meal replacements found at grocery stores or pharmacies, which are meant to substitute for one or two meals a day. Under the proper medical supervision, VLCDs can help jump-start weight loss in a moderately to extremely obese person at the rate of 3 to 5 pounds (1.3 to 2.2 kilograms) per week. Studies show that the long-term effectiveness of VLCDs varies widely, but weight regain is common. Combining a VLCD with behavior therapy, physical activity, and active follow-up treatment may help increase weight loss and prevent weight regain.

To be successful with weight management for the long term, people need to find and adopt a healthy eating and activity plan that addresses dietary intake, eating behavior, and physical activity. The plan should avoid leaving people feeling deprived so that they can maintain the plan for the long term.

Healthy Weight-Control Programs

Weight-loss and weight maintenance programs should encourage healthy behaviors that you can stick with every day. Safe and effective weight-loss programs should have these components (National Institute of Diabetes and Digestive and Kidney Diseases [NIDDK] 2008):

- Healthy eating plans that reduce calories but don't forbid specific foods or food groups.
- Tips to increase moderate-intensity physical activity.
- Tips on healthy behavior changes that also keep your cultural needs in mind.
- Slow and steady weight loss. Depending on your starting weight, experts recommend losing weight at a rate of .5 to 2 pounds (.2 to .9 kilogram) per week. Weight loss may be faster at the beginning of a program.
- Medical care if you are planning to lose weight by following a special-formula diet, such as a VLCD.
- A plan to keep the weight off after you have lost it.

To determine if a weight-control program meets those guidelines, gather as much information as possible about the program before you start. The five questions that follow will help you be a smart consumer and gather information so you can separate good weight-control programs from bad programs.

1. What does the weight-loss program consist of?
    - Does the program offer one-on-one counseling or group classes?
    - Do you have to follow a specific meal plan or keep food records?
    - Do you have to purchase special food, drugs, or supplements?
    - Does the program help you be more physically active, follow a specific activity plan, or provide exercise instruction?
    - Does the program teach you to make positive and healthy behavior changes?
    - Is the program sensitive to your lifestyle and cultural needs?
2. What are the staff qualifications?
    - Who supervises the program?
    - What type of weight management training, experience, education, and certifications do staff members have?
3. Does the program carry any risks?
    - Could the program hurt you?
    - Could the recommended drugs or supplements harm your health?
    - Do participants talk with a doctor?
    - Does a doctor run the program?
    - Will the program doctors work with your personal doctor if you have a medical condition such as high blood pressure or are taking prescribed drugs?
4. How much does the program cost?
    - What is the total cost of the program?
    - Are there other costs, such as weekly attendance fees, food and supplement purchases, and so on?
    - Are there fees for a follow-up program after you lose weight?
    - Are there other fees for medical tests?

5. What results do participants typically have?
    - How much weight do participants lose on average and how long do they keep the weight off?
    - Does the program offer publications or materials that describe what results participants typically have?

WEIGHT-LOSS MAINTENANCE

Keeping weight off after you've lost it is often a bigger challenge than losing it in the first place. Many people repeatedly lose weight and gain weight; the majority of people who lost weight typically return to their baseline weight within 3 to 5 years (Wadden et al. 1989). Some people do keep the weight off, though. How do they do it?

Founded in 1994, the National Weight Control Registry (NWCR; see www.nwcr.ws) maintains a database of people who have intentionally lost at least 30 pounds (13.5 kilograms) and

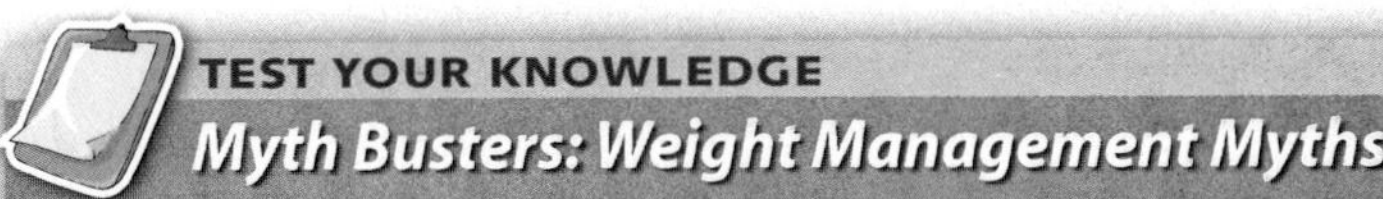

TEST YOUR KNOWLEDGE

Myth Busters: Weight Management Myths

With so much information about food, nutrition, and weight loss out there, it is sometimes difficult to separate myth from fact. Here are a few common myths about weight management.

Myth: Natural or herbal products are safe and effective for weight loss.

Busted: A weight-loss product that claims to be natural or herbal is not necessarily safe. These products don't undergo the rigorous scientific testing and evaluation by the FDA, so they aren't usually scientifically tested to prove that they're safe or that they work. Some herbal products containing ephedra (a substance now banned in the United States) have caused serious health problems and even death. Talk to a health care provider before deciding to take any weight-loss product.

Myth: It's impossible to lose weight if you eat fast food.

Busted: Fast food can fit into a healthy meal plan if you choose wisely and watch portion size. Most fast-food restaurants offer healthier options on their menus; look for special icons signifying reduced-fat or reduced-calorie items. Also, avoid value sizes. It's tempting to try to maximize the amount of food you get for your money, but you'll pay a lot in terms of calories. Various Web sites offer a wealth of information for how to eat healthy at fast-food restaurants.

Myth: Lifting weights is not good exercise if you want to lose weight, because it will make you bulk up.

Busted: Lifting weights or doing strengthening activities such as push-ups and crunches on a regular basis can actually help you maintain or lose weight. Those activities can help you build muscle, and muscle burns more calories than body fat does. So if you have more muscle, you burn more calories. Doing strengthening activities 2 or 3 days a week will not bulk you up. Only intense strength training is likely to put on a large amount of muscle mass.

More myths: Now that you have expanded your understanding of health, nutrition, and physical activity, see if you can debunk some of these other common myths:

- Eating late in the evening causes weight gain.
- Dairy products are fattening and unhealthy.
- Becoming a vegetarian ensures that you will lose weight and be healthier.

maintained that weight loss for at least 1 year. Researchers have examined what behaviors and strategies those people use to maintain their weight loss (Wing and Hill 2001). Studies consistently show that people have to decrease calorie intake and increase physical activity in order to lose weight and maintain the loss. Almost all NWCR participants (89 percent) have reported changing their diet and activity level, and many regularly monitor their body weight.

Dietary Intake

The average NWCR participant consumes slightly fewer than 1,400 calories (24 percent from fat, 19 percent from protein, and 56 percent from carbohydrate) eating about 4.87 meals or snacks a day. Despite the popularity of low-carbohydrate diets, only 7.6 percent of participants reported eating fewer than 90 grams of carbohydrate a day. Thus, the low-fat, high-carbohydrate, low-calorie eating pattern characterizes most registry participants. Those people also avoid fried foods and substitute low-fat foods for high-fat foods.

Physical Activity

People who are successful at weight loss engage in high levels of physical activity. Over three-quarters of all NWCR registrants use a combination of both lifestyle activity (e.g., taking the stairs) and programmed exercise. On average, women registered with the NWCR expend about 2,500 calories through physical activity each week, and men expend about 3,300 calories each week. Those amounts equate to about 1 hour of moderate-intensity physical activity, such as brisk walking, each day. That amount is much greater than what is recommended in national guidelines, which is 30 minutes of moderate-intensity physical activity at least 3 days a week.

Weight Monitoring

NWCR participants monitor their weight. About three-quarters of all registrants reported that they weighed themselves at least once a week. Frequent **weight monitoring** seems to help people detect small increases in weight and lets them adjustment weight management techniques before they have a major relapse.

Overall, the findings from the NWCR help combat the idea that it's impossible to maintain weight loss. Additionally, it appears that over time, weight maintenance becomes easier; once weight loss is maintained past 2 to 5 years, the likelihood of long-term success increases greatly.

CRITICAL MOMENTS FOR WEIGHT MANAGEMENT

It might be easier to prevent weight gain than to lose weight. Research has suggested that there are some critical points in the life course that are associated with unwanted weight gain.

College

Everyone has heard warnings about the dreaded freshman 15, in which most freshmen pack on double-digit pounds, but is it real? In college, you can come and go as you please, eat and drink how you like, and go to as many parties as you can stand. For many new college students, this freedom comes with a price, although it may not be as high as some think. In a large study of undergraduate students, researchers discovered that the freshman 15 (7 kilograms) was closer to the freshman 5 to 7 (2.2 to 3.1 kilograms), followed by the sophomore 2 or 3 (.9 to 1.3 kilograms). Possible reasons for weight gain include more drinking (particularly added calories from alcoholic beverages), more socializing that involves eating, greater availability of high-fat foods in dorm cafeterias, and less physical activity. However, weight gain during the first year of college isn't a requirement!

Marriage

When you say "I do" to loving, honoring, and cherishing your partner, are you also unknowingly committing to gaining a few extra pounds? Studies suggest that starting a marriage is associated with weight gain among both women and men. Reasons for this postnuptial poundage include taking on increased responsibilities inside and outside the home, having children, retaining postpregnancy pounds, cooking bigger meals, sharing mealtimes (people eat more when in larger numbers), eating out more often, and having fewer opportunities to exercise. However, the news is not all bad. Research from 2008 has shown that when one spouse upgrades his or her health habits, the other spouse is likely to do so as well (Falba and Sindelar 2008).

Pregnancy and Postpregnancy

Pregnant women who gain a lot of weight and don't lose it after giving birth may face long-term health consequences. The recommended amount of weight gain with a pregnancy is 25 to 35 pounds (11 to 16 kilograms) for a woman of normal weight, less for an overweight woman and more for an underweight woman. Many women who gain too much weight have difficulty returning to their prepregnancy weight after the child is born. The USDA has released MyPyramid for Moms with specific advice for healthy eating and activity during and after pregnancy. See www.mypyramid.gov/mypyramidmoms/ to learn more.

Holidays

Holidays are times of celebration and festivities, many of which involve food. Holidays can be especially challenging for people trying to manage their weight. Studies have shown that it's fairly common for people to gain weight during holiday seasons. One study found that, on average, people in the United States gained about 0.37 kilogram (just under a pound) during the 6 weeks between Thanksgiving and New Year (Roberts and Mayer 2000). Weight gain was even greater among people who were overweight or obese, and 14 of them gained more than 3 kilograms (5 pounds). Watching portion sizes, sampling energy-dense foods in moderation, and exercising regularly can help prevent packing on the pounds over the winter holiday season. Additionally, frequent monitoring of body weight has been shown to be effective in helping some avoid the holiday weight gain (Boutelle, Kirschenbaum, Baker, and Mitchell 1999).

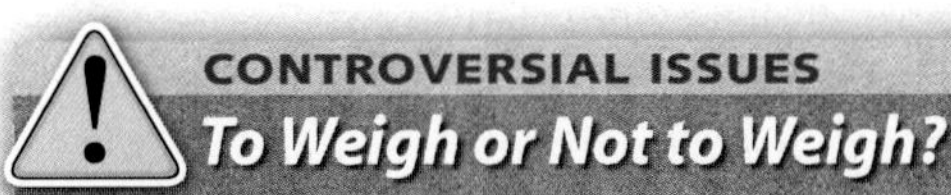

A controversy exists about whether it's beneficial or harmful to use scales and self-weighing for weight management. Proponents suggest that regularly monitoring body weight can show short-term changes in weight, permitting early behavioral adjustment (O'Neil and Brown 2005). However, others suggest that regular weighing can lead to an unhealthy and even obsessive focus on weight (Dionne and Yeudall 2005). Think about how much you monitor your body weight. Do you use a scale, or do you rely on other methods, such as how your clothes fit, to keep tabs on how much you weigh? Do you think your method helps you manage your weight?

SIZE ACCEPTANCE

Several social, professional, and academic size-acceptance organizations have emerged in response to the pervasive stigmatization of overweight people and the conflicting information about body weight and health consequences, including the National Association to Advance Fat Acceptance (NAAFA; www.naafaonline.com/dev2/), Council on Size and Weight Discrimination (CSWD; www.cswd.org), Weight Realities Division of the Society for Nutrition Education (SNE; www.sne.org), and Center for Weight and Health at the University of California at Berkeley (www.cnr.berkeley.edu/cwh). Many other organizations and Web sites exist to combat the challenges that overweight and obese people face.

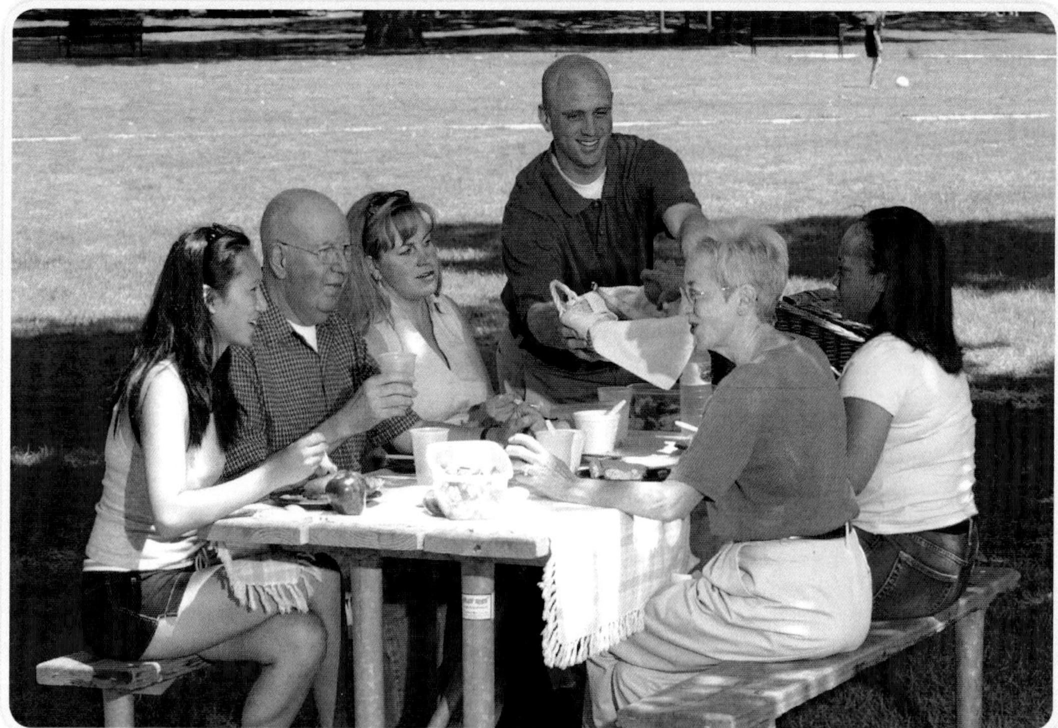

It's fun to celebrate holidays and other special occasions with family and friends, but remember to watch your portion sizes during the festivities.

© Human Kinetics

Health at Any Size

Health at Any Size (HAAS) is a size-acceptance, **nondiet movement** that attempts to help overweight and obese people decrease or eliminate thoughts associated with negative body image while highlighting the importance of accepting themselves and resolving issues related to eating and exercise that hinder long-term weight maintenance. This movement replaces the question "How can fat people lose weight?" with "How can people who are large be healthy?"

There are nine tenets of the size-acceptance, nondiet movement:

- Human beings come in a variety of sizes and shapes. It's good to celebrate this diversity as a positive characteristic of the human race.
- There is no ideal body size, shape, or weight that every person should strive to achieve.
- Every body is a good body, whatever its size or shape.
- Self-esteem and body image are strongly linked. Helping people feel good about their bodies and who they are can help motivate them to maintain healthy behaviors.
- Appearance stereotyping is inherently unfair because it is based on superficial factors that people have little or no control over.
- It's necessary to respect the bodies of others even though they might be different from our own.
- Each person is responsible for taking care of his own body.
- Good health is not defined by body size; it is a state of physical, mental, and social well-being.
- People of all sizes and shapes can reduce their risk of poor health by adopting healthy lifestyles.

Self-acceptance is important in improving self-esteem and general satisfaction with life. People with high self-regard have a vested interest in taking good care of themselves. Conversely, those with low self-esteem may have little motivation to engage in healthy behaviors. It can be destructive to focus too much on the importance of achieving a supposedly ideal body weight or to have unattainable appearance goals. Self-acceptance isn't the same as complacency or ignoring health concerns.

Fat Versus Fit

Many known health risks are associated with overweight and obesity, but not every overweight or obese person is unhealthy. A large study of more than 25,000 men conducted at the Cooper Institute for Aerobics Research found that cardiorespiratory fitness was a better predictor of heart disease than body weight was (Barlow, Kohl, Gibbons, and Blair 1995). Another study found that obese men who exercised regularly had death rates only slightly higher than those of unfit men of normal weight, whereas obese men who did not work out had death rates two to three times those of normal-weight men. Such findings suggest that exercise offers protection even to very heavy men (Wei et al. 1999).

Similar associations have been observed among women. For almost 4 years, researchers tracked heart attacks and other cardiovascular events among 906 women who had taken a test to assess the extent of clogged coronary arteries (Wessel et al. 2004). Women's lack of physical activity was a better predictor of having a heart attack or a cardiovascular event than weight was. Although this body of literature is fairly controversial, it suggests that some people can be both fat and fit. Despite differences in these studies, they all suggest that physical activity will offset some of the effects of excess weight. So apart from any weight-loss goals, it is vital to make exercise a part of your daily routine.

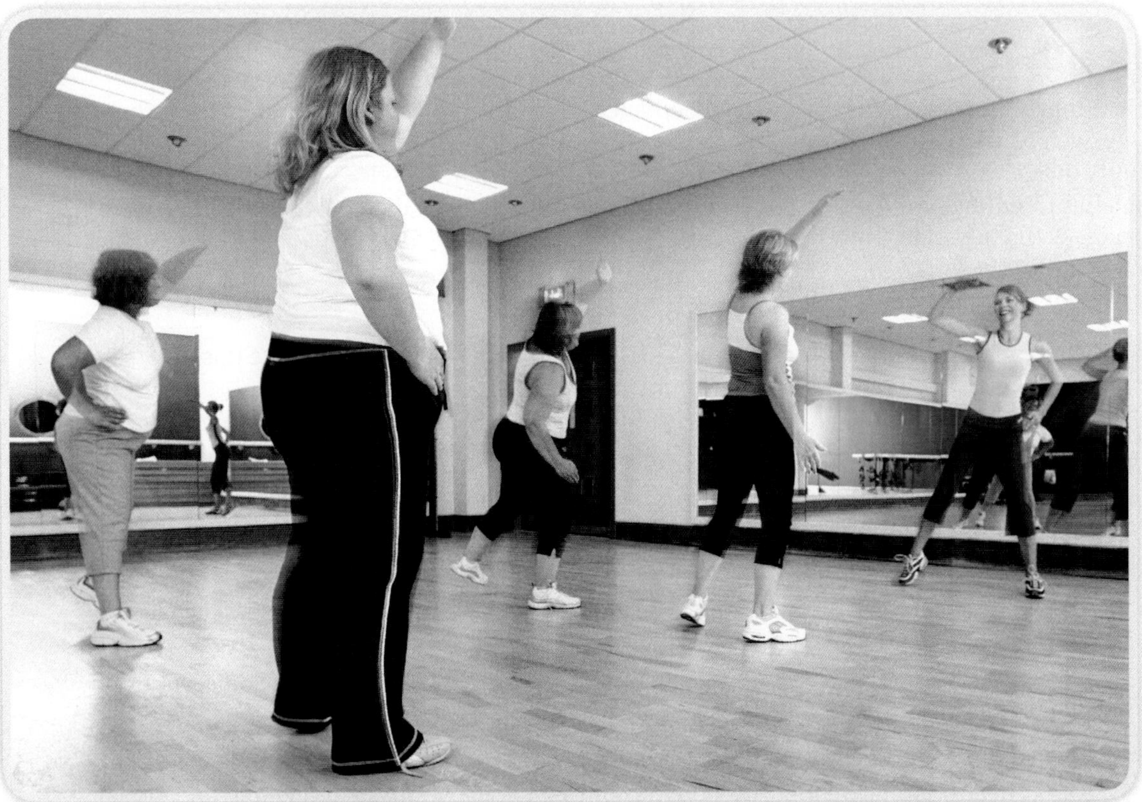

People who are overweight or obese can improve their health through cardiorespiratory exercise even if they don't lose much weight in the process.

© Bananastock

MANAGING TOO LITTLE BODY WEIGHT (UNDERWEIGHT)

Just as people who are overweight find it hard to lose weight, those who are underweight find it hard to gain. It's imperative to understand and treat the underlying causes of underweight. The goal is to create a positive energy balance so that the amount of calories consumed exceeds the calories expended. Underweight people should attempt to increase their daily calorie intake by 500 to 1,000 calories above what is needed to meet basic energy needs. They should increase their intake gradually to avoid stomach discomfort. These strategies help facilitate weight gain:

- Consuming small, frequent meals and snacks of energy-dense foods and beverages
- Consuming beverages at the end of the meal or between meals
- Using high-calorie weight-gain beverages, powders, and foods
- Getting social support to encourage food consumption even when not hungry
- Taking a basic vitamin and mineral supplement to help fill nutritional gaps associated with inadequate dietary intake
- Checking with a medical professional to see if any medications are interfering with weight status

If weight-gain strategies aren't successful, additional intervention could be necessary. Prescription appetite stimulants are available and may help increase dietary intake. Some medications help speed stomach emptying, which may improve appetite for subsequent meals. If underweight is perpetuated by poor digestion or absorption, digestive enzyme replacements are also available.

CHANGING THE OBESOGENIC ENVIRONMENT

It is becoming exceedingly clear that both biology and the environment play major roles in determining a person's body weight and body composition. However, the field of weight control has focused on why people are overweight or obese and how to change individual behaviors rather than focusing on why society is overweight or obese and trying to develop societal fixes. Here are some environmental strategies and policy recommendations to encourage healthy behavior and weight (Hill, Story, and Jeffery 2001).

Community Organizing and Action

- Develop community-wide councils to organize and direct activities that promote healthy eating and physical activity.
- Establish standards for foods served at cafeterias, vending machines, and snack stands on city or county property and in government buildings.

Schools and Worksites

- Eliminate sales of soda, candy, and other high-fat, high-sugar foods in schools.
- Require that foods that compete with school meals be consistent with national nutrition guidelines.
- Provide exercise and locker-room facilities at work.
- Open school gyms and swimming pools to the community during nonschool hours.

Food Packaging and Labeling

- Reward manufacturers for marketing foods in smaller portion sizes.
- Require warning labels on high-calorie, low nutrient-dense foods.

Media and Advertising

- Increase mass media promotion of healthy foods and physical activity.
- Promote walking and biking as a means of transportation.
- Promote water as the main daily drink choice.
- Regulate advertising and marketing practices to balance positive and negative media messages about food and physical activity.

Financial and Economic Incentives

- Use pricing strategies to promote purchase of healthy foods.
- Remove sales taxes or provide incentives for purchase of exercise equipment or for use of active forms of transportation such as walking or riding a bike to work.
- Levy state or local taxes on soda, candy, and high-fat, high-sugar snacks to fund subsidies for fruits and vegetables.

Transportation and Urban and Rural Development

- Construct safe walkways and cycle paths.
- Modify building design to encourage taking the stairs.
- Create pedestrian zones in cities.
- Add more water fountains in public buildings and outdoor areas.

WEIGHT MANAGEMENT 101

We are in the midst of an obesity epidemic with ramifications that go beyond the physical health of the individual. Too much or too little body weight is associated with morbidity and mortality, but there are social, political, and economic ramifications as well. With the myriad influences on each side of the energy balance equation, managing a healthy body weight is a challenge.

Research hasn't yet found a magic solution to help people manage their weight throughout the life span. As a result, the weight-loss industry has exploded, responding with hundreds of plans to aid in weight control. Some approaches are safe and potentially effective, but many others are based on gimmicks and weak science and lead to discouragement and short-term success. They might even damage the health of users. Learning to become a critical consumer is essential.

Effective, healthy, long-term solutions for weight management are likely going to involve multiple factors, addressing both the individual and the environment. At the individual level, long-term lifestyle change that incorporates basic principles of healthy eating, portion control, and regular exercise is the key to success. Environmental changes such as limiting marketing of unhealthy foods to children or providing exercise facilities in the workplace may make it easier for people to maintain a healthy body weight. Surgical and pharmaceutical options, though not without serious risk, have become increasingly popular and may aid those who struggle with substantial amounts of excess body fat and related diseases.

There probably will never be a magic bullet for weight loss or obesity prevention, and the pressure to achieve the ideal body is likely to continue. However, it is important to respect the body you have and treat it well, whatever size you are. Self-esteem, body image, and the behaviors you choose to engage in are related. People of all shapes and sizes can improve their health and well-being by adopting and maintaining a healthy lifestyle—a lifestyle that doesn't involve three payments of $49.99.

REVIEW QUESTIONS

1. What does it mean to say that people are exposed to a toxic food environment and a toxic activity environment? Give examples of each.
2. Describe the main factors that determine energy expenditure.
3. Explain three ways that people can use to assess how fat they are and how much body weight they carry.
4. Research suggests that there are numerous consequences of excess body fatness. Discuss three physical health and two mental health consequences.
5. How does socioeconomic status play a role in obesity?
6. Describe two treatment options for someone who is overweight and two treatment options for someone who is underweight.
7. Explain the dieter's cycle and how it can affect someone trying to lose weight.
8. What are the components of a healthy weight management program?
9. Describe how the Health at Any Size movement tries to help overweight and obese people, including at least three of its tenets in your explanation.
10. What is the difference between hunger, satiation, satiety, and appetite?

CRITICAL THINKING

1. Define *healthy weight* in a way that makes the most sense to you. Be sure to support your definition.
2. Do you think the obesity epidemic is caused by individual behavior, environmental factors, both, or other factors? Support your position regarding the root causes of the obesity epidemic.

APPLICATION ACTIVITIES

1. Create a food and physical activity diary form. Include space to write what foods you eat (including how much) and what exercise you engage in (including duration). Include space to record other factors you think might be important influences on eating and exercise behavior (e.g., time, feelings, accompanying activity while eating). For two weekdays and one weekend day, complete the self-monitoring form. Review your forms and search for patterns pertaining to your eating and exercise behavior. Did your eating cluster around certain times of the day? Did you eat when you were depressed, bored, anxious, or angry? Did you tend to eat when doing other activities (e.g., driving)? Did you eat more of certain foods when you were stressed? Did certain circumstances or situations influence how, when, and how much you ate or exercised? Write a two- to three-page reflective paper on your findings.
2. Become a diet detective. Delve into a self-help book or program for weight control. In an essay, describe the fundamental principles of the program, the rules, and the reported rationale as to how the program facilitates weight loss. Now apply a critical eye. From reading this chapter, you should have learned what every weight-control program should include, along with questions to ask. Discuss the strengths and weaknesses of the program you chose, including any red flags that come to mind. Finally, draw some conclusions—would you recommend this weight-control program to others? Why or why not?

GLOSSARY

anorexia nervosa—Psychological eating disorder characterized by a distorted body image with an extreme fear of gaining weight and refusal to stay in a healthy body composition zone.

appetite—Psychological desire to eat; may or may not be associated with physical hunger. Typically related to the pleasant sensations often associated with food.

appetite suppressants—Drugs that promote weight loss by decreasing appetite or increasing the feeling of being full. They function in the body by increasing one or more brain chemicals that affect mood and appetite. Phentermine and sibutramine are the most commonly prescribed FDA-approved drugs of this type in the United States.

bariatric surgery—Operations (e.g., gastroplasty, gastric bypass) performed to treat obesity by modifying the size of the stomach and sometimes the gastrointestinal tract to reduce the amount of food consumed and, with some procedures, the amount of nutrients that can be absorbed by the body.

basal metabolic rate (BMR)—Energy needed to sustain the metabolic activities of cells and tissues and to maintain vital body systems and processes; rate of metabolism that occurs when a person is awake but at rest in a warm environment and has not eaten for at least 12 hours. Accounts for 60 to 70 percent of total energy use.

behavior therapy—Approach to improving human behavior through the reinforcement of acceptable behavior and suppression of undesirable behavior.

bioelectrical impedance analysis (BIA)—Body composition method that measures the conductivity of a low-level electrical current as it passes through the body to estimate total body water, fat-free mass, and fat mass.

body image—Internal representation of one's outer appearance, influenced by biological, social, and interpersonal factors.

body mass index (BMI)—Measure of body weight relative to height that is calculated by dividing weight in kilograms by height in meters squared. Used to screen for weight categories that may indicate future health problems.

bulimia nervosa—Illness characterized by repeated episodes of eating large quantities of food in a short time followed by inappropriate compensatory methods such as purging (e.g., self-induced vomiting or misuse of laxatives, diuretics, or enemas). Fasting and excessive exercise also often follow a binge.

chain breaking—Breaking the link between two or more behaviors (e.g., snacking while watching television).

cholecystokinin (CCK)—Hormone released from the epithelial cells of the small intestine. Primarily responsible for stimulating the digestion of fat and protein while also helping to slow gastric emptying and regulate appetite.

cognitive-behavioral therapy—Therapy in which maladaptive thoughts and behaviors are modified and problem-solving and coping skills are enhanced.

cognitive restructuring—Changing one's frame of mind regarding eating, activity, and weight control to be more positive and to promote health rather than being negative and overly critical.

contingency management—Forming a plan of action in order to respond to a situation where overeating or inactivity might be likely.

direct calorimetry—Direct measurement of energy expenditure by assessing the amount of heat produced by the body.

dual-energy X-ray absorptiometry (DXA)—Radiographic body composition method used to estimate bone mass as well as lean tissue mass and fat mass.

eating disorders—Conditions characterized by severe disturbances in eating behavior, such as extreme reduction of food intake or extreme overeating, or feelings of extreme distress or concern about body weight or shape (i.e., anorexia nervosa, bulimia nervosa, binge-eating disorder). It is possible for a person to exhibit disordered eating patterns without having a clinical eating disorder.

energy density—Amount of energy (in calories) in a weighed amount of food, generally presented as calories per gram. Foods with a lower energy density provide fewer calories per gram than foods with a higher energy density do; thus consumption of foods low in energy density may help manage hunger and control body weight.

energy intake—Energy (calorie) content of food provided by fat (9 calories per gram), carbohydrate (4 calories), protein (4 calories), and alcohol (7 calories).

energy output—Use of energy (calories) for basic bodily functions and processes, physical activity, TEF, and thermogenesis.

estimated energy requirements (EER)—Average dietary energy intake that is predicted to maintain energy balance in a healthy person of a defined age, gender, weight, height, and level of physical activity consistent with good health.

fat-absorption inhibitors—Drugs that reduce the ability to absorb body fat by about 30 percent by blocking the dietary fat digesting enzyme lipase; also known as *lipase inhibitors*. Orlistat is an FDA-approved drug of this type.

fat cell theory—Theory that the quantity of fat stored in the body is the result of the number and size of fat cells.

fen-phen—Combination of the appetite-suppressing drugs fenfluramine and phentermine. The FDA recommended the withdrawal of this combination therapy from the market in 1997 because of its link to the development of serious heart valve problems.

ghrelin—Hormone produced primarily by the stomach; acts on the hypothalamus to stimulate hunger and feeding.

hunger—Physiological need for food often accompanied by discomfort, weakness, or pain.

hydrodensitometry—Body composition method used to estimate body volume by submersion underwater; also known as *underwater weighing* or *hydrostatic weighing*.

hyperplastic obesity—When a person reaches a body weight that is about 40 percent overweight or more, fat tissue is likely to contain both bigger fat cells and more of them.

hypertrophic obesity—Greater-than-average number of fat cells.

hypothalamus—Region of the brain involved in regulating hunger and satiety, respiration, body temperature, water balance, and other bodily functions.

indirect calorimetry—Measures energy expenditure by determining the oxygen consumption and carbon dioxide production of the body over a given time.

leptin—Hormone secreted by adipose tissue that is correlated with body-fat percentage and thought to have a role in regulating body weight and appetite.

negative energy balance—Energy output exceeds energy intake, resulting in weight loss.

neuropeptide Y—Neurotransmitter distributed throughout the brain and peripheral nervous tissue that is linked with eating behavior, depression, anxiety, and cardiovascular function.

nondiet movement—Approach to food that centers on learning to recognize and follow internal hunger and fullness cues, to follow guidelines for healthy food choices, to increase physical activity levels, and to worry less about body shape and size and focus more on self-acceptance.

nonexercise activity thermogenesis (NEAT)—Energy expended during activities of daily living.

normal weight—Having a BMI between 18.5 and 24.9.

obese—State of adiposity in which body fatness is above the ideal for health; a BMI of 30 and above.

obesogenic environment—Environment conducive to the development and maintenance of nutrition and physical activity behaviors that generate obesity.

overweight—State of adiposity in which body weight exceeds a standard based on height; a BMI of 25 to 29.9.

positive energy balance—Energy intake exceeds energy output, resulting in weight gain.

Prader-Willi syndrome—Genetic condition caused by the absence of chromosomal material from chromosome 15 occurring in about 1/10,000 to 1/25,000 live births. The classic feature of this syndrome is the development of an insatiable appetite that often results in obesity.

resting metabolic rate (RMR)—Similar to BMR except that it measures energy expenditure when the body is not completely rested and in a fasting state; typically about 6 percent higher than BMR.

satiation—Feeling of satisfaction and fullness that terminates a meal.

satiety—Effect of food that delays subsequent intake of food; feeling of satisfaction and fullness following eating that diminishes the desire for food.

self-acceptance—Level of satisfaction or happiness with oneself that is thought to be necessary for good mental health.

self-monitoring—Tracking foods eaten and conditions affecting eating (e.g., location, time, state of mind), usually in a diary or by using an online diet tracking tool; may also be used to track physical activity behavior and body weight.

serotonin—Neurotransmitter that serves many functions, including regulation of emotions, mood, sleep, and appetite.

set-point theory—Theory that a regulatory mechanism operates to keep body weight and body fatness at a certain level.

skinfold measurements—Method of estimating body fatness by using calipers to measure the thickness of two layers of skin and the underlying subcutaneous fat at various points on the body.

social support—Network of family, friends, neighbors, and community members that can be called on to give psychological, physical, social, and financial help during times of need.

stimulus control—Changing the environment to minimize the stimuli for unhealthy eating behavior and maximize the stimuli for healthy eating behavior and physical activity.

thermic effect of food (TEF)—Increase in energy expenditure associated with the digestion, absorption, and metabolism of food.

thermoregulation—Body system for maintaining an appropriate temperature.

underweight—Body weight that is 15 to 20 percent below ideal weight; a BMI below 18.5.

very-low-calorie diet (VLCD)—Doctor-supervised diet that typically uses commercially prepared formulas to promote rapid weight loss among obese people by providing 800 calories per day or less.

waist circumference—Distance around the smallest part of the waist (below the rib cage and above the umbilicus); circumference above a certain measure is considered to be a risk factor for the development of weight-related diseases.

waist-to-hip ratio (WHR)—Measurement of fat distribution that is associated with risk of some weight-related diseases, such as heart disease.

weight cycling—Repeated cycles of weight gain and weight loss.

weight monitoring—Process of tracking body weight; may be conducted by a medical professional, within a weight-loss group setting, or using a personal scale.

weight stigmatization—Stereotypes and prejudice toward children and adults who are overweight or obese. People who are stigmatized because they are overweight or obese are ascribed negative stereotypes that increase vulnerability to unfair treatment, prejudice, and discrimination.

REFERENCES AND RESOURCES

Balkau, B., J.E. Deanfield, J.P. Despres, J.P. Bassand, K.A. Fox, S.C. Smith Jr., P. Barter, C.E. Tan, L. Van Gaal, H.U. Wittchen, C. Massien, and S.M. Haffner. 2007. International Day for the Evaluation of Abdominal Obesity (IDEA): A study of waist circumference, cardiovascular disease, and diabetes mellitus in 168,000 primary care patients in 63 countries. *Circulation* 116 (17): 1942-1951.

Barlow, C.E., H.W. Kohl III, L.W. Gibbons, and S.N. Blair. 1995. Physical fitness, mortality and obesity. *International Journal of Obesity* 19 (Suppl. 4): S41-44.

Barsh, G.S., I.S. Farooqi, and S. O'Rahilly. 2000. Genetics of body-weight regulation. *Nature* 404 (6778): 644-651.

Bell, E.A., V.H. Castellanos, C.L. Pelkman, M.L. Thorwart, and B.J. Rolls. 1998. Energy density of foods affects energy intake in normal-weight women. *American Journal of Clinical Nutrition* 67 (3): 412-420.

Bell, E.A., and B.J. Rolls. 2001. Energy density of foods affects energy intake across multiple levels of fat content in lean and obese women. *American Journal of Clinical Nutrition* 73 (6): 1010-1018.

Boutelle, K.N., D.S. Kirschenbaum, R.C. Baker, and M.E. Mitchell. 1999. How can obese weight controllers minimize weight gain during the high risk holiday season? By self-monitoring very consistently. *Health Psychology* 18 (4): 364-368.

Brownson, R.C., T.K. Boehmer, and D.A. Luke. 2005. Declining rates of physical activity in the United States: What are the contributors? *Annual Review of Public Health* 26: 421-443.

Burton-Freeman, B., P.A. Davis, and B.O. Schneeman. 2002. Plasma cholecystokinin is associated with subjective measures of satiety in women. *American Journal of Clinical Nutrition* 76 (3): 659-667.

Cassady, D., K.M. Jetter, and J. Culp. 2007. Is price a barrier to eating more fruits and vegetables for low-income families? *Journal of the American Dietetic Association* 107 (11): 1909-1915.

Centers for Disease Control and Prevention (CDC). 2005. CDC Behavioral Risk Factor Surveillance System 2005 data. http://apps.nccd.cdc.gov/brfss/index.asp.

Chen, E.Y., and M. Brown. 2005. Obesity stigma in sexual relationships. *Obesity Research* 13 (8): 1393-1397.

Committee on Physical Activity, Health, Transportation, and Land Use, ed. 2005. *Does the built environment influence physical activity? Examining the evidence.* Washington, DC: Transportation Research Board.

de Castro, J.M., and E.M. Brewer. 1992. The amount eaten in meals by humans is a power function of the number of people present. *Physiology & Behavior* 51 (1): 121-125.

Dionne, M.M., and F. Yeudall. 2005. Monitoring of weight in weight loss programs: A double-edged sword? *Journal of Nutrition Education and Behavior* 37 (6): 315-318.

Falba, T.A., and J.L. Sindelar. 2008. Spousal concordance in health behavior change. *Health Services Research* 43 (1 Pt 1): 96-116.

Food and Nutrition Board. 2005. *Dietary Reference Intakes for energy, carbohydrate, fiber, fat, fatty acids, cholesterol, protein, and amino acids (macronutrients).* Washington, DC: National Academies Press.

Frazao, E., ed. 1999. *America's eating habits: Changes and consequences.* Washington, DC: USDA/Economic Research Service.

Friedman, M.A., and K.D. Brownell. 2002. Psychological consequences of obesity. In *Eating disorders and obesity,* ed. C.G. Fairburn and K.D. Brownell, 393-398. New York: Guilford Press.

Gallagher, D., S.B. Heymsfield, M. Heo, S.A. Jebb, P.R. Murgatroyd, and Y. Sakamoto. 2000. Healthy percentage body fat ranges: An approach for developing guidelines based on body mass index. *American Journal of Clinical Nutrition* 72 (3): 694-701.

Hill, S.F., M. Story, and R.W. Jeffery. 2001. Environmental influences on eating and activity. *Annual Review of Public Health* 22: 309-335.

Jebb, S.A. 2002. Energy intake and body weight. In *Eating disorders and obesity,* ed. C.G. Fairburn and K.D. Brownell, 37-42. New York: Guilford Press.

Johnson, C. 2002. Obesity, weight management, and self-esteem. In *Handbook of obesity treatment,* ed. T.A. Wadden and A.J. Stunkard, 480-493. New York: Guilford Press.

Kahn, B.E., and B. Wansink. 2004. The influence of assortment structure on perceived variety and consumption quantities. *Journal of Consumer Research* 30: 519-533.

Latner, J.D., and A.J. Stunkard. 2003. Getting worse: The stigmatization of obese children. *Obesity Research* 11 (3): 452-456.

Mafeis, C., G. Talamini, and L. Tato. 1998. Influence of diet, physical activity, and parents' obesity on children's adiposity: A four-year longitudinal study. *International Journal of Obesity* 22: 758-764.

National Institute of Diabetes and Digestive and Kidney Diseases (NIDDK). 2008. Choosing a safe and successful weight-loss program. http://win.niddk.nih.gov/publications/choosing.htm.

Nielsen, S.J., and B.M. Popkin. 2003. Patterns and trends in food portion sizes, 1977-1998. *Journal of the American Medical Association* 289 (4): 450.

Ogden, C.L., M.D. Carroll, M.A. McDowell, and K.M. Flegal. 2007. *Obesity among adults in the United States: No change since 2003-2004.* NCHS data brief no 1. Hyattsville, MD: National Center for Health Statistics.

O'Neil, P.M., and J.D. Brown. 2005. Weighing the evidence: Benefits of regular weight monitoring for weight control. *Journal of Nutrition Education and Behavior* 37 (6): 319-322.

Paddon-Jones, D., E. Westman, R.D. Mattes, R.R. Wolfe, A. Astrup, and M. Westerterp-Plantenga. 2008. Protein, weight management, and satiety. *American Journal of Clinical Nutrition* 87 (5): 1558S-1561S.

Puhl, R., and K.D. Brownell. 2001. Bias, discrimination, and obesity. *Obesity Research* 9 (12): 788-805.

Ravussin, E., and B.A. Swinburn. 1992. Effect of caloric restriction and weight loss on energy expenditure. In *Treatment of the severely obese patient,* ed. T.A. Wadden and T. Van Itallie, 163-189. New York: Guilford Press.

Richardson, S.A., N. Goodman, A.H. Hastorf, and S.M. Dornbusch. 1961. Cultural uniformity in reaction to physical disabilities. *American Sociological Review* 26: 241-247.

Roberts, S.B., and J. Mayer. 2000. Holiday weight gain: Fact or fiction? *Nutrition Reviews* 58 (12): 378-379.

Rolls, B.J., E.L. Morris, and L.S. Row. 2002. Portion size of food affects energy intake in normal-weight and overweight men and women. *American Journal of Clinical Nutrition* 76 (6): 1207-1213.

Schwartz, M.B., and K.D. Brownell. 2002. Obesity and body image. In *Body image: A handbook of theory, research, and clinical practice,* ed. T.F. Cash and T. Pruzinsky, 200-209. New York: Guilford Press.

Schwartz, M.W., D.G. Baskin, K.J. Kaiyala, and S.C. Woods. 1999. Model for the regulation of energy balance and adiposity by the central nervous system. *American Journal of Clinical Nutrition* 69 (4): 584-596.

Sobal, J. 1991. Obesity and nutritional sociology: A model for coping with the stigma of obesity. *Clinical Sociology Review* 9: 125-141.

Sobal, J., V. Nicolopoulos, and J. Lee. 1995. Attitudes about overweight and dating among secondary school students. *International Journal of Obesity* 19 (6): 376-381.

St. Jeor, S.T., B.V. Howard, T.E. Prewitt, V. Bovee, T. Bazzarre, and R.H. Eckel. 2001. Dietary protein and weight reduction: A statement for healthcare professionals from the Nutrition Committee of the Council on Nutrition, Physical Activity, and Metabolism of the American Heart Association. *Circulation* 104 (15): 1869-1874.

Taylor, P., C. Funk, and P. Craighill. 2006. *Americans see weight problems everywhere but in the mirror.* A social trends report. Washington, DC: Pew Research Center.

U.S. Department of Health and Human Services (USDHHS) and U.S. Department of Agriculture (USDA). 2005. *Dietary Guidelines for Americans 2005.* www.health.gov/dietaryguidelines/dga2005/document/pdf/DGA2005.pdf.

Wadden, T.A., J.A. Sternberg, K.A. Letizia, A.J. Stunkard, and G.D. Foster. 1989. Treatment of obesity by very low calorie diet, behavior therapy, and their combination: A five-year perspective. *International Journal of Obesity* 13 (Suppl. 2): 39-46.

Wansink, B., and M.M. Cheney. 2005. Super bowls: Serving bowl size and food consumption. *Journal of the American Medical Association* 293 (14): 1727-1728.

Wansink, B., J.E. Painter, and Y.K. Lee. 2006. The office candy dish: Proximity's influence on estimated and actual consumption. *International Journal of Obesity* 30 (5): 871-875.

Wansink, B., J.E. Painter, and J. North. 2005. Bottomless bowls: Why visual cues of portion size may influence intake. *Obesity Research* 13 (1): 93-100.

Wansink, B., and K. van Ittersum. 2005. Shape of glass and amount of alcohol poured: Comparative study of effect of practice and concentration. *British Medical Journal* 331 (7531): 1512-1514.

Wansink, B., K. van Ittersum, and J.E. Painter. 2006. Ice cream illusions: Bowls, spoons, and self-served portion sizes. *American Journal of Preventive Medicine* 31 (3): 240-243.

Wardle, J., S. Carnell, C.M. Haworth, and R. Plomin. 2008. Evidence for a strong genetic influence on childhood adiposity despite the force of the obesogenic environment. *American Journal of Clinical Nutrition* 87 (2): 398-404.

Wei, M., J.B. Kampert, C.E. Barlow, M.Z. Nichaman, L.W. Gibbons, R.S. Paffenbarger Jr., and S.N. Blair. 1999. Relationship between low cardiorespiratory fitness and mortality in normal-weight, overweight, and obese men. *Journal of the American Medical Association* 282 (16): 547-553.

Wessel, T.R., C.B. Arant, M.B. Olson, B.D. Johnson, S.E. Reis, B.L. Sharaf, L.J. Shaw, E. Handberg, G. Sopko, S.F. Kelsey, C.J. Pepine, and N.B. Merz. 2004. Relationship of physical fitness vs. body mass index with coronary artery disease and cardiovascular events in women. *Journal of the American Medical Association* 292 (10): 1179-1187.

Wing, R.R., and J.O. Hill. 2001. Successful weight loss maintenance. *Annual Review of Nutrition* 21: 323-341.

Young, L.R., and M. Nestle. 2002. The contribution of expanding portion sizes to the U.S. obesity epidemic. *American Journal of Public Health* 92 (2): 246-249.

Yusuf, S., S. Hawken, S. Ounpuu, L. Bautista, M.G. Franzosi, P. Commerford, C.C. Lang, Z. Rumboldt, C.L. Onen, L. Lisheng, S. Tanomsup, P. Wangai Jr., F. Razak, A.M. Sharma, and S.S. Anand. 2005. Obesity and the risk of myocardial infarction in 27,000 participants from 52 countries: A case-control study. *Lancet* 366 (9497): 1640-1649.

Zhang, Q., and Y. Wang. 2004. Trends in the association between obesity and socioeconomic status in U.S. adults: 1971 to 2000. *Obesity Research* 12 (10): 1622-1632.

Other helpful resources include the following.

Allison, D.B., V.C. Basile, and H.E. Yuker. 1991. The measurement of attitudes toward and beliefs about obese persons. *International Journal of Eating Disorders* 10: 599-607.

American Dietetic Association (ADA) Evidence Analysis Library. www.adaevidencelibrary.com. The evidence analysis library contains the most relevant nutritional research on important dietetic practice questions.

Brownell, K.D., R. Puhl, M.B. Schwartz, and L. Rudd. 2005. *Weight bias: Nature, consequences, and remedies.* New York: Guilford.

Dietary Guidelines for Americans 2005. www.healthierus.gov/dietaryguidelines/. This site contains a wealth of information about the dietary guidelines released every 5 years by the U.S. government.

FDA Food Labeling and Nutrition. www.cfsan.fda.gov/~dms/lab-gen.html. This site offers a wealth of information on nutrition facts labels.

MyPyramid. www.mypyramid.gov. The USDA developed this site to help people put the dietary guidelines into practice.

National Association to Advance Fat Acceptance (NAAFA). www.naafaonline.com/dev2/. NAAFA works to eliminate discrimination based on body size and to provide fat people with the tools for self-empowerment through public education, advocacy, and member support.

National Weight Control Registry. www.nwcr.ws. Learn more about how people who have successfully lost weight have managed to keep it off.

Nutrient Data Laboratory. www.nal.usda.gov/fnic/foodcomp/search/. This site from the USDA will help you learn more about what's in the foods you eat.

Portion Distortion! http://hp2010.nhlbihin.net/portion/index.htm. Learn more and test your knowledge of portion sizes and serving sizes at this site.

Rudd Center for Food Policy and Obesity. www.yaleruddcenter.org. The Rudd Center is a nonprofit research and public policy organization devoted to improving the world's diet, preventing obesity, and reducing weight stigma.

USDA Food and Nutrition Information Center. http://fnic.nal.usda.gov/. This site provides credible, accurate, and practical resources about dietary guidance, nutrition, diet and disease, and much more.

Wansink, B. 2006. *Mindless eating: Why we eat more than we think.* New York: Bantam Dell.

Weight-Control Information Network. www.win.niddk.nih.gov. This site provides up-to-date, science-based information on weight control, obesity, physical activity, and related nutritional issues.

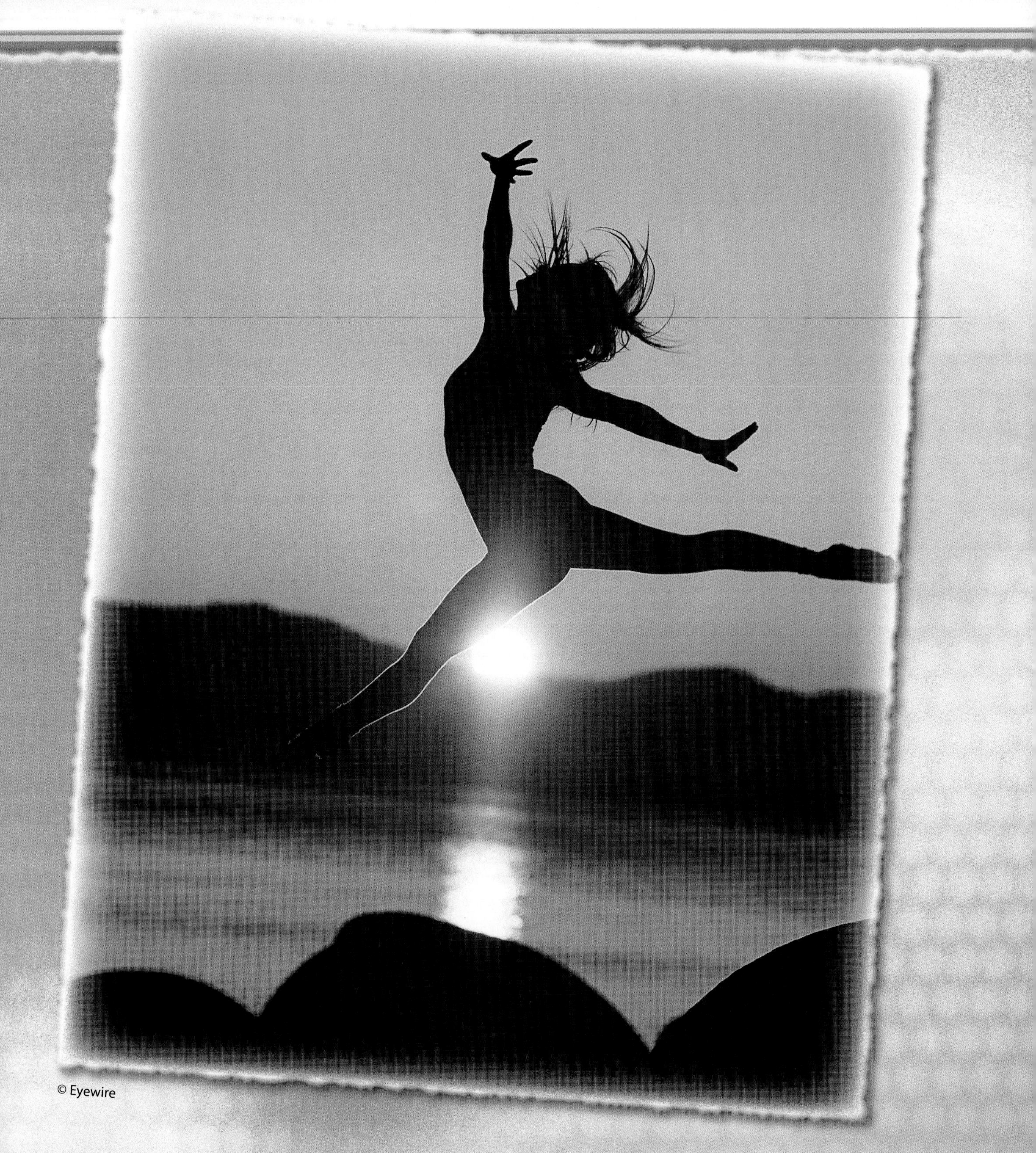

© Eyewire

CHAPTER 5

MENTAL HEALTH

DIANA MEIER, MSW, MPH
Director of Health Education

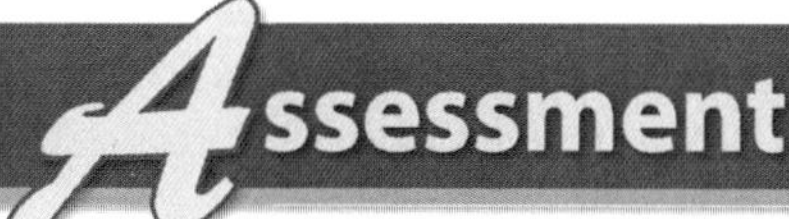

Assessment

- How would you define mental health and mental illness?
- Did you know that suicide is the second leading cause of death among college students?
- Why are some people reluctant to seek treatment for mental illness?
- How do antipsychotic, antimanic, antidepressant, and antianxiety medications work?
- What warning signs might you see in a friend who is suffering from mental illness?
- What's the difference between a psychiatrist and a psychologist?

Objectives

- Define *mental health* and understand what constitutes both good mental health and poor mental health.
- Understand the magnitude of mental illness and the changing perspective on mental illness and treatment of the mentally ill.
- Understand the effects of genetics and environment on mental health.
- Identify the major theories of mental health that guide treatment of mental disorders.
- Explain how the *Diagnostic and Statistical Manual of Mental Disorders (DSM)* is used to diagnose mental illness.
- Recognize signs that people may be a danger to themselves or others.

Before we can talk about mental health, we need to define the concept. Think about it like this: When you're physically healthy, your body works so you can do what you need to do to carry out normal activities of daily living. If you're not physically healthy, it's more challenging to function. You can rack up medical bills, feel more stress, and find it difficult to do things you used to enjoy. Similarly, when you're mentally healthy, your brain is well and you're able to take care of your daily activities and relationships. You experience emotions such as sadness and anxiety and yet you are still able to handle your job, studies, and interpersonal relationships. If you have poor mental health, your response to those normal emotions might impair your daily functioning.

Mental health can be described as not only the absence of mental disorders but also the mental functioning that allows for productive activities, interpersonal relationships, and adaptability. Generally, people with good mental health have an overall sense of well-being, the ability to enjoy life, resiliency, and a sense of being able to manage difficult situations. They're able to participate in life to its fullest, adapt to change, maintain balance in all areas of life, take care of themselves, exhibit self-confidence, and pay appropriate attention to mind, body, spirit, creativity, education, and health (Helpguide 2007).

Mental illness is defined by abnormal brain processes that lead to impaired function. The labels that describe the status of mental health as a disorder, disease, or illness aren't specifically defined, change as knowledge of mental status increases, and are often used interchangeably.

It's much harder to determine the status of mental health than physical health. If someone's arm hurts, an X ray can easily confirm whether his arm is broken. If he's fatigued, a blood test can determine if he has anemia. But if he feels fatigued, unmotivated, and anxious, no blood test or X ray will substantiate what is going on in his brain. A physician or counselor can ask some questions or give the person some self-report tests, but it's hard to come to definite conclusions in this relatively new field of study. As researchers learn more about the brain and behavior, diagnosis and treatment will likely become more accurate and definitive.

In the United States, an estimated 26.2 percent of Americans aged 18 and older, or about one in four adults, suffer from a diagnosable mental disorder in a given year, making mental disorders the leading cause of disability in the United States in the 15- to 44-year-old age group. Six percent of adults, or 1 in 17, are diagnosed with serious mental illness, and nearly half of those with a mental disorder have two or more disorders (National Institute of Mental Health [NIMH] 2007b).

In addition, estimates suggest that 20 percent of children under the age of 18 have mental disorders with at least minimal functional impairment (U.S. Surgeon General 2007). Among children and adolescents, federal guidelines define a subcategory of serious emotional disturbance (SED) that includes young people with more severe functional limitations. Estimates suggest that approximately 5 to 9 percent of children aged 9 through 17 meet the guidelines for SED.

The American Psychological Association Practice Organization (APAPO) reports that indirect costs of untreated mental health disorders result in a $79 billion annual loss to businesses due to absenteeism and loss of productivity. Indirect costs of poor employee health, such as absenteeism, disability, and lost performance at work, are two to three times higher than the direct medical costs. Furthermore, the total cost of presenteeism (productivity loss resulting from on-the-job employee health problems) is estimated to be more than $150 billion a year. Mood disorders alone are estimated to cost more than $50 billion per year in lost productivity. It is estimated that American employees used about 8.8 million sick days in 2001 due to untreated or mistreated depression (APAPO 2008).

This chapter will overview the history of the study of mental health and mental disorders and explain how treatment methods have changed over time. You'll learn how the brain and the environment influence mental health and what behaviors help professionals diagnose a mental illness. The most important part of the chapter is information about how you can get help for yourself or your friends if you suspect that intervention from a mental health professional would be beneficial.

GENDER ISSUES

Hysterical Wandering Womb

The term *hysteria* is derived from the Greek word for womb, *hystera*. The concept of the wandering womb surfaced as early as sixth century BCE to explain health problems such as headaches and coughs among women. The theory was later used to explain madness among women. According to the theory, a woman's womb would wander around the body if it wasn't stabilized through frequent intercourse. If the uterus wandered off and lodged near the brain, it was thought to cause hysteria. Treatment included having the woman sniff a foul scent to repel the womb back to where it belonged. Another treatment was to place something sweet smelling by the vulva to lure the womb back.

YOUNG ADULTS AND MENTAL HEALTH

Mental health problems can develop from both environmental and biological causes. People in college have high rates of mental health problems and the beginnings of mental health disorders. The college experience brings with it multiple transitions, including new responsibilities and increased independence. Stressful transitions include shifting roles within the immediate family, developing new friendships and relationships, maintaining a course load of college-level classes, and taking on adult responsibilities such as paying rent and other bills. Without good mental health and coping skills, managing all these new responsibilities can become overwhelming and lead to destructive coping behaviors.

According to the American Psychological Association, one out of four young adults will experience a depressive episode by age 24, with nearly half of all college students reporting that at some point during college they've been so depressed they've had trouble functioning (Benton et al. 2003). Untreated depression can lead to suicide, which is the second leading cause of death among college students. A 2004 study by the American College Health Association (ACHA) indicated that of the students who reported being diagnosed with depression, 25 percent were in mental health therapy and 38 percent were taking medication for depression. Of all the students in the study, more than 60 percent reported feeling that things were hopeless one or more times, and 40 percent of the men and 50 percent of the women reported they'd had difficulty functioning because of depression. Additionally, 10 percent of students in the study reported seriously considering suicide at least once (Benton et al. 2003).

Alcohol abuse can mask underlying psychological illness, because a person might use alcohol to temporarily alleviate feelings of depression or anxiety. Forty-six percent of young adults (12.4 million) engaged in drinking that exceeded the recommended daily limits at least once in the past year, and 14.5 percent (3.9 million) had an average consumption that exceeded the recommended weekly limits (National Institute on Alcohol Abuse and Alcoholism [NIAAA] 2006). College students have higher rates of clinically significant alcohol-related problems than people the same age who don't attend college; 24 percent of college men and 13 percent of college women suffered from these problems, compared with 22 percent of men and 9 percent of women who weren't attending college (Benton et al. 2003). The NIAAA reported that alcohol-related unintentional fatal injures increased from 1,500 to 1,700 from 1998 to 2001 (NIAAA 2005). During that time, national surveys indicate that the number of students who drove under the influence of alcohol increased from 2.3 million to 2.8 million (Substance Abuse and Mental Health Services Administration [SAMHSA] 2004).

Harm to others through drinking and driving is not the only potential consequence to nondrinkers. A study supported by the U.S. Department of Education found the following secondary effects among nondrinkers and light drinkers who live on campus: 60 percent had

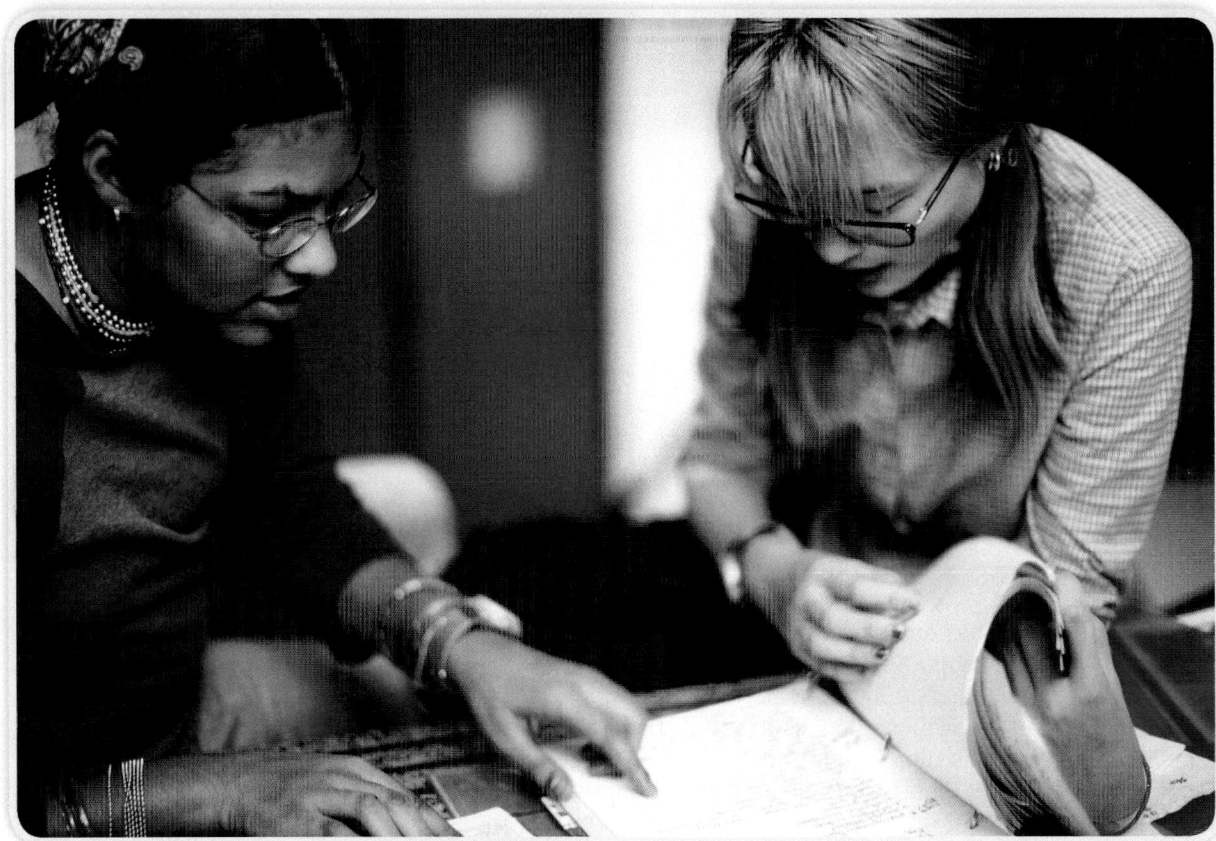

College can be a stressful time for students, and pressure to complete academic work is only one of the factors that contribute to their overall mental health.

© Photodisc

their study or sleep interrupted, 47 percent had to take care of a drunk student, 30 percent had been insulted or harassed by a heavy drinker, 20 percent of women experienced unwanted sexual advances, 15 percent had property damaged, 9 percent had been assaulted, and 1 percent had been sexually assaulted or raped (Kapner 2003).

HISTORY AND STIGMA

During the 1700s, people who behaved unconventionally because they had a mental illness were assumed to be possessed by demons or to be influenced by the devil. Those people were often tortured in an attempt to drive the demons out of the body. Views on mental illness began to change in the early 1800s. At that time, mental illness began to be viewed as a disease of the brain; it wasn't something a person could control, and it wasn't the result of demon possession. As a result, thousands of dungeon prisoners were released from torturous conditions and moved into asylums where experimental medical interventions were done (Torrey 1997). Just the transition to more humane care improved patient well-being and behavior. Even so, many of the experimental methods for treating mental illness were ethically questionable and would be considered inhumane by today's standards (Frick 2002).

In the early 1900s, people with mental illness, mental retardation, and other developmental disabilities received care in large public institutions or at home by families who didn't have governmental financial support. By 1955, when deinstitutionalization began, more than 550,000 people were in public mental hospitals (Torrey 1997). **Deinstitutionalization** refers to the policy of moving severely mentally ill people out of large, state-supported institutions and then closing some or all of those institutions. Deinstitutionalization was based on the belief that mental illness should be treated in the least restrictive setting.

Deinstitutionalization didn't ensure that medication, rehabilitation, and transitional services were in place for people who were discharged from institutions. It has redefined the state of crisis for the mentally ill, because many of them can't access appropriate treatment. A disproportionate number of people with mental illness are in jails, shelters, and substance abuse rehabilitation facilities.

Despite huge advances in medical understanding of mental illness, the stigma persists. Research indicates that the likelihood of violence is low among the mentally ill, but many people continue to believe that people who have a mental illness are violent. The media likely contribute to this negative perception because they feature only the most severe cases of people with mental illness. Those sensational cases include murder–suicides such as those at Columbine and Virginia Tech, women with postpartum depression and co-occurring disorders who murder their children, or sociopaths who murder. These extreme cases don't represent even a significant fraction of those with mental illness, but they perpetuate the social stigma. Because of the social stigma for mental illness and the limitations in care, nearly two-thirds of people with diagnosable mental disorders don't seek treatment (U.S. Surgeon General 2007).

TREATMENT METHODS OVER TIME

Back when people with mental illness were committed to mental institutions, one of the few therapeutic options was the **lobotomy**, also known as *leucotomy*. The procedure involved drilling holes into the skull and using a blade to sever nerve fibers that run from the frontal lobes to the rest of the brain. The treatment was developed in 1935 by a neurologist who contended that psychiatric symptoms were caused over time by faulty nerve connections. He believed that if these nerves were severed and new connections formed, patients' symptoms would improve. By the late 1950s, when neurologic medications started to be used, tens of thousands of lobotomies had been performed in the United States (ScienceWeek 2005). Lobotomy seems barbaric by current treatment standards, but it was highly regarded in its time. Approaches to mental health treatment and understanding of the brain and behavior are still developing, so it's likely that the treatment methods used today will be obsolete in the decades to come.

What Do You Do?

Watch one of the following movies and then write a short paper to discuss your opinion about the portrayal of the particular mental disorder, the accuracy of the portrayal, and the overall impact the movie had on its viewers. Does the movie perpetuate healthy or unhealthy stereotypes of mental illness?

- *Trainspotting* (1996)
- *One Flew Over the Cuckoo's Nest* (1975)
- *A Beautiful Mind* (2001)
- *Girl, Interrupted* (1999)
- *Sybil* (1976)
- *Kalifornia* (1993)
- *Good Will Hunting* (1997)
- *Rain Man* (1988)
- *Fight Club* (1999)

Another controversial treatment from the past is **electroconvulsive therapy (ECT)** for depression. A person who is going to receive ECT treatment undergoes general anesthesia and receives a muscle relaxer. Therapists place electrodes on the scalp and apply a finely controlled electric current, which causes a brief seizure in the brain. Because the patient received muscle relaxers, the seizure causes only slight limb movement. When the patient wakes up minutes later, she doesn't remember the treatment. The therapy is typically administered three times a week for 2 to 4 weeks, and it's usually followed by therapy and medication management. ECT earned a less-than-reputable reputation during the 1940s and 1950s because poorly trained staff misused equipment and incorrectly administered treatment. ECT is still used today, though, when other methods aren't successful in treating severe depression or when a patient is a threat to himself or others (WebMD 2008). This procedure involves milder, more directive shocks for treatment with side effects of mild memory impairment.

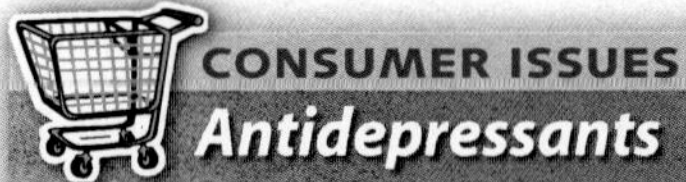

Between 1995 and 2002 (the most recent year for which statistics are available), the use of antidepressant drugs rose 48 percent (Centers for Disease Control and Prevention [CDC] 2004), making them the most commonly prescribed drugs in the United States. They're prescribed more than drugs to treat high blood pressure, high cholesterol, asthma, or headaches. Are we decreasing stigma and finally recognizing an unmet need, or has the pharmaceutical industry created a market of consumers from people who are experiencing the expected highs and lows of daily living?

Next time you visit your physician or dentist, take a look around the office at paperweights, pens, notepads, and posters. You will note pharmaceutical gifts that are part of a push to sell, and have the doctor prescribe, a particular medication.

MEDICATION

Medication replaced the lobotomies in the 1950s. In the same way that there is stigma associated with having mental illness, there is also a stigma associated with accessing treatment, including taking medicine for mental illness, even though medications have made marked strides in the treatment of mental illness.

A person with a headache probably doesn't think twice about taking ibuprofen. A person with diabetes probably has the support of family and friends as she takes her insulin. But a person with hallucinations or recurrent depression who could find relief by taking psychiatric medications often encounters a societal stigma, and that stigma serves as a barrier to seeking treatment and taking medication.

Medications target maladaptive brain functioning. The brain contains more than 100 billion nerve cells, or neurons, that control energy level, appetite, sleep, and sex drive. Neurons both send and receive neurotransmitters as chemical signals to activate or inhibit the function of neighboring cells. Their effective release and uptake are essential in the functioning of the brain and resulting behavior. Psychotropic medications help targeted neurons to either uptake or release appropriate levels of neurotransmitters. Due to complexity, the development of effective treatments is difficult. In addition, improvement of efficacy and reduction of side effects continues to be a goal of medication development.

The effects of psychotherapeutic medications differ for each person, as does the duration of treatment. One person might need medication for a defined length of time and never need medication again to stay healthy. Another person, though, might need to take medication indefinitely (NIMH 2007a). People with severe illnesses such as schizophrenia need to take medications for the rest of their lives to stay mentally stable.

Classes of medication include antipsychotics, antimanics, antidepressants, and antianxiety medication. **Antipsychotic medications** are used to treat a person who is **psychotic**, or has lost contact with reality and may be having auditory or visual hallucinations or delusions. Antipsychotic medications counter these symptoms but don't cure them. This class of medications blocks neurotransmitters, particularly dopamine, which relieves the psychotic symptoms in a marked way. Side effects, though, can include stiff muscles, tremors, and abnormal movement. Newer medications with added potency and reduced side effects have entered the market, but they have the potential to cause other side effects that require patients to regularly monitor their blood level of the drugs.

Antimanic medications are used to treat bipolar disorder, which is a brain disorder that causes unusual shifts in a person's mood, energy, and ability to function (NIMH 2008a). Lithium is the drug most commonly used to treat bipolar symptoms (NIMH 2007a). It regulates severe mood swings; however, its severe side effects—nausea, weakness, fatigue, and significant weight gain—have led many patients to stop lithium treatment.

Antidepressant medications are used to treat major depression—depression far beyond what might be considered normal sadness or melancholy. These medications aren't stimulants. Instead, they restore brain activity to a functional level. Some people experience relief from symptoms within a few weeks of beginning treatment; for others, the medicine doesn't begin to work until as many as 8 weeks have passed. Different antidepressant medications target different neurotransmitters, so it's hard for doctors to figure out what medication will be most effective for a particular person or to determine if he needs more than one medication to improve symptoms. For that reason, patients need to stick with a regimen for at least 6 months to see if it's effective (NIMH 2007a). If it's not effective, they need to discuss discontinuing an antidepressant with the prescribing doctor because they might experience severe side effects if the medication isn't decreased and removed from the system properly.

Antianxiety medications are used to treat prolonged states or high levels of anxiety symptoms, including irritability, uneasiness and feelings of apprehension, rapid heartbeat, nausea, and breathing problems. Antianxiety medication is useful for treating panic disorders, phobias, and obsessive-compulsive disorder. Some antidepressant medications can treat anxiety disorders, too. Antianxiety medications provide immediate relief of symptoms and fall under the classification of benzodiazepines (NIMH 2007a).

Medication research is expanding to meet the needs of special groups, including children, the elderly, and pregnant and nursing women. Doctors have to take additional factors into consideration when they're treating special populations. For example, children aren't as verbal as adults, so they're less likely to report negative side effects. The elderly metabolize medication more slowly. They're also more likely to forget their regimen and to take excessive quantities of medication. Both over- and undermedicating can result in negative health consequences. When doctors prescribe medicine for pregnant or nursing women, they have to be sure the medicine won't result in birth defects or have negative effects on breast-feeding children.

PSYCHOLOGICAL THEORIES

Earlier in the chapter, you learned that treatment methods have changed over time. In the same way, theories about what causes healthy or unhealthy mental states have also changed over time.

Psychodynamic Theory

Psychodynamic theory developed from a belief that behavior results from subconscious conflicts in the psyche. Sigmund Freud (1856-1939) was a renowned psychiatrist who was the first to develop many psychodynamic theories, and his work is still studied today. Freud developed **psychoanalytic theory**, which asserts that much of mental life is unconscious and that past experiences, notably in early childhood, shape how one feels and behaves in life. Freud divided the personality into three parts: the id (the unconscious part of the brain that seeks pleasure from food, comfort, attention, and so on), the ego (the rational part of the brain), and the superego (the conscience). His theory held that when all three parts of the personality are in equilibrium, a person is mentally healthy (see figure 5.1). When a person's id is in conflict

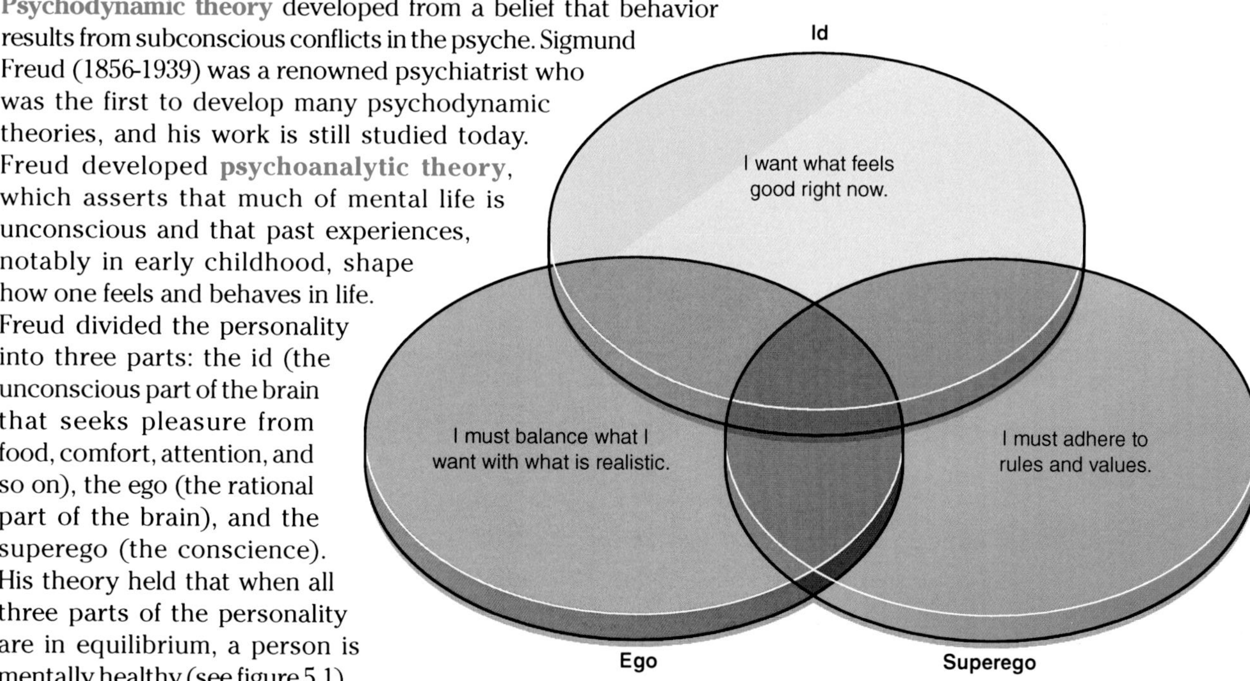

Figure 5.1 Freud theorized that people must achieve balance between the id (the unconscious), the ego (the rational), and the superego (the conscience).

with the superego and the ego cannot mediate the two, the imbalance will lead to mental disorders (U.S. Surgeon General 2007).

Behaviorism and Social Learning

Behaviorism, pioneered by J.B. Watson and B.F. Skinner in the early part of the 20th century, rejects psychodynamic theories and asserts that behaviors are learned from the environment and the positive or negative consequences of a person's behavior. For example, when a child cries because he skinned his knee and is soothed by a cookie from his mother, he is likely to cry when he simply wants a cookie or his mother's attention. Because behaviorists believe that maladaptive behavior is learned, they also believe it can be unlearned through behavior modification.

Social learning theory, led by Albert Bandura in the late 1960s, emphasizes the importance of observing and modeling the behaviors, attitudes, and emotional reaction of others as the key component of psychological development. According to this theory, people don't need to experience a consequence for behavior but can learn by observing the behaviors and consequences of behavior of those around them (American Psychiatric Association [APA] 1994).

Cognitive-behavioral therapy uses these theories of learning. Its approach to helping someone with a psychological problem is based on the belief that people have the ability to make changes in their lives without having to understand why the change occurs. (This approach is in contrast to psychodynamic theory, which attributes behavior to unconscious motivation.) Because cognitive-behavioral therapy isn't focused on a person's past, it is less time consuming and less costly than psychotherapy.

Albert Ellis is an important contributor to the field of cognitive-behavioral theorists. He used both theories to develop **rational emotive behavior therapy (REBT)** in 1955. The premise of REBT is that it's not an event that creates emotions but rather a person's thoughts and beliefs about the event that leads to her feeling anxious, or angry, or depressed (Health and Human Development Programs [HHD] 2007). REBT, then, challenges a person's belief systems and helps her develop healthier perceptions about life events. For example, if you believe that you're stupid and that you'll never succeed in life because you scored a low grade on a test, you'll be depressed. The resulting emotions probably won't be as powerful, though, if you learn to reframe the belief, such as "I may not have scored as highly as I would have liked, but I'll look for ways to achieve a higher score next time."

Proponents of behavioral and social learning developed theories about stages of development that help people achieve mental health. Lawrence Kohlberg defined stages of moral development that include the preconvention level, or self-focused morality (ages birth to 9); the conventional level, or other-focused morality (ages 9 to adolescence); and the postconventional level, or higher-focused morality (adulthood) (U.S. Surgeon General 2007).

Erik Erikson defined **stages of psychosocial development** (see table 5.1). He asserted that successful completion of each these stages would result in a healthy personality and healthy interactions with others. A person who didn't master these stages would be unhealthy. These are the stages that Erikson defined (Richmond 2008):

1. Trust versus mistrust (birth to age 1)
2. Autonomy versus shame and doubt (ages 1 to 3)
3. Initiative versus guilt (ages 3 to 6)
4. Industry versus inferiority (ages 6 to puberty)
5. Identity versus role confusion (adolescence through early adulthood)
6. Intimacy versus isolation (during young adulthood)
7. Generativity versus stagnation (middle adulthood)
8. Ego integrity versus despair (older adulthood)

TABLE 5.1 Erikson's Stages of Psychosocial Development

Stage	Age	Result of successful completion	Result of unsuccessful completion
Trust vs. mistrust	Birth to age 1	Learn to trust others	Feel anxiety and mistrust
Autonomy vs. shame and doubt	1 to 3	Learn confidence and independence	Remain overly dependent on others; lack self-esteem
Initiative vs. guilt	3 to 6	Learn to assert control and make decisions	Feel guilt; become inhibited
Industry vs. inferiority	6 to puberty	Learn confidence in your skills	Lack confidence in your skills
Identity vs. role confusion	Adolescence through early adulthood	Learn to be independent and in control	Feel unsure and doubtful about yourself
Intimacy vs. isolation	Young adulthood	Develop strong relationships with others	Lack close relationships; feel isolated
Generativity vs. stagnation	Middle adulthood	Feel useful in making good contributions to the world	Feel little involvement with the rest of the world
Ego integrity vs. despair	Older adulthood	Feel assured that your life was successful and fulfilling	Feel dissatisfied with your life; regret the choices you made

WHAT DETERMINES MENTAL HEALTH?

The question of what influences mental health remains controversial. Is it nature or nurture? Does the mind affect the body, or does the body affect the mind? What role does environment play?

Brain and Behavior

Advances in technology since the 1990s have allowed physicians to take pictures of the living brain, and those pictures have offered insight into mental health. The images indicate that functions of the brain affect mental outcomes, but those functions aren't necessarily predetermined or genetic. The brain and how it works are influenced by both genetics and interaction with environment.

For some time, mental health treatment was based on what scientists knew about how neurotransmitters in the brain function. They thought that levels of neurotransmitters in the brain, such as serotonin, were the primary determinants of depression or aggression. Science has expanded its understanding beyond the role of neurotransmitters, and now researchers are looking at the effects of genes, molecules, and environmental and social experiences on neural circuits (U.S. Surgeon General 2007).

Research suggests that mental disorders are the product of multiple genes, yet none has been identified for common mental disorders. The complexity of such studies is enormous because the human genome contains somewhere close to 80,000 genes. Family studies of mental illness have been beneficial in determining that genes do play a role in the predisposition to disorders. Though some diseases, such as cystic fibrosis, occur as a result of the transmission of a single mutation, it appears that mental illnesses are more genetically complex and arise from the interaction of multiple genes and environmental factors (Walker 2005).

Psychosocial Influences

The brain alone doesn't determine mental health functioning. Stress, mood, personality, and gender all influence mental health, as do parents, socioeconomic status, race, culture, religious affiliation, and social groups. Biology of the illness, risk factors, barriers to treatment, and factors that facilitate recovery all influence mental health and make it hard to identify a prognosis or outcome (U.S. Surgeon General 2007).

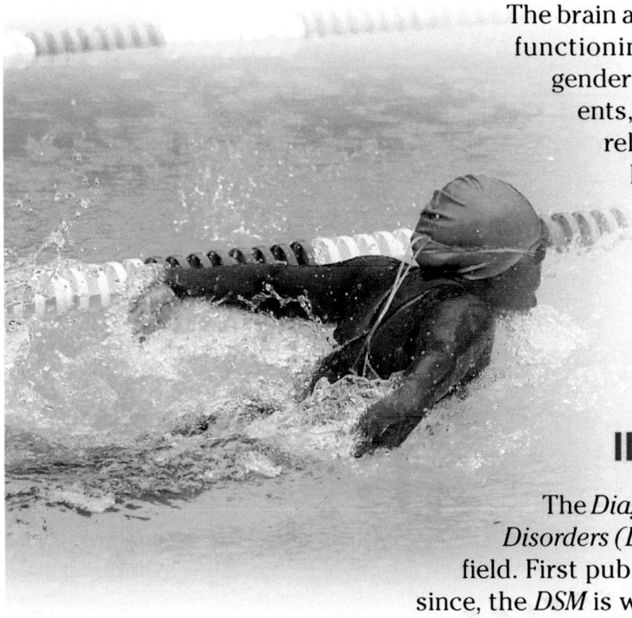

Working out by doing an activity you enjoy can help relieve stress.

© iStockphoto/dswebb

DIAGNOSING MENTAL ILLNESS

The *Diagnostic and Statistical Manual of Mental Disorders (DSM)* is the bible for the mental health field. First published in 1952 and revised four times since, the *DSM* is written by the APA. The manual helps mental health professionals identify whether a person's state of mind is normal. For example, it's normal for a person to experience grief following a significant loss. The *DSM* can help distinguish if the person's pattern of grief is normal and will resolve on its own with some support, or if it has become pervasive and requires additional intervention.

The *DSM* has five axes:

- Axis I: Clinical disorders
- Axis II: Developmental disorders and personality disorders
- Axis III: General medical conditions
- Axis IV: Psychosocial or environmental factors
- Axis V: Global assessment functioning

Axis I disorders are conditions that need clinical attention. Axis II records developmental and personality disorders so the clinician can take these diagnoses into consideration for additional intervention and treatment options.

Axis III defines current physical health problems that might be affecting mental health. This could include a life-threatening illness such as cancer, a chronic health illness such as hepatitis or HIV, a permanent physical disability, or a temporary health impairment such as undergoing chemotherapy.

Axis IV defines key psychosocial and environmental factors that might be affecting the client's mental health. Psychosocial factors include going through a divorce, moving from home to college, losing a job, or breaking off a relationship. Environmental factors could include an overcrowded living situation, lack of occupational opportunity, or perhaps an environment that triggers drug use.

Axis V estimates how well a person is functioning. There's a scale for people under age 18 and a scale for adults. The scale measures factors such as the ability to complete daily tasks independently and to participate in social interaction and activity. This scale allows the clinician to develop realistic treatment goals based on the client's functioning and to measure improvement or deterioration over time.

This section of the chapter will focus on axis I and axis II disorders because they're the most prevalent. Following are summaries of the disorders; they don't represent detailed diagnostic criteria.

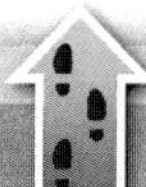

STEPS FOR BEHAVIORAL CHANGE

Mind Maintenance

It's hard to change behavior, but when it comes to managing daily stress, replacing negative coping skills with healthy habits can be well worth the effort. Poorly managed stress can lead to poor physical and mental health. Managing academic, social, and personal aspects of life is essential for your well-being and success. Here are some tips identified on a great resource, www.campusblues.com.

1. Add a workout to your schedule at least every other day. You don't have to consider yourself athletic or be in great shape to begin to jog; power walk; use stair-climbing, rowing, or biking machines; swim; or do any other form of exercise. Don't categorize these workouts as recreational time that you can blow off; instead, prioritize the time as a way to ensure that minor stresses don't build.
2. Identify and write down long-term (this semester or this year) and short-term (this day or this week) goals. Make them part of your time management schedule.
3. Develop a time management schedule that provides time for academic, social, and physical activities. Follow the schedule! Seek the help of an adviser in developing better time management skills.
4. Find 20 minutes of alone time to relax each day. Take a walk, write in a journal, or meditate.
5. Don't sweat the small stuff. When an issue arises, always ask yourself if it is worth getting upset about. If it isn't affecting your goal achievement, it may not be worth stressing over.
6. Keep a sense of humor and try to think positive.
7. Most important, communicate! Talking to a trusted friend, roommate, classmate, family member, professor, significant other, or coworker about issues of concern can be helpful. We all need someone to listen.

If this list seems overwhelming or unrealistic, you may already be overly stressed or depressed. Find other resources that can help you to work through current challenges and begin to achieve and maintain a fulfilling college career.

Axis I: Clinical Disorders

Clinical disorders include disorders usually first diagnosed in infancy, childhood, or adolescence (mental retardation, learning disorders, motor skill disorder, communication disorder, attention-deficit/hyperactivity disorder, tic disorders); anxiety disorders (obsessive-compulsive disorder, acute stress disorder); psychotic disorders (schizophrenia, schizo-affective disorder, phobias, post-traumatic stress disorder); mood disorders (bipolar disorder, depressive disorder); somatoform disorders (pain disorder, body dysmorphic disorder); eating disorders (anorexia, bulimia); impulse disorders (kleptomania, trichotillomania, pyromania); and substance-related disorders (alcohol-related disorders, amphetamine-related disorders, inhalant-related disorders, and so on).

Disorders Diagnosed in Infancy, Childhood, or Adolescence

This classification is for convenient diagnosis and treatment rather than to suggest differences between childhood and adult disorders. These disorders are present during childhood or adolescence, though sometimes they are not diagnosed until adulthood. In addition, a child might be diagnosed with an adult disorder, though this is not typical.

One such disorder is mental retardation, characterized by an IQ under 70 before age 18 and concurrent impairments in adaptive functioning. Learning disorders are characterized by academic performance significantly lower than expected for age and education. Attention-deficit/hyperactivity disorder (ADHD) is characterized by symptoms of inattention, hyperactivity, and impulsivity. Tic disorders, such as Tourette's syndrome, are characterized by vocal and motor tics.

Anxiety Disorders

Anxiety is a normal reaction to stress. It can be beneficial when it motivates you to focus attention and energy to study for exams or prepare for a job interview, for example. When anxiety loses its positive impact and becomes irrational or excessive, though, it may become a disorder. Anxiety disorders include generalized anxiety disorder, panic disorder, phobias, obsessive-compulsive disorder, and post-traumatic stress disorder.

Generalized anxiety may lead to excessive worry and anxiety regarding such events as work or school. This may lead to fatigue, irritability, difficulty concentrating, or sleep disturbances. Those with panic disorder suffer recurrent, unexpected panic attacks followed by concern, worry, or behavioral change related to the attacks. Obsessive-compulsive disorder (OCD) is characterized by recurrent, unwanted thoughts (obsessions) or repetitive behaviors (compulsions). Repetitive behaviors such as hand washing, counting, checking, or cleaning are often performed with the hope of preventing obsessive thoughts or making them go away. Performing the rituals provides only temporary relief, but not performing them markedly increases anxiety.

Post-traumatic stress disorder (PTSD) has received increased attention because it has been frequently diagnosed in veterans returning from the Iraq War. This disorder develops following personal exposure to an extremely traumatic event such as experiencing serious injury, witnessing a death, or learning about the violent death or injury of a close relation. It is characterized by recurrent symptoms resulting from exposure to the trauma and persistently reexperiencing the event for over a month. This experience is also known as a *flashback* and may result in prolonged distress and heightened arousal. Flashbacks are often extreme when the person is exposed to reminders of the traumatic event, also known as *triggers*.

Psychotic Disorders

Major symptoms of psychotic disorders are delusions and hallucinations. The major diagnoses are schizophrenia and schizoaffective disorders.

Contrary to common belief, people with schizophrenia don't have more than one personality. Multiple personality disorder is a different disorder and is quite rare. **Schizophrenia** is a chronic, severe, and disabling brain disorder. It often develops between the late teens and mid-30s and rarely occurs before adolescence, and it affects about 1.1 percent of the U.S. population aged 18 and older. In addition to hallucinations and delusions, symptoms can include disorganized speech, bizarre behavior, and inappropriate emotional responses. There is no cure for schizophrenia, treatments are less than optimal, and it is considered the most debilitating mental illness.

Schizoaffective disorder is characterized by hallucinations and delusions common to schizophrenia and by mood disorder symptoms. Though not as severe as schizophrenia, this illness is significantly debilitating.

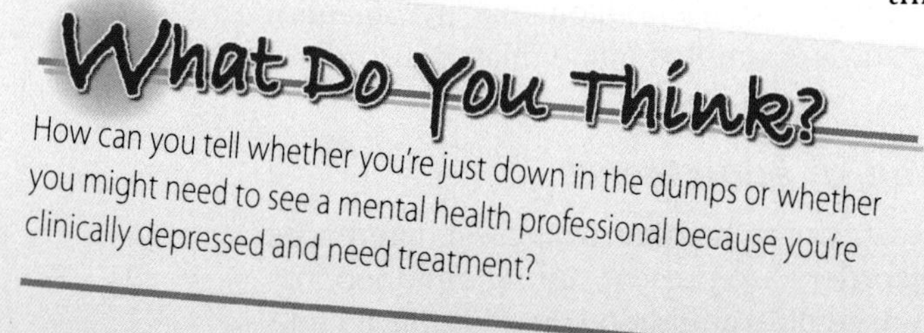

Mood Disorders

The primary symptom of mood disorders is a disturbance in mood. Similar to anxiety, sadness is a normal emotion that helps you cope with difficult situations. Excessive and debilitating sadness, though, might be diagnosed as depression. Some mood disorders include major depression and bipolar disorder.

CONTROVERSIAL ISSUES

Prison Interventions

According to a 2006 report by the U.S. Department of Justice, 55 percent of males and 73 percent of females in state prisons have mental health problems. The numbers are slightly lower in federal prisons and slightly higher in local jails. The rate of reported mental illness in the prison population is five times greater than in the general adult population (56.2 percent compared with 11 percent). Life in prison, needless to say, is not conducive to improved mental health. Not surprisingly, suicide is the leading cause of death among inmates, and almost all of those who commit suicide have a major psychiatric disorder.

Almost 90 percent of prisons have mental health services, and 1 in 8 prisoners receives mental health therapy. About 60 percent of prisoners who have been diagnosed with mental illness are receiving psychotropic medications for their condition.

The effectiveness of prison interventions is questionable. The Bureau of Justice Statistics report states that 58 percent of state prisoners with mental problems have been charged with violating prison rules and 24 percent have been charged with physical or verbal assault. Those statistics compare to 43 percent and 12 percent of their counterparts without mental health problems.

Last, 1 in 5 state prisoners with mental health problems has been injured in a prison fight, compared with 1 in 10 of state prisoners without mental health problems. Discrepancies in behavior between mentally ill and mentally healthy inmates continue despite interventions.

Signs of **depression** include persistent sadness, hopelessness, and feelings of guilt, worthlessness, and helplessness. People who are depressed often lose interest in things that once brought joy and may begin to isolate themselves from others. If not treated, depression can lead to suicide. The Centers for Disease Control and Prevention (CDC 2007) indicates that suicide emerges as a significant problem during the teen years, increases among young adults aged 20 to 24, and continues to marginally increase over the following two decades.

Bipolar disorder is also known as *manic depression*. It's a mental illness in which a person's moods swing from an elevated high (mania) to a severe low (depression). The periods of mania and depression last for different amounts of time, and they also vary in their severity.

Somatoform Disorders

Somatoform disorders have symptoms of medical conditions, but no medical condition can be found by a physician. Disorders in this category include somatization disorder, pain disorder, and hypochondriasis.

Somatization disorder is characterized by a pattern of recurring, multiple, and clinically significant somatic complaints that result in medical treatment or cause impairment in functioning before the age of 30. The complaints cannot be fully explained by a known condition, and if a medical condition exists, the complaints are excessive to what is normal. To meet criteria for this diagnosis, there must be pain symptoms that include two gastrointestinal symptoms, one sexual symptom, and one report of physical impairment. Pain disorder is similar but includes reported pain that is the predominant focus of clinical intervention, as well as a history of psychological factors related to the onset, severity, exacerbation, or maintenance of the pain. Features of hypochondria include a preoccupation with fears of having a serious disease based on misinterpreting signs and symptoms of the body. Hypochondriacs are able to acknowledge the possibility that the disease does not exist, but the worry causes impairment.

Eating Disorders

Eating disorders are defined by extremes: eating or not eating an extreme amount of food and having an extreme obsession with body shape or size. Eating disorders are complex, and despite research to understand them, the biological, behavioral, and social underpinnings of these illnesses remain elusive (NIMH 2008b).

People with **anorexia nervosa** usually have a body image disorder and refuse to maintain a healthy weight because they're intensely afraid of gaining weight. A person with anorexia will typically weigh herself excessively, have strict food rituals, and keep her weight down through excessive exercising or purging. Anorexia can affect the body in many ways. Menstruation may stop, osteoporosis might develop, the hair and nails may become brittle, and body temperature and blood pressure could drop. Many people with anorexia have other psychological disorders at the same time.

Bulimia nervosa is characterized by recurrent episodes of bingeing and purging. A binge is when a person eats a large amount of food in a short amount of time and feels a lack of control over the eating. After the binge, the person feels guilt and compensates by purging, fasting, or exercising excessively. A person with bulimia nervosa often has a normal weight but, similar to people with anorexia, he hates his body and body weight. The health impact of bulimia includes swollen neck glands, reflux disorder, dehydration, and worn tooth enamel that leads to sensitive and decaying teeth. People with bulimia often have other psychological disorders, too.

Binge eating disorder falls under the category of eating disorder not otherwise specified. The disorder is characterized by binge eating similar to that described for bulimia nervosa. However, binge eating is not followed by purging, excessive exercise, or fasting. As a result, people with binge eating disorder often are overweight or obese (NIMH 2008b). As in bulimia nervosa, the person feels out of control during the eating episode and feels guilt and shame after a binge. Health problems accompanying binge eating disorder include cardiovascular disease and hypertension. People with binge eating disorder often have co-occurring psychological disorders.

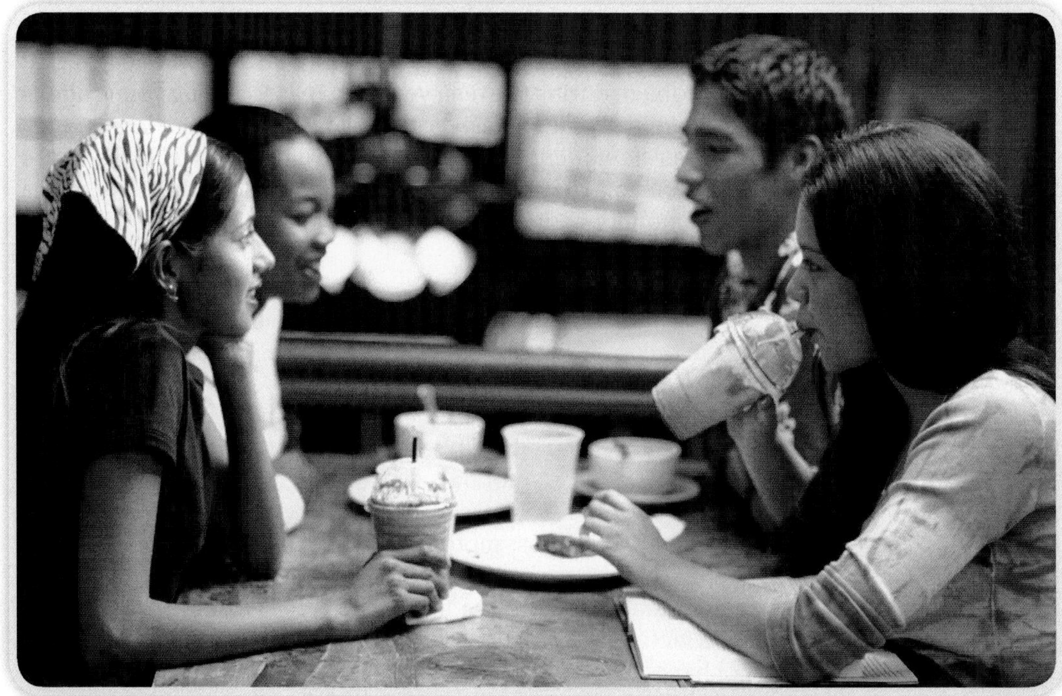

Socializing with friends often involves food, but sometimes the stress and responsibilities of college life can result in the development of an eating disorder.

© Photodisc

Impulse Disorders

Impulse disorders are characterized by the failure to resist the impulse to perform a harmful act. Most of the disorders result in the person feeling increased tension before the act, followed by pleasure or relief following the act. There may or may not be regret or guilt.

- Kleptomania involves the failure to resist impulses to steal items that are not of need or value. Tension rises before the theft and is relieved upon the theft. These thefts are typically unplanned and might be delayed if immediate arrest is possible.
- Trichotillomania involves the recurrent pulling out of one's own hair that results in noticeable hair loss. The place of hair pulling may include the scalp, eyebrows, or eyelashes. It often occurs in states of relaxation or distraction, such as watching television. Attempting to resist the urge to pull the hair often results in tension.
- Pyromania is diagnosed among people who experience arousal before setting a fire as well as a fascination with fire. They may watch fires, set off false alarms, and derive pleasure from people or equipment associated with fire.

What Do You Do?

The Internet is a great resource for communication, exploration, and having fun, but some people have trouble controlling the amount of time they spend surfing the Web. Some activities such as gaming or social networking kill time, but others such as online gambling and cybersex can cause serious problems. Some have proposed categorizing it as an impulse disorder and adding it to the next edition of *DSM* (Block 2008). However, others maintain that the disorder is mainly theoretical; for one analysis, see the Internet Addiction Guide at http://psychcentral.com/netaddiction.

If you want to take a nonscientific look at your own surfing habits, take the Internet Addiction Test. You can find it at www.netaddiction.com/resources/internet_addiction_test.htm.

Substance Use Disorders

The World Health Organization (WHO) estimates that 76.3 million people worldwide have an alcohol use disorder, and the United Nations Office on Drugs and Crime estimates that 200 million people use illicit drugs. According to the NIH, whites abuse alcohol more than other racial and ethnic groups, men abuse more than women, and youths abuse more than adults. The National Institute on Drug Abuse (NIDA) indicates that 74 percent of illicit drug users are white, but blacks have higher rates of use than other groups. These differences in gender and racial or ethnic groups do not differ for youths aged 12 to 17 (HHD 2007).

Levels of substance abuse are categorized in the *DSM* as *substance abuse* and *substance dependence*. **Substance abuse** is classified as use of a substance to the point where it is having a negative impact on the person's life. Negative impacts could include being arrested for drunk driving, having trouble maintaining healthy personal relationships, missing work or school, or going to work or school under the influence. In 2006, an estimated 22.6 million people (9.2 percent of the U.S. population aged 12 or older) were classified with substance abuse or dependence; 3.8 million abused or were dependent on illicit drugs; and 15.6 million abused or were dependent on alcohol but not illicit drugs. A little more than 3 million people were classified with abuse of or dependence on both alcohol and illicit drugs (SAMHSA 2007).

Substance dependence, often called *addiction*, means that a person builds tolerance and must increase the level of use to induce the same effect, the person continues use despite negative consequences and the desire to quit, and physical withdrawal symptoms occur when the level of the substance is not maintained in the body. Examples of withdrawal include potentially fatal symptoms such as delirium tremens or symptoms such as anxiety or headaches. If you drink a lot of coffee every day, you've probably gotten a headache when you forgot your morning dose. The headache is an example of a withdrawal symptom; however, that example doesn't qualify as a *DSM* diagnosis of substance dependence, because coffee drinking is unlikely to be causing severe negative consequences in relationships or social life.

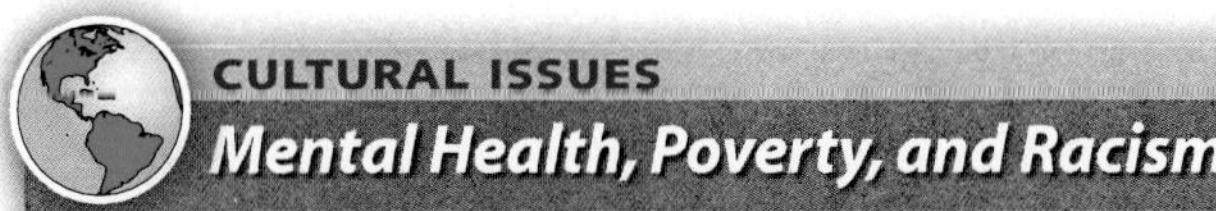

CULTURAL ISSUES

Mental Health, Poverty, and Racism

According to the U.S. Surgeon General's report on mental health (2007), living in poverty has a measurable effect on mental health. Those in the lowest strata of income, education, and occupation are two to three times more likely than those in the highest strata to have a mental disorder. Minority populations in the United States are overrepresented in the lower income brackets. Poverty rates in 2006 were as follows: non-Hispanic whites (8.2 percent), Hispanics (20.6 percent), Blacks (24.3 percent), and Asians (10.3 percent) (U.S. Census Bureau 2007).

Other factors affect mental health outcomes among minorities:

- Stress arises from discrimination and racism, predisposing people to depression and anxiety.
- Clinicians who are biased, who apply stereotypes, and who lack cultural competency deter minority populations from using mental health services.
- Many people who live in poverty do not have insurance to cover mental health services.
- Lack of services can lead to self-medication, which can initiate cycles of substance abuse and dependence.

A National Health Interview Survey (NHIS) following the aftermath of Hurricane Katrina serves as an alarming example of how racism can affect mental health. Before the hurricane, Louisiana had some of the worst health statistics in the country, with large health disparities between minorities and Caucasian residents. In the aftermath, uninsured people and Medicaid enrollees were more than twice as likely as those with private insurance to report fair or poor mental health, and 12 percent of the uninsured reported depression, which was twice the average in that area. The economically disadvantaged, the uninsured, and African Americans were significantly more likely to report a decline in health status following the hurricane than those who were financially secure, white, and insured. Of note, the most economically disadvantaged people were least likely to return to the area and participate in the survey (Hurricane Katrina Community Advisory Group and Kessler 2007).

Axis II: Development Disorders and Personality Disorders

As mentioned earlier, axis II disorders include childhood disorders, mental retardation, and personality disorders such as borderline personality disorder, narcissistic personality disorder, and paranoid personality disorder. The diagnosis of personality disorders is based on clinical syndromes with long-lasting and pervasive symptoms that affect the way people interact with their environment. People with personality disorders have more difficulty in every aspect of their lives because of maladaptive traits that cause discomfort and impair the ability to participate in everyday functions. Personality disorders include borderline, antisocial, histrionic, and narcissistic disorders.

Borderline personality disorder (BPD) is a serious mental illness characterized by pervasive instability in moods, interpersonal relationships, self-image, and behavior. A person with BPD may have intense bouts of anger and depression; cognitive distortions that lead to unstable goals, friendships, and values; chaotic relationships; and feelings of emptiness and lack of identity. People with BPD often try to injure themselves, and they have high rates of suicide attempts. BPD patients often need extensive mental health services, and they account for 20 percent of psychiatric hospitalizations. A fairly new cognitive treatment, dialectical behavioral therapy (DBT), has demonstrated promising results. This therapy allows patients to reexamine their thoughts and beliefs in order to challenge their reality and replace the thoughts with realistic ones. Though still in the experimental phase, it has shown promising results with deescalating destructive behavior.

Antisocial personality disorder is a pattern of disregard for and violation of the rights of others. This behavior begins in childhood or early adolescence and continues into adulthood. As a child, this behavior may be diagnosed as conduct disorder; however, the diagnosis of antisocial personality disorder can only be given to someone 18 years of age or older. Additional symptoms include behaviors that fail to conform to social norms and laws and may be grounds for arrest, deceitfulness, irritability and aggressiveness, reckless regard for safety of self or others, and lack of remorse for having hurt, mistreated, or stolen from another.

Histrionic personality disorder involves a pattern of emotionality and attention seeking. People with this disorder feel uncomfortable when they are not the center of attention and are often lively and dramatic to draw attention to themselves. They may gain attention through provocative or seductive behavior, display rapid shifting of shallow emotions, be easily influenced by the behavior of others, and consider relationships to be more intimate than they actually are.

Narcissistic personality disorder includes a pattern of grandiosity, need for admiration, and lack of empathy. People with this disorder often inflate their accomplishments and abilities and underestimate those of others. They may be surprised when others do not view them the same way. They tend to be preoccupied with fantasies of unlimited success, power, brilliance, beauty, or love.

TREATMENT MODALITIES

The stereotypical image of therapy for mental health is a person reclined on a couch telling the therapist about childhood traumas. Therapy has come a long way over the years, and a multitude of approaches exist to improve mental health. The methods for treating mental illness are referred to as **modalities**. Different treatments may work for a person based on current circumstances, beliefs, prejudices, and willingness. The therapist is only a facilitator of change; without a willing party, progress is unlikely (Richmond 2008).

Individual therapy uses the relationship between the therapist and client to examine and overcome current challenges. Clinicians use different therapy modalities, such as psychotherapy or cognitive-behavioral therapy. Many therapists use an eclectic model, selecting interventions from varying treatment modalities based on what will be most beneficial for the client. A client in individual therapy may benefit by concurrent family therapy, group therapy, or support group participation.

A family therapist is well trained in family systems, recognizing that all members play a part in triggering or sustaining a mentally disordered person's behavior. Group therapy incorporates both therapeutic guidance and peer feedback for improving mental health. Participants in a group can offer support, share ideas, learn social skills, and alleviate isolation during their treatment. Support groups are made up of people who face common challenges such as grieving, having an ill child, having a shared medical diagnosis, or undergoing mental health and addiction recovery. Support groups are typically facilitated by a layperson who shares the common issue of the participants. The mutual support is beneficial to participants and can lead to long-term change. People with mental illness and addictions benefit most from support groups after they have stabilized their condition.

What Do You Do?

Find the treatment options for mental health on your campus. Does the student health center provide counseling or diagnosis and treatment for mental health problems? Are campus support groups available for different situations, such as grief, stress, or anxiety?

GETTING HELP

All the information in the world about the history of mental health treatment, how mental health disorders are diagnosed, and how they're treated won't do any good if people don't know how to get help when they need it. This section covers how to get help for yourself or for friends who may need it.

When You Need Help

If you need help for mental illness, you might not know where to find it or might not want to find it because you're afraid of the stigma that goes along with treatment. When an emotional problem strikes, you might feel as if you should be able to deal with it on your own. Seeking professional services or medical treatment, getting support from others going through the same experience, and having the understanding of someone in your personal life can all be essential to getting through rough times or mental health concerns.

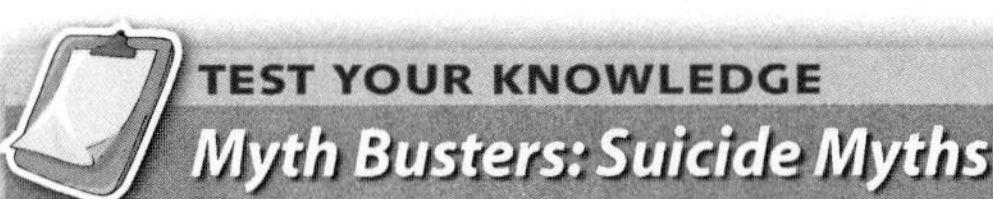

When it comes to a sensitive topic like suicide, it can be hard to separate myths from facts. Check out the following common myths about suicide and learn the truth.

Myth: People who commit suicide don't warn others.
Busted: Eight out of 10 people who kill themselves have given definite clues about their intentions.

Myth: People who talk about suicide are only trying to get attention. They won't really do it.
Busted: Most people who commit suicide let someone know their intention as a cry for help. More than 70 percent of people who threaten suicide either attempt or complete a suicide.

Myth: Nothing can keep a person who really wants to commit suicide from going through with the plan.
Busted: Most people who commit suicide are torn between wanting to live and wanting to die. They want their pain to end and see no other way to make it stop other than to take their own life. What they really want is a way to live, but without the relentless suffering. With intervention and support, they may be able to overcome their depression and lead a fulfilling life.

Myth: After a suicidal person begins to feel better, the risk of suicide is over.
Busted: The highest rates of suicide occur within 3 months of improvement from a severely depressed state. It is essential that the person continue to be monitored and be given psychological care and support.

Myth: After a person has attempted suicide, he is unlikely to try again.
Busted: Eighty percent of all people who die from suicide have made at least one previous attempt. A previous attempt is the strongest predictor of another attempt.

Myth: A drunk person who talks about suicide should not be taken seriously.
Busted: Over half of students who committed suicide were intoxicated, and a large percent were thought to have significant substance use problems. Anyone who discusses suicide should be taken seriously.

Myth: Mentioning suicide to someone who is severely depressed will increase the chance of her committing suicide.
Busted: Many depressed people have considered suicide, and mentioning it will not plant the idea in their head. Early discussion can help people feel understood and supported and allow them to better explore their feelings and get help.

When deciding to seek help, remember that mental health and physical health are closely related, that mental health problems can be treated, that mental health is complex, and that mental health problems are not a sign of weakness or something you can overcome with a quick attitude adjustment or surge of willpower (American Psychological Association Help Center 2004).

Sometimes entering a counseling session can be intimidating. The classic vision of a tweed-suited psychiatrist evoking deep secrets from a hypnotized client may even be a deterrent to making an appointment. The truth is, therapy has come a long way, but professionals have their own style and approach. If you are not comfortable in the atmosphere, you may want to select a different professional.

When you first enter the office, you will likely be asked for your insurance card or proof of student status. Next, there will be paperwork to complete, perhaps regarding the reason for your visit and some family history.

The goal of the first session is to become acquainted and to give the counselor a better idea of why you have sought counseling. Family history and your current psychosocial situation will offer insight into factors that may be contributing to your current status. Some people become frustrated that the real problem is not being immediately addressed. However, the only way a therapist can assist you is by having a complete picture of your circumstances.

These first sessions are also an opportunity for you to assess your therapist's ability to work with your particular issues. If you are not comfortable with the therapist's approach or history of working with similar clients, find a new therapist! Therapists are invested in your well-being and want you to find the right person to facilitate your progress.

Friends in Crisis

People who suffer from mental illness frequently exhibit signs that they are suffering. Mental health problems are often stigmatized, and your friends might not want to admit that they are having a difficult time coping. Being aware of warning signs and assisting someone in need can make the difference between life and death.

These behaviors might indicate underlying problems:

- Avoidance of friends, family, and social events
- Fixation on a problem
- Outbursts of anger or crying
- Sleep disturbances
- Change in eating habits or weight
- An outgoing person becoming withdrawn or a shy person becoming uncharacteristically active or erratic
- Excessive substance use

To help troubled friends, you have to talk to them (don't lecture, though). Take them seriously. Saying, "It's not a big deal" will only make things worse. Encourage them to seek help and offer to go with them. Let them know they can reach out to you. Joyce Walker (2005) coined the acronym *CLUES* to help people remember the five steps to helping a troubled person—**c**onnect, **l**isten, **u**nderstand, **e**xpress concern, and **s**eek help.

If a friend shows signs that he is in immediate danger, you need to take a more proactive approach. The warning signs for suicide include threats or talk of killing oneself; preparing for death by giving away prized possessions, saying good-byes, and writing good-bye letters; and saying that there is no hope. At least 75 percent of people who commit suicide demonstrate distinct warning signs (Governor's Suicide Prevention Advisory Commission 1998).

Violence

Not only are the warning signs for suicide apparent, but there are also behaviors that strongly signal when someone intends to harm others. Indicators of a person's propensity to violence

ISSUES IN THE NEWS

School Violence: Pointing the Finger

April 20, 1999, Littleton, Colorado: Eric Harris, 18, and Dylan Klebold, 17, both students at Columbine High School, shot and killed 14 students and 1 teacher, wounded 23, and then committed suicide. The two students had plotted for a year to kill at least 500 and blow up their school.

February 29, 2000, Mount Morris Township, Michigan: A 6-year-old boy at Buell Elementary School used a .32-caliber handgun to shoot and kill 6-year-old classmate, Kayla Rolland.

March 5, 2001, Santee, California: Charles Andrew Williams, 15, a student at Santana High School, shot and killed 2 and wounded 13 by firing from a bathroom at the high school.

March 21, 2005, Red Lake, Minnesota: Jeff Weise, 16, a Red Lake Senior High School student, shot and killed his grandfather and his companion. He then arrived at school where he killed a teacher, a security guard, five students, and himself.

April 16, 2007, Blacksburg, Virginia: Cho Seung-Hui, a 23-year-old Virginia Tech student, shot and killed two in a dorm. Two hours later, he went into a classroom building where he killed 30 more, wounded 15, and then shot himself, making this the most deadly shooting rampage in U.S. history.

February 14, 2008, DeKalb, Illinois: At Northern Illinois University, former student Stephen Kazmierczak walked into a lecture hall and began firing several guns into the crowd, killing 5 students and wounding 16, before shooting himself.

These are extreme cases of school violence that were highly publicized by the media. Are they isolated incidents, or are they indicative of a trend among young people toward violence? U.S. public schools experiencing violent incidents increased from 71 to 81 percent between 1999 and 2004, and 8 percent of teachers are threatened with violence on school grounds at least once a month (Constitutional Rights Foundation [CRF] 2008). What's causing this increase of violence? Two contributing factors are access to firearms and media influence.

In a 1996 study, 42 percent of 7th through 10th graders in large cities claimed they could get a gun if they wanted, and 28 percent reported handling a gun without an adult knowing (Bergstein et al. 1996). More than 35 percent of households with a minor have at least one firearm, so those statistics seem realistic.

According to the Center for Media Education, by the time the average American child reaches seventh grade, she will have witnessed 8,000 murders and 100,000 acts of violence on television (CRF 2008). Some studies suggest that violence in television shows, films, video games, and music increases aggressive behaviors among young people. Additionally, technology has allowed bullying and threats to expand beyond campus through text messaging and e-mail. Such behavior is called *cyberbullying*.

include losing her temper frequently, getting in physical fights, vandalizing property, using illegal substances more than usual, taking more risks, carrying a weapon, injuring animals, and making threats. Watch for these signs that a person may have immediate plans to harm others (Isothermal Community College 2008):

- Any direct statements about the intention to harm self or other people.
- Hints of intent to harm, such as saying, "I might not be around after the weekend," or "You may not want to be in class tomorrow," or "People might get hurt if they're not careful."
- Behaviors that suggest a person is planning his affairs, such as saying good-byes and telling others what he'd like done should something happen to him.
- Fascination with violence in music or games or admiration for violent media figures.

- Extreme difficulty adjusting to college life.
- Significant changes in behavior, appearance, moods, or activities.
- Statements about access to firearms and having them on campus.

Trust your instincts if you get the sense that someone might be planning violence. If you're wrong about somebody's intentions, the consequences are minimal. If you're right, you may prevent extreme damage. Talk to the person about your concerns and seek assistance from your on-site counseling department, a knowledgeable adult, a crisis hotline, or if necessary, the police.

What Do You Think?

Do the media glamorize school violence, making violent rampages a way for young people to seek fame? Do parents make such rampages possible through their ownership of weapons? Should schools be held accountable for preventing violence on campus, or should the media be more responsible regarding television, film, and video game production? Should YouTube and other Web sites be responsible for screening potential threats, or does responsibility ultimately lie with parents?

Prevention

The Institute of Medicine defines prevention in the mental health field in terms of three core activities: prevention, treatment, and maintenance. The goal of **prevention** is to intervene in ways that ward off the onset of a mental disorder. The goal of **treatment** is to identify people with existing mental illness, administer treatment, and try to prevent co-occurring disorders. The goal of **maintenance** is to reduce the likelihood of recurrence and to provide rehabilitation from the effects of mental disorders.

Prevention interventions must take into consideration risk factors for mental disorders as well as protective factors. **Risk factors** are variables that increase the likelihood that a particular person will develop a disorder. Risk factors include variables that are predetermined, such as gender or brain chemistry. They also include variables that can be modified through intervention. Living environment, lack of social support, and low self-esteem are examples of risk factors that can be modified.

Protective factors are variables that reduce the impact of risk factors. The role of protective factors is new and mental health professionals are doing research to learn more. Most intervention research identifies a risk factor among a population and then identifies interventions that might reduce the risk factor or increase protective factors. If the risk factor decreases or the protective factors increase, the intervention could be judged successful and it's less likely that the problem will continue. Some common risk factors to be targeted in research include neurophysiological deficits, family relation factors, chronic illness, and low socioeconomic status.

One example of figuring out a possible intervention strategy might be to look at suicide risk among a high-risk population such as college students. An identified risk could be social isolation among transfer students. In order to intervene, mental health professionals would attempt to reduce isolation through programs and groups targeted to assimilate transfers into their new campus setting. In addition, the campus could institute a 24-hour crisis line and develop ongoing activities targeting these students.

MENTAL HEALTH PROFESSIONALS

There are many diverse jobs within the field of mental health. Employee qualifications may be a specialty certificate, undergraduate degree, doctorate, or simply life experience. Opportunities exist in many settings, including community-based organizations, nonprofit organizations, hospitals, treatment centers, schools, colleges, private practice, and consulting firms. Education in the field of mental health provides a foundation for any career that involves working within the community or with clients.

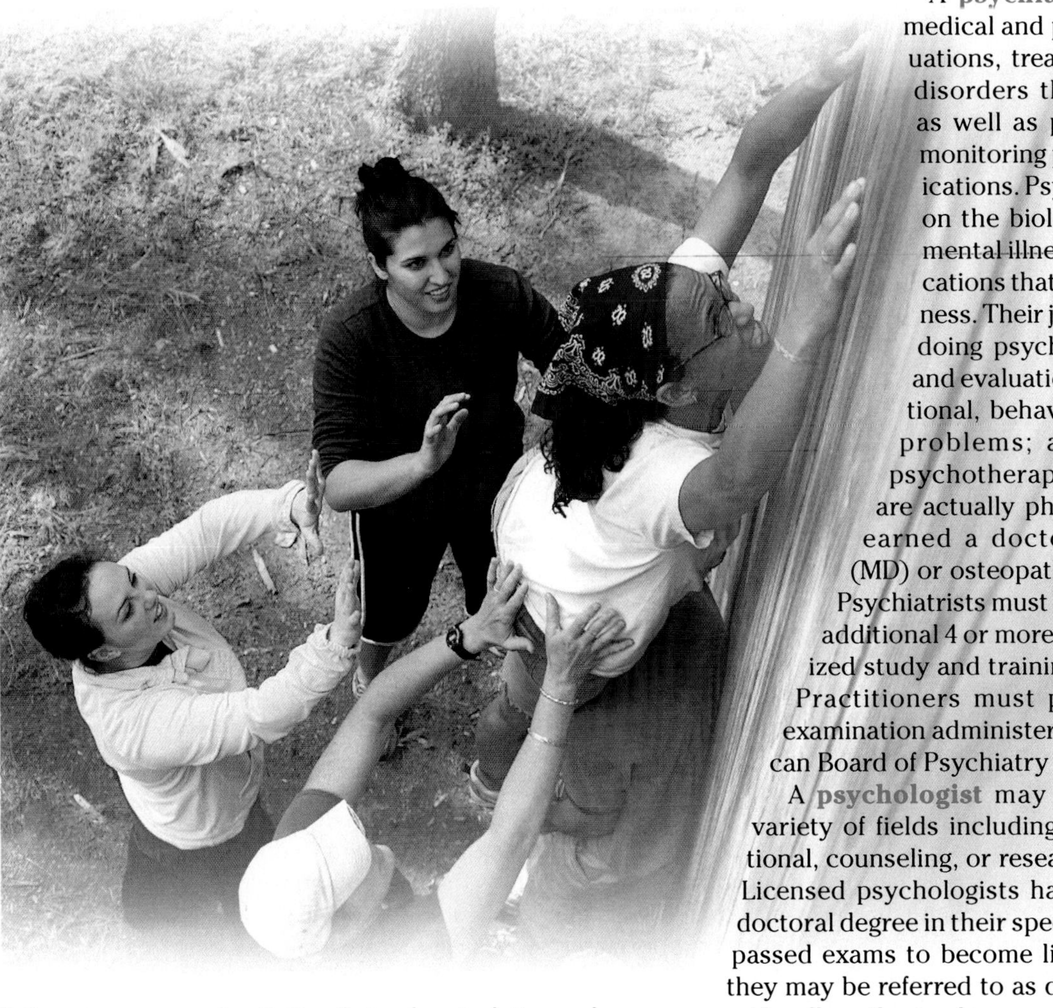

College programs and activities that reduce isolation and encourage students to form bonds can improve students' mental health.

© iStockphoto/Mark Rose

A **psychiatrist** conducts medical and psychiatric evaluations, treating psychiatric disorders through therapy as well as prescribing and monitoring psychiatric medications. Psychiatrists focus on the biological causes of mental illness and the medications that best treat the illness. Their job might include doing psychological testing and evaluation; treating emotional, behavioral, or mental problems; and practicing psychotherapy. Psychiatrists are actually physicians, having earned a doctor of medicine (MD) or osteopathic (DO) degree. Psychiatrists must also complete an additional 4 or more years of specialized study and training in psychiatry. Practitioners must pass a national examination administered by the American Board of Psychiatry and Neurology.

A **psychologist** may specialize in a variety of fields including clinical, educational, counseling, or research psychology. Licensed psychologists have completed a doctoral degree in their specialized field and passed exams to become licensed. Though they may be referred to as doctors, they are not legally authorized to prescribe medication. Psychologists generally work in hospitals, schools, clinics, or private practice.

A **licensed clinical social worker (LCSW)** may also specialize in a variety of fields, including treatment and assessment, case management, hospital social work, psychotherapy, or program oversight. The focus of the work usually revolves around psychosocial factors such as economic struggles, relationships, physical health, and social stressors. A 2-year master's degree in social work (MSW), an additional 2 years of supervised training, and the passing of state board examinations are required to be licensed. These professionals work in public and private settings that include schools, hospitals, mental health care facilities, community-based organizations, substance abuse treatment centers, court systems, and correctional institutions.

A **marriage and family therapist (MFT)** works with individuals and families. MFTs work with people who are experiencing problems with family relationships or other aspects that affect the family, such as divorce, family violence, and parenting. MFTs may work in clinics, hospitals, community-based organizations, schools, or private practice. Licensure requires a 2-year master's program and 2 years of experience under the supervision of an MFT.

A **mental health technician** and **mental health aide** work with emotionally disturbed or impaired people, usually in psychiatric hospitals or mental health clinics. They serve as part of an interdisciplinary team that usually includes psychiatrists, psychologists, and registered nurses. Job duties include helping patients with personal care and organizing or overseeing educational and recreational activities. Technicians and aides tend to spend more time with clients than other professionals on-site. A technician has more training than an aide and might assist with record keeping, administering medication, and planning and implementing treatment plans. Formal education includes postsecondary coursework at a vocational technical center or community college.

A **substance abuse counselor** trains to work with people who have substance abuse problems. Counselors may work in mental health agencies, hospitals, correctional institutions, or treatment facilities. Educational requirements to work as a substance abuse counselor range from a 2-year associate degree to a graduate degree, depending on the job responsibilities.

What Do You Do?

Below are some suggestions for maintaining mental health. Mark the ones that you think might help you stay mentally healthy during college. Then, write down what you can do to work on them. For example, if you marked "Get enough rest," write a phrase or two that describes what you'll do to get more sleep. You might write, "Make a weekly to-do list to ensure I can get all my work done without pulling more than one all-nighter in a month."

- Get enough rest.
- Eat a balanced diet.
- Avoid or moderate your intake of caffeine, alcohol, tobacco, or other drugs.
- Engage in physical activity, take time to do something fun, or relax.
- Meet your spiritual needs.
- Prioritize challenges and responsibilities.
- Develop a strong support network.

MENTAL HEALTH 101

Good mental health gives you an overall sense of well-being and the ability to adapt, maintain balance, and manage difficult situations. However, in the United States, about one in four adults suffers from a diagnosable mental disorder in a given year, and about half of all college students report that they've had trouble functioning due to depression. Despite advances in medical understanding over the years, the persistent stigma of mental illness and its limited care options prevent many people from seeking treatment, even though effective medications are available.

The APA's *Diagnostic and Statistical Manual of Mental Disorders (DSM)* helps professionals categorize a person's state of mind according to five axes. The most prevalent disorders fall under axis I (clinical disorders, which include anxiety disorders, psychotic disorders, mood disorders, substance abuse disorders, and others) and axis II (development and personality disorders, such as mental retardation, borderline personality disorder, antisocial personality disorder, and others).

It's important to recognize the signs of mental illness and seek the appropriate treatment. Professional counselors have different approaches, so choose a therapist that you're comfortable with. Watch for warning signs from friends and encourage them to get help, and take more direct action if you see signs of suicide or impending violence. Trust your instincts and be prepared to seek assistance or alert authorities as needed.

The goal of prevention is intervening to ward off the onset of mental illness, and it takes into account both risk factors and protective factors. Many diverse occupations exist in the field of mental health, including psychiatrists, psychologists, licensed clinical social workers, marriage and family therapists, mental health technicians and aides, and substance abuse counselors.

REVIEW QUESTIONS

1. How many Americans aged 18 and older suffer from a diagnosable mental disorder in a given year?
2. In the 16th century, what did society view as the cause of mental illness?
3. What is deinstitutionalization?
4. What kind of drugs are the most commonly prescribed medications in the United States?
5. According to Freud's psychoanalytic theory, what parts of the personality must be in balance for mental health?
6. What is the *DSM*, and what is it used for?
7. The *DSM* has five axes. Briefly describe two of those axes and give examples of the types of disorders in each.
8. Which psychotic disorder is considered the most debilitating mental illness, and why?
9. What is the strongest indicator that a person might try to commit suicide?
10. Give three signs that a person might have immediate plans to harm others through violence.

CRITICAL THINKING

1. Look at your own school and surrounding environment. What factors support good mental health? What factors put a person at risk for mental health problems? Think of stressors and pressures as well as systems in place to assist students.
2. Say you have a friend with bipolar disorder and the medicine she takes is effective at treating her symptoms but has made her gain 30 pounds (13.5 kilograms). She wants to stop taking the medicine because she's disgusted by the way she looks. What would you say to encourage her to keep taking the medicine?

APPLICATION ACTIVITIES

1. Create an intervention that will decrease the incidence of unhealthy behavior, such as smoking, drug use, alcohol abuse, or eating disorders, among young adults. Design a prevention intervention model. Describe how you will determine whom to target, how you will target them, and how you will select an intervention model. How will you measure the success of your model?
2. The Holmes-Rahe Life Social Readjustment Rating Scale, developed in 1967, assesses your risk of developing a stress-related illness based on events (such as divorce or personal injury) that have occurred during the past year of your life. Each event is worth a certain number of points, and you get your final score by summing the points for the events you've experienced. The Student Stress Scale, a recent adaptation of the Holmes-Rahe scale, includes more events (such as getting low grades or having car trouble) that are familiar to college students. Find both scales online and rate yourself. For each scale, your final score will give a rough estimate of how your stress might affect your health.

GLOSSARY

anorexia nervosa—An eating disorder in which a person is intensely afraid of gaining weight.

antianxiety medications—Medications used to treat prolonged states or high levels of anxiety symptoms, including irritability, uneasiness and feelings of apprehension, rapid heartbeat, nausea, and breathing problems.

antidepressant medications—Medications used to treat major depression (depression far beyond what might be considered normal sadness or melancholy).

antimanic medications—Medications used to treat bipolar disorder.

antipsychotic medications—Medications used to treat a person who is psychotic.

anxiety—A normal reaction to stress.

behaviorism—The theory that behaviors are learned from the environment and the positive or negative consequences of a person's behavior.

binge eating disorder—An eating disorder characterized by binge eating similar to that described for bulimia nervosa. However, binge eating is not followed by purging, excessive exercise, or fasting.

bipolar disorder—A mental illness in which a person's moods swing from an elevated high (mania) to a severe low (depression); also known as *manic depression*.

borderline personality disorder (BPD)—A serious mental illness characterized by pervasive instability in moods, interpersonal relationships, self-image, and behavior.

bulimia nervosa—An eating disorder characterized by recurrent episodes of bingeing and purging.

cognitive-behavioral therapy—The approach to helping someone with a psychological problem that is based on the belief that people have the ability to make changes in their lives without having to understand why the change occurs.

deinstitutionalization—The policy of moving severely mentally ill people out of large, state-supported institutions and then closing some or all of those institutions.

depression—Mood disorder characterized by excessive and debilitating sadness.

electroconvulsive therapy (ECT)—This method for treating depression involves giving a patient general anesthesia and a muscle relaxer, placing electrodes on the scalp, and applying a finely controlled electric current, which causes a brief seizure in the brain.

licensed clinical social worker (LCSW)—A mental health professional who may specialize in a variety of fields, including treatment and assessment, case management, hospital social work, psychotherapy, or program oversight. The focus of the work usually revolves around psychosocial factors such as economic struggles, relationships, physical health, and social stressors.

lobotomy—This method for treating mental illness involves drilling holes into the skull and using a blade to sever nerve fibers that run from the frontal lobes to the rest of the brain. Also known as *leucotomy*.

maintenance—Reducing the likelihood of recurrence and providing rehabilitation from the effects of mental disorders.

marriage and family therapist (MFT)—A mental health professional who works with individuals and families who are experiencing problems with family relationships or other aspects that affect the family, such as divorce, family violence, and parenting.

mental health—The absence of mental disorders and the mental functioning that allows for productive activities, interpersonal relationships, and adaptability.

mental health aide—A mental health professional who works with emotionally disturbed or impaired people, usually in psychiatric hospitals or mental health clinics. Job duties include helping patients with personal care and organizing or overseeing educational and recreational activities.

mental health technician—A mental health professional who works with emotionally disturbed or impaired people, usually in psychiatric hospitals or mental health clinics. Job duties include helping patients with personal care and organizing or overseeing educational and recreational activities. A technician might assist with record keeping, administering medication, and planning and implementing treatment plans.

mental illness—Abnormal brain processes that lead to impaired function.

modalities—The methods for treating mental illness.

prevention—Intervening in ways that ward off the onset of a mental disorder.

protective factors—Variables that reduce the impact of risk factors.

psychiatrist—A mental health professional who conducts medical and psychiatric evaluations, treating psychiatric disorders through therapy as well as prescribing and monitoring psychiatric medications.

psychoanalytic theory—The theory that much of mental life is unconscious and that past experiences, notably in early childhood, shape how one feels and behaves in life. When the id, ego, and superego are in equilibrium, a person is mentally healthy, but when a person's id is in conflict with the superego and the ego cannot mediate the two, the imbalance will lead to mental disorders.

psychodynamic theory—The theory that behavior results from subconscious conflicts in the psyche.

psychologist—A mental health professional who may specialize in a variety of fields including clinical, educational, counseling, or research psychology. Though they may be referred to as doctors, they are not legally authorized to prescribe medication.

psychotic—Describes a person who has lost contact with reality and may be having auditory or visual hallucinations or delusions.

rational emotive behavior therapy (REBT)—The approach to helping someone with a psychological problem that is based on the belief that it's not an event that creates emotions but rather a person's thoughts and beliefs about the event that lead to her feeling anxious, angry, or depressed.

risk factors—Variables that increase the likelihood that a particular person will develop a disorder.

schizophrenia—A chronic, severe, and disabling brain disorder. Symptoms can include hallucinations and delusions, disorganized speech, bizarre behavior, and inappropriate emotional responses.

social learning theory—The theory that emphasizes the importance of observing and modeling the behaviors, attitudes, and emotional reaction of others as the key component of psychological development. According to this theory, people don't need to experience a consequence for behavior but can learn by observing the behaviors and consequences of behavior of those around them.

stages of psychosocial development—The theory that describes eight developmental steps a person goes through, the completion of which results in a healthy personality and healthy interactions with others. A person who doesn't master these stages is unhealthy.

substance abuse—The use of a substance to the point where it is having a negative impact on the person's life.

substance abuse counselor—A mental health professional who works with people who have substance abuse problems.

substance dependence—The use of a substance to the point that a person builds tolerance and must increase the level of use to induce the same effect. The person continues use despite negative consequences and the desire to quit, and physical withdrawal symptoms occur when the level of the substance is not maintained in the body. Also known as *addiction*.

treatment—Identifying people with existing mental illness, administering treatment, and trying to prevent co-occurring disorders.

REFERENCES AND RESOURCES

American College Health Association. 2004. American College Health Association survey shows increase of depression among college students over four-year period. www.acha.org/newsroom/pr_ncha_11_18_04.cfm.

American Psychiatric Association (APA). 1994. *Diagnostic and statistical manual of mental disorders.* 4th ed. Washington, DC: Author.

American Psychological Association Help Center. 2004. Change your mind about mental health. www.apahelpcenter.org/featuredtopics/feature.php?id=37&ch=9.

American Psychological Association Practice Organization (APAPO). 2008. Congress should enact the Senate Mental Health Parity Bill. www.apapractice.org/apo/pracorg/legislative/mental_health_parity1.html#.

Benton, S.A., J.M. Robertson, W.-C. Tseng, F.B. Newton, and S.L. Benton. 2003. Changes in counseling center client problems across 13 years. *Professional Psychology: Research and Practice* 34 (1): 66-72.

Bergstein, J.M., D. Hemenway, B. Kennedy, S. Quaday, and R.J. Ander. 1996. Guns in young hands: A survey of urban teenagers' attitudes and behaviors related to handgun violence. *Journal of Trauma* 41 (5): 794-798.

Block, J.J. 2008. Issues for *DSM-V*: Internet addiction. *The American Journal of Psychiatry* 165: 306-307.

Centers for Disease Control and Prevention (CDC). 2004. Almost half of Americans use at least one prescription drug annual report on nation's health shows. Press release. www.cdc.gov/od/oc/media/pressrel/r041202.htm.

———. 2007. Suicide trends among youths and young adults aged 10-24 years—United States, 1990-2004. www.cdc.gov/mmwr/preview/mmwrhtml/mm5635a2.htm.

Constitutional Rights Foundation (CRF). 2008. Causes of school violence. www.crf-usa.org/school-violence/causes-of-school-violence.html.

Frick, K.L. 2002. Women's mental illness: A response to oppression. www.cwrl.utexas.edu/~ulrich/femhist/madness.shtml.

Governor's Suicide Prevention Advisory Commission. 1998. State of Colorado suicide prevention and intervention plan. www.sprc.org/stateinformation/PDF/stateplans/plan_co.pdf.

Health and Human Development Programs (HHD). 2007. Topics: Alcohol, tobacco, and other drug prevention. www.hhd.org/abouthhd/whatwedo_topics_alcohol.asp.

Helpguide. 2007. Improving emotional health: Strategies and tips for good mental health. www.helpguide.org/mental_emotional_health.htm.

Hurricane Katrina Community Advisory Group, and R.C. Kessler. 2007. Hurricane Katrina's impact on the care of survivors with chronic medical conditions. *Journal of General Internal Medicine* 22 (9): 1225-1230.

Isothermal Community College. 2008. Warning signs: How you can help prevent campus violence. www.isothermal.edu/publications/Warning%20Signs.pdf.

Kapner, D.A. 2003. InfoFacts resources: The Higher Education Center for Alcohol and Other Drug Abuse and Violence Prevention: Secondary effects of heavy drinking on campus. www.higheredcenter.org/files/product/secondary-effects.pdf.

National Institute on Alcohol Abuse and Alcoholism (NIAAA). 2005: College alcohol problems exceed previous estimates. www.nih.gov/news/pr/mar2005/niaaa-17.htm.

———. 2006. Young adult drinking. *Alcohol Alert* 68. http://pubs.niaaa.nih.gov/publications/aa68/aa68.htm.

National Institute of Mental Health (NIMH). 2007a. Medications. www.nimh.nih.gov/health/publications/medications/complete-publication.shtml.

———. 2007b. Mental health topics. www.nimh.nih.gov/health/topics/index.shtml.

———. 2008a. Bipolar disorder. www.nimh.nih.gov/health/publications/bipolar-disorder/complete-publication.shtml.

———. 2008b. Eating disorders. www.nimh.nih.gov/health/publications/eating-disorders/complete-publication.shtml.

Richmond, R.L. 2008. A guide to psychology and its practices: Types of psychological treatment. www.guidetopsychology.com/txtypes.htm.

ScienceWeek. 2005. History of medicine: On lobotomy. http://scienceweek.com/2005/sw050812-6.htm.

Substance Abuse and Mental Health Services Administration (SAMHSA). 2004. *Overview of findings from the 2003 National Survey on Drug Use and Health* (Office of Applied Studies, NSDUH Series H-24, DHHS Publication No. SMA 04-3963). Rockville, MD: U.S. Department of Health and Human Services. www.oas.samhsa.gov/NHSDA/2k3NSDUH/2k3OverviewW.pdf.

———. 2007. Illicit drug use. www.oas.samhsa.gov/NSDUH/2k6NSDUH/2k6results.cfm#Ch2.

Torrey, E.F. 1997. *Out of the shadows: Confronting America's mental illness crisis.* New York: Wiley. Excerpts are available online at: www.pbs.org/wgbh/pages/frontline/shows/asylums/special/excerpt.html.

U.S. Census Bureau. 2007. Poverty: 2006 highlights. www.census.gov/hhes/www/poverty/poverty06/pov06hi.html.

U.S. Department of Justice, Bureau of Justice Statistics. 2006. Study finds more than half of all prison and jail inmates have mental health problems. www.ojp.usdoj.gov/bjs/pub/press/mhppjipr.htm.

U.S. Surgeon General. 2007. Mental health: A report of the Surgeon General. www.surgeongeneral.gov/library/mentalhealth/home.html.

Walker, J. 2005. Helping friends in trouble: Stress, depression, and suicide. University of Minnesota Extension. www.extension.umn.edu/distribution/youthdevelopment/DA2787.html.

WebMd. 2008. Electroconvulsive and other depression therapies. www.webmd.com/depression/guide/electroconvulsive-therapy.

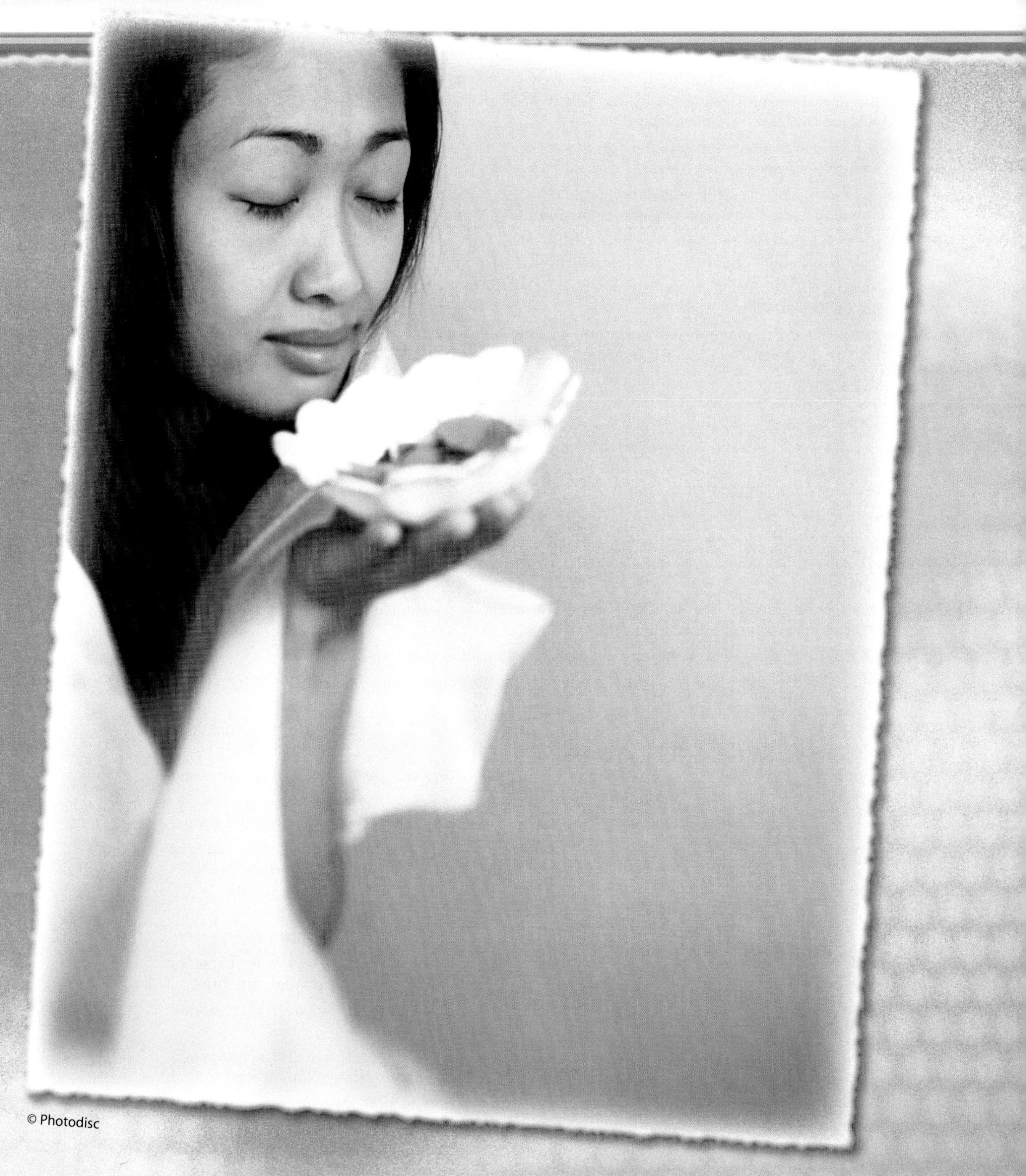

© Photodisc

CHAPTER 

STRESS MANAGEMENT

CHRISTINE PENDON, MPH, CHES
Los Angeles Air Force Base

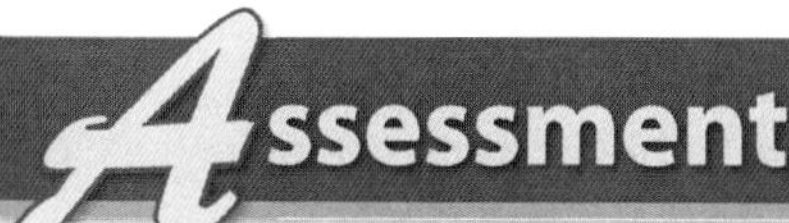

Assessment

- What is the fight-or-flight response?
- Is stress always negative, or can it be positive?
- In the United States, how many employees are absent from work each day because of stress?
- What role does stress play in cardiovascular disease, ulcers, cancer, and diabetes?
- Have you ever tried to relieve stress through deep breathing or muscle relaxation?
- How much sleep is needed to help relieve stress?
- Everyone manages stress differently. Do you think that you use positive or negative coping techniques?

Objectives

- Understand the effects of stress.
- Define *stress*, *stressor*, and *stress response*.
- Comprehend the four types of stress and the five types of stressors.
- Describe at least three diseases associated with stress.
- Identify at least three stress management techniques.
- Identify stressors in your life and learn coping mechanisms to deal with them.

Stress seems to be a way of life for college students. Relationships, school, work, decisions—everything piles up. If you don't know how to cope with stress, your body begins to feel the effects over time, and too much stress for too long can actually make you sick and even shorten your life. When you're stressed, your outlook and behavior also change.

Stress can be defined in many ways. According to Hans Selye, the father of modern research on stress and people's responses to it, stress is the "non-specific response of the body to any demand for change" (American Institute of Stress [AIS] 2007e). Since the early 1930s, researchers have struggled to define and understand stress. In 1932, Walter Cannon discovered the **fight-or-flight response** to stress in which the body automatically reacts to threatening situations by either confronting or fleeing the situation (Neimark n.d.). But it was not until 1956 that Selye identified and defined stress.

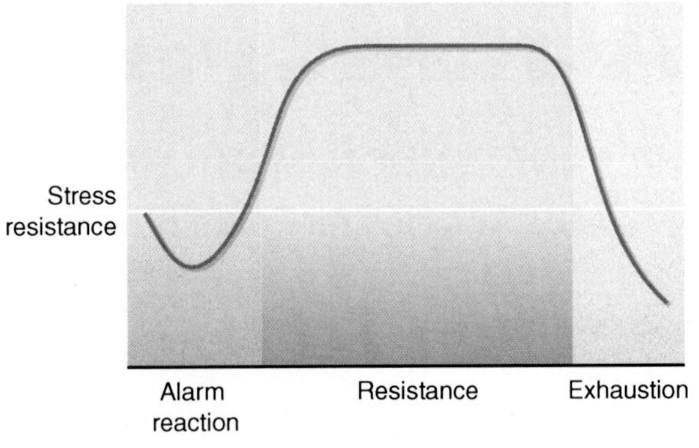

Figure 6.1 The general adaptation syndrome involves three stages of a person's response to stress.

Selye hypothesized that people exhibit physiological and behavioral changes in response to stressful situations. He expanded Cannon's theory and developed the **general adaptation syndrome (GAS)**. GAS consists of three stages: alarm reaction, resistance or adaptation, and exhaustion (see figure 6.1). Alarm reaction is similar to the fight-or-flight response. Resistance or adaptation is when the stressor is not removed and the body adjusts to function under the stressful condition. Once the body reaches its peak, it automatically goes into the exhaustion phase, in which the body begins to deteriorate and the person has a high risk for developing an illness (Holistic Online 2007).

According to Selye, stress is the body's nonspecific response to any demand of change (AIS 2007e). The term **stress** is typically used to describe a situation that causes a physical or an emotional reaction, as well as describing the reaction itself. For this chapter, stress defines a person's reaction to a situation or event. **Stressor**, on the other hand, refers to the situation causing the stress. **Stress response** describes any physiological changes associated with stress. For example, let's say you're focused intently on a TV show and your roommate bursts into the room and yells, "Boo!" You jump and yell, and you feel your heart racing. In that case, the surprise is the stressor, jumping and screaming is the stress, and the increased heart rate is the stress response.

Stress can't always be avoided. Trying to understand stress, its causes, and how to manage it can be difficult because there are several factors that can be associated with it. The purpose of this chapter is to provide an introduction to stress and stress management. It will cover key terms, types of stress and stressors, effects of stress on the body, the association of stress with diseases, and stress management techniques. If you understand the dynamics of stress and how to manage it, you might be able to reduce stress in your life and avoid developing poor health as a result of stress.

TYPES OF STRESS

Stress is complex because it consists of various causes, symptoms, and treatment. Although most people perceive stress as negative, it can also be positive. Getting into a car accident, studying for finals, breaking up with a boyfriend or girlfriend, or experiencing a death in the family are some examples of negative stressors, or **distress**. On the other hand, being promoted at work, going on vacation, or having a baby are examples of positive stress, or **eustress**. Stress is divided into four categories: acute stress, episodic acute stress, chronic stress, and traumatic stress.

Acute Stress

Acute stress is the most common form of stress. Some causes of acute stress include studying for an exam, caring for a sick child, or having a disagreement in a relationship. Acute stress lasts for a short time and is easy to manage. If you're dealing with acute stress, you might have emotional distress, headaches, nausea, and increased blood pressure and heartbeat (American Psychological Association [APA] 2007).

Episodic Acute Stress

Episodic acute stress is when you consistently experience acute stress. As acute stress for one situation fades, another stressor appears. Some causes of episodic acute stress include working on a project that has several deadlines or planning a wedding. Episodic acute stress will typically cause you to be disorganized, anxious, short tempered, or irritable. In most cases, people who experience episodic acute stress believe nothing is wrong with them, and they blame others for their behavior. Some common symptoms of episodic acute stress are headaches, migraines, hypertension, and chest pain. Treating episodic acute stress requires professional help, and it might take months to resolve it (APA 2007).

What Do You Do?

Following is a list of common stresses and stressors. How do you feel in each situation? Match each stress with a stressor.

Stress	Stressor
1. Happy	a. Car accident
2. Angry	b. Graduation
3. Scared	c. Planning a wedding
4. Frustrated	d. Earning an *A* on a final exam
5. Sad	e. Working a double shift
6. Confused	f. Finding out class is cancelled
7. Surprised	g. Relatives visiting
8. Calm	h. Going out on a first date
9. Excited	i. Riding on an airplane
10. Tired	j. Waking up late for class

Chronic Stress

Chronic stress is the result of constantly experiencing stressors. Unlike acute stress, chronic stress doesn't go away. Because the body is constantly at an elevated state (e.g., high blood pressure, increased heart rate), it is difficult for the body to relax and it's hard to bring its systems back to normal. Chronic stress is dangerous because it can put you at a high risk for adverse health effects. Some symptoms of chronic stress are high blood pressure, increased heart rate, irritability, and restless sleep. Treating chronic stress requires professional help and may take months to cure. If left untreated, people are at risk for committing suicide, becoming violent, having a heart attack or stroke, or getting cancer (APA 2007).

Post-Traumatic Stress Disorder

Post-traumatic stress disorder (PTSD) happens when a person experiences a dangerous or life-threatening event, such as rape, child abuse, war, car accidents, and so on. Each year, approximately 5.2 million Americans develop PTSD—it's something that could happen to anyone. Signs of PTSD may develop as early as 3 months after the event or take years to develop. Some signs are terror, loss of pleasure in activities related to the traumatic event, nightmares, insomnia, and social withdrawal. Treating PTSD requires professional help, and it can take months to cure. Several types of therapy are available to treat PTSD. If left untreated, it puts sufferers at a high risk for committing suicide, becoming violent, and developing psychological problems (APA 2007; MedlinePlus 2008).

TYPES OF STRESSORS

As you read in the introduction to this chapter, a stressor is the source of stress. Almost anything can be a stressor, including something that occurred in the past, something that's happening now, or something that will occur in the future. A stressor could be a person or an event. Stressors affect people differently. For example, preparing a dinner party for 15 guests could be stressful for one person, but another might find it enjoyable. This section will provide an overview of the five major categories of stressors: work, school, family, financial, and life changes.

Work Stress

Your parents or school counselors have probably told you that if you find a job in a field you love, it won't feel like work. That's not always the case. Work is one of the main stressors for many people. The increasing demands of work have resulted in an increase in employees reporting that they feel stress. According to the 2000 Attitudes in the American Workplace VI Survey, 80 percent of employees reported that they felt stress at work, and 40 percent reported that they needed assistance in learning how to manage their stress (AIS 2007b). Another survey found that one-fourth of workers view their jobs as the number one stressor in their lives (National Institute for Occupational Safety and Health [NIOSH] 2008). Stress is the second leading cause of employees reporting poor health at work.

Furthermore, according to the American Institute of Stress (AIS), every day approximately 1 million American employees are absent from work due to stress (AIS 2007b).

Some employers think that stress comes with the job and employees should learn how to manage it. However, with the increasing number of employees calling in sick because they are stressed, companies are losing money. Approximately $300 billion is spent by businesses annually on preventing or treating stress, dealing with reduced productivity and absenteeism as a result of stress, and increasing health insurance costs because of stress-related illness (AIS 2007b).

A study published in 2007 examined factors associated with job stress. The three variables examined were external resources (gender, age, type of employment), personal resources (extrovert or introvert, emotional stability, autonomy), and stressors (pressure from work). People (409 men and 346 women) who worked at least 20 hours a week participated in the study. Participants completed a questionnaire focusing on their personality, workload, work pressure, coping mechanisms, social support, and emotional exhaustion. The study found that employees' workload and pressure are strongly associated with their stress level, regardless of their external or personal resources (Michielsen et al. 2007). Still, the NIOSH model of job stress suggests that individual factors can affect the degree to which stressors cause stress in employees (see figure 6.2). For example, a worker who is worried about a sick child may have a harder time coping with stressors from his job, while the same pressures may have less effect on another employee who just won a big cash prize in a contest.

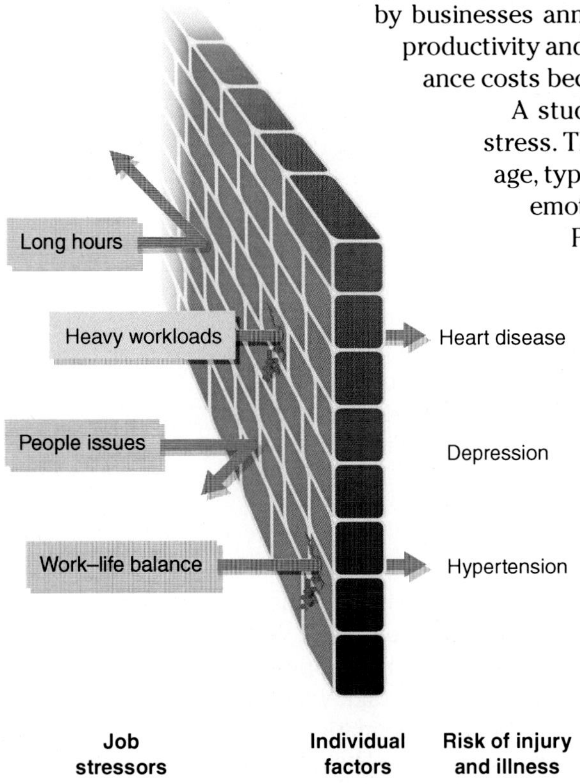

Figure 6.2 Employees with different individual factors in their lives can be affected differently by the same stressors at work.

National Institute for Occupational Safety Social Health 2008.

ISSUES IN THE NEWS
Technostress

Within the last 15 years, technology has become more and more a part of daily life. For example, computers, the Internet, and cell phones are some devices that have increased productivity and communication. But with the rapid pace of new technology developments, people are becoming overwhelmed and technostress has become more prevalent. Technostress is a negative reaction when people are fearful and resistant to change or adapting to new technology that is introduced at home, at work, and in recreational activities. Technostress develops because of the fast pace of technological change, lack of proper training, increased workload, lack of standardization within technologies, and reliance on hardware and software to function properly.

People who develop technostress are at an increased risk for poor job performance and judgments. Common symptoms of technostress include anxiety, headaches, mental fatigue, or feelings of helplessness. In order to cope with technostress, people can purchase more user-friendly equipment, enhance communication skills, be patient, and increase their awareness and education level (Weil and Rosen 2004).

Working longer hours, having heavy workloads, dealing with interpersonal issues, and trying to balance work and personal life are the four major areas causing stress in the workplace. The average work week in the United States is now 47 hours. According to the International Labor Organization, American employees work an extra month compared with Japanese employees and three extra months compared with German employees (AIS 2007b).

Work stress occurs when there's a mismatch between the job requirements and the employee's capabilities, resources, or needs. Each occupation has its own stressors. For example, teachers may feel stress from preparing lesson plans, ensuring that their students are learning the material, meeting the expectations of parents and administrators, and so on. Military members may feel stress that comes from intense training, working long hours, or being deployed. Studies have found that, regardless of the occupation, work stressors put employees at a high risk for experiencing burnout and for developing adverse health effects such as heart disease, depression, and hypertension (AIS 2007b; NIOSH 2008).

According to surveys conducted by private and governmental agencies, there has been a dramatic increase in workplace stress. The responses vary from self-reports to carefully worded questionnaires. We know that stress is worse now compared with the past because absenteeism has increased (800,000 employees call in sick every day, triple the number from 1996 to 2000), Americans are working longer hours (on average 47 hours per week), homicides occurring in the workplace are the second leading cause of death at work (20 U.S. employees are murdered each week), $300 billion is spent annually by businesses due to stress, and job turnover is 40 percent due to stress. These surveys were conducted from 1990 through 2000.

Employers can do some things to reduce or prevent workplace stress. Identifying potential stressors, compromising with employees to balance work and life, implementing stress management courses, increasing support from management, and providing incentives to employees for their hard work are all ways to manage the effects of stress at work. Because most adults spent the majority of their time at work, it is important to create a healthy work environment to keep employees healthy and productive (AIS 2007b; Kelly and Colquhoun 2005; NIOSH 2008).

School Stress

School is another place where people spend a lot of time. Until the past few years, researchers didn't think school caused a lot of stress, but students are reporting that they're experiencing more stress than in past years. Robotham and Julian (2006) conducted a study that reviewed previous research on students' stress levels in higher education. The review found that students were not considered to be a high priority in stress research, and it is believed that the increase in students reporting that they are stressed is due to their increased awareness of the signs and symptoms of stress. Financial pressures, studying, and the transition to college life were the three areas that were examined.

In a 2007 study of 350 college freshmen, researchers asked participants to complete a survey that consisted of questions focusing on their physical health, alcohol use and smoking, perfectionism, optimism or pessimism, psychological adaptation, self-esteem, coping tactics, and personality. The results concluded that it was difficult for freshmen to cope with their stressors. Participants reported that they experienced more negative moods (anger, anxiety, depression, and tension) compared with positive moods. Also, participants reported that instead of using positive coping techniques, they increased their alcohol consumption (Pritchard, Wilson, and Yamnitz 2007).

School stress isn't limited to college students, either. Elementary and high school students report that they feel stress, too. For example, one study found that high school students who lived in low socioeconomic areas felt more distress than students who lived in high socioeconomic areas (Solberg, Carlstrom, Howard, and Jones 2007). Lack of school materials, overcrowding in classrooms, and poor educational curriculum were some of the identified stressors.

Regardless of the educational level, the demands of school have increased from previous years and students feel more stress. For example, in the 1970s American teachers and parents did not put a lot of pressure on children regarding their education. In the 1980s, American teachers and parents increased the pressure because children's reading skills were not at the same level as that of students in other countries. Today, teachers, parents, and school boards are increasing the pressure and stress on children by requiring students to learn more material and participate in extracurricular activities without increasing the time frame of the school day or year (Davis 2000). A study was conducted in 2005 to find out what worried kids most about going back to school. The study found that 600 students between the ages of 14 and 17 reported schoolwork (32 percent), social issues (30 percent), appearance issues (25 percent), nothing (10 percent), and extracurricular issues (3 percent) (KidsHealth 2005). Transitional changes, lack of support from teachers and family members, and lack of resources are some of the things that cause students to feel stress (Solberg et al. 2007). To reduce school stress, teachers, administrators, and family members need to be aware of the signs and symptoms of stress and encourage students to practice stress management techniques to relieve their stress.

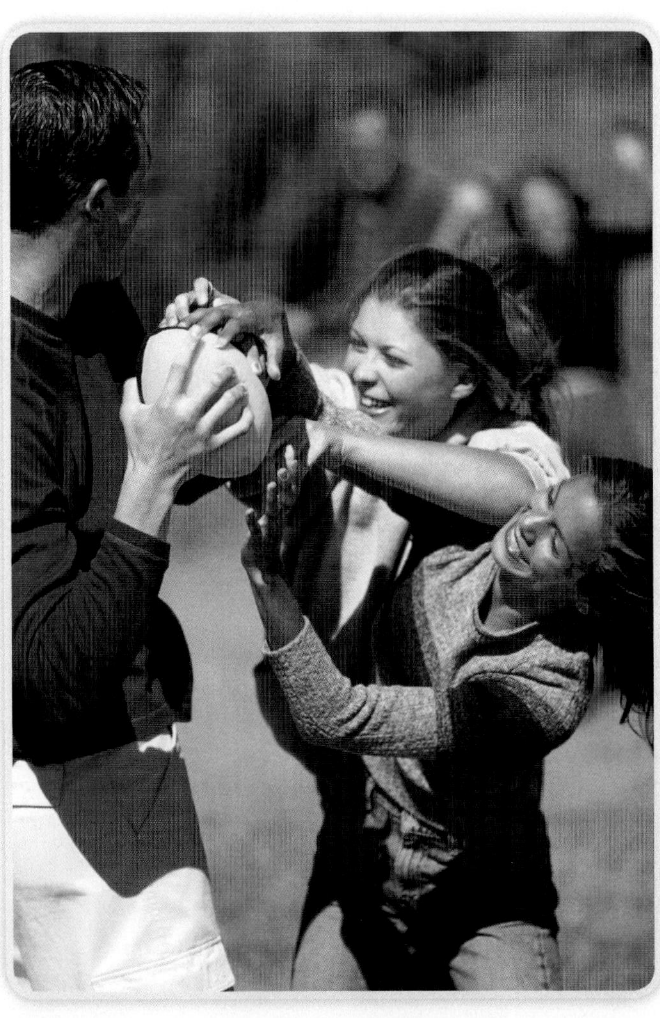

Getting exercise and playing games with friends can help students relieve stress.

© Photodisc

CULTURAL ISSUES

School Six Days a Week?

Earning an education plays a vital role in being successful in life. However, the stress that is associated with academia differs for each country. For example, stress levels differ between American students and Japanese students because of the time that is spent at school and studying. The duration of a school year in the United States is 180 days, or 5 days a week, whereas in Japan it is 240 days, or 6 days per week (Harper 2008). Japanese students in elementary and junior high schools have approximately half a day of classes on Saturdays, and students in high schools attend classes on Saturdays for about 5 hours (Frasz and Kato n.d.). In addition, many Japanese students attend cram schools several nights a week to prepare for entrance exams, further reducing their free time (Weisman 1992). Due to the amount of time spent in school and studying, Japanese students have little time to relax and enjoy their youth.

Family Stress

Along with stress from work and school, family members can also be sources of stress. According to the 2006 APA survey, mothers felt more stress compared with fathers, because mothers reported they were primarily responsible for taking care of the household, children, grandparents, and other family responsibilities (APA 2007).

Each person feels family stress differently. Some of the common stressors within a family include completing household chores, handling financial concerns, getting an education, and negotiating living arrangements. Caring for an ill family member is one of the major stressors within families. Having to make decisions about the type of treatment that should be given, health insurance, and living arrangements is stressful. Additionally, family members must try to balance work, take care of household and school obligations, and keep up with their normal activities and responsibilities.

Studies have shown, though, that support from family members has a positive effect as ill family members go through the recovery process. For example, a study that examined family members' roles during rehabilitation found that when people who are ill view the illness as a family problem rather than as an individual problem, they have a more successful recovery. Dealing with the illness together as a family provided a sense of comfort and reduced the stress level for all family members (Rosenthal, Ferrin, Wilson, and Frain 2005).

It's almost impossible to avoid stress from family members, and trying to cope with family stressors can be hard. In most instances, the stressor affects more than one person, and others in the family might handle the situation differently. Learning to cope with family stressors could prevent the situation from getting worse. One of the most effective techniques for dealing with family stressors is honest and open communication among family members.

Financial Stress

Financial issues are a major contributor to a person's stress level. It does not matter if you are single or married; the idea that making more money will bring more happiness and reduce stress is false. More money does provide the ability to do more things, but research has found that most people do not adjust their lifestyles in ways that would increase their overall happiness and reduce their stress level. According to the 2006 APA survey, money was the top source of stress for adults and approximately 60 percent of participants associated their stress with money and work (APA 2007).

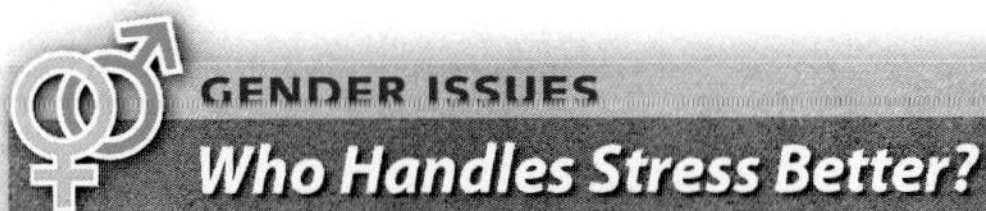

Is there a real difference in how men and women cope with stressors? Men and women have different coping mechanisms because of their biological makeup. Cortisol, epinephrine, and oxytocin are the three hormones that affect how men and women handle stress. Both men and women produce all three types of hormones, but oxytocin is the key to the difference in how men and women handle stress. When a stressful situation occurs, the brain releases a large amount of oxytocin in women, making them feel more relaxed, whereas oxytocin is released only in small amounts in men.

Along with trying to manage your own money, research has found that financial concerns are one of the top reasons why married couples fight and divorce. Since the 1960s, the divorce rate has been increasing in the United States. In the 1960s, the divorce rate per 1,000 people was 2.6 percent, and the rate rose to 5.2 percent in the 1980s. Based on the current trend, it is estimated that 40 to 50 percent of all first marriages in the United States will end in divorce (Psychology Encyclopedia 2007). In order to avoid arguments and divorce, it is important to recognize that financial issues are not just about the numbers. Clearly communicate your philosophies about money management, spending habits, and financial planning. When discussing financial concerns, make sure you discuss them at an appropriate time and place where you are less likely to be distracted. It is not appropriate to talk about financial issues when you are shopping at the mall, for instance. And lastly, understand that talking about finances can cause some debate. If the conversation becomes too heated, take a time-out. Let your partner know how you feel and that you may need some time to think about what is being said, and continue to discuss the issue when both of you are calm (Equality in Marriage Institute 2008).

Financial stress can cause people to develop unhealthy coping strategies such as drinking alcohol, smoking, insomnia, hostility, anxiety, depression, and so on. In order to prevent or reduce financial stress, it is important to review your expenditures. Make a list of all financial obligations. Try to cut down on your debt. For example, limit the number of times you go out to eat at restaurants or buy new clothes. And lastly, be a smart shopper. Before you buy something new, consider whether that item is a necessity and will benefit your overall quality of life. In many instances, spending less will reduce your stress level (Scott 2007b).

Major Life Changes

Many situations happen every day that can cause stress. Events that change a person's life can be some of the most stressful. Dealing with change is difficult for most people, and learning to adjust behavior to accommodate changes can bring on stress.

Major life changes can be positive or negative. Getting married, graduating from college, or moving out of your parents' home are examples of life-changing events that are usually positive. Being raped, developing a chronic illness, or losing your job are examples of negative life events. Whether the life changes are positive or negative, you need to learn how to cope during these times because they have been associated with the development of adverse health effects such as hypertension and heart disease (Cromer and Sachs-Ericsson 2006). Learning how to handle stressors, especially during major life changes, could prevent you from getting sick in the future. The next section describes what happens to the body when it experiences stress.

EFFECTS OF STRESS ON BODY SYSTEMS

Stress affects the systems in the body and puts you at risk for adverse health effects. Everybody responds differently to stressors, so stress effects vary from person to person. For example, stressors could bring on a migraine in one person and depression in another.

Stress can affect you on many levels. Here are some of the symptoms that are associated with stress (Insel and Roth 2002):

- **Cognitive symptoms:** Headaches, insomnia, difficulty remembering things, inability to concentrate
- **Physiological symptoms:** Ulcers, increased heart rate, hypertension, sexual problems, gastrointestinal problems, frequent illnesses, increased respiratory rate, disruption in glucose production and breakdown
- **Behavioral symptoms:** Crying, disrupted eating habits, grinding of teeth, hostility, increased use of substances, difficulty communicating with others, social isolation
- **Emotional symptoms:** Crying, fatigue, anxiety, depression, hypervigilance, impulsiveness, irritability

This section describes how stress affects the systems in the body and the health risks associated with stress, which are summarized in table 6.1. Each system (cardiovascular, nervous, digestive, and immune) has a specific function, and stress can affect all of them because they are all connected. For example, if stress caused a heart attack, all four systems would suffer. The cardiovascular system would be affected because the heart couldn't pump blood. The nervous system would be affected because the heart attack would cause low blood flow to the brain. The digestive system would be affected because the lack of oxygen to the brain would impair its ability to tell the body how to properly break down food. And the immune system would be affected because with the heart unable to pump blood, the body couldn't react quickly to fight off illness or infection.

Cardiovascular System

The cardiovascular system consists of the heart and blood vessels (arteries, capillaries, and veins). Pulmonary circulation connects the heart and the lungs in a loop, and systemic circulation sends blood from the heart to other parts of the body.

Several studies have examined the association between stress and cardiovascular disease (CVD). For example, one study examined the relationship between burnout and CVD. The study found that burnout puts people at a higher risk of CVD and cardiovascular-related events, even if the stressor disappears. Because the body adapted to function under stressful conditions, it was difficult for it to go back to working at normal levels (Melamed et al. 2006).

The effects of stress on the cardiovascular system could cause major health problems. When the body is under stress, blood vessels constrict, causing heart rate and blood pressure to increase. People who experience chronic stress are at a higher risk of developing CVD, hypertension, and atherosclerosis, a disease that blocks blood vessels with fatty deposits (Insel and Roth 2002).

TABLE 6.1 Effects of Stress on Body Systems

System	Possible effects of stress
Cardiovascular	CVD, hypertension, atherosclerosis
Nervous	Reduced ability to perform essential tasks
Digestive	Inflammatory bowel disease, ulcers, irritable bowel movement, gastroesophageal reflux disease, intestinal barrier function
Immune	Lowered immune functions, potentially leading to autoimmune disorders, immunodeficiency disorders, allergies, or cancers

Nervous System

The nervous system consists of the brain, spinal cord, and nerves. It functions both under voluntary control and under the autonomic nervous system. When your brain signals your feet to run up the stairs, you're experiencing an example of voluntary control. Your heart beating, on the other hand, is an example of the autonomic system at work. The autonomic nervous system has a parasympathetic division and a sympathetic division. The parasympathetic division is at work when people are relaxed and the sympathetic division is at work when they are aroused (APA 2008).

One study examined people who feel they have a purpose in life and the effects of that feeling on the nervous system. Participants (32 men and women) were asked to complete the Manifest Anxiety Scale, the Cornell Medical Index, and the Youth and Adulthood Experiences Inventory. Afterward, they were asked to watch a video of a roller coaster, which would be used to measure the effects of stress on the nervous system. The study concluded that participants who had a positive childhood and who believed they had a purpose in life were less likely to experience stress and had better coping strategies. Participants who didn't believe that they had a purpose in life were more likely to experience stress (Ishida and Okada 2006).

Because the nervous system plays a vital role in the body, its inability to function properly could alter a person's life. The nervous system is the main communication line to every part of the body. The effects of stress on the nervous system can damage the ability of the body to perform essential tasks, such as walking, reaching for a cup, and so on.

Digestive System

The digestive system consists of the alimentary canal (digestive tract), liver, and pancreas. The alimentary canal includes the stomach, intestines, and esophagus. The digestive system absorbs food into the body. Food is broken down into nutrients, vitamins, and minerals and is distributed throughout the body. Waste is removed from the body as feces.

Several studies have examined the association between stress and the digestive system. A review of past literature determined that people develop inflammatory bowel disease (an inflammation of the intestines that can lead to ulcerative colitis and Crohn's disease) due to the effects of stress on the neurotransmitters, hormones, and immune cells. As a result, the digestive system can't properly produce acids to break down the food and get rid of waste (Niess et al. 2002).

People who don't learn how to manage their stress are at risk for developing trouble with the digestive system. Stress, especially chronic stress, could cause the body to create more acid and slow down gastric emptying. Stress has been known to cause ulcers, irritable bowel movements, gastroesophageal reflux disease, intestinal barrier function, and inflammatory bowel disease (AIS 2007a).

Immune System

The immune system consists of tissues, cells, and organs. Its purpose is to protect the body from anything that could cause illnesses. There are two types of immunity: innate (or natural) and acquired (or adaptive). Innate immunity is found naturally in the body; skin and mucous membranes are two examples. Acquired immunity is immunity that is developed throughout life. It can be either *active* or *passive*. Hepatitis shots and tuberculosis shots are examples of active immunity. Passive immunity is immunity that is taken from another source, such as when babies receive antibodies from their mother's breast milk.

In a study that examined the effects of stress on the immune system and aging, researchers examined stress levels during the stages of life. The study found that acute or chronic stress early in life lowered people's immune functions. In other words, the effects of stress early in life aren't necessarily observable at the time, but as people grow older, their ability to fight off illnesses and infections decreases (Graham, Christian, and Kiecolt-Glaser 2006).

Having a strong immune system is important for maintaining a healthy life. Although there are several defense mechanisms to protect the body, experiencing stressors throughout life reduces the ability of the immune system to fight off illnesses or infections. If the immune system is unable to fight, stress could put a person at risk for developing autoimmune disorders (when the body mistakenly attacks healthy organs and tissues), immunodeficiency disorders (when the immune system is not working properly), allergies, and cancers.

STRESS AND DISEASE

Many studies over the years have examined the association between stress and various diseases. Stress is one of the most common underlying factors associated with diseases. Several studies have found that stress is linked to all leading causes of death, which include cardiovascular disease, cancer, accidents, and suicides. Stress caused or complicated 90 percent of diseases (Smith, Jaffe-Gill, and Segal 2008). The purpose of this section is to provide an overview of the association between stress and diseases. This section will discuss five of the major health problems that currently affect many Americans' lives: hypertension, CVD, cancer, obesity, and diabetes.

Hypertension and Stress

Blood pressure is the strength with which the blood pushes against the artery walls (see figure 6.3). The systolic measure of blood pressure is when the heart beats, and the diastolic measure is when the heart is at rest. Both the systolic and diastolic pressures are used to measure blood pressure, with the systolic pressure presented over the diastolic pressure. Normal blood pressure is less than 120 over 80 mmHg. A measure of 140 over 90 is considered high (MedlinePlus 2007b). Because the nervous system plays a vital role in the body, its inability to function properly could alter a person's life. The nervous system is the main communication line to every part of the body. Chronic exposure to stress can cause the body to create a large amount of unhealthy hormones, such as adrenaline and cortisol, which contributes to hypertension.

Hypertension (high blood pressure) is known as the silent killer because it usually has no symptoms. Although hypertension is most common in adults, people of any age can develop it. According to the CDC, one out of three American adults has hypertension. In 2002, hypertension was the leading contributor to 277,000 deaths in the United States, and in 2006, the United States spent approximately $65 billion to prevent and treat hypertension (CDC 2007b).

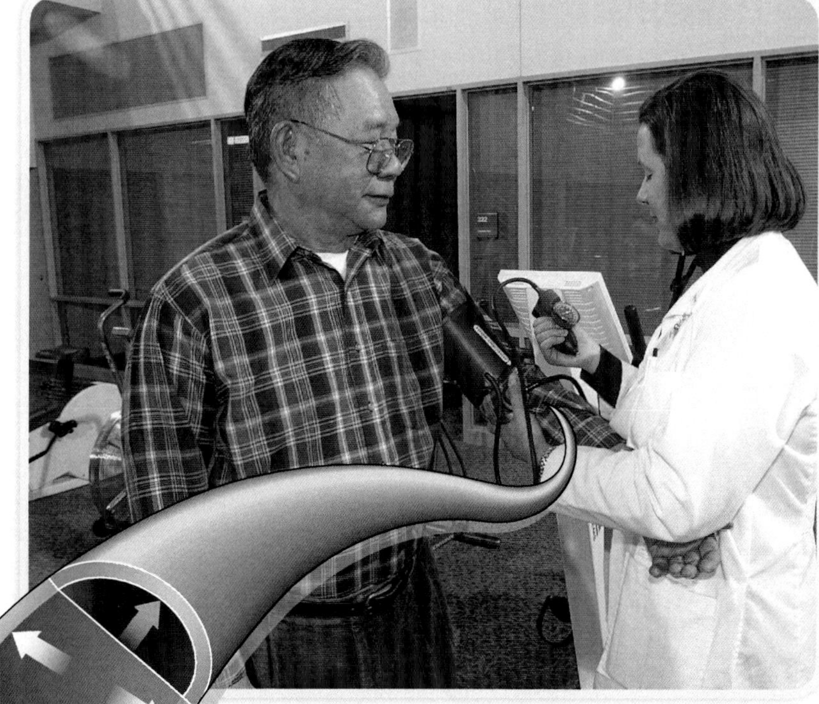

Figure 6.3 When a doctor checks your blood pressure, she's checking just that—literally, the pressure that your blood exerts against the walls of your arteries.

Stress is a major contributor to the development of hypertension. A study examined whether there was a difference in stress levels among several occupations and the development of hypertension. The study found that although each job had a different stress level, there was no difference in the development of hypertension (Rau 2006). In other words, it's true that different jobs have different levels of stress, but job stress contributes to the development of hypertension regardless of the occupation.

Cardiovascular Disease and Stress

Any disorder that develops in the heart or blood vessels could cause CVD. This group of diseases includes coronary heart disease (CHD), atherosclerosis, cerebrovascular disease, hypertension, peripheral artery disease, rheumatic heart disease, congenital heart disease, and heart failure. Cardiovascular disease is the leading cause of death for Americans, killing approximately 700,000 Americans each year. In 2005, 17.5 million people died from cardiovascular disease worldwide (World Health Organization [WHO] 2007).

Several studies show that constant stressors, such as job stress or parental stress, activate the stress response, causing the heart rate and blood pressure to rise (AIS 2007c; Morelius, Lundh, and Nelson 2002). Researchers have found that people who react to stressors in a hostile manner have a higher risk for developing CVD than people who respond to stressors calmly (AIS 2007c). Both acute stress and chronic stress put a strain on the heart and increase the risk of developing CVD.

When the body is under stress, blood vessels constrict, causing heart rate and blood pressure to increase. People who experience chronic stress are at a higher risk of developing CVD, hypertension, and atherosclerosis (Insel and Roth 2002).

Cancer and Stress

Cancer develops when cells grow abnormally. There are many types of cancers, including breast cancer, lung cancer, prostate cancer, and others. According to the National Cancer Institute (NCI), approximately 1,444,920 Americans got cancer in 2007, and approximately 559,650 Americans died from the disease (NCI 2007).

Stress can cause the body to activate the endocrine system to create unhealthy hormones that can affect the immune system. Although it is not a known fact that the effects of stress on the immune system are a direct cause of cancer, the body's inability to properly fight off illnesses or diseases does contribute to the development of cancer cells.

Having cancer causes an enormous amount of stress for patients and their families and friends. One study was conducted to determine if stress had different effects on people of various races who had breast cancer. A total of 200 women who were diagnosed with breast cancer participated in the study. Half of the participants were Caucasian and half were African American. Participants were asked to complete the Stress Symptom Checklist. The study concluded there was no difference between race and the level of stress among cancer patients. However, participants who were able to manage their stress and accept the challenges of cancer had a more successful recovery than the participants who had unhealthy levels of stress.

Regardless of the type of cancer, the stress that patients experience could lead to the development of other health problems. Therefore, learning how to cope with cancer is one of the simplest and most effective tools for ensuring a healthy recovery and preventing the development of other health problems.

CONSUMER ISSUES

Stress Insurance?

Most health insurance doesn't cover stress prevention or treatment options. Should these options be covered given the health effects of chronic stress? Where would the line of coverage be drawn? For example, should health insurance cover getting a massage or taking a vacation because those activities can relieve stress? Would you pay extra for health insurance that offered coverage?

Obesity and Stress

Obesity describes people who have a body mass index (BMI) of 30 or higher. An adult who has a BMI between 18.5 and 24.9 is considered to be in a healthy weight range. A

BMI of 25.0 to 29.9 indicates overweight. According to the CDC, approximately one-third of American adults are obese (CDC 2007a). In 2002, the United States spent approximately $117 billion on the direct and indirect costs of obesity.

Although several factors are associated with obesity, such as diet and exercise, stress is also a major contributing factor to its development. For example, stress can alter the ability of the digestive system to break down foods, and it can also cause fatigue, which might keep people from exercising (Insel and Roth 2002).

A lot of people use food as a coping mechanism for stressors. For example, one study found that job stress increased eating among employees (Nishitani and Sakakibara 2005). Overeating contributes to obesity. When people encounter a lot of stressors, they typically consume more food at a faster pace. As a result, the body doesn't have enough time or energy to properly break down the food and release it, which causes the excess food to be stored in the body (CDC 2007a, 2008a).

Diabetes and Stress

Throughout the United States, 20.8 million children and adults have diabetes. Diabetes is a disease that prevents the body from properly producing or using insulin. Insulin is a hormone that converts sugars, starches, and other foods into energy. There are two major types of diabetes: Type 1 diabetes is when the body cannot produce insulin, and type 2 diabetes is when the body cannot properly use insulin.

Stress affects people who have diabetes because it alters their blood glucose levels. Under stress, the ability to utilize the fight-or-flight response is ineffective because the body is unable to produce the insulin that is needed to create the extra energy to take action. Chronic stress plays a major role in diabetes because the body is continually releasing stress hormones. Whether it is physical stress, such as recovering from a surgery, or mental stress, the stress hormones that are produced directly alter blood glucose levels (American Diabetes Association 2008).

STRESS MANAGEMENT TECHNIQUES

Everyone experiences stressors daily, and everyone responds to them differently. Some people feel that dealing with their stress will cost thousands of dollars. However, several inexpensive and effective stress management techniques are available, such as exercise or yoga. This section describes some of the easiest and most effective stress management techniques available.

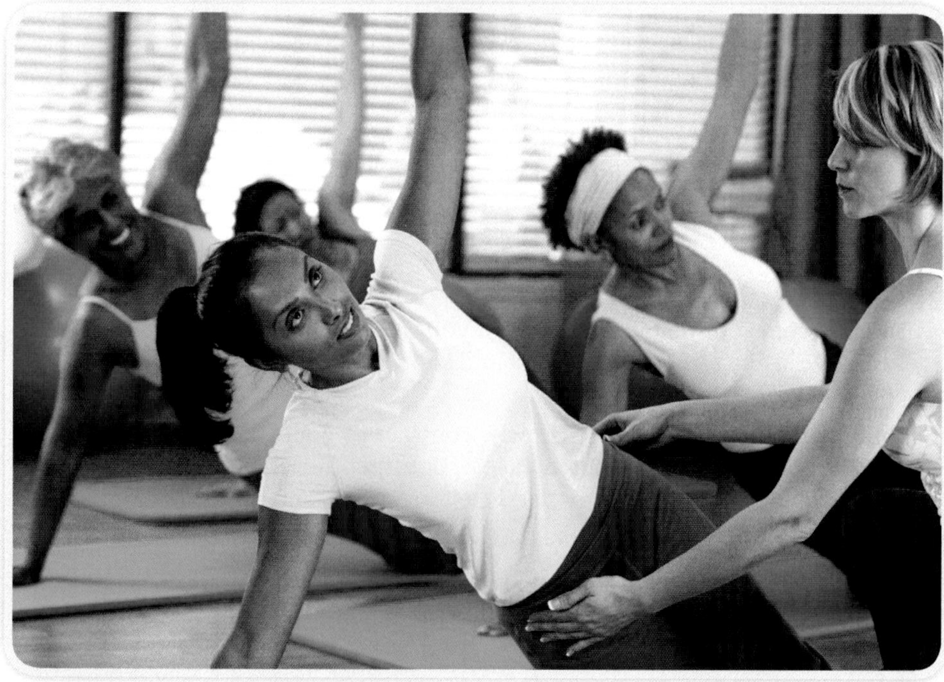

Taking a yoga class will not only increase your balance, strength, and flexibility, but it can also help you learn to manage your stress.

© John Feingersh/Blend Images/Getty Images

Meditation

Meditation originated in Eastern religions and has been adopted by Western culture. Meditation doesn't require formal training or education. The purpose of meditation is to clear your mind, calmly thinking about what's causing your stress and regaining a sense of peace by focusing on calming yourself.

Different forms of meditation have developed over the years. Two common forms of meditation are **mindfulness** and **concentration meditation**. You can practice mindfulness by sitting alone in a quiet room and focusing your attention on any object or process, such as a sound or breathing. Concentration meditation is used in religious and spiritual practices. People who practice concentration meditation typically focus their attention on a prayer. Both forms of meditation are effective and simple, and you can practice either technique anywhere.

Deep Breathing and Muscle Relaxation

Breathing is associated with stress level. For example, deep, slow breathing demonstrates that you're relaxed and calm; fast, shallow breathing indicates that you might be feeling stress. Practicing **deep breathing** can help you slow your breathing pattern, quiet your mind, and relax your body (Lewis 2007).

It's important to practice deep breathing correctly. To practice deep breathing correctly, you need to breathe from the diaphragm, not from the chest (see figure 6.4). Practicing deep breathing can be beneficial to your health because the diaphragm is connected to the heart, lungs, and other internal organs. Breathing diaphragmatically allows more oxygen to enter the body.

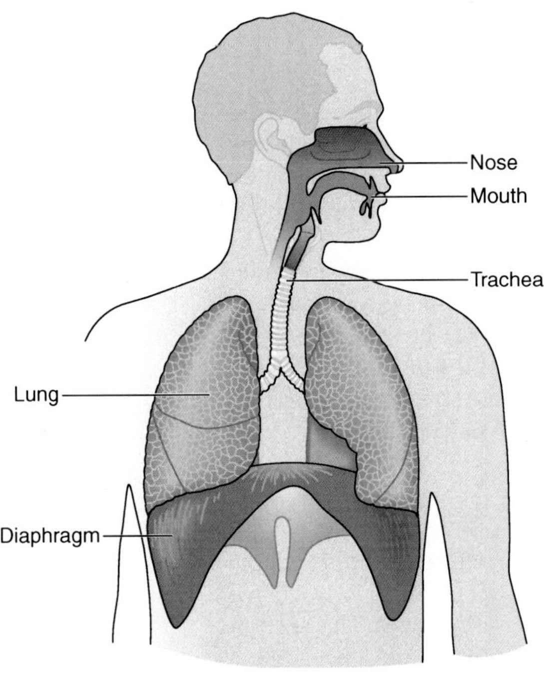

Figure 6.4 When you breathe deeply from your diaphragm, it contracts, drawing the lungs down and allowing more air to enter your body.

In 1930, Edmund Jacobson developed the **progressive muscle relaxation technique** to help relieve stress and anxiety. He believed that relieving tension from the muscles would calm the mind and relieve stress. Many physicians use the progressive muscle relaxation technique in combination with other therapies to help patients experiencing stress. The technique is simple; you don't need formal training or education to use it. Simply tense and relax various muscle groups while sitting or lying in a relaxed position.

Try the following exercise that combines deep breathing and muscle relaxation. Take your pulse for 1 minute before you begin and again when you're finished to see if your heart rate changes as a result of using these techniques.

- Sit back with your feet flat on the ground, relax your arms, and close your eyes.
- Inhale deeply, hold your breath for a few seconds, and slowly exhale. Make sure that you're breathing from your diaphragm and not your chest. If you're doing it right, your stomach will move in and out, but your chest and shoulders will stay still. Continue deep breathing two or three times.
- As you continue to breathe in and out slowly, contract or squeeze the muscles of the right leg, hold it for a few seconds, and release it. Contract the leg muscles two or three times, and then move on to other body parts (left leg, right arm, left arm, shoulders).
- After you've gone through the major muscles of the body, inhale deeply, hold it for a few seconds, and slowly exhale.
- Repeat two or three times and then open your eyes.

Deep breathing and muscle relaxation might not work for everyone. Did you see a difference in your pulse after the exercise?

Nutrition

Coping with stressors by eating isn't necessarily a healthy practice, because a combination of poor diet and stress can increase the risk of developing adverse health effects. However, using good nutritional practices to manage stress is effective (Holistic Online 2007).

Maintaining a healthy diet is one of the most effective ways to reduce and relieve stress. Incorporating more whole foods, nutrients, and vitamins into your diet will help reduce stress because the body will be more prepared to handle stress when it occurs. Studies have found that when people experience stress, their nutrients and vitamins are depleted. Limit or avoid these foods to reduce stress levels (Holistic Online 2007):

- Caffeine: It affects the nervous system and can cause insomnia if you consume too much.
- Sugar: It doesn't provide any nutrients. Although sugar provides an immediate high, it's followed by a prolonged low.
- Alcohol: It depletes vitamins and nutrients. It can cause insomnia and impairs judgment.

Exercise

Exercise is an effective tool for reducing stress. Several studies have examined the relationship between exercise and stress management. For example, one study found that exercise increases the ability of the body to mobilize energy and prepares the body to better cope with stress when it occurs. Another study found that exercise puts people in a more relaxed state because it reduces anxiety and blood pressure (Exercise and Stress Connection 2007).

Although exercise helps you stay healthy and reduces stress, it's not always an easy habit to incorporate into daily life. With increasing demands from work, family, school, and so on, trying to fit in some time to work out can be hard. A gym workout is one avenue to reduce stress, but it isn't the only one. Just being more active in your daily activities can add light to moderate exercise to your day. For example, using the stairs instead of the elevator and washing your car by hand instead of going through the automatic car wash are two examples of ways to add a little exercise into your day. Regardless of the exercise you choose, the simple fact that you're being active will reduce your stress level and improve your overall well-being (Exercise and Stress Connection 2007).

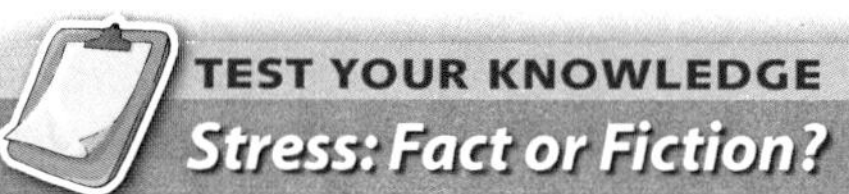

TEST YOUR KNOWLEDGE

Stress: Fact or Fiction?

Read each of the following statements and determine if it is fact or fiction.

1. It's common for people who return from war to experience PTSD.
2. Different stressors affect people differently.
3. Most people can't cope with acute stress.
4. Meditation is the best stress management technique.
5. Stress can alter body functions.
6. Writing a class paper is not a stressor.
7. Learning how to manage your time will reduce stress.
8. Lack of sleep could cause stress.
9. Professional help is available to reduce stress.
10. You can't always avoid stressors.

Answers:

1) fact; 2) fact; 3) fiction; 4) fiction; 5) fact; 6) fiction; 7) fact; 8) fact; 9) fact; 10) fact

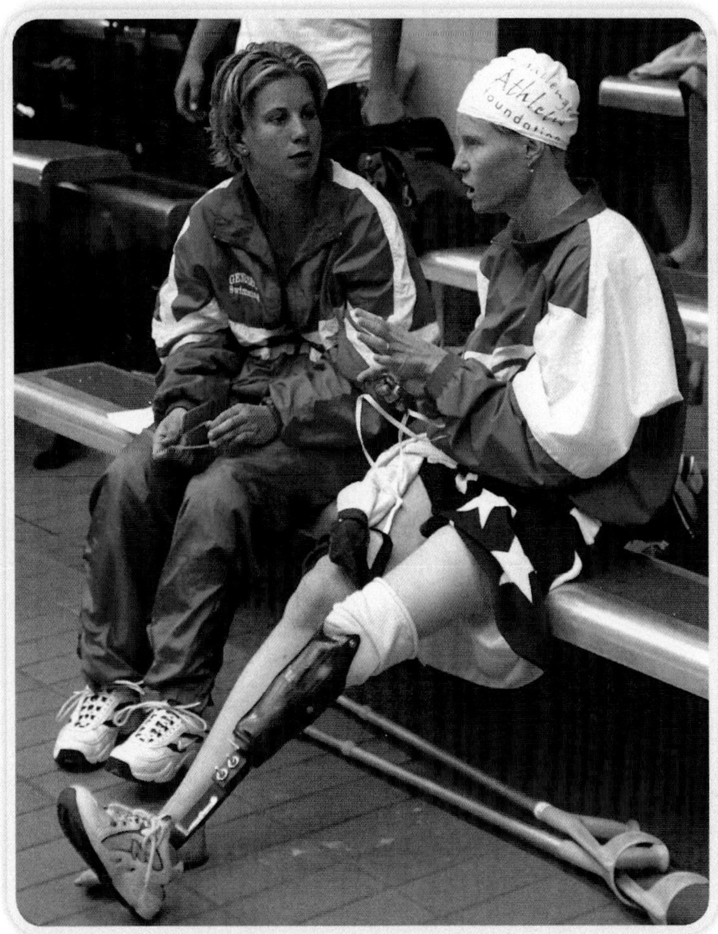

Having friends who will listen to you and support you makes it easier to deal with anxiety and stress.

©Human Kinetics

Social Support

Having a strong social support system makes it easier to cope with stress. One of the most effective ways to reduce stress is through the support of others. A study found that people who have a strong social support system are less likely to be stressed. Knowing that there are people who will empathize with what you're going through, who will listen to you, and who can provide advice on how to overcome stressors will reduce your anxiety and stress.

Communication

Do you find yourself upset when things aren't done the way you'd like them to be done? Do you find yourself sitting quietly when everyone is expressing their ideas for a project or trip? People who have a hard time communicating how they feel are putting themselves in a stressful situation. Learning how to be a good listener and clearly communicating your ideas and feelings is an effective way to reduce stress. Being able to communicate well with others demonstrates assertiveness and can be beneficial in the workplace and in developing social relationships.

Sleep

Getting the proper amount of sleep every night is important, because it allows the body to recharge and relieve stress that might have occurred during the day. The CDC recommends that adults get 7 to 9 hours of sleep each night (CDC 2008b). Sleep affects your mental and physical abilities to accomplish daily tasks. Lack of sleep could cause headaches, forgetfulness, and inability to focus, and it can put you at risk of developing an illness.

A good night's sleep typically consists of 8 full hours of sleep. There are two main phases of sleep: **rapid eye movement (REM) sleep** and **non-REM sleep**. You're in REM sleep when you're dreaming and your closed eyes move back and forth. Non-REM sleep has four phases in which you fall into deeper sleep. As you enter each new phase, your heart rate, temperature, and breathing rate decline.

Almost everyone has nights when they can't fall asleep. However, experiencing **insomnia**, or consistent trouble sleeping, puts you at risk for developing health problems. Some common causes of insomnia are high caffeine intake, alcohol consumption before going to bed, and stress. Try these tips for getting a good night's sleep:

- Maintain a regular sleep schedule. Going to bed and waking up at about the same time every day will help reinforce your body's sleep–wake cycle, which can help you to sleep better.
- Establish a bedtime routine. Doing the same relaxing activities every night before sleep, such as reading a book for 15 minutes or listening to relaxing music, will teach your body to associate those activities with sleep.
- Use your bedroom only for sleep and sex. Don't eat, study, talk on the phone, or watch TV while in bed. The fewer activities you do in bed, the more your body will associate the bed with sleep.

- Exercise regularly. Regular physical activity helps you fall asleep faster, and the sleep you get is better. You shouldn't exercise within 3 hours of your bedtime, though, as your increased body temperature will make it harder to fall asleep.
- Limit napping. Napping can make it harder to fall asleep if you nap too long or too close to bedtime. Try not to nap any later than midafternoon and for no longer than 30 minutes.
- Avoid caffeine, nicotine, and alcohol in the evenings. Caffeine and nicotine are stimulants that can make it harder to fall asleep. Alcohol can make you fall asleep faster, but it lowers your sleep quality.
- Finish eating at least 2 or 3 hours before bedtime. You should also avoid a lot of drinking before bed, as your sleep could be disrupted by frequent trips to the bathroom.
- Create a cool, dark, quiet, and comfortable sleep environment. Use curtains, fans, ear plugs, extra blankets, humidifiers, or other devices to create an environment that allows you to sleep comfortably.

What Do You Do?

It can be hard to talk to other people about the stress you feel. Writing in a journal is a good way to let your thoughts out. Journaling can provide a safe way to vent, because no one will hear you. Writing your thoughts down is also a great way to clearly see the stressors you experienced throughout the day, and it gives you a chance to come up with a plan for avoiding similar situations in the future. Try keeping a journal for a week to see if it helps you manage stress.

Time Management

"There's just not enough time in the day to get everything done!" Sound familiar? Time management can be one of the most difficult tasks to incorporate into your busy life. But being able to manage time actually reduces stress. Three of the most common reasons people have trouble managing their time include perfectionism, overcommitment, and procrastination. Here are some suggestions that could help you manage time:

- Set priorities.
- Set realistic goals.
- Schedule enough time for each task.
- Break down long-term goals into short-term goals.
- Keep track of the tasks you put off.
- Consider completing your least favorite tasks first.
- Consolidate tasks when possible.
- Delegate responsibility when possible.
- Say no when necessary.
- Give yourself a break.

Biofeedback

Biofeedback is a relatively new technique for stress management. It is a form of alternative medicine that monitors bodily processes. For example, biofeedback technicians can monitor heart rate, skin temperature, or muscle tension. One of the main benefits of biofeedback is that it allows people to physically view and monitor their stress level. The purpose of biofeedback is to teach people how it feels to be relaxed, how to induce relaxation, and how to incorporate relaxation into daily life (Scott 2007a).

Several instruments can be used for biofeedback. The three most common are electromyography (EMG), peripheral skin temperature, and electroencephalography (EEG). EMG

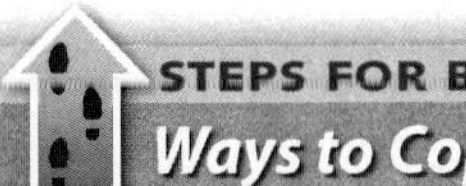

STEPS FOR BEHAVIORAL CHANGE

Ways to Cope With Stress

Following are some coping mechanisms for dealing with stress.

Learn how to cope. Use stress inoculation to mentally prepare ahead of time for potential stressors. Stress inoculation is a technique developed by a psychologist named Donald Meichenbaum to teach people to mentally prepare themselves to cope with stressors that may occur in the future. It consists of three phases. During phase I (conceptualization and education), people learn important terminology, concepts, and theories. In phase II (skills rehearsal and application), people learn skills and apply them to possible scenarios that could occur (practice is done in a classroom setting). In phase III (real-life application), people apply their knowledge and skills in society (Schiraldi 2007).

Work on responses. Train yourself to change your responses to stressful situations. Try to go with the flow of life and be flexible. It is important to understand and be accepting of events that occur in life that you may not have the ability to change. Try to forgive yourself and others of their faults. Enjoy life in the present and try to avoid basing your happiness on a goal that may be achieved in the future. When challenges occur, perceive them as learning opportunities and not as stressors. Improving your responses to stressful situations will improve your overall well-being (Insel and Roth 2002).

Recognize and evaluate stressors. Feeling that you are not in control of the situation often adds more stress. When this occurs, it is important to take charge and regain control by setting realistic goals. Be confident in your actions and focus on the things that you can control. Here is a simple approach that could be used to identify and evaluate stressors (Insel and Roth 2002):

1. Identify the problem and its cause.
2. Identify at least two solutions to overcome the stressor.
3. Weigh the pros and cons for each solution.
4. Decide which solution you will use.
5. Make a list of things that need to be done in order to overcome the stressor.
6. Begin to do the listed actions.
7. Evaluate the outcome and revise your approach if needed.

Downsize lifestyle stressors. Take a step back and consider simplifying. Your outlook on life can contribute to your stress level. For example, meeting expectations, whether they are your own or someone else's, is exhausting. When you or others set high expectations that are not fulfilled, it is easy to feel stressed and disappointed. By modifying your expectations to a realistic goal, you can reduce your stress and pursue a happy life. Along with modifying expectations, keeping a positive mind-set and not holding on to stressful situations that occurred in the past is another way to reduce stress levels (Insel and Roth 2002).

is the most common instrument used in biofeedback. EMG electrodes or other types of sensors are placed on the body to measure muscle tension. Using EMG allows people to quickly see their stress level, practice techniques to reduce their stress level, and determine which stress management technique is most effective. The peripheral skin temperature technique attaches sensors to a person's fingers or feet to measure skin temperature. When the person is stressed, the body temperature will drop. A low skin temperature reading will inform the person to use a relaxation technique to increase body temperature. EEG monitors brain waves during different mental states, such as sleep, calmness, or wakefulness. A person who is stressed will have an EEG reading that is an abnormal frequency and amplitude (Scott 2007a).

Unlike the other stress management techniques, biofeedback requires proper training and knowledge. No matter which instrument provides the biofeedback, the technique lets people physically see their stress level. Using biofeedback can be expensive, but it's effective.

Visualization

Stress affects every part of the body, but the mind is the first place where stress is felt. One of the main functions of the mind is to perceive whether a situation is stressful. If a situation appears to be stressful, the mind sends a warning to the other body parts. Common warning signs include forgetfulness, headaches, agitation, nervous habits, and muscle tension.

Changing the way you perceive a situation can be a good way to cope with stress. Visualization is a mental technique that helps change a stressful situation into a positive one. Practicing visualization doesn't require formal training, and it doesn't take a lot of time. Here's an example of how to practice visualization:

- Sit or lie down and relax your body. Close your eyes and take a couple of deep breaths. Mentally scan your body for any muscle tension and try to relax those muscles. When you feel relaxed, imagine yourself at your favorite place where you feel safe and calm and where you can make all of your worries disappear.
- Look around your favorite place. How do you feel? What do you hear? What do you smell? Look all around your favorite place and notice how it makes you feel. Tell yourself, "I am relaxed. My worries are gone and all the stress has left my body." You are safe.
- You can return to your favorite place anytime. Using your imagination is an effective way to cope with stress. Learning how to use visualization as a coping technique will increase your overall well-being.

NEGATIVE COPING TECHNIQUES

Trying to manage stress can be stressful in itself. The previous section described some common stress management techniques. Unfortunately, some people resort to unhealthy behaviors to deal with their stress. Using tobacco, consuming alcohol, and binge eating are three of the most common unhealthy behaviors people use to cope with stress. Using any of those behaviors can be dangerous, because it's easy for them to become habits that can last for the rest of your life.

Tobacco Use

Many people use tobacco as a quick stress reliever. The nicotine in tobacco provides a relaxed feeling. Unfortunately, using tobacco products has more negative effects than positive. Nicotine is one of the most addictive drugs (National Institute on Drug Abuse [NIDA] 2007). Nicotine is a chemical that absorbs quickly into the body, causing an immediate response. It affects the brain to make it want it more. Each year nearly 5 million people die as a result of using tobacco. By 2010, that number is estimated to increase to 10 million deaths each year (CDC 2008c).

Alcohol Consumption

Consuming alcohol to reduce stress is common. Alcohol allows people to feel more relaxed and forget about the stressors experienced during the day. Although alcohol consumption is legal for people over the age of 21, drinking irresponsibly could lead to lifelong health problems, such as alcohol abuse or dependency. Alcohol consumption also makes people more likely to take risks, and those risks have consequences. The risks of motor vehicle accidents, falling, and drowning increase when alcohol is involved. People who drink too much alcohol are more likely to commit suicide or homicide or engage in risky sexual activities that can result in unintended pregnancies. Continued alcohol use or abuse could also lead to a person having a baby with fetal alcohol syndrome or getting chronic liver disease or cancer (CDC 2007a; MedlinePlus 2007a). Although drinking alcohol might provide short-term stress relief, it doesn't eliminate the cause of the stress, and its long-term consequences are serious.

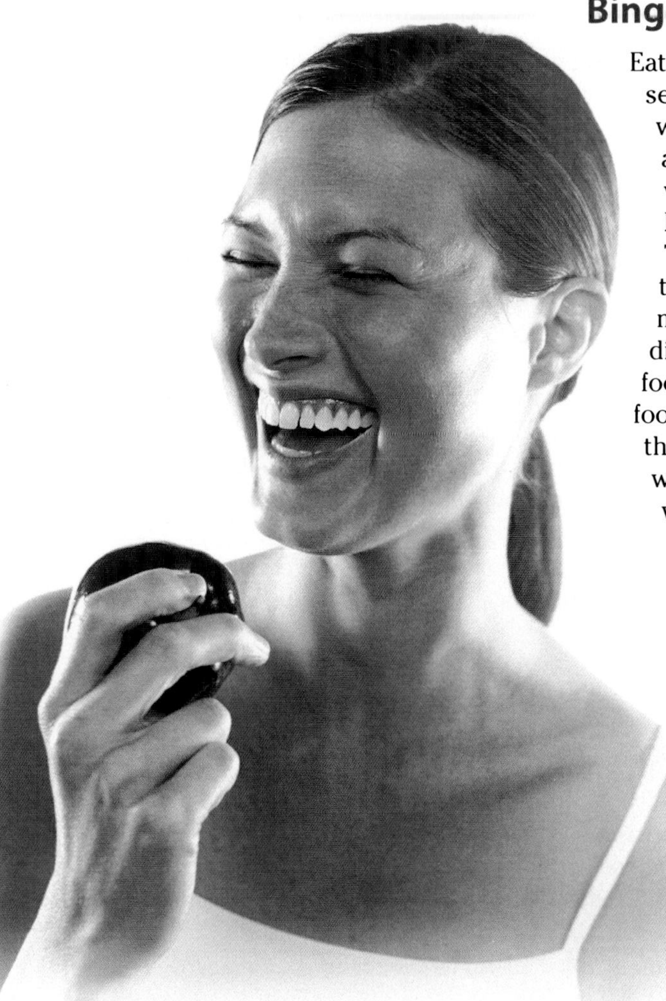

Eating healthy foods helps you handle stress by providing good nutrition and reducing your chances of developing a serious health problem.

© Photodisc

Binge Eating

Eating provides a sense of self-reward and a feeling of sedation afterward. Although food provides the body with the proper vitamins and nutrients to function and to deal with stress, eating too much or eating the wrong kinds of food leads to other health problems. Most people eat unhealthy foods to cope with stress. Those foods might make you feel better in the short term, but over the long term they lead to the development of major health problems, such as obesity and diabetes. Rather than binge eating or eating unhealthy foods to deal with stress, try to incorporate healthy foods into your diet and eat earlier in the day rather than later. Eating earlier in the day prepares the body with the proper vitamins and nutrients to help cope with stress (Insel and Roth 2002).

STRESS MANAGEMENT 101

Stress can be defined in many ways, and it consists of various causes, symptoms, and treatments. Stressors—sources of stress—can come from work, school, family, financial issues, and major life changes. The associated health risks can affect the body's cardiovascular, nervous, digestive, and immune systems, and stress is a common underlying factor associated with diseases, including hypertension, cancer, and obesity. Stress can come from a variety of sources and can last for as little as a day to as long as several years. Although stress can't always be avoided, learning how to manage it can reduce the risks of developing adverse health effects (AIS 2007d, 2007e).

Positive stress management techniques include meditation, deep breathing, muscle relaxation, healthy eating, exercise, having a social support system, getting enough sleep, and more. However, the methods that help you cope with stress won't necessarily be the same as those that help someone else. The things that you find stressful to begin with might not even be a big deal to another person. The most successful technique for managing stress is to be in tune with your body. Figure out what causes you to feel stress, and find the stress management techniques that work best for you. Look around you for resources in your area that specialize in helping with specific stressors. You can't avoid all stressors, but they don't have to control the way you live. Developing a stress management plan will allow you to pursue a healthy life (Insel and Roth 2002; Wallace 2007).

CHAPTER REVIEW

REVIEW QUESTIONS

1. What is the difference between stress and stressors?
2. Describe the four types of stress.
3. What are the five types of stressors? Provide an example of each type.
4. What can employers do to reduce or prevent stress in the workplace?
5. Stress is associated with cognitive symptoms, physiological symptoms, behavioral symptoms, and emotional symptoms. Name two examples of each.
6. Explain how stress affects two body systems.
7. Why is stress an underlying factor in the development of diseases? Provide two examples of diseases that are associated with stress.
8. Compare and contrast two positive stress management techniques.
9. What are some negative techniques for coping with stress, and why do people turn to them?
10. To reduce stress levels, what foods should be avoided, and why?

CRITICAL THINKING

1. Each person responds to stress differently. With the growing number of employees reporting that they feel stressed, do you think that being stressed is a valid reason for not fulfilling job obligations? Why or why not? Do you think it is a manager's responsibility to ensure that each employee is not stressed? Why or why not? If yes, what preventive techniques would you use?
2. Your best friend, who is in the army, returns from war. She confides in you that she can't sleep and has nightmares and thoughts of hurting herself. Your friend asks you not to tell anyone about how she is feeling because she's afraid of the repercussions. What would you do? What advice would you give your friend?

APPLICATION ACTIVITIES

1. The purpose of this activity is to demonstrate how muscle tension is associated with stress. Pair up with another student and massage your partner's shoulders and upper back for 3 minutes. The person who is receiving the massage can tell the other person if the massage is too hard or too soft. Then switch roles. (If you don't feel comfortable giving and receiving a massage on your shoulders and upper back, you do not have to participate.) Afterward, discuss the following topics as a class or in small groups.

   - Did the massage relieve muscle tension and stress?
   - Why do you think muscle tension is associated with stress?
   - What other stress management techniques do you think are effective?

2. In pairs or in small groups of three or four people, answer the following questions and share any personal experiences that you may have encountered. This is a fun way to see how people respond to stress differently.

   - Do you feel stress when you have to ride in an airplane? How do you cope with the stress?
   - Do you feel stress before you take a final exam? How do you cope with the stress?
   - Do you feel stress when you have to speak in front of a crowd? How do you cope with the stress?

- Do you feel stress when you almost get into a car accident? How do you cope with the stress?
- Do you feel stress when you have to take care of your younger brother or sister? How do you cope with the stress?
- Do you feel stress when you engage in extreme sports such as bungee jumping? How do you cope with the stress?
- Do you feel stress when you have to finish five different things by the end of the day? How do you cope with the stress?
- Do you feel stress when you first start to date someone? How do you cope with the stress?
- Do you feel stress before you go on a job interview? How do you cope with the stress?
- Do you feel stress when you have to buy a present for your significant other? How do you cope with the stress?

GLOSSARY

acute stress—The most common form of stress. Causes include studying for an exam, caring for a sick child, or having a disagreement in a relationship. Acute stress lasts for only a short time and is easy to manage and treat.

biofeedback—Form of alternative medicine that monitors bodily processes to help manage stress.

chronic stress—The result of constantly experiencing stressors. Unlike acute stress, chronic stress doesn't go away. Because the body is constantly at an elevated state, it is difficult for the body to relax and to bring its systems back to normal.

concentration meditation—Meditation that involves focusing attention on a prayer.

deep breathing—Deep, slow breathing can help slow your breathing pattern, quiet your mind, and relax your body.

distress—Negative stress.

episodic acute stress—When you consistently experience acute stress. As acute stress for one situation fades, another stressor appears.

eustress—Positive stress.

fight-or-flight response—The body's automatic reaction to fight or flee a perceived threatening situation.

general adaptation syndrome (GAS)—The body's reaction to stress in long-term stressful situations. It consists of three phases: alarm reaction, resistance or adaptation, and exhaustion.

insomnia—Consistent trouble sleeping.

meditation—The purpose of meditation is to clear your mind, calmly think about what's causing the stress, and regain a sense of peace by focusing on yourself.

mindfulness—Sitting alone in a quiet room and focusing your attention on any object or process, such as a sound or breathing.

non-REM sleep—Sleep stage with four phases in which you fall into deeper sleep.

post-traumatic stress disorder (PTSD)—Occurs when people experience a dangerous or life-threatening event, such as rape, child abuse, war, car accidents, and so on.

progressive muscle relaxation technique—Tensing and relaxing various muscle groups while sitting or lying calmly in a relaxed position.

rapid eye movement (REM) sleep—Sleep stage when you're dreaming and when your closed eyes move back and forth.

stress—Physiological and emotional responses to any disturbing stimulus.

stressor—Any physical or psychological event or condition that produces stress.

stress response—The physiological changes associated with stress.

REFERENCES AND RESOURCES

American Diabetes Association. 2008. Stress. www.diabetes.org/type-1-diabetes/stress.jsp.

American Institute of Stress (AIS). 2007a. Effects of stress. www.stress.org/topic-effects.htm.

———. 2007b. Job stress. www.stress.org/job.htm.

———. 2007c. Stress and heart disease, type A behavior and heart disease, prevention and treatment of heart disease, heart disease and job stress. www.stress.org/topic-heart.htm.

———. 2007d. Stress reduction, stress relievers. www.stress.org/topic-reduction.htm.

———. 2007e. Stress, definition of stress, stressor. What is stress? Eustress? www.stress.org/topic-definition-stress.htm.

American Psychological Association (APA). 2007. Stress: The different kinds of stress. http://apahelp-center.org/articles/article.php?id=21.

———. 2008. Stress: How does stress affect your body? http://apahelpcenter.org/articles/article.php?id=141.

Centers for Disease Control and Prevention (CDC). 2007a. Defining overweight and obesity. www.cdc.gov/nccdphp/dnpa/obesity/defining.htm.

———. 2007b. High blood pressure facts. www.cdc.gov/bloodpressure/facts.htm.

———. 2008a. Overweight and obesity: Contributing factors. www.cdc.gov/nccdphp/dnpa/obesity/contributing_factors.htm.

———. 2008b. Sleep and sleep disorders. www.cdc.gov/features/sleep/.

———. 2008c. Smoking and tobacco use. www.cdc.gov/tobacco/basic_information/index.htm.

Cromer, K.R., and N. Sachs-Ericsson. 2006. The association between childhood abuse, PTSD, and the occurrence of adult health problems: Moderation via current life stress. *Journal of Traumatic Stress* 19: 967-971.

Davis, J. 2000. Schools piling on too much homework, psychologists say. www.rense.com/general5/hm.htm.

Equality in Marriage Institute. 2008. Marriage and money: Talking about money. www.equalityinmarriage.org/bmtalk.html.

Exercise and Stress Connection. 2007. Exercise as a stress management modality. www.imt.net/~randolfi/ExerciseStress.html.

Frasz, C., and K. Kato. n.d. The educational structure of the Japanese school system. www.ed.gov/pubs/Research5/Japan/structure_j.html.

Graham, J.E., L.M. Christian, and J.K. Kiecolt-Glaser. 2006. Stress, age, and immune function: Toward a lifespan approach. *Journal of Behavioral Medicine* 4: 389-400.

Harper, J. 2008. Some thoughts on why Japanese students are better than U.S. students on international mathematics assessments. www.nctm.org/resources/content.aspx?id=1560.

Holistic Online. 2007. Stress, the silent killer: Nutrition. www.holisticonline.com/Stress/stress_nutrition.htm.

Insel, P.M., and W.T. Roth. 2002. *Core concepts in health.* 9th ed. San Francisco: McGraw-Hill.

Ishida, R., and M. Okada. 2006. Effects of a firm purpose in life on anxiety and sympathetic nervous activity caused by emotional stress: Assessment by psycho-physiological method. *Stress and Health* 22: 275-281.

Kelly, P., and D. Colquhoun. 2005. The professionalization of stress management: Health and well-being as a professional duty of care. *Critical Public Health* 15: 135-145.

KidsHealth. 2005. What stresses you out about school? www.kidshealth.org/teen/school_jobs/school/school_stress.html.

Lewis, D. 2007. Deep breathing. www.authentic-breathing.com/deep_breathing.htm.

MedlinePlus. 2007a. Alcohol use. www.nlm.nih.gov/medlineplus/ency/article/001944.htm.

———. 2007b. High blood pressure (hypertension). www.nlm.nih.gov/medlineplus/ency/article/000468.htm.

———. 2008. Post-traumatic stress disorder. www.nlm.nih.gov/medlineplus/posttraumaticstressdisorder.html.

Melamed, S., A. Shirom, S. Toker, S. Berliner, and I. Shapira. 2006. Burnout and risk of cardiovascular disease: Evidence, possible causal paths, and promising research directions. *Psychological Bulletin* 132: 327-353.

Michielsen, H.J., M.A. Croon, T.M. Willemsen, J. de Vries, and G.L. van Heck. 2007. Which constructs can predict emotional exhaustion in a working population? A study into its determinants. *Stress and Health* 23: 121-130.

Morelius, E., U. Lundh, and N. Nelson. 2002. Parental stress in relation to the severity of congenital heart disease in the offspring. *Pediatric Nursing* 28: 28-32.

National Cancer Institute (NCI). 2007. Cancer statistics. www.cancer.gov/statistics/.

National Institute for Occupational Safety and Health (NIOSH). 2008. Stress at work. www.cdc.gov/niosh/topics/stress/.

National Institute on Drug Abuse (NIDA). 2007. Tobacco/Nicotine. www.drugabuse.gov/DrugPages/Nicotine.html.

Neimark, N.F. n.d. The fight or flight response. Mind/Body Education Center. www.thebodysoulconnection.com/EducationCenter/fight.html.

Niess, J.H., H. Monnikes, A.U. Dignass, B.F. Klapp, and P.C. Arck. 2002. Review on the influence of stress on immune mediators, neuropeptides and hormones with relevance for inflammatory bowel disease. *Digestion* 65: 131-140.

Nishitani, N., and H. Sakakibara. 2005. Relationship of obesity to job stress and eating behavior in male Japanese workers. *International Journal of Obesity* 30: 528-533.

Pritchard, M., G. Wilson, and B. Yamnitz. 2007. What predicts adjustments among college students? A longitudinal panel study. *Journal of American College Health* 56: 15-22.

Psychology Encyclopedia. 2007. Divorce. http://psychology.jrank.org/pages/191/Divorce.html.

Rau, R. 2006. The association between blood pressure and work stress: The importance of measuring isolated systolic hypertension. *Work and Stress* 20: 84-97.

Robotham, D., and C. Julian. 2006. Stress and the higher education student: A critical review of literature. *Journal of Further and Higher Education* 30: 107-117.

Rosenthal, D.A., J.M. Ferrin, K. Wilson, and M. Frain. 2005. Acceptance rates of African American versus white consumers of vocational rehabilitation services: A meta-analysis. *Journal of Rehabilitation* 71: 36-74.

Schiraldi, G. 2007. Stress inoculation training. Centre For Teaching Excellence. www.otal.umd.edu/wiki/cte/index.php?title=Stress_Inoculation_Training.

Scott, E. 2007a. Biofeedback and stress relief. http://stress.about.com/od/programsandpractices/a/biofeedback.htm.

———. 2007b. Money stress: Making smart money choices for less stress and more happiness. http://stress.about.com/od/financialstress/a/money.htm.

Smith, M., E. Jaffe-Gill, and J. Segal. 2008. Understanding stress: Signs, symptoms, causes, and effects. www.helpguide.org/mental/stress_signs.htm.

Solberg, V.S.H., A.H. Carlstrom, K.A.S. Howard, and J.E. Jones. 2007. Classifying at-risk high school youth: The influence of exposure to community violence and protective factors on academic and health outcomes. *Career Development Quarterly* 55: 313-327.

Wallace, E.V. 2007. Managing stress: What consumers want to know from health educators. *American Journal of Health Studies* 22: 56-58.

Weil, M.M., and L.D. Rosen. 2004. A conversation with TechnoStress authors. www.technostress.com/tsconversation.htm.

Weisman, S.R. 1992. How do Japan's students do it? They cram. *New York Times*, April 27: A1.

World Health Organization (WHO). 2007. Cardiovascular diseases. www.who.int/topics/cardiovascular_diseases/en/.

Other helpful resources include the following.

American Institute of Stress (AIS). 2007a. Stress and cancer: Diseases of civilization, communication, and control. www.stress.org/topic-cancer.htm.

———. 2007b. Stress in the workplace, job stress, occupational stress, job stress questionnaire. www.stress.org/topic-workplace.htm.

American Psychological Association (APA). 2004. Exercise fuels the brain's stress buffers. www.apahelpcenter.org/articles/article.php?id=25.

Discovery Health Stress Management Center. http://health.discovery.com/centers/stress/stress.html. This site is full of information on stress management, including tips and tricks for overcoming stress, quizzes, a tool kit, blogs, and more.

Healthline: Stress Health Channel. www.healthline.com/channel/stress.html. This site offers links to articles and videos about managing stress.

Meditation Center. 2007. Online meditation center. www.meditationcenter.com.

MedlinePlus. 2008. Stress management. www.nlm.nih.gov/medlineplus/ency/article/001942.htm. This site provides assessment suggestions, individual stress management plan ideas, and links to other resources.

National Institute for Occupational Safety and Health (NIOSH). 2008. Stress at work. www.cdc.gov/niosh/topics/stress/.

WebMD: Stress Management Health Center. www.webmd.com/balance/stress-management/default.htm. This page offers links to articles about stress management, as well as blogs and message boards. You can also find an interactive tool for measuring your stress level by following the "Topic Overview" link.

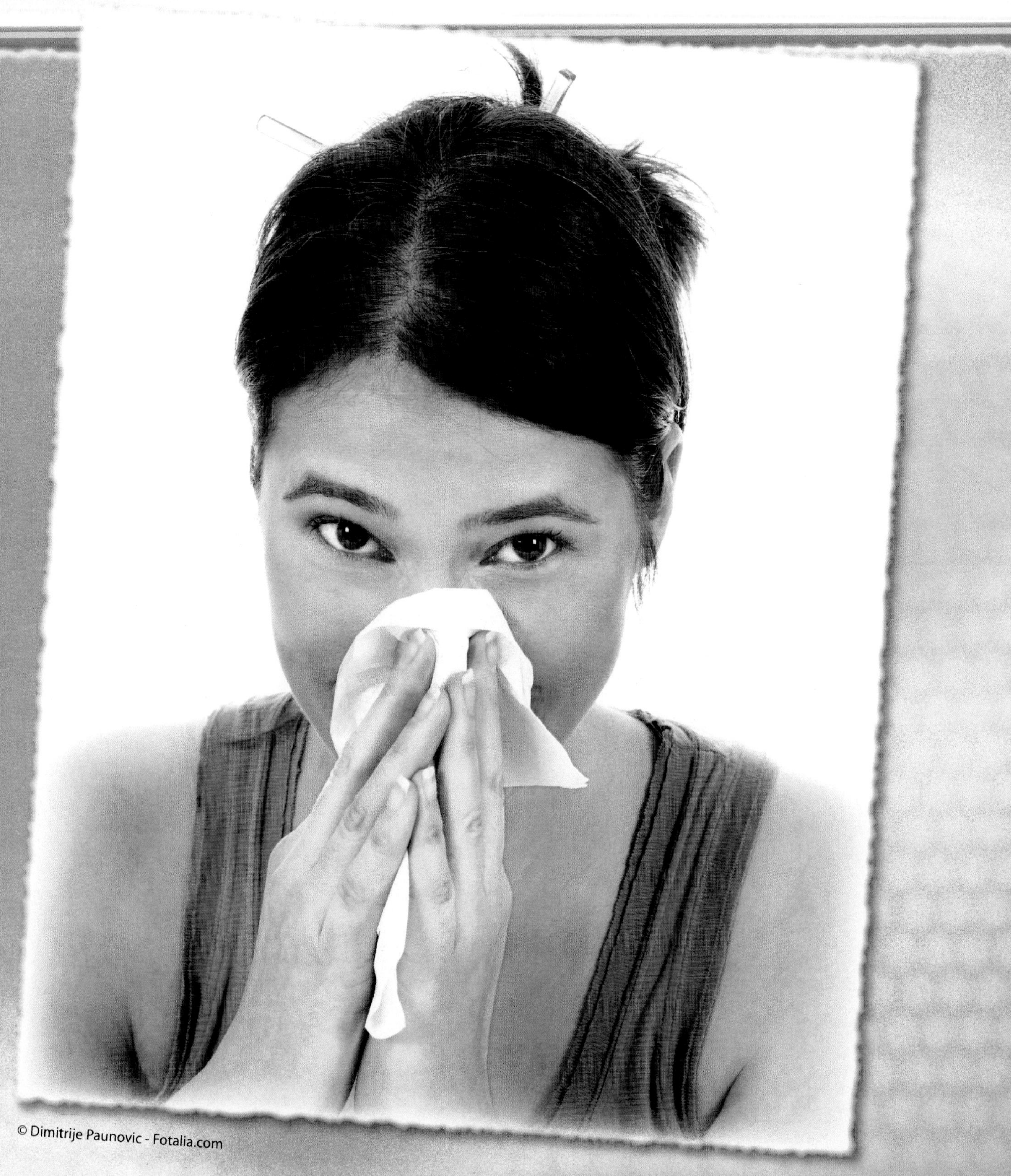
© Dimitrije Paunovic - Fotalia.com

CHAPTER 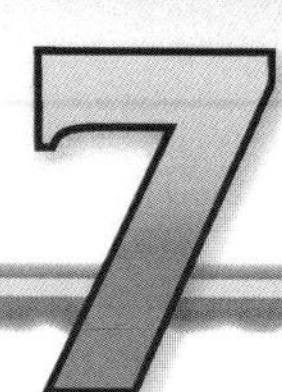

INFECTIOUS DISEASES

BHIBHA DAS, MPH
University of Illinois

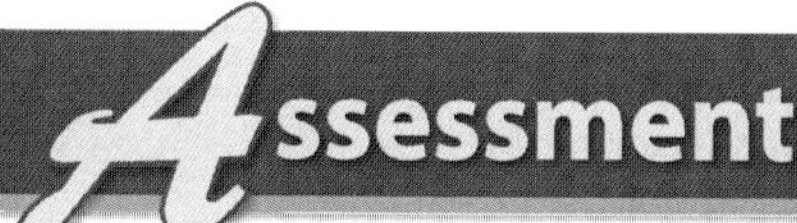

Assessment

- What's the easiest and most common way to be infected by a pathogen?
- Can using alcohol and tobacco reduce your chances of warding off disease?
- Why do many people catch colds in the winter?
- Why are college students at an increased risk of contracting meningitis?
- Do you know any of the signs or symptoms of AIDS?
- What's the difference between syphilis, gonorrhea, and herpes?
- What immunizations should college students get?
- Do you know the proper way to wash your hands to stop outbreaks of disease?

Objectives

- Define *infectious disease*.
- Understand the chain of infection.
- Understand the transmission methods of infectious agents.
- Identify the six major causes of infectious diseases.
- Understand the difference between controllable and uncontrollable risk factors.
- Understand the components of the external defenses and immune system of the body.
- Identify common infectious diseases and their causes, symptoms, and treatments.
- Define *acquired immunodeficiency syndrome* (AIDS) and the virus that causes it.
- Identify ways to protect yourself from infectious diseases.

Mary Mallon was a poor Irish immigrant to the United States who worked as a cook in the homes of wealthy New Yorkers during the early 20th century. In 1906, Mary was hired to be a cook at the summer cottage of Charles Henry Warren. Soon after Mary started, the Warren family became sick with typhoid fever, a serious, often fatal illness characterized by headaches, loss of energy, upset stomach, and high fever. An investigation traced the contamination to Mary. Investigators traced Mary's employment history back to 1900 and discovered that typhoid outbreaks followed Mary from job to job. Between 1900 and 1907, Typhoid Mary, as she came to be called, worked in seven homes and infected 22 people with typhoid fever (Leavitt 1997).

Salmonella Typhi, the bacteria that cause typhoid fever, can survive only in a human host. The bacteria can be found in the fecal matter of people who have the disease and carriers (people who have the pathogen but do not experience full-blown symptoms; people who have the disease are carriers, but vice versa is not always true). People who have been infected often carry the bacteria within the bloodstream and intestinal tract. Some carriers have such a slight case of the disease that they show only flulike symptoms (Centers for Disease Control and Prevention [CDC] 2005b). Historians suppose that Typhoid Mary had a weak case of typhoid fever that was never diagnosed, and through her career as a cook, she infected dozens of people. Typhoid Mary was sent into isolation at North Brother Island where she died in November of 1938 (Leavitt 1997). Typhoid Mary's story highlights the importance of understanding and recognizing infectious diseases and practicing prevention methods.

An **infectious disease**, or communicable disease, can be spread easily from one person to another (Donatelle and Ketcham 2007). This chapter will discuss how communicable diseases are spread and what causes them. You'll learn about the risk factors that you can and can't control and also how your body defends against the diseases. We'll cover the most common infectious diseases, and you'll learn how to protect yourself from them so you can stay strong and healthy.

CHAIN OF INFECTION

The method by which a pathogen transmits a disease is the **chain of infection** (Payne 2007). There are six distinct links in the chain of infection (see figure 7.1). Each link represents a step in the transmission of an infection, and each link has to be present for an infection to occur.

The first link is the **agent** (Payne 2007). The agent is any disease-causing microorganism. Agents are also called *pathogens* or *germs*. The agent is capable of causing disease, or is virulent. Agents can be bacteria, viruses, fungi, protozoa, parasitic worms, and prions, and we'll discuss them in more detail later in the chapter. Some agents are more virulent than others and can lead to serious infectious diseases such as tuberculosis. Other agents may not be virulent to begin with but can mutate into more virulent forms, such as the influenza virus. Public health officials are afraid of a worldwide influenza pandemic in the future because of the ability of the influenza virus to mutate.

Agents search for viable environments in which to survive. An optimal environment where an agent can live, grow, and reproduce is known as the **reservoir**, which is the second link in the chain of infection (Payne 2007). Often, the reservoir is the body of an infected person. Within the reservoir, the agents continue to live and grow before they're transmitted to others. Animals can also be reservoirs. For example, the door mouse is a reservoir for the hantavirus, a virus that can cause kidney and circulatory problems. The final type of reservoir is a nonliving environment. Soil, for example, is the reservoir for bacteria such as *Clostridium tetani*, which causes tetanus.

The third link in the chain of infection is the **portal of exit** (Payne 2007). The portal of exit is the route agents take out of the reservoirs on their way to causing disease in others. The main portals of exit are blood and the respiratory, digestive, urinary, and reproductive systems. The mouth and nose are often the portals of exit for respiratory infections, such as cold and

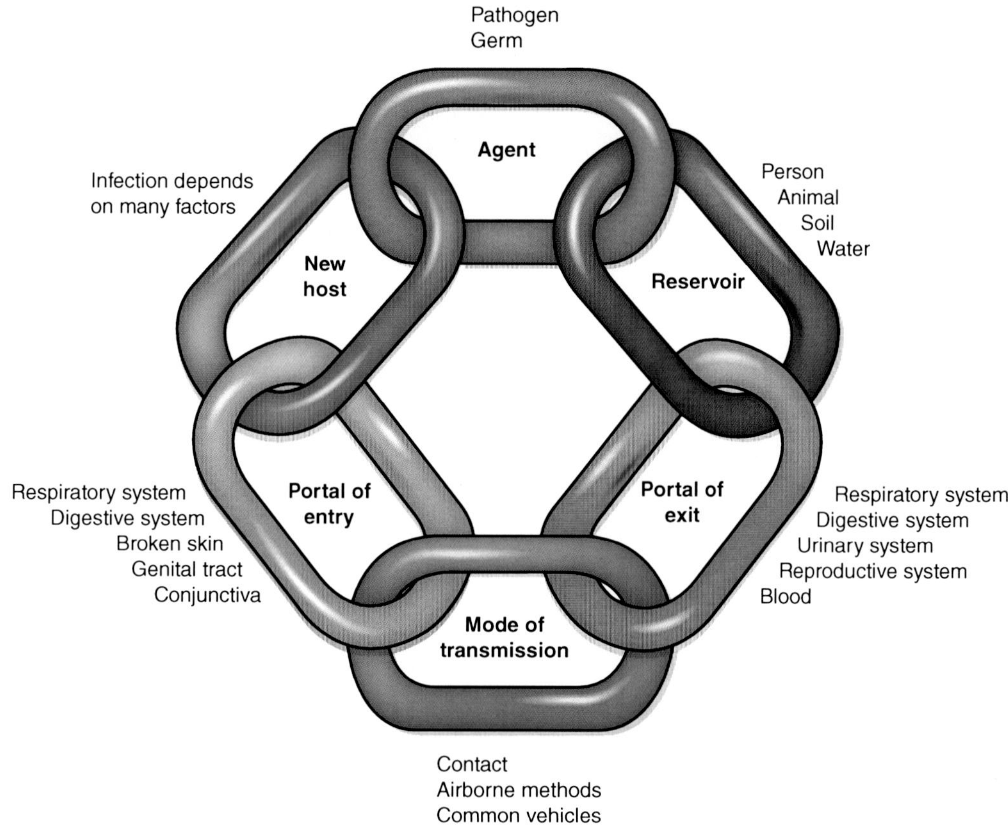

Figure 7.1 The six links in the chain of infection show how a pathogen transmits a disease.

flu viruses. Digestive infectious illnesses, such as hepatitis A and typhoid fever, use feces or saliva as portal exits. Sexually transmitted infections (STIs) such as syphilis generally exit the body through the urethra or genital region. Blood-borne diseases, such as human immunodeficiency virus (HIV), leave the reservoirs through needles (e.g., hypodermic syringes), bleeding wounds, or insects (e.g., mosquitoes).

The fourth link in the chain of infection is the **mode of transmission**, which is the method that agents use to move from reservoirs through portals of exit into potential hosts (Payne 2007). Modes of transmission include direct and indirect contact, air, and common vehicles and will be covered in the next section.

The **portal of entry** is the fifth link in the chain of infection (Payne 2007). There are three main and two secondary portals of entry through which agents can enter potential hosts. The three primary portals of entry are the respiratory system, the digestive system, and a break in the skin. The two secondary portals of entry are the genital tract and the conjunctiva (the thin membrane that covers the surface of the inner eyelid and the white part of the eyeball). There are three ways for an agent to gain entry to a potential host. An agent can infect cells in the portal of entry, or if the skin has been broken through trauma, bite, or injection, the agent can enter that way. Finally, the infection can be congenital. A congenital infection is acquired during development in the uterus and is not due to heredity. An example of a congenital infection is congenital syphilis. In this instance, syphilis is transferred from mother to baby before the baby is born.

The sixth and final link in the chain of transmission is the **new host**. The new host is a person who can get sick when exposed to a disease-causing microorganism.

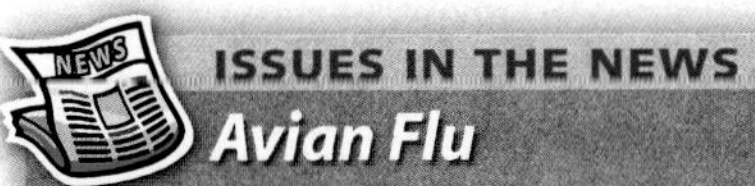

ISSUES IN THE NEWS

Avian Flu

Avian influenza, or bird flu, is caused by avian influenza viruses. Common signs and symptoms of avian influenza include cough, fever, sore throat, muscle aches, and conjunctivitis. Those with a severe case of avian flu may have viral pneumonia along with respiratory distress. Avian influenza viruses are very contagious and are responsible for the deaths of both wild and domestic birds, along with some human deaths. Fortunately, it is very difficult for humans to develop bird flu. The majority of people who developed bird flu symptoms were in close contact with sick birds. The avian influenza virus, H5N1, concerns public health officials because if it were to mutate into a type that could be transmitted from person to person more easily, we could face a global pandemic, similar to the one that occurred in 1918 and 1919 (Mayo Clinic 2008a).

METHODS OF TRANSMISSION

Germs can be transferred from an infectious body to a person in several ways. Transmission methods include contact, air, and common vehicle (Mayo Clinic 2007h).

Contact

Direct contact is the easiest way for pathogens to infect someone. There are three types of direct contact: person to person, animal to person, and mother to unborn child (Mayo Clinic 2007h).

People most commonly become infected with a disease through person-to-person contact. Kissing, sharing straws, exchanging bodily fluids through sexual contact, or even receiving a blood transfusion from an infected person are some ways that diseases pass from one person to another. Animals, especially household pets, are also common carriers of infectious agents. People can become infected from animals while hiking in dense woods, petting a dog, or scooping litter out of a cat box. The final type of direct contact transmission is from mother to unborn child. Pathogens can pass through the placenta from a pregnant woman to her fetus. For example, a mother can transmit HIV to her unborn child, and that virus can later lead to acquired immunodeficiency syndrome (AIDS) (CDC 2007f).

Indirect contact is another method of transmission to humans. Disease-causing organisms can live on doorknobs, telephones, and computer keyboards, among other things. When you use the computer keyboard in a computer lab, you risk becoming infected with germs that the previous user left behind. It is very much a game of chance when it comes to becoming infected.

Airborne

Droplets and particles are airborne methods of transmission. Anytime people sneeze or cough, they spread **droplets** throughout the air. If they are sick, germs are in the droplets, and if your mouth, nose, or eyes become exposed to these droplets, you might get sick (Mayo Clinic 2007h).

Germs can also travel through the air in **particles**, which are much smaller than droplets. Because particles are smaller than droplets, they tend to stay in the air longer and can also travel in airstreams. Tuberculosis and influenza are two types of infectious diseases that have the ability to spread both through droplet and particle transmission (Mayo Clinic 2006c, 2007i).

Common Vehicle and Vector

Unfortunately, contact with a sick person and intercepting an airborne transmission aren't the only ways you can become infected with a nasty bug. Infectious diseases can also be spread through insect carriers and even through food (Mayo Clinic 2007h). Mosquitoes, lice, and ticks are some of the more common carriers of infectious diseases. Insect carriers are often referred to as **vectors** and can transmit germs to humans by landing on or by biting them. Common infectious diseases that are spread by vectors are malaria and West Nile virus by mosquitoes and Lyme disease by ticks (CDC 2007b).

Germs also can spread through contaminated food and water. Uncooked meat and unwashed fruits and vegetables are often carriers of infectious germs. Unclean, unpurified water—often the type of water found in underdeveloped countries—is another source of infectious diseases.

CAUSES OF INFECTIOUS DISEASES

After pathogens have entered the body, they can multiply, causing an infection and ultimately a disease. The six major causes of infectious disease are bacteria, viruses, fungi, protozoa, parasitic worms, and prions (Payne 2007) (see table 7.1).

Bacteria

Bacteria are microscopic, single-celled organisms that can be found practically anywhere. There are three types of bacteria, and each is named for its shape: cocci (spherical), bacilli (rodlike), and spirilla (spiral) (Payne 2007). Many types of bacteria live in the body without causing harm. An example is *Escherichia coli*, which is more commonly known as *E. coli*. This

TABLE 7.1 Six Major Causes of Infectious Diseases

Cause	Description	Disease(s)
Bacteria	Microscopic, single-celled organism	Pertussis (*Bordetella pertussis*), Lyme disease (*Borrelia burgdorferi*), peptic ulcers (*Helicobacter pylori*), tuberculosis (*Mycobacterium tuberculosis*), pneumonia (*Mycoplasma*)
Viruses	Infectious parasites	The common cold (rhinovirus), genital warts (human papillomaviruses), influenza (influenza A and B), chicken pox (varicella zoster), genital herpes (herpes simplex 1 and 2)
Fungi	Single-celled or multicelled organisms that replicate by budding or making spores	Yeast infections (*Candida albicans*), athlete's foot (dermatophyte fungi), histoplasmosis (*Histoplasma capsulatum*)
Protozoa	Simple, one-celled organisms that usually can live independently of a host	Diarrhea, urethritis, vaginitis, malaria (*Plasmodium falciparum*), toxoplasmosis (Toxoplasma *gondii*), giardiasis (*Giardia lamblia*), trichomoniasis (*Trichomonas vaginalis*), amoebic dysentery (*Entamoeba histolytica*)
Parasitic worms	Wormlike parasites (helminths) that live on or in a host	Pinworm infections (*Enterobius vermicularis*), hookworm infections (*Necator americanus*), roundworm infections (*Ascaris lumbricoides*)
Prions	Infectious agents that researchers believe consist solely of protein material but lack DNA and RNA	Bovine spongiform encephalopathy (BSE), or mad cow disease

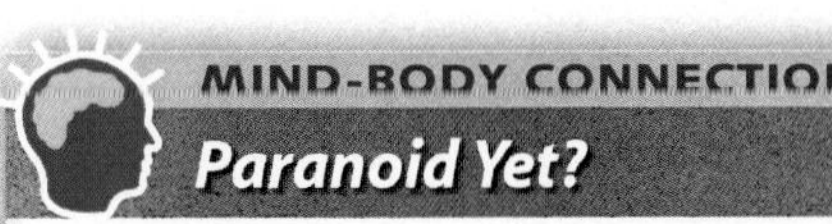

The information about how diseases are transmitted is enough to make a person paranoid. Germs live on everything, and some people take extreme measures to avoid them. For example, actress Jessica Alba has said that she shines a black light on hotel beds to check them for stains and germs, and the TV series *Monk* follows a former detective who struggles with many phobias, including a fear of germs. How do you walk the line between keeping yourself safe and being obsessive about avoiding contact with anything that might make you sick?

type of bacteria is found naturally in the large intestine, where its function is to help digest food. However, it can cause a urinary tract infection if it enters the urinary tract. Infectious diseases caused by bacteria include pertussis *(Bordetella pertussis)*, Lyme disease *(Borrelia burgdorferi)*, peptic ulcers *(Helicobacter pylori)*, tuberculosis *(Mycobacterium tuberculosis)*, and pneumonia *(Mycoplasma)*.

Viruses

So small that they are visible only with an electron microscope, **viruses** are infectious parasites made up of a protein shell that encloses either deoxyribonucleic acid (DNA) or ribonucleic acid (RNA) (Teague, Mackenzie, and Rosenthal 2006). Because viruses were not identified until the 20th century, there's still a lot we don't know about the role they play in the development of diseases. Viruses can't reproduce by themselves, so they're dependent on other living beings for reproduction. As a result, viruses can't survive for long outside of a host. After a virus has entered a living host, its genetic material (either the DNA or RNA) replicates continuously, until the cell bursts. At that time, thousands of cell viruses are released to continue the process of cell invasion and replication. Due to the unique makeup of viruses, diseases caused by them are among some of the most contagious (Teague et al. 2006). Infectious diseases caused by viruses include the common cold (rhinovirus), genital warts (human papillomaviruses), influenza (influenza A and B), chicken pox (varicella zoster), and genital herpes (herpes simplex 1 and 2).

Fungi

A **fungus** is a single-celled or multicelled organism (Teague et al. 2006). Many fungi have valuable functions, but some types can cause infections. Fungi replicate by either budding or making spores, and many fungal infections come from environmental exposure to the spores. Types of fungi include yeast and mold. Infectious diseases caused by fungi include yeast infections *(Candida albicans)*, athlete's foot (dermatophyte fungi), and histoplasmosis *(Histoplasma capsulatum)* (Teague et al. 2006).

Protozoa

Protozoa, the simplest life forms, are one-celled organisms that usually can live independently of a host (Payne 2007). Infectious diseases caused by protozoa often afflict people in developing countries because of undeveloped sanitation systems. Protozoa can be transmitted by feces or contaminated water or food. Mosquitoes and air transmit protozoa that cause diseases such as malaria and *Pneumocystis jiroveci* pneumonia, respectively (Payne 2007). Infectious diseases caused by protozoa include diarrhea, urethritis, vaginitis, malaria *(Plasmodium falciparum)*, toxoplasmosis (Toxoplasma *gondii*), giardiasis *(Giardia lamblia)*, trichomoniasis *(Trichomonas vaginalis)*, and amoebic dysentery *(Entamoeba histolytica)*. In addition, a type of pneumonia that strikes people who have weak immune systems (such as people with HIV) is caused by the protozoa *Pneumocystis jiroveci*. (In addition, viruses cause pneumonia in young children, and bacteria cause it in older children and adults.)

Parasitic Worms

Parasitic worms, or helminths, are another type of pathogen that spreads infectious diseases (Insel 2005). The largest of the pathogens, parasitic worms live on or in a host. Parasitic worms can infect people who unintentionally consume worm eggs either in food or water. In addition, worm larvae can break through and burrow into the skin. Parasitic worms cause pinworm infections *(Enterobius vermicularis)*, hookworm infections *(Necator americanus)*, and roundworm infections *(Ascaris lumbricoides)* (Insel 2005).

Prions

Prions are infectious agents that researchers believe consist solely of protein material but lack DNA and RNA (Insel 2005). Relatively little is known about prions, but it is clear that they are responsible for the spread of bovine spongiform encephalopathy (BSE), or mad cow disease. Prions normally are found within brain tissue, so they infect people who eat the cows' infected brain or nerve tissue. Due to their unique composition and ability to self-replicate, prions that infect a cell often change the function or shape of the cell's proteins into an abnormal and damaging form (Insel 2005). As a result, the infected person suffers a degeneration of brain and nervous system functions.

In clinical settings, prions are often called *transmissible spongiform encephalopathies* (TSEs). Diseases caused by prions are usually characterized by spongelike holes in the brain, dementia, and weakness. These symptoms usually kill the infected person.

RISK FACTORS

All diseases have risk factors that increase the chances of becoming ill. Some factors you can control and some you can't, but with proper knowledge, skills, and awareness, you can minimize your risks.

Controllable Risk Factors

Some risk factors are controllable. You can significantly reduce the chances of becoming infected by adopting a healthy lifestyle, which supports the immune system, the main mechanism for fighting off infectious diseases (Donatelle and Ketcham 2007). When your immune system is weakened, it is easier for pathogens to enter the body (Microbytes 2004).

You can do several things to acquire and maintain a strong immune system. For example, engage in daily moderate-intensity physical activity and eat a well-balanced diet that is full of whole grains, fruits, and vegetables (National Institutes of Health [NIH] 2003). Getting adequate sleep is important to keeping your immune system strong. In addition, don't smoke or use illegal drugs and do limit your alcohol consumption, manage your stress levels, and get vaccinations when needed. By choosing whether to take these actions, you are deciding whether you want a strong immune system.

Additionally, practicing good hygiene helps reduce the chance of contracting infectious diseases (Mayo Clinic 2007e). For example, by washing your hands before you eat, you are less likely to be exposed to pathogens.

You can also regulate your environment. For example, if you already have a weakened immune system, you should avoid places such as hospitals and doctors' offices, which are full of infectious pathogens. Furthermore, determining where you live and what conditions you live in affects your susceptibility to infectious diseases. An unclean environment may invite unwanted guests in your home that can be carriers of infectious diseases.

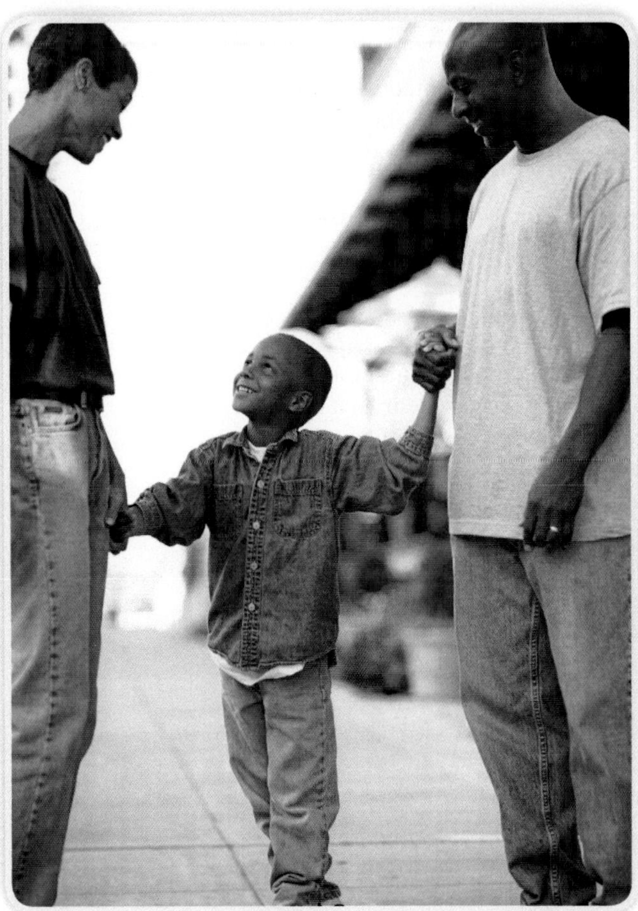

Your heredity and the living conditions of your environment can affect your susceptibility to infectious diseases.

© Photodisc

Uncontrollable Risk Factors

Some risk factors you have no influence over. One of the greatest uncontrollable risk factors is heredity. For example, you have no control over whether your mother will be infected with AIDS or syphilis. If she is, you are at a risk of having the disease passed to you when you are born. Heredity can cause chronic diseases, which can lead to weakened immune systems that make you more susceptible to infectious diseases. Age can also play a role in your chances of contracting an infectious disease. Newborns and younger children are at a higher risk for contracting an infectious disease than older children because they have not developed a strong immune system and have not been vaccinated against illnesses such as polio or measles (CDC 2007m). Furthermore, as the body ages, the immune system becomes more and more susceptible to infectious illnesses. For this reason, an older person may experience more severe signs and symptoms of an illness than a younger person would. Often, an infectious illness that may simply be a nuisance to a younger person may be fatal to the elderly.

The environment you live in also can affect your risk of getting infectious diseases. As mentioned, your environment can be a controllable risk factor in that you can decide where you want to live. However, it is also uncontrollable to some degree because if you live in a certain area, there are elements of the environment that you can't control. For instance, if you live in Los Angeles, you can't do much about the air quality in the area. Pollutants such as drugs, chemicals, and waste in food and water can greatly increase susceptibility to infectious diseases. Socioeconomic status also plays a role in infectious disease immunity. Crowded living conditions often make it easier for communicable diseases to be passed from person to person.

YOUR BODY'S DEFENSES

Even though the world is full of potentially damaging pathogens, the body has the remarkable ability to ward them off through a set of external barriers and the immune system. Working together, these defenses help keep the body healthy and pathogen free.

External Barriers

The first line of defense against invading pathogens is the external barriers of the body, which include both physical and chemical barriers (NIH 2003). The largest organ, the skin, is one of the most important physical barriers. The skin is home to many bacteria and fungi, but it's hard for those pathogens to enter the body unless there is a cut or break in the skin. Sometimes an insect bite can help pathogens get into the body, such as when mosquitoes help transfer the West Nile virus.

The body also has openings that are not covered by skin, and those openings can become portals of entry. The body protects itself in those instances through mucous membranes, which help trap pathogens attempting to enter the body and so protect the respiratory and gastrointestinal tracts along with other portals of entry. The body also uses hair and cilia as a means of protecting itself. **Cilia** are hairlike projections in the lungs and respiratory tract. They propel any pathogens toward openings in the body where they are released into the external environment (NIH 2003).

Not only does the body have physical defenses, but it has chemical ones as well. Secretions such as saliva and stomach acid provide another line of defense against infectious pathogens. Those secretions are often filled with enzymes, or special proteins, that destroy invading pathogens (NIH 2003).

Unfortunately, the external barriers can be damaged. One of the most common sources of damage to the external barriers is tobacco smoke, which can cause significant damage to the cilia protecting the airway. As a result, smokers often have a prominent cough, which expels pathogens from the airways. Medications and alcohol abuse are other sources of damage to the external defenses. Prolonged use of certain medications and alcohol can weaken mucous membranes, decreasing the ability of the membranes to keep pathogens out of the body.

Immune System

If pathogens do breach the external defense system, your body is armed with an immune system to protect itself. The immune system is highly complex, and its primary goal is to remove pathogens and other foreign materials after they've entered the body. Components of the immune system include the tonsils, lymph nodes, lymphatic vessels, thymus, spleen, Peyer's patches, appendix, and bone marrow (see figure 7.2).

The immune system has two parts: the **innate immune system** and **acquired immune system** (NIH 2003). Both systems are similar in function, but there are significant differences between the two.

The innate immune system is a fast-response system that is present from birth and that is designed to remove any foreign matter. When a pathogen breaches the external defenses, the innate immune system causes inflammation at the site. The inflammation causes redness, pain, warmth, and swelling. The innate system also helps the body identify bacteria, and it activates cells to clear dead cells because an overabundance of dead cells can prevent the body from functioning properly. Finally, the innate system identifies foreign substances in the organs, tissues, blood, and lymph and removes them by the use of macrophages. Macrophages are white blood cells that ingest foreign material and remove it from the body (NIH 2003).

The acquired immune system is composed of two types: active and passive. Active immunity targets specific foreign particles. The active immune system grows as you are exposed to a variety of disease-causing pathogens. Every time a cell of the active immune system is exposed to a disease-causing pathogen, it creates a memory of the pathogen. As a result, the next time the cell encounters the same pathogen, it can launch a faster, more aggressive response (NIH 2003). For example, when the body is exposed to the chicken pox virus, it creates a memory of the virus. The next time the body is exposed to the virus, the active immune system remembers it and launches an aggressive attack before the virus becomes a full-blown infection (Baron 1996).

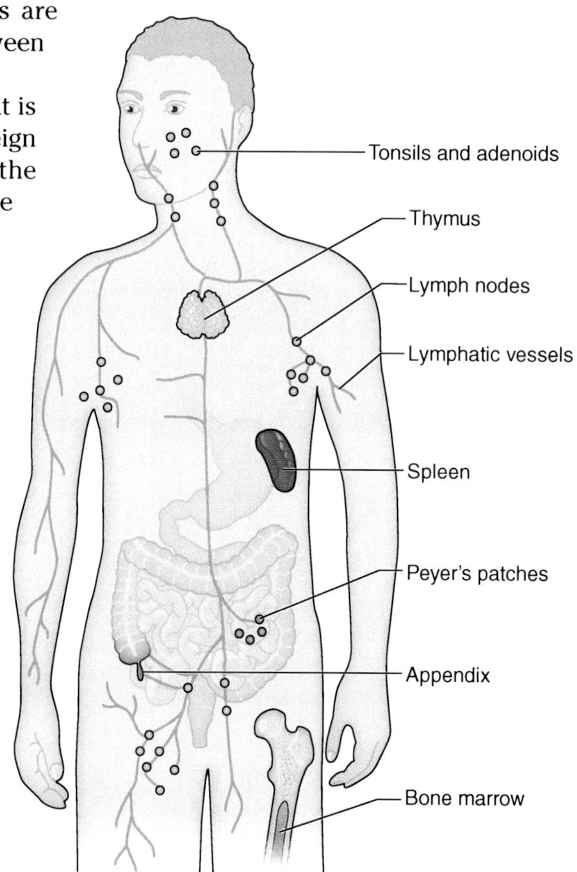

Figure 7.2 The immune system, which consists of numerous components, works to fight pathogens and foreign materials that enter your body.

Vaccinations, or immunizations, are also considered part of the active immune system. A vaccination requires small doses of an antigen, usually dead or weakened live viruses. These small doses of antigen activate immune system memory, allowing the body to react efficiently to any future exposure (Microbytes 2004).

Passive immunity is immunity that is received from another source. For example, most babies receive immunity from their mother through the placenta. Newborns also can acquire passive immunity through their mother's breast milk. This passive immunity helps protect the newborn until his or her body can actively establish its own immunity.

Autoimmune diseases occur when the body launches the immune system against its own cells and tissues. This occurs because the body cannot recognize those cells and tissues as part of it. In a normally functioning immune system, the white blood cells of the immune system protect the body from disease-causing pathogens. However, in an immune system affected by an autoimmune disease, the immune system cannot differentiate between healthy cells and tissues and disease-causing pathogens (MedlinePlus 2007). Because the immune system cannot differentiate between the two, it destroys perfectly healthy body cells.

The causes behind autoimmune disorders are still unknown, although researchers hypothesize that genetics, sex, and environmental factors may play a role in causing these diseases. Examples of autoimmune diseases are lupus, multiple sclerosis, Graves' disease, and rheumatoid arthritis. Women are more likely than men to be affected by autoimmune disorders (MedlinePlus 2007).

Allergies

Allergies, also known as *hypersensitivity*, occur when the immune system reacts to something that does not cause reactions in other people. When you experience an allergic reaction, your immune system is responding to a false alarm. Common causes of allergies include pollen, pet dander, mold, food, and medications. Allergies are due to your genetics along with your environment. Symptoms of allergies include sneezing, itching, rashes, swelling, and a runny nose, depending on the type of allergy (MedlinePlus 2008).

Although most allergies are simply inconveniences, severe allergic reactions can occur. These severe and sometimes fatal allergic reactions are known as *anaphylaxis*. Anaphylactic reactions are often sudden and severe and can involve the whole body. When a person experiences anaphylactic, histamine is released into the body, which causes airways to constrict. As a result, it is difficult for the person to breathe normally. Signs and symptoms of anaphylaxis include difficulty breathing, weakness, rapid pulse, and mental confusion. If a person is having an anaphylactic reaction, immediate professional medical attention is required. Call emergency medical services (911) immediately, and if the person having the reaction has an epinephrine needle nearby, the epinephrine should be injected immediately into the thigh in order to open airways and lower blood pressure (MedlinePlus 2008).

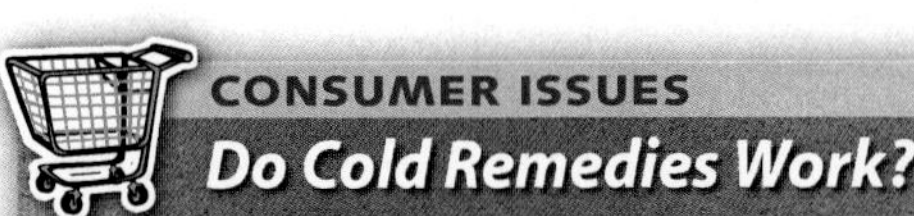

CONSUMER ISSUES

Do Cold Remedies Work?

Several products on the market claim to help you avoid catching colds or recover from a cold faster and make it less severe. For example, Airborne is one product that claims to help you avoid catching colds. Created by a school teacher, Airborne is a dietary supplement composed of 17 types of vitamins, minerals, and herbs that are claimed to work together to help your body's immune system fight off colds (Airborne Health 2007). Another product, Zicam, is a homeopathic medicine that claims to reduce both the duration and severity of a cold if it is taken when symptoms are first noticed (Zicam 2008).

As always, talk with your health care provider if you have questions about these or other products or if you have extenuating medical conditions that may be compromised by using such products.

COMMON INFECTIOUS DISEASES

There are scores of infectious diseases. This chapter can't cover them all, so we'll focus on the ones that you're most likely to encounter during your college career: the common cold, influenza, bacterial meningitis, pertussis, tuberculosis, mononucleosis, pneumonia, and West Nile virus (see table 7.2).

TABLE 7.2 Eight Common Infectious Diseases

Disease	Symptoms or effects	Treatment	Vaccination
Common cold (acute rhinitis)	Mild muscle aches, mild weakness, a runny or stuffy nose, a sore throat, nasal discharge	Drink plenty of fluids, get plenty of rest, and eat well to help bolster your weakened immune system; take over-the-counter medications to ease muscle aches or to help with a runny nose, fatigue, or fever.	None
Influenza (the flu)	Headaches; severe muscle aches; sudden onset of fatigue and weakness; sudden onset of a high fever, chills, sore throat, and cough	Drink plenty of fluids, get plenty of rest, take aspirin when needed, take antiviral prescription medication if needed.	Yes; recommended for those with compromised or weakened immune systems
Bacterial meningitis	Sudden onset of a high fever, sudden onset of a severe headache, acute fatigue, nausea, and stiff neck; purple rash and seizures may occur if the disease progresses; can lead to brain damage or death	Seek early diagnosis via a spinal tap; treat with antibiotics.	Yes; required by many colleges and universities
Pertussis (whooping cough)	Runny nose, slight fever, nasal congestion, dry coughs that can last for several minutes and end with a whooping sound	Treat with antibiotics.	Yes; most American infants are vaccinated, but immunity decreases over time
Tuberculosis	Fever, weight loss, weakness, night sweats, chest pain, coughing, coughing of blood	Treat with antibiotics.	Not given routinely in the United States
Mononucleosis (mono)	Sore throat, fever, swollen glands, headache, chills, nausea, severe and persistent fatigue and weakness; spleen may become enlarged and rupture	Get plenty of bed rest (a month or two), eat a balanced diet, drink adequate fluids, and use over-the-counter medications such as aspirin and lozenges.	None
Pneumonia	High fever, severe chest pains, shortness of breath, chills, productive cough	Treat with antibiotics.	Yes, for bacterial pneumonia (the most common form)
West Nile virus	Headache, fever, diarrhea, nausea, vomiting, skin rash, backache, swollen lymph glands, lack of appetite; rarely, inflammation of the brain or spinal cord (which can cause paralysis)	For severe cases, treat with intravenous fluids combined with pain relievers.	None

Common Cold

Everyone has caught a **cold** at one time or another. It's the most prevalent infectious disease of all. Even though a cold usually lasts a short time and is generally harmless, it's irritating and gets in the way of your daily activities.

The common cold, also known as *acute rhinitis*, can be caused by any of the more than 200 types of rhinoviruses (Mayo Clinic 2007a). It's a contagious viral infection that is generally spread by person-to-person contact. That's why many people catch colds in the winter: They have to stay indoors more.

The cold is characterized as a severe infection of the upper respiratory tract. Symptoms of acute rhinitis in the early stages include mild muscle aches, mild weakness, a runny or stuffy nose, a sore throat, and nasal discharge (Mayo Clinic 2007a). Symptoms usually become less noticeable after a few days. Although there is no known cure for colds, there are things you can do to alleviate your symptoms. When you first notice symptoms, drink plenty of fluids, get plenty of rest, and eat well to help bolster your weakened immune system (Mayo Clinic 2007a). Because colds are caused by viruses, antibiotics are not effective in alleviating symptoms. To alleviate symptoms, you can take over-the-counter medications to ease muscle aches or to help with a runny nose, fatigue, or fever. You can find the appropriate medication by talking to a pharmacist at your local drugstore. You can also gargle with hot water and salt and use lozenges to help a sore throat.

Influenza

Another acute infectious disease caused by viruses is **influenza**, or the flu (Mayo Clinic 2007i). The flu is an infection of the respiratory tract caused by the influenza virus and is usually transmitted by way of droplets. Because influenza is highly contagious, it has spawned several outbreaks. The infamous Spanish flu in 1918 and 1919 caused approximately 50 million deaths worldwide (CDC 2007j).

Similar to the common cold, the flu is especially prevalent during winter months because people are in close contact in crowded environments. The flu is characterized by headaches, severe muscle aches, sudden onset fatigue and weakness, and sudden onset of a high fever, chills, sore throat, and cough (CDC 2007j). People tend to fully recover from the flu within 1 to 2 weeks.

To help reduce flu symptoms, you should get plenty of rest, drink lots of fluids, and take aspirin when needed. Antiviral prescription medications are available to shorten the duration of the illness. In otherwise healthy people, the flu usually isn't life threatening (CDC 2007j). However, in people with an immune system that is already compromised, the flu can be fatal. Sometimes people with the flu can develop complications, such as pneumonia. People with compromised or weak immune systems should get an annual influenza vaccination (Mayo Clinic 2007i).

What Do You Do?

Try to track the chain of infection for the flu. Identify the agent, the reservoir, the portal of the exit, the mode of transmission, the portal of entry, and the new host.

Bacterial Meningitis

Meningitis is an inflammation of the meninges, the membranes covering the brain and spinal cord. Meningitis can be caused by both a virus and bacteria (CDC 2007h). Viral meningitis is often mild, but bacterial meningitis requires immediate attention because it can be fatal.

The close, cramped quarters of college dormitories are excellent places for bacterial meningitis to spread. It spreads through air droplets or by direct contact with someone who is infected. Although bacterial meningitis is rare, it can have serious consequences. In cases of bacterial meningitis, early diagnosis and treatment are crucial because the disease can attack the organs, creating brain damage and resulting in amputations and even death (CDC 2007h).College students are at an increased risk of contracting meningococcal meningitis, a virulent form of meningitis, because of their lifestyle. Not only do many college students live in a dormitory setting, but they are in contact with students from all over the world, have irregular sleep patterns, smoke and share cigarettes, and share food and beverages. Because the early signs and symptoms of meningococcal meningitis are similar to those of the common cold or influenza, people don't seek immediate treatment (CDC 2007h).

Signs and symptoms of meningococcal meningitis include sudden onset of a high fever, sudden onset of a severe headache, acute fatigue, nausea, and a stiff neck. A purple rash and seizures may occur if the disease progresses (Mayo Clinic 2007j). Definite diagnosis of meningococcal meningitis can only be done by analyzing a sample of spinal fluid, which is obtained through a spinal tap. After the bacterium has been identified, meningococcal meningitis can be treated with antibiotics. Fortunately, a vaccine (Menactra) is now available for meningococcal meningitis and the other three types of bacterial meningitis (Mayo Clinic 2007j). It is more than 80 percent effective, and more and more colleges and universities are requiring students to be immunized for bacterial meningitis.

Pertussis

Pertussis, more commonly known as *whooping cough*, is a highly communicable disease that can last for many weeks (CDC 2005a). An infection of the respiratory tract, pertussis is spread through droplets by *Bordetella pertussis* bacteria. Symptoms of pertussis include runny nose, slight fever, and nasal congestion—symptoms that are similar to those of the common cold. However, unlike the common cold, whooping cough sufferers have a dry cough, resulting in coughing bouts that can last for several minutes and end with a whooping sound. Most Americans are vaccinated for pertussis as infants, but as they reach adolescence and adulthood, their immunity decreases over time (Mayo Clinic 2007n). If you do get pertussis, it can be treated with antibiotics.

Tuberculosis

Tuberculosis is one of the most common infectious diseases in the world; it affects about 30 percent of the global population. In the 1800s, tuberculosis was a major killer in the United

ISSUES IN THE NEWS

The 2007 Tuberculosis Scare

Does the name *Andrew Speaker* ring a bell? In the early summer months of 2007, it seemed you couldn't turn on the news without hearing his name.

Andrew Speaker is an American citizen who flew to Europe in May 2007 for his wedding and honeymoon even though he knew he had tuberculosis. Speaker's ordeal started in January 2007 when he went to the doctor after a fall and a chest X ray revealed tuberculosis. On May 11, public health officials met with Speaker to recommend that he not travel. Despite this recommendation, Speaker flew to Europe. While he was abroad, the CDC contacted him and told him not to travel because recent test results revealed he had XDR-TB, a dangerous, drug-resistant strain of tuberculosis. Despite the warning, on May 24th Speaker traveled to Canada because he was on a no-fly list for the United States. He crossed the Canadian–United States border and checked in to a New York hospital, where he was immediately placed in isolation. On May 28th, he flew on a CDC airplane to Atlanta, where he became the first American since 1963 to be placed into CDC-ordered isolation. From there, he was flown to the National Jewish Hospital in Denver (Bluestein and Barrett 2007; Hartenstein 2007).

What would you have done if you were in Speaker's situation? How would you have felt if you had been one of the passengers on the airplanes whose health was compromised?

States (Mayo Clinic 2006c). Known as *consumption* or *white death*, tuberculosis was easily spread due to crowded living conditions, poor sanitation, and lack of quarantine measures. However, by the 1980s, tuberculosis was thought to be under control in the United States (CDC 2007l). As more immigrants enter the United States and more people from the United States travel to other countries, though, the incidence of tuberculosis is on the rise again (Fauci 2004).

Tuberculosis is a chronic bacterial infection caused by *Mycobacterium tuberculosis*. It is spread from person to person through the air when an infected person coughs, sneezes, or even speaks. Tuberculosis most often affects the lungs, but it can also affect the brain, kidneys, and spine. Symptoms of tuberculosis include fever, weight loss, weakness, night sweats, chest pain, coughing, and coughing of blood (Mayo Clinic 2006c).

Fortunately, tuberculosis can be treated with medication. People who are diagnosed with tuberculosis are considered highly contagious and are often quarantined. They aren't allowed to attend school or work and can't visit with friends or family without the protection of a precautionary face mask (CDC 2007l).

Unfortunately, certain strains of the tuberculosis bacterium have become resistant to antibiotics. Multidrug-resistant (MDR) tuberculosis is becoming more and more prevalent in the United States. Factors leading to the increase in MDR tuberculosis include patients failing to take medications properly, improper care and treatment of the disease by health care providers, and weakened immune systems of susceptible people. Public health workers are once again reminding the public to take precautions, get screened, and get treatment if necessary to help combat this reemerging communicable disease.

Mononucleosis

Mononucleosis, also known in the vernacular as *kissing disease* or *mono,* is a communicable disease caused by the Epstein-Barr virus. Mono is spread by contact with the saliva of an infected person. Symptoms of mono are sore throat, fever, swollen glands, headache, chills, nausea, and severe and persistent fatigue and weakness. Occasionally, the spleen may become enlarged and rupture, in which case prompt medical attention is required (Mayo Clinic 2006a).

The persistent fatigue and weakness associated with mono often requires at least a month or two of rest (Mayo Clinic 2006a). That's a significant amount of time for a college student to be out of commission, so it's important to maintain a healthy and strong immune system to fend off the illness. The best ways to boost immunity are to eat a well-balanced diet, get plenty of sleep, and exercise regularly.

Treatment for mononucleosis involves getting lots of bed rest, eating a balanced diet, drinking adequate fluids, and using over-the-counter medications such as aspirin and lozenges. Eventually, the body will develop immunity to the disease and normal activities can resume (Mayo Clinic 2006a).

Pneumonia

The leading cause of death in the United States in the early 1900s was pneumonia. Today, it's ranked eighth overall, but it's the leading cause of death from infectious disease (CDC 2007g).

Pneumonia is an infection of the lungs and lower respiratory tract, and it's caused by bacteria, viruses, or fungi. The most common form is bacterial pneumonia. Pneumonia generally follows a bout of another illness, such as a cold or the flu. Characteristics of pneumonia are high fever, severe chest pains, shortness of breath, chills, and a productive cough. It is easily transmittable from person to person. Bacterial pneumonia is generally treated with antibiotics. People with compromised immune systems such as the very young, the very old, and those with AIDS are at a higher risk of contracting pneumonia than the general population is (Mayo Clinic 2007l). Fortunately, vaccinations are available for bacterial pneumonia, and people who are at a higher risk should be vaccinated.

West Nile Virus

The **West Nile virus** is transmitted by mosquitoes that have bitten wild birds—usually crows and jays—that serve as reservoirs for the virus (CDC 2006e). The virus is endemic to Africa, West Asia, and the Middle East, and it was introduced to the United States during the summer of 1999. Since then, all 48 contiguous states have reported cases of the virus (CDC 2007b).

The majority of people who have become infected with West Nile virus don't display any signs or symptoms or develop only a mild infection known as *West Nile fever.* Signs and symptoms include headache, fever, diarrhea, nausea, vomiting, skin rash, backache, swollen lymph glands, and a lack of appetite (CDC 2006e). On rare occasions, the virus can cause **encephalitis**, or inflammation of the brain, along with inflammation of the membranes surrounding the brain, or **meningoencephalitis**. An inflammation of the spinal cord due to the West Nile virus is known as **West Nile poliomyelitis** and causes weakening of the arms and legs, severe headache, lack of coordination and balance, and paralysis (Mayo Clinic 2007m). The symptoms of West Nile fever generally last for no more than a week, but the neurological infections can last for weeks and can even be permanent.

The risk of getting West Nile virus depends on several variables. First, the time of year is a factor. The West Nile virus follows a seasonal pattern in the temperate regions of the United States. The high-risk season begins in the late spring and peaks in the late summer and early fall. However, people who live in southern climates are at risk throughout the year, and living in or visiting areas of the United States that are more prone to mosquito-borne illnesses can increase the risk of developing West Nile virus. Finally, the amount of time spent outside increases the risk of becoming infected because the likelihood of being bitten by an infected mosquito is higher when you're outside a lot (CDC 2007b).

People are more likely to become severely ill from the virus if they are older than 50 or have a weakened immune system. Blood tests can determine whether a person has been infected with the West Nile virus. If a clinician suspects a more serious condition than West Nile fever,

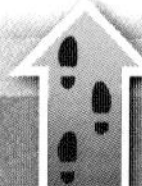

STEPS FOR BEHAVIORAL CHANGE

Fight the Bite

The first and foremost thing you can do to protect yourself from West Nile virus is prevent mosquito bites. Use insect repellent containing DEET, Picaridin, oil of lemon, eucalyptus, or IR3535. Insect repellents with these active ingredients have been proven to provide long-lasting protection and are safe for humans. Because mosquitoes are most active at dawn and dusk, consider staying inside during these times. If you have to be outside, make sure you use insect repellent and wear long-sleeved shirts and long pants. Repair or replace broken screens on your windows and doors so that mosquitoes stay out. Also, eliminate standing water and debris near your home so mosquitoes don't have a chance to reproduce:

- If you have a birdbath, make sure it is cleaned weekly.
- If you have an ornamental pond, stock it with fish that eat mosquito larvae, such as minnows or goldfish.
- Empty water from containers where mosquitoes might breed.
- Empty your pet's water bowl daily so mosquitoes don't have a chance to repopulate in the standing water.
- If your property has tree-rot holes or hollow stumps, fill those in so they do not accumulate water.
- Unclog roof gutters and empty unused swimming pools.

spinal taps, CAT scans, and magnetic resonance imaging (MRI) can determine if encephalitis or West Nile poliomyelitis are present.

Most people who have been infected with West Nile virus recover on their own. For those with more severe cases, intravenous fluids combined with pain relievers are recommended (Mayo Clinic 2007m).

SEXUALLY TRANSMITTED INFECTIONS

Many infectious diseases are transmitted through sexual contact and fall under the category of **sexually transmitted infections (STIs)**. The symptoms, severity, and treatment differ for each. The risk of getting an STI increases when people don't practice safe sex. In other words, people with multiple sexual partners, those whose sexual partners have many sexual partners, and those who don't use latex or polyurethane condoms increase their risk of getting an STI. This section describes the transmission, symptoms, and treatment of eight common STIs.

HIV and AIDS

Acquired immunodeficiency syndrome (AIDS) is a chronic, life-threatening infectious disease that is one of the most significant public health threats globally (CDC 2007f). The virus that causes AIDS is the human immunodeficiency virus (HIV), and it affects millions worldwide. HIV damages the immune system, making it difficult for the body to fight disease-causing organisms. Approximately 39 million people worldwide are living with HIV, and nearly half of them are women between the ages of 15 and 24 (CDC 2007f).

Similar to most STIs, HIV does not usually display any signs or symptoms in its early stages. One symptom that may present itself is a flulike illness that lasts anywhere from 2 to 6 weeks. Other symptoms of initial infection are similar to symptoms of many other illnesses, so people

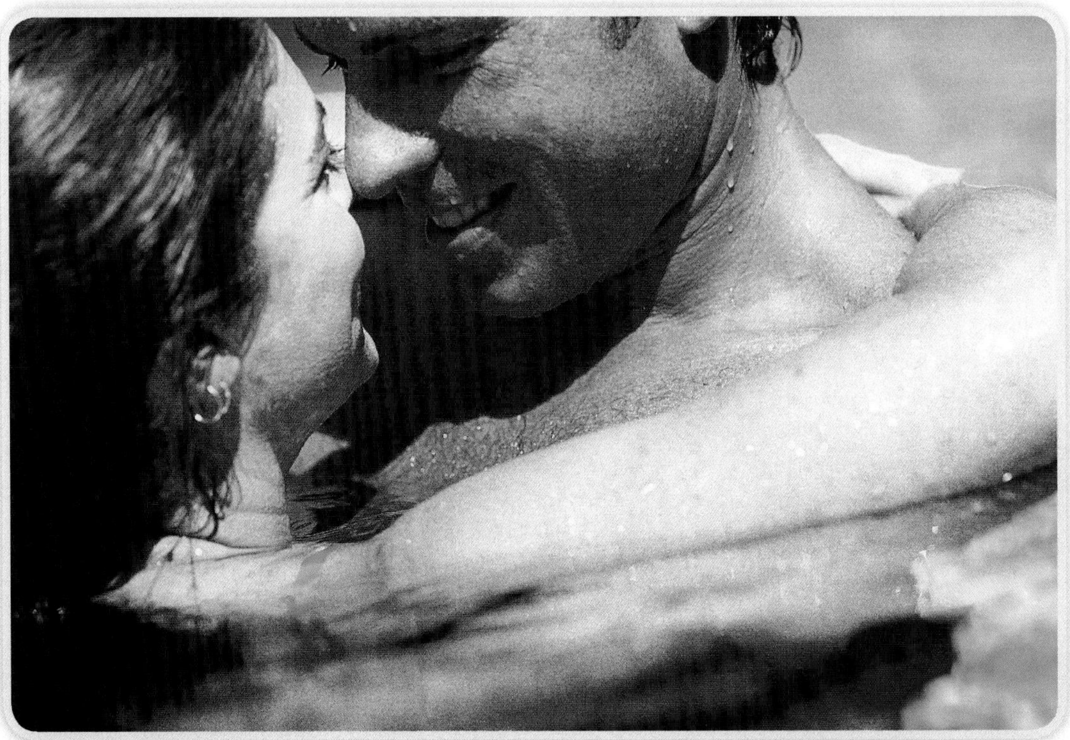

Practice safe sex to reduce your chances of developing or spreading a sexually transmitted infection.

© Stewart Cohen / Digital Vision

might not realize they have HIV. It's crucial to practice safe sex, because even if partners don't seem sick, they might still have the virus and be able to pass it on (CDC 2007f).

After HIV has entered the body, the virus multiplies in the lymph nodes, destroying **helper T cells**, the white blood cells that oversee the immune system. HIV can be at work in the body destroying the immune system for as long as 8 years before an infected person notices any signs or symptoms of illness. When signs and symptoms do appear, they include swollen lymph nodes, diarrhea, weight loss, fever, cough, and shortness of breath (CDC 2007f). More serious signs begin to appear in the last phase of the infection, which can happen 10 or more years after the initial infection. At this point, the infection often becomes full-blown AIDS.

With AIDS, the immune system has become very compromised, leaving the afflicted person susceptible to a variety of infections. At this stage, a person with AIDS has many unpleasant symptoms (Mayo Clinic 2007g):

- Profuse night sweats
- Chills that last for several weeks
- A fever higher than 100 degrees Fahrenheit (38 degrees Celsius) that lasts for several weeks
- Dry cough
- Shortness of breath
- Persistent diarrhea
- Lesions on the tongue or in the mouth
- Headaches
- Blurred vision
- Chronic fatigue
- Swollen lymph nodes
- Rapid weight loss

HIV can be transmitted in several ways. The most common method is sexual transmission. Blood, semen, and vaginal secretions carry HIV and can infect anyone who comes into contact with them. Another method of transmission is through infected blood. The virus can live in blood and blood products that are given during blood transfusions. Before 1985, hospitals and blood banks didn't do any blood screening for HIV, so people who received blood transfusions before 1985 were at risk of becoming infected with the virus. Now, blood is tested and donors are screened to better protect the public (Mayo Clinic 2007g).

People who share needles are also at a higher risk of contracting HIV. Intravenous drug users need to either sterilize their needles or participate in needle exchange programs in which they can trade used needles and syringes for new, sterile ones. Health care workers are also at risk of becoming infected with HIV through accidental needle sticks. An infected mother can pass the virus to her unborn child or to her newborn through breast-feeding. Transmission through those methods is much more prevalent in underdeveloped countries, such as those in sub-Saharan Africa, than in developed nations. In rare instances, HIV can be transmitted through organ transplants or the use of unsterilized medical equipment (CDC 2007f).

HIV is an equal-opportunity infector. The virus can infect anyone regardless of age, gender, race, or sexual orientation. However, certain behaviors make the risk of developing HIV even higher. Unprotected sex with multiple partners is a major risk factor for contracting HIV, and so is having unprotected sex with someone who is HIV-positive. Having another STI also increases the risk of contracting HIV (CDC 2007f).

HIV is diagnosed by testing for the presence of antibodies in the blood. The CDC recommends that every adult be tested at least once for HIV and that people who have a high risk for infection be tested more frequently (CDC 2007f). Because it takes time for the body to create antibodies against HIV, tests are not reliable immediately after infection. In the early days of HIV screening, only one test existed and the results often took several weeks. However, as

What Do You Do?

In 2006, the CDC reported that 33.7 percent of adult men in the United States had been tested for HIV, and 37.8 percent of adult women had been tested. Furthermore, the CDC believes that approximately 180,000 to 280,000 people nationwide are infected with HIV but do not know it (CDC 2008b; National HIV Testing Day [NHTD] n.d.). What can you do? Visit www.hivtest.org/search/result.cfm to find an HIV testing clinic near you. By taking the test, you can take control of your life.

technology has advanced, a rapid test has been developed that can give results in as little as 20 minutes.

The most common complication from HIV is susceptibility to various infections. Because the immune system is greatly weakened, the body is more vulnerable to disease-causing pathogens. Bacterial pneumonia is one of the most common infections found in people with HIV. In underdeveloped nations, tuberculosis is another opportunistic infection that develops in those who are HIV-positive. Additionally, people with HIV are at a higher risk of developing viral infections such as herpes, viral hepatitis, and human papillomavirus (HPV) (CDC 2007f). Furthermore, people who are HIV-positive are at a greater risk of developing certain types of cancer than those who are not.

A type of cancer commonly found in HIV-infected people is Kaposi's sarcoma, a tumor in the walls of the blood vessels. This cancer is characterized by pink or red lesions in the skin or mouth. People with HIV are also at a higher risk of developing non-Hodgkin's lymphoma, a cancer of the white blood cells that is characterized by painless swelling in the lymph nodes of the neck, groin, or armpit (CDC 2007f).

When HIV and AIDS were first diagnosed in the early 1980s, clinicians could do little for people who were infected. Remarkable medical advances now allow people who have access to medications and proper medical care to live longer, healthier lives. Antiretroviral medications now exist that allow HIV-positive people to live almost normal lives. These medications allow them to attend college, maintain full-time jobs, and have relationships. Though the drugs can extend lives, they can't completely cure the illness and they often have severe side effects. Plus, the antiviral drugs are expensive. Researchers are currently working on developing more pharmaceuticals that will further extend the lives of people with HIV and AIDS. They're also working on a vaccine to help prevent the spread of the disease (CDC 2007f).

Because there's still no vaccine for HIV or cure for AIDS, practicing safe sex is essential. Using a condom during sex is one of the most effective and efficient methods of preventing the spread of HIV. It's important to know the HIV status of all potential sexual partners. In addition, intravenous drug users shouldn't share needles and need to be sure to use a clean, sterile needle every time. Many communities provide needle exchange programs. People traveling overseas should be cautious of receiving tainted blood products because many countries don't have rigorous blood screening. Finally, any sexually active person should get tested for HIV (CDC 2007f).

Hepatitis

Hepatitis B, a serious liver disease, is caused by the hepatitis B virus (HBV). HBV can be transmitted from one person to another through sexual contact, through shared needles, and from mother to child during pregnancy (Mayo Clinic 2007f). It's highly contagious and can also be spread through close, nonsexual contact by exposure to infected blood and by contact with mucous membranes. Although hepatitis B can be fatal and has no cure, a vaccine is available. Any health care worker who has frequent contact with blood and other bodily fluids should be vaccinated (CDC 2006c).

People infected with hepatitis B often are asymptomatic, but if an infected person does display symptoms, they include nausea, fever, chills, fatigue, loss of appetite, dark urine, abdominal pain, jaundice, and joint pain (CDC 2006c). Because hepatitis B is a viral infection, those who become infected carry HBV their entire lives. As a result, they are at a higher risk for developing liver cancer, liver failure, and cirrhosis.

Blood tests can be used to diagnose someone with HBV. No treatment exists for acute cases of HBV infections, but those with chronic infections can use antiviral drugs. But, it's better to avoid the disease than to treat it. The CDC recommends the HBV vaccination for all infants, unvaccinated children and adolescents, and unvaccinated adults. In addition, people who are sexually active should use protection such as condoms (CDC 2006c). Intravenous drug users should never share needles or syringes. Finally, people getting a tattoo or body piercing need to make sure that all the needles and equipment are sterile.

Syphilis

Caused by the bacterium *Treponema pallidum*, **syphilis** is an STI with signs and symptoms similar to those of other diseases (CDC 2007k). Syphilis used to cause death and disability, but now it can be treated with antibiotics. It is transmitted through direct contact with a syphilis sore during oral, vaginal, or anal sex. Infected women can also pass syphilis to their children in utero (CDC 2007k).

Syphilis has three stages: primary, secondary, and tertiary. In the primary (first) stage of the disease, a chancre sore develops, usually at the site of the initial infection (see figure 7.3). The sore in males can usually be found near the penis or scrotum. The site of infection in women is often internal, usually on the cervix or vaginal wall. The sore can also be found in the mouth or throat if a person got the infection through oral sex. The chancre sore usually develops within 10 to 90 days of initial exposure. Because chancres have large amounts of bacteria, they make syphilis highly contagious when they're present. Often painless, the chancre sores heal on their own in a few weeks (Mayo Clinic 2006b).

If the infection isn't treated during the primary stage, it will progress to the secondary stage. The secondary stage appears anywhere from 3 weeks to 1 year after the chancre disappears. This stage is characterized by white patches on the skin, lesions on mucous membranes, hair loss, fever, headache, fatigue, weight loss, and swollen lymph nodes (Mayo Clinic 2006b). As in the primary stage, signs of secondary syphilis will heal with or without treatment. However, if no treatment is obtained during this stage, syphilis will progress to the latent, or tertiary, stage of the disease, which is the final stage.

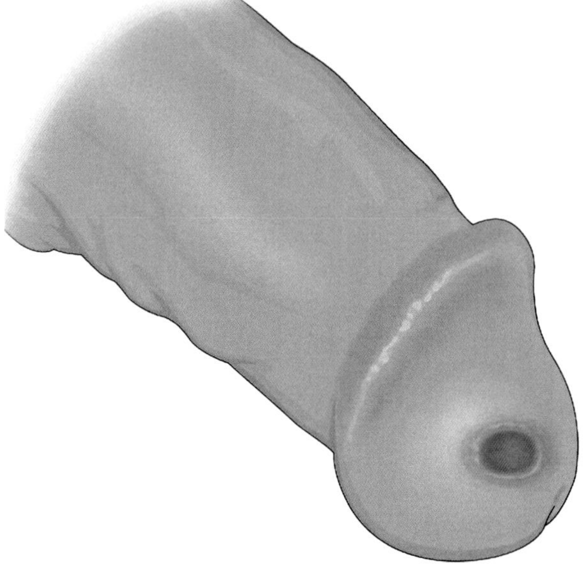

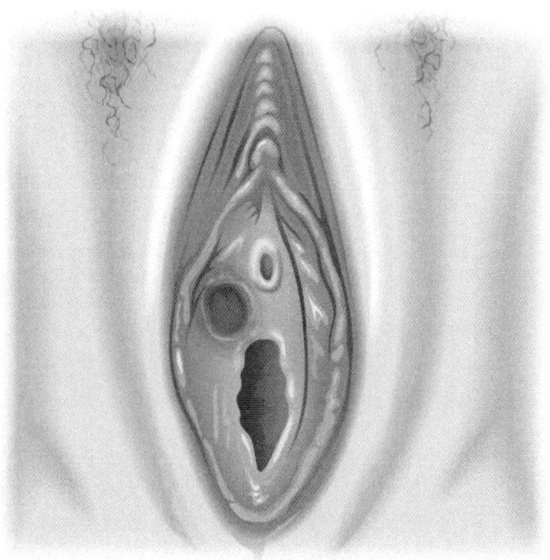

Figure 7.3 With syphilis, a chancre sore can develop on the penis or on the cervix or vaginal wall. The bacteria-laden sores make syphilis highly contagious.

During the latent, or hidden, stage of the disease, the disease is still present even though there are no signs and symptoms. During the latent stage, infection is usually not transmitted to others except from mother to child (congenital syphilis) (Mayo Clinic 2006b). Congenital syphilis often results in mental and physical problems for the newborn, including blindness, deafness, disfigurement, and even death. In the tertiary stage, severe internal damage to the organs can occur. There is often damage to the central nervous system, causing difficulty in muscle movement, numbness, and paralysis. In addition, sufferers in the tertiary stage may experience blindness, senility, dementia, and cardiovascular damage.

Syphilis is diagnosed by analyzing infected tissue and blood tests. Antibiotics can treat syphilis in all its stages, but it is easiest to cure in the early stages. Penicillin is the most common antibiotic for treatment, but others can be used by people who are allergic to penicillin. Although penicillin will kill *Treponema pallidum* and prevent further damage, it can't repair damage already done. People undergoing treatment for syphilis must not engage in sexual contact in order to avoid spreading the disease to their partners (Mayo Clinic 2006b).

Chlamydia

Chlamydia, an infection of the urogenital tract caused by the bacteria *Chlamydia trachomatis*, is the most frequently reported bacterial STI in the United States. *Chlamydia trachomatis* can be transmitted from one infected person to another through oral, vaginal, or anal sex. Infected mothers can also pass the bacteria to their babies during vaginal childbirth (CDC 2006a).

Because approximately 75 percent of infected women and 50 percent of infected men do not experience any signs or symptoms, chlamydia is known as the silent disease. Women who do experience symptoms may experience a burning sensation when urinating or abnormal vaginal discharge. As the infection spreads, women may experience lower back pain and abdominal pain, fever, bleeding between menstrual periods, and painful intercourse. Infected men can experience penile discharge, a burning sensation when urinating, and burning around the opening of the penis (CDC 2006a).

Serious consequences for women can occur if they leave chlamydia untreated. They can develop pelvic inflammatory disease (PID), which can damage the reproductive organs. In addition, women may experience chronic pelvic pain and infertility as a result of untreated chlamydia. These women also have an elevated risk of ectopic (tubal) pregnancy, a potentially life-threatening form of pregnancy where implantation of the fertilized egg occurs outside the uterus (CDC 2006d). The Centers for Disease Control and Prevention (CDC) recommends annual screenings for all sexually active women aged 25 and younger. The CDC also recommends screenings anytime a woman changes sex partners or has multiple sex partners (CDC 2006a). Men have few consequences from untreated chlamydia. They may experience fever and pain and, on rare occasions, sterility.

Fortunately, laboratory tests are available to diagnose chlamydia. Some tests use urine samples and others require a specimen from the cervix or penis. When chlamydia has been diagnosed, it can be treated and cured with antibiotics (CDC 2006a). All sexual partners of an infected person should be tested. It's possible for sexual partners to become reinfected, so people with chlamydia shouldn't have sexual intercourse until treatment is complete.

Gonorrhea

Gonorrhea is another common STI. Caused by the bacterium *Neisseria gonorrhoeae,* it is spread by contact with the mouth, vagina, penis, or anus. It can also be transmitted from an infected mother to her baby during delivery. Gonorrhea affects the linings of the urethra, genital tract, pharynx, and rectum. Although any sexually active person is at risk for becoming infected with gonorrhea, sexually active teenagers, young adults, and African Americans are at higher risk (CDC 2006b). As is the case with all STIs, the more sexual partners a person has, the greater the risk of developing gonorrhea.

CULTURAL ISSUES

Risks for African Americans

According to the CDC, in 2005, African Americans were 18 times more likely than Caucasians to be infected with gonorrhea (CDC 2007i). This is due in part to a lack of culturally appropriate television, print, billboard, and radio ads informing African Americans about the risk of gonorrhea, along with the lack of culturally appropriate educational materials. However, gonorrhea is not the only sexually transmitted disease African Americans have a greater risk of acquiring. For instance, in 2005, African Americans were 49 percent of the new HIV/AIDS cases in the United States. The primary method of transmission for African American men with HIV/AIDS was sexual relationships with other men. The next most common form of transmission was intravenous drug use, followed by high-risk sexual relationships between heterosexuals. For African American women, the most common method of transmission was high-risk sexual relationships, followed by intravenous drug use. It's not just adults who are disproportionately affected by HIV/AIDS—65 percent of all infants who were infected with HIV perinatally were African American (CDC 2008a).

African Americans face several obstacles to prevention and treatment of sexually transmitted diseases. First, many African Americans who are in poverty often live day to day, which means that medical care is not a priority for them, and they often lack health insurance, which can delay possible treatment and care. Because of the lack of health care, those who become infected might not realize it and might pass the disease to others. Another challenge faced by the African American community is denial. Because HIV/AIDS was initially seen in white homosexual males, some African Americans mistakenly believe the disease afflicts only those individuals. Finally, intravenous drug use is a very common method of HIV infection (CDC 2007i). Individuals who are intravenous drug users are also risk takers, causing them to engage in risky behaviors such as unprotected sex or exchanging sex for drugs.

Similar to chlamydia, some women are asymptomatic when they have been infected with gonorrhea. Those women who do have symptoms usually have a burning sensation when they urinate, vaginal discharge, painful intercourse, and severe menstrual cramping. Men can display symptoms 2 to 5 days after infection, although occasionally it can take up to a month for symptoms to appear. Symptoms in men include a burning sensation when urinating; white, yellow, or green penile discharge; and painful testicles.

If left untreated, gonorrhea can cause problems in both men and women. Women can develop PID, which can cause internal abscesses and chronic pelvic pain. Women with PID are more likely to be infertile or have ectopic pregnancies (Mayo Clinic 2007d). If men are not treated, they can develop epididymitis, an inflammation of the small tube (epididymis) behind the testicles, which causes pain and swelling in the scrotum and testicles. Children born to infected women can develop conjunctivitis, which is treated with silver nitrate drops in the eye (Mayo Clinic 2007d). If the *Neisseria gonorrhoeae* was transmitted orally, the infected person may experience soreness and redness in the throat.

Screenings are recommended for women who are under the age of 25, have had multiple sex partners in a single year, exchange sex for money or drugs, or have a history of several gonorrhea infections. In 2005, the U.S. Preventive Services Task Force found insufficient evidence to recommend for or against screening for men. Men usually have symptoms that lead to diagnosis and treatment. Asymptomatic infections are rare in men, whereas women often do not experience any clinical symptoms such as pain while urinating or discharge (CDC 2006b). Urine samples or an analysis of an infected area can be used to diagnosis gonorrhea.

Gonorrhea can be successfully treated with antibiotics. Many strains of gonorrhea are becoming drug-resistant, so it is vital that an infected person take the full course of medication prescribed. People infected with gonorrhea often also have chlamydia, so antibiotics for both infections are usually administered simultaneously. Because gonorrhea is highly contagious even when there are no signs or symptoms, precautions when engaging in any type of sexual activity are important (CDC 2006b). As with any STI, condom use is vital to deterring the spread of gonorrhea. People with gonorrhea should avoid any form of sexual contact until they have finished the course of medication and the infection has been cured.

Genital Herpes

A highly contagious STI, **genital herpes** is caused by a strain of the herpes simplex virus types 1 and 2 (HSV-1 and HSV-2). Most cases of genital herpes are caused by HSV-2 when it enters the body through tiny breaks in the skin or mucous membranes during either sexual contact or skin-to-skin contact. Often there are no signs or symptoms of genital herpes, but when they do occur they include pain, itching, a burning sensation when urinating, and sores (small, red bumps or blisters) in the genital area (see figure 7.4). The first outbreak is often the most painful. In addition to sores, the outbreak is characterized by a headache, fever, muscle aches, and swollen lymph nodes in the groin (CDC 2007c). Subsequent outbreaks can occur weeks or even months after the initial outbreak and are generally less severe. However, the number of outbreaks usually declines over the years. Both herpes viruses are found in the genital sores, but they can also be released between outbreaks. Therefore, it is important to practice safe sex methods even when no outbreak is apparent. In addition, HSV-1, which causes fever blisters, can cause genital herpes when there is oral–genital contact (Mayo Clinic 2007b).

For most healthy adults, there are no other complications from genital herpes. Nevertheless, being infected with genital herpes increases the risk of contracting other STIs. Studies have linked genital herpes combined with the presence of the HPV to an increased risk of cervical cancer. People with weakened immune systems may also experience more severe outbreaks than their healthier counterparts. Outbreaks can be triggered by stress, illness, surgery, and fatigue. A mother who has open sores can pass the infection to her newborn, who may be afflicted with brain damage, blindness, and even death. Because of the risk to the newborn, many physicians recommend that women with herpes deliver by cesarean section (CDC 2007c).

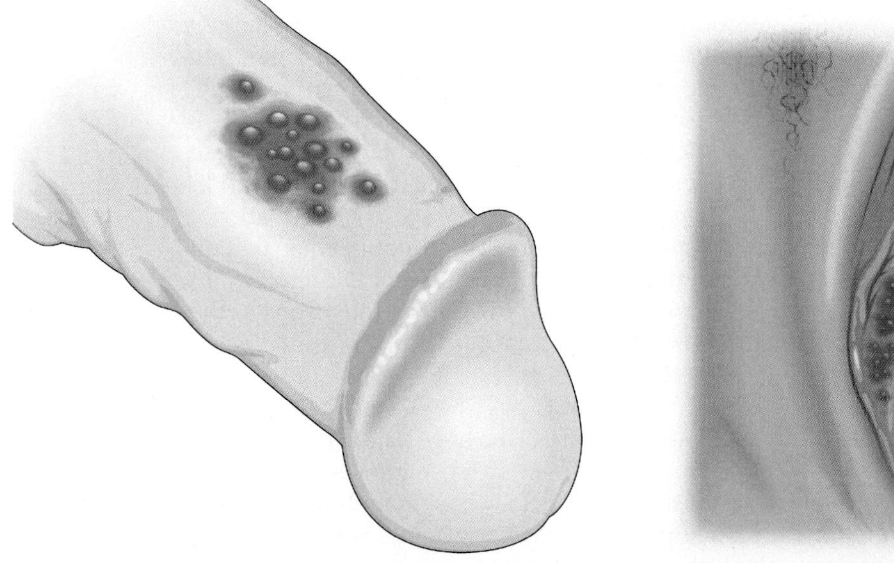

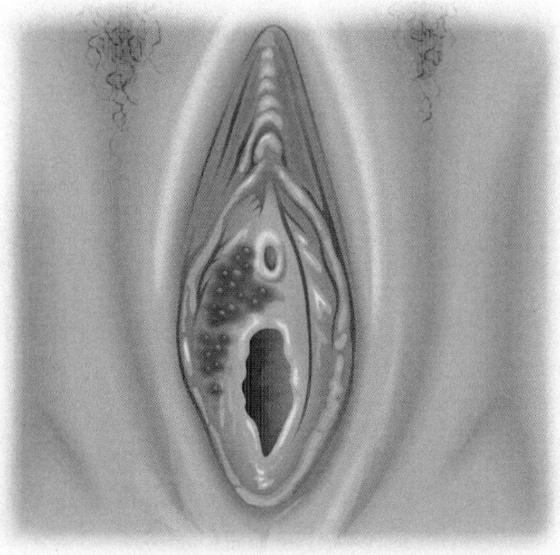

Figure 7.4 Symptoms of genital herpes can include small, red bumps or blisters on the penis or the vagina. Medications can shorten and prevent outbreaks, but currently no cure for herpes exists.

A health care provider can do a visual inspection of the genital area to diagnose genital herpes. In addition, diagnosis can be done by examining a sample or culture of the blisters. Blood tests are also available to detect herpes.

No treatment is available to cure herpes. However, antiviral medications can help shorten and prevent outbreaks. If the medications are taken daily, they can reduce the chance of infecting partners. Using condoms, limiting the number of sexual partners, and avoiding intercourse if either partner has a herpes outbreak are all ways to prevent the transmission of genital herpes. Although there is no vaccine for genital herpes on the market currently, several pharmaceutical companies are in the process of researching and developing them (CDC 2007c).

Genital Warts

Genital warts is an STI caused by the human papillomavirus (HPV). Genital warts can be found in the vagina, cervix, or rectum. In addition, genital warts can be found in the mouth or throat if there has been oral sexual contact.

HPV is transmitted mainly by genital contact. It affects 20 million people, and half of the sexually active population in the United States has had genital HPV at least once in their lives. Because most HPV infections don't show any signs or symptoms, infected people don't know they've been infected and can unwittingly transmit the infection to their partners. Occasionally, a pregnant woman may pass HPV to her child during a vaginal birth (CDC 2007d).

The warts can appear as flesh-colored bumps or have a cauliflower-like appearance. Genital warts are typically soft, moist, and pink (Mayo Clinic 2007c). They can be as small as a millimeter in diameter, but they can also increase into large clusters. Genital warts can also cause itching in the genital area along with bleeding and pain during intercourse.

Genital warts can be diagnosed by a visual exam. Often, the presence of HPV will cause an abnormal Pap smear in women (Mayo Clinic 2007c). HPV is of concern because it has been linked to cervical cancer. Because cervical cancer is preventable, it is vital for sexually active women to receive an annual gynecological exam including a Pap smear.

There is no cure for genital warts, but the warts can be removed by medications, such as topical creams. Health care workers can remove the warts by treatments such as freezing with liquid nitrogen or surgical removal. Even after the warts are removed, the virus will always remain in the body.

Having unprotected sex can increase the risk of developing genital warts. In addition, being diagnosed with another STI, becoming sexually active before age 20, having three or more sexual partners before age 35, and having sex with partners who have had three or more partners all increase the odds of contracting HPV (CDC 2007d).

The U.S. Food and Drug Administration (FDA) approved the Gardasil vaccine in June 2006 to offer protection from the most dangerous strains of HPV. The CDC recommends the vaccination for all 11- and 12-year-old girls, along with females aged 13 to 26 who have not already been vaccinated (CDC 2007d). To be most effective, the vaccine should be administered to girls before they become sexually active.

What Do You Do?

It's hard to make rational, well-considered decisions about your sexual behavior when you're unprepared and you find yourself in the heat of the moment. Take a few minutes now to decide how you'll talk with a potential sex partner about sexual history and health. How will you start the conversation? When will you bring it up? What will you want to ask and share about your own history?

Pelvic Inflammatory Disease

Pelvic inflammatory disease (PID) is an infection of the female reproductive organs, including the uterus and fallopian tubes. PID is a frequent and serious complication from untreated STIs such as gonorrhea and chlamydia. Similar to most STIs in women, there are few signs and symptoms. Women often do not realize they have PID until they attempt to become pregnant or begin to experience chronic pelvic pain.

PID is caused when bacteria, such as those that cause gonorrhea and chlamydia, move from the vagina or cervix to the reproductive organs. Women under the age of 25 are at a higher risk of developing PID because their cervixes are not fully mature (Mayo Clinic 2007k). Women who have multiple sex partners, who have sexual partners who have had multiple sexual partners, who douche, and who use an intrauterine device for contraception are all at higher risk of developing PID.

Most women with PID are asymptomatic, but some women do experience symptoms, which include painful intercourse, painful urination, heavy and odorous vaginal discharge, pain in the lower back and abdomen, and irregular menstrual bleeding (Mayo Clinic 2007k). Because PID often doesn't produce symptoms, it is difficult to diagnose, but clinical exams, such as a pelvic exam, can diagnose the disease. In addition, health care providers may do an analysis of vaginal discharge and cervical cultures and do pelvic ultrasounds (CDC 2004).

Fortunately, PID can be treated with antibiotics, either orally or by injection. Women should take the full course of the medication, even if symptoms have disappeared, to prevent the infection from recurring. If an infected woman shows signs of nausea, vomiting, or fever; is pregnant; doesn't respond to the medications; has an abscess in the fallopian tube or ovary; or is HIV-positive, she may need to go to the hospital.

Untreated PID results in scar tissue and abscesses, which can damage the reproductive organs. As a result, women with PID are more likely to have ectopic pregnancies, be infertile, and suffer from chronic pelvic pain (CDC 2004). Most cases of PID can be prevented by

CONTROVERSIAL ISSUES

Vaccinations and Autism

Some parents believe that vaccinations can cause children to develop autism, a developmental disability that can cause social interaction and communication problems (CDC 2007a). In February 2009, three U.S. families who claimed that vaccines had caused autism in their children were denied compensation by a special federal court ruling that found the vaccines weren't to blame. The rulings are the first test cases out of more than 5,000 claims that have been filed.

Scientists have conducted studies on whether a link exists between vaccinations and autism—you can read about past and current studies at www.cdc.gov/ncbddd/autism/documents/vaccine_studies.pdf—but they have found no scientific evidence showing a link between any vaccine or series of vaccinations and autism (National Institute of Child Health and Human Development 2006). Despite these results, some parents are choosing not to have their children vaccinated, which has the potential to create a serious public health problem.

To give you an idea of the magnitude of this problem, imagine a world in which people did not vaccinate. For example, before the development of the polio vaccine, 13,000 to 20,000 cases of polio occurred annually in the United States. In 2006, there were only 2,000 cases of polio globally (CDC 2007n). If people stop vaccinating before polio is eliminated, however, we could see a significant resurgence of the disease. Mumps is another communicable disease that has seen a decline in cases because of the introduction of the mumps vaccine, which is part of the mumps, measles, rubella (MMR) vaccination combination. In 1964, before the development of the mumps vaccine, there were approximately 212,000 cases of the disease in the United States (CDC 2007n). After the introduction of the vaccine, cases of mumps decreased. Because mumps is a highly contagious disease, even a few unvaccinated individuals can create an outbreak.

Vaccines are an important part of preventive care. Highly communicable diseases still exist and can become commonplace if we don't all do our part to protect ourselves and others.

following safe sex practices, such as having a monogamous sexual relationship and using latex condoms. Because PID is closely linked to chlamydia and gonorrhea, it is important for women to get treated immediately if they know they have been infected. Women should also get regular screenings for STIs if they have high-risk sexual behavior.

HOW TO PROTECT YOURSELF

Despite the numerous infectious diseases, pathogens, and transmittal methods, there are steps you can take to protect yourself. These include immunizations, hand washing, and safe sex.

Immunization

One of the most important things you can do to protect yourself against infectious diseases is to get timely vaccinations. Many of the infectious diseases that were widespread in the past have been controlled in the United States through the use of vaccinations. Vaccine-preventable diseases are at an all-time low (CDC 2007m). However, some children, adolescents, and adults remain underimmunized. Because some people haven't been vaccinated, it's even more important for you to receive all of your vaccinations and keep them up to date. Get a copy of your immunization records and make sure you're up to date. If you aren't, make an appointment with the health clinic to get the vaccinations you're missing.

College students especially should get the meningitis vaccine due to their close living quarters. In addition, women who haven't become sexually active or don't have HPV should consider getting the HPV vaccine to prevent genital warts and possibly cervical cancer (CDC 2007m). (The HPV vaccine is still effective for someone who is sexually active, but only if she hasn't been infected by HPV already from a previous partner.) Furthermore, although some illnesses, such as polio, have been completely eradicated in the United States, they're still prevalent in other countries. If you travel or participate in study abroad programs you might put yourself at risk for these diseases. Make sure you're up to date and compliant with vaccination schedules to eliminate any unnecessary risk.

Figure 7.5 shows the recommended adult immunization schedule for people over 18 years old. You can find the schedule for teens and college students who are 18 or younger at the

	Age group				
Vaccine	19–26 years	27–49 years	50–59 years	60–64 years	≥65 years
Tetanus, diphtheria, pertussis (Td/Tdap)*	Substitute 1-time dose of Tdap for Td booster; then boost with Td every 10 years				Td booster every 10 years
Human papillomavirus (HPV)*	3 doses (females)				
Varicella*	2 doses				
Zoster				1 dose	
Measles, mumps, rubella (MMR)*	1 or 2 doses		1 dose		
Influenza*	1 dose annually				
Pneumococcal (polysaccharide)	1 or 2 doses				1 dose
Hepatitis A*	2 doses				
Hepatitis B*	3 doses				
Meningococcal*	1 or more doses				

** Covered by the Vaccine Injury Compensation Program*

☐ For all persons in this category who meet the age requirements and who lack evidence of immunity (e.g., lack documentation of vaccination or have no evidence of prior infection)

■ Recommended if some other risk factor is present (e.g., on the basis of medical, occupational, lifestyle, or other indications)

Figure 7.5 College students should follow the CDC's recommended immunization schedule for people over 18 years of age.

Adapted from CDC 2007m.

Web site of the Centers for Disease Control and Prevention (www.cdc.gov/vaccines/recs/schedules). No matter which schedule you follow, be sure to read the CDC's detailed footnotes about various immunizations, which you can find in the full schedules on their Web site.

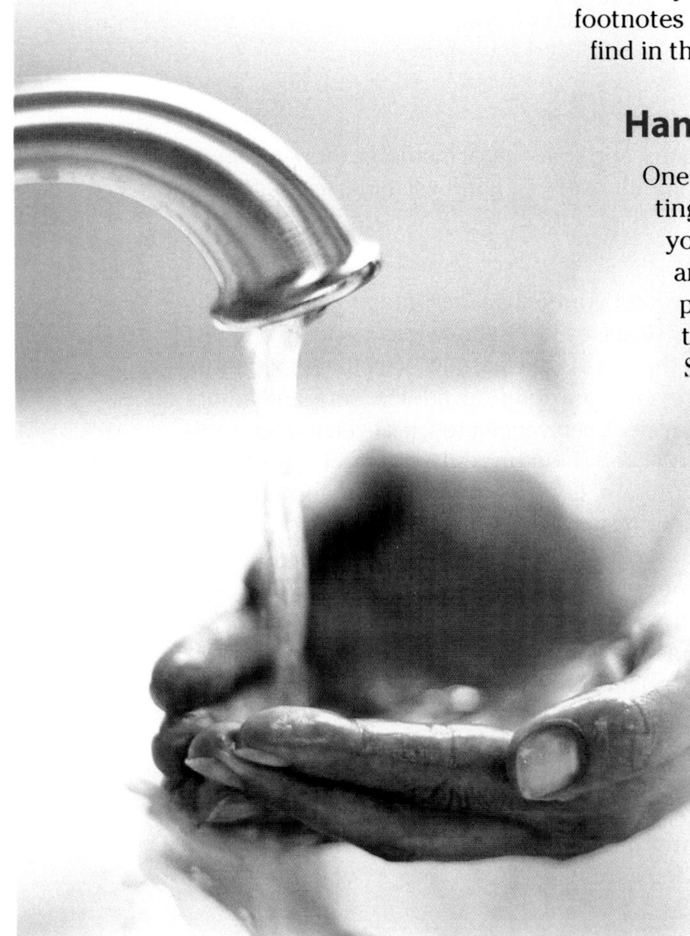

Wash your hands for about as long as it takes you to sing "Happy Birthday" twice.

© Photodisc

Hand Washing

One of the best things you can do to keep from getting sick or spreading germs to others is to wash your hands. You'd think that would be simple, but an observational study discovered that only 75 percent of people (only 66 percent of men) wash their hands after using the restroom (American Society for Microbiology 2007).

Hand washing and the use of alcohol-based hand rubs have been proven to stop outbreaks of disease. Certain circumstances require hand washing (Mayo Clinic 2007e). Pets can transfer disease-causing pathogens to their owners, so wash your hands after touching or cleaning up after your pets. Always wash your hands after using the toilet, after changing a diaper, before and after preparing food, before eating, after sneezing, after coughing, after blowing your nose, before and after treating cuts and wounds, and after touching garbage (CDC 2007e). When in doubt, wash your hands!

The CDC recommends washing hands with soap and clean, warm water for at least 20 seconds. If soap and clean water aren't readily available, use alcohol-based hand hygiene products until you can wash your hands with soap and clean water (CDC 2007e). If your hands are visibly dirty, they should be washed immediately with soap and water. Failure to wash hands can lead to the spread of the common cold and flu, which are caused by viruses that can live on surfaces for hours. In addition, poorly washed hands lead to nearly half of all foodborne illnesses.

Here's the proper way to wash your hands. First, wet your hands with warm, running water and apply soap to them. Make sure to lather well. Vigorously scrub your hands for approximately 20 seconds (or about the length of singing "Happy Birthday" twice in a row). Scrub all surfaces, including hands, wrists, between fingers, under watches, and under rings. Use a nail brush to get under fingernails if possible. After scrubbing, rinse your hands. Dry your hands with a towel, and then use the towel to turn off the faucet.

STEPS FOR BEHAVIORAL CHANGE

Inked: Tattooing Safety

College is a time when a lot of young adults decide to get tattoos. Although getting a tattoo may just take a few hours, it is a decision you will live with for the rest of your life. Taking steps to protect yourself will serve you well in the future.

Although there are usually few complications from receiving a tattoo, there is still the potential for infection because a tattoo breaks the skin barrier, your body's most protective barrier. Risks from tattoos include bloodborne diseases, skin disorders, skin infections, allergic reactions, and MRI complications.

What can you do to protect yourself? Before getting a tattoo, find out if the tattoo parlor has a state or local license. The regulation requirements vary from state to state, so check with the county or state health department for tattoo regulations. Make sure you select a parlor that is clean and professional and has trained staff. Make sure equipment is sterilized using an autoclave, or heat sterilization machine. Equipment that cannot be sterilized, such as tables and sinks, should be disinfected using a bleach solution after each use. When receiving your tattoo, make sure the tattoo artist removes the needle from a sealed, sterile package. Your tattoo artist should use clean, unused trays and containers. Finally, make sure your tattoo artist has washed his or her hands and wears a new pair of latex gloves when applying your tattoo (Mayo Clinic 2008b).

Safe Sex Practices

If you're sexually active, you need to know the basics of safe sex to protect yourself from STI-causing organisms. The best method of avoiding transmission of any STI is to practice abstinence. However, if that it is not possible, it is best to be in a long-term, mutually monogamous relationship with a partner who has been tested and is uninfected. It is also important to use a latex condom during any type of sexual activity in which bodily fluids, such as semen or vaginal secretions, can be exchanged. In addition, limit the number of sexual partners you have, and avoid sexual activity with any partner whose sexual history you don't know. Finally, limit excessive use of alcohol or other drugs, because studies have proven that use of alcohol and drugs can impair judgment, leading to risky sexual practices (Mayo Clinic 2007h).

INFECTIOUS DISEASES 101

Infectious diseases are an everyday part of life. Everything we do, from shaking hands with a person with the flu to having unsafe sexual relations, puts us at risk of developing an infectious disease. Some diseases, such as the common cold, are mild and can be treated with rest and medication, whereas others, such as AIDS, are serious and require a lifetime of care and medication. Understanding what infectious diseases are is an important step to being healthy.

Pathogens, or germs, are the agents in the chain of infection that transmit diseases. Methods of transmission include direct or indirect contact, airborne droplets and particles, insect carriers, and contaminated food and water. You can control some of your risk factors for becoming infected by making healthy lifestyle choices to keep your immune system strong and practicing good hygiene. Be sure to get timely vaccinations, wash your hands when needed, and practice safe sex. Understanding how infectious diseases are spread can help you become and stay healthy.

CHAPTER REVIEW

REVIEW QUESTIONS

1. Describe how a pathogen transmits a disease through the chain of infection.
2. Germs can enter a host through five portals of entry. What are they?
3. Name the three types of direct contact, and give an example of each.
4. What are the six major causes of infectious diseases?
5. Describe some things you can do to acquire and maintain a strong immune system.
6. Name the two parts of the immune system, and compare how they work.
7. How can you alleviate the symptoms of colds or the flu?
8. What is the leading cause of death from infectious disease?
9. How can HIV (the virus that causes AIDS) be transmitted?
10. Name and describe the symptoms of two sexually transmitted infections.

CRITICAL THINKING

1. Why are college students at an increased risk for contracting meningococcal meningitis? What are some steps you can take to protect yourself from this disease?
2. In 2006, the CDC approved a vaccination for HPV. What is the optimal age range during which women should receive this vaccination and why? Why is it important for females to receive this vaccination? Discuss both short-term and long-term effects.

APPLICATION ACTIVITIES

1. Visit your local health care provider or campus health center. Get tested for sexually transmitted diseases and HIV/AIDS. Discuss the results with your health care provider.
2. Make a list of topics that you would like to discuss with your current or future sexual partner to help prevent infectious diseases. Include such things as past drug behavior and previous sexual encounters.

GLOSSARY

acquired immune system—Part of the immune system grows as you are exposed to a variety of disease-causing pathogens by creating a memory of the pathogens when you are exposed to them.

acquired immunodeficiency syndrome (AIDS)—Chronic, life-threatening infectious disease caused by HIV that is a significant global public health threat. Damages the immune system, thereby making it difficult for the body to fight disease-causing organisms.

agent—Any disease-causing microorganism; also known as *pathogens* or *germs*. First link in the chain of infection.

bacteria—Microscopic, single-celled organisms that can be found practically anywhere; some cause diseases.

chain of infection—Method by which a pathogen transmits a disease. There are six distinct links: agent, reservoir, portal of exit, mode of transmission, portal of entry, and new host.

chlamydia—Infection of the urogenital tract caused by *Chlamydia trachomatis*. One of the most prevalent STIs, it can be transmitted sexually or from mother to child during pregnancy.

cilia—Hair projections in the lungs and respiratory tract.

cold—Disease caused by any of the more than 200 types of rhinoviruses; also known as *acute rhinitis*.

droplets—Tiny drops that can contain germs and lead to illness from airborne transmission.

encephalitis—Inflammation of the brain; a rare symptom of West Nile virus.

fungus—Single-celled or multicelled plant that may cause disease.

genital herpes—Highly contagious STI caused by a strain of the herpes simplex virus; characterized by pain, itching, and small, red bumps or blisters in the genital area.

genital warts—STI caused by HPV; characterized by flesh-colored bumps or cauliflower-like warts.

gonorrhea—STI caused by bacterium *Neisseria gonorrhoeae*; spreads sexually or from mother to child during delivery.

helper T cells—White blood cells that oversee the immune system; can be destroyed by HIV.

hepatitis B—Serious liver disease caused by HBV; can be transmitted by sexual contact, by shared needles, or from mother to child during pregnancy.

infectious disease—Disease that is easily spread from one person to another; also known as *communicable disease*.

influenza—Infection of the respiratory tract, also known as the flu, that is caused by the influenza virus and usually transmitted by droplets. Characterized by headaches, severe muscle aches, sudden fatigue and weakness, and a high fever.

innate immune system—Part of the immune system that is present from birth; fast-response system designed to remove any foreign matter.

meningitis—Inflammation of the meninges, the membranes covering the brain and spinal cord; can be caused either by a virus or bacteria and is characterized by a sudden high fever, sudden severe headache, nausea, and stiff neck.

meningoencephalitis—Inflammation of the membranes surrounding the brain; a rare symptom of the West Nile virus.

mode of transmission—Method agents use to move from reservoirs through portals of exit into potential hosts; fourth link in the chain of infection.

mononucleosis—Caused by the Epstein-Barr virus; symptoms include sore throat, fever, headache, chills, nausea, fatigue, and weakness. Also known as *kissing disease* or *mono*.

new host—Person who can get sick when exposed to the agent; sixth and final link in the chain of transmission.

parasitic worms—Parasites that live on or in a host; also known as *helminths*.

particles—Airborne method of transmission that are smaller than droplets and can contain germs.

pelvic inflammatory disease (PID)—Infection of the female reproductive organs, including the uterus and fallopian tubes; a frequent and serious complication from untreated STIs such as gonorrhea and chlamydia.

pertussis—Infectious disease that can last for many weeks and is spread by droplets; characterized by coughing bouts that last several minutes and end with a whooping sound. Also known as *whooping cough*.

pneumonia—Infection of the lungs and lower respiratory tract that is caused by bacteria, viruses, or fungi (most common form is bacterial); symptoms include high fever, severe chest pains, shortness of breath, chills, and a productive cough.

portal of entry—Method agents use to gain entry into a potential host; fifth link in the chain of infection.

portal of exit—Path agents take out of the reservoirs on their way to causing disease in others; third link in the chain of infection.

prions—Infectious agents that researchers believe to consist solely of protein material but that lack DNA and RNA.

protozoa—One-celled organisms that can live independently of a host.

reservoir—Ideal environment where an agent can live, grow, and reproduce; second link in the chain of infection.

sexually transmitted infections (STIs)—Infectious diseases that are transmitted through sexual contact.

syphilis—STI caused by bacterium *Treponema pallidum*; can be transmitted during sexual contact or from mother to child during pregnancy.

tuberculosis—Bacterial disease caused by bacteria that affect the lungs but can also affect the brain, kidneys, and spine; also known as *consumption* or *white death*.

vectors—Insects that carry infectious diseases.

viruses—Infectious parasites made up of a protein shell that encloses either DNA or RNA.

West Nile poliomyelitis—Inflammation of the spinal cord due to West Nile virus; can cause weakening of the arms and legs, severe headache, lack of coordination and balance, and paralysis.

West Nile virus—Viral infection transmitted by mosquitoes; symptoms include headache, fever, diarrhea, nausea, vomiting, skin rash, swollen lymph glands, and a lack of appetite.

REFERENCES AND RESOURCES

Airborne Health. 2007. What's in Airborne. www.airbornehealth.com/about_whatsinside.php.

American Society for Microbiology. 2007. Clean Hands Campaign. www.washup.org.

Baron, S. (ed.). 1996. *Medical microbiology.* 4th ed. Galveston, TX: University of Texas Medical Branch at Galveston.

Bluestein, G., and D. Barrett. 2007. What was TB guy thinking? *Seattle Times,* June 1. http://seattletimes.nwsource.com/html/nationworld/2003730475_tb01.html.

Centers for Disease Control and Prevention (CDC). 2004. Pelvic inflammatory disease. www.cdc.gov/std/PID/STDFact-PID.htm.

———. 2005a. Pertussis. www.cdc.gov/ncidod/dbmd/diseaseinfo/pertussis_t.htm.

———. 2005b. Typhoid fever. www.cdc.gov/ncidod/dbmd/diseaseinfo/typhoidfever_g.htm.

———. 2006a. Chlamydia fact sheet. www.cdc.gov/std/chlamydia/STDFact-chlamydia.htm.

———. 2006b. Gonorrhea fact sheet. www.cdc.gov/std/gonorrhea/STDFact-gonorrhea.htm.

———. 2006c. Hepatitis B FAQs for health professionals. www.cdc.gov/hepatitis/HBV/HBVfaq.htm.

———. 2006d. Risk of ectopic pregnancy after tubal sterilization fact sheet. www.cdc.gov/reproductivehealth/UnintendedPregnancy/EctopicPreg_factsheet.htm.

———. 2006e. West Nile virus: What you need to know. www.cdc.gov/ncidod/dvbid/westnile/wnv_factsheet.htm.

———. 2007a. Autism spectrum disorders overview. www.cdc.gov/ncbddd/autism/overview.htm.

———. 2007b. Fight the bite. www.cdc.gov/ncidod/dvbid/westnile/.

———. 2007c. Genital herpes. www.cdc.gov/std/herpes/default.htm.

———. 2007d. Genital HPV infection fact sheet. www.cdc.gov/std/HPV/STDFact-HPV.htm.

———. 2007e. Hand hygiene in health care settings. www.cdc.gov/handhygiene/.

———. 2007f. HIV/AIDS. www.cdc.gov/hiv/.

———. 2007g. Leading causes of death. www.cdc.gov/nchs/fastats/lcod.htm.

———. 2007h. Meningitis (meningococcal disease). www.cdc.gov/meningitis/bacterial/faqs.htm.

———. 2007i. Prevention challenges. www.cdc.gov/hiv/topics/aa/challenges.htm.

———. 2007j. Seasonal flu. www.cdc.gov/flu/.

———. 2007k. Syphilis. www.cdc.gov/std/syphilis/default.htm.

———. 2007l. Tuberculosis information for employees in non-healthcare settings. www.cdc.gov/tb/pubs/tbfactsheets/nonhealthcare_employers.htm.

———. 2007m. Vaccinations and immunizations. www.cdc.gov/vaccines/.

———. 2007n. What would happen if we stopped vaccinations? www.cdc.gov/vaccines/vac-gen/whatifstop.htm.

———. 2008a. Fact sheet: HIV/AIDS among African Americans. www.cdc.gov/hiv/topics/aa/resources/factsheets/aa.htm.

———. 2008b. HIV: Get tested and know your status. www.cdc.gov/features/dsHIVtest/.

Donatelle, R.J., and P. Ketcham. 2007. *Access to health.* 10th ed. San Francisco: Benjamin Cummings.

Fauci, A. 2004. The NIH response to emerging and re-emerging infectious diseases: Implications for global health. www.hhs.gov/asl/testify/t040428a.html.

Hartenstein, M. 2007. Timeline of Speaker's TB odyssey. http://abcnews.go.com/US/story?id=3235763.

Insel, P. 2005. *Core concepts in health.* 10th ed. New York: McGraw-Hill.

Leavitt, J.W. 1997. *Typhoid Mary.* Boston: Beacon Press.

Mayo Clinic. 2006a. Mononucleosis. www.mayoclinic.com/health/mononucleosis/DS00352.

———. 2006b. Syphilis. www.mayoclinic.com/health/syphilis/DS00374.

———. 2006c. Tuberculosis. www.mayoclinic.com/health/tuberculosis/DS00372.

———. 2007a. Common cold. www.mayoclinic.com/health/common-cold/DS00056.

———. 2007b. Genital herpes. www.mayoclinic.com/health/genital-herpes/DS00179.

———. 2007c. Genital warts. www.mayoclinic.com/health/genital-warts/DS00087.

———. 2007d. Gonorrhea. www.mayoclinic.com/health/gonorrhea/DS00180.

———. 2007e. Hand washing: An easy way to prevent infection. www.mayoclinic.com/health/hand-washing/HQ00407.

———. 2007f. Hepatitis B. www.mayoclinic.com/health/hepatitis-b/DS00398.

———. 2007g. HIV/AIDS. www.mayoclinic.com/health/hiv-aids/DS00005.

———. 2007h. Infectious disease: How they spread, how to stop them. www.mayoclinic.com/health/infectious-disease/ID00004.

———. 2007i. Influenza (flu). www.mayoclinic.com/health/influenza/DS00081.

———. 2007j. Meningitis. www.mayoclinic.com/health/meningitis/DS00118.

———. 2007k. Pelvic inflammatory disease. www.mayoclinic.com/health/pelvic-inflammatory-disease/DS00402.

———. 2007l. Pneumonia. www.mayoclinic.com/health/pneumonia/DS00135.

———. 2007m. West Nile virus. www.mayoclinic.com/health/west-nile-virus/DS00438.

———. 2007n. Whooping cough. www.mayoclinic.com/health/whooping-cough/DS00445.

———. 2008a. Bird flu (avian influenza). www.mayoclinic.com/health/bird-flu/DS00566.

———. 2008b. Tattoos: Risks and precautions to know first. www.mayoclinic.com/health/tattoos-and-piercings/MC00020.

MedlinePlus. 2007. Autoimmune disorders. www.nlm.nih.gov/medlineplus/ency/article/000816.htm.

———. 2008. Allergy. www.nlm.nih.gov/medlineplus/allergy.html.

Microbytes. 2004. Innate and acquired immunity. www.microbiologybytes.com/iandi/1b.html.

National HIV Testing Day (NHTD). n.d. NHTD main page. www.hivtest.org/press_files/whatis.cfm.

National Institute of Child Health and Human Development. 2006. Why do people think that vaccines can cause autism? www.nichd.nih.gov/publications/pubs/autism/mmr/sub2.cfm.

National Institutes of Health (NIH). 2003. Understanding the immune system: How it works. www.niaid.nih.gov/publications/immune/the_immune_system.pdf.

Payne, W.A. 2007. *Understanding your health.* 9th ed. New York: McGraw-Hill.

Teague, M.L., S.L.C. Mackenzie, and D.M. Rosenthal. 2006. *Your health today: Choices in a changing society.* New York: McGraw-Hill.

Zicam. 2008. Frequently asked questions. www.zicam.com/products/faqs.

Other helpful resources include the following.

Centers for Disease Control and Prevention (CDC). 2004. All about hantaviruses. www.cdc.gov/ncidod/diseases/hanta/hps/noframes/glossary.htm.

National Institutes of Health (NIH). 1999. Understanding emerging and re-emerging infectious diseases. http://science.education.nih.gov/supplements/nih1/diseases/guide/understanding1.htm.

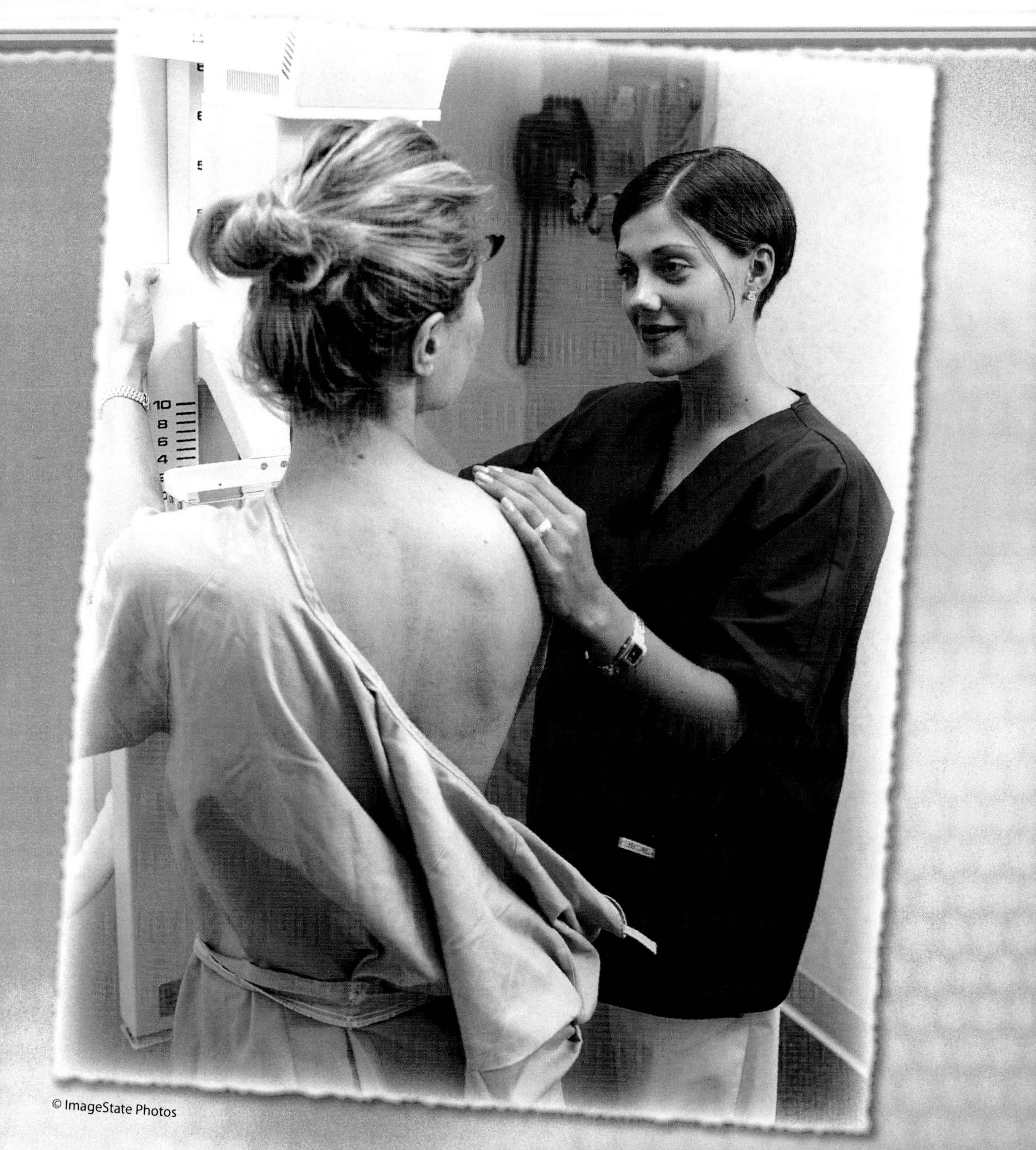

© ImageState Photos

CHAPTER 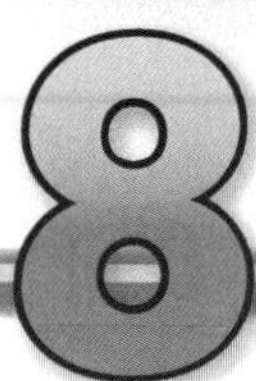

CHRONIC DISEASES

PAMELA DOUGHTY, PHD, CHES
Institute for Obesity Research and Program Evaluation, Texas A&M University

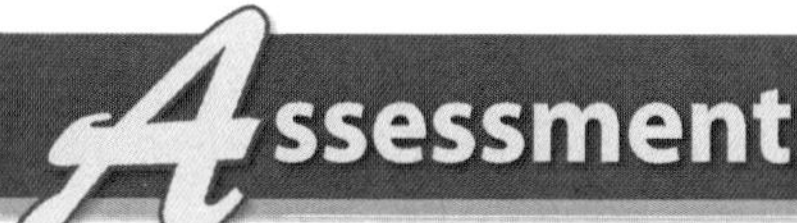

Assessment

- Did you know that chronic diseases account for 7 out of 10 deaths in the United States?
- If your blood pressure is 160 over 100, is that good or bad?
- What exactly happens to the heart during a heart attack?
- Does using tobacco affect your chances of developing bronchitis, emphysema, and other chronic obstructive pulmonary diseases?
- Do you know the warning signs of breast cancer?
- What are the two leading causes of cancer deaths in men?
- Did you know that about 25 percent of people with diabetes don't realize that they have the disease?

Objectives

- Define *chronic disease*.
- List behaviors that increase the likelihood of getting a chronic disease.
- Explain the relationship between chronic disease and medical care dollars.
- Discuss preventive measures for chronic disease.
- Describe the symptoms of cardiovascular disease, diabetes, and arthritis.
- Discuss the treatments for various cancers.
- Describe the diagnosis of cancers.

You know how it feels when you're sick. Even a simple cold can make you miserable. You feel drained and achy, you can't breathe, your head and stomach probably hurt, it's hard to keep doing what you need to do at school or work, and you just want to feel well again. Eventually, though, after shelling out a few dollars for some cold medicine and resting for a few days, you get better and your life returns to normal. When you get the flu or catch a cold, you have an acute illness, or one that you get over within a relatively short time.

Imagine, though, if those symptoms never went away, and if the limitations they put on your activities never let up. Imagine if, instead of a spending few dollars and a little time to get over being sick, you were facing thousands of dollars of medical bills and a lifetime of illness. This chapter discusses **chronic diseases**—those that last a long time—and what you can do now to try to avoid them.

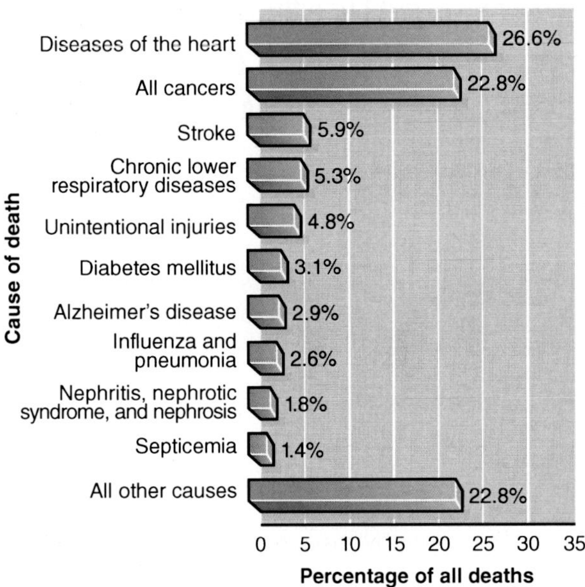

Figure 8.1 Percent of deaths in the United States.

Chronic diseases are diseases such as cancer, diabetes, arthritis, heart disease, autoimmune diseases, and a host of others. The National Institutes of Health (NIH) categorizes an illness that lasts more than 3 months as chronic. Cancer, heart disease, and diabetes are the most prevalent chronic diseases, and they are also the most costly for both the patient and the U.S. government (Centers for Disease Control and Prevention [CDC] 2007b).

Chronic diseases account for 70 percent of all deaths in the United States—that's 7 out of 10 deaths, or 1.7 million deaths a year. These diseases cause prolonged suffering and pain and place major limitations on activity for more than 25 million people in the United States (CDC 2007b). As you can see in figure 8.1, heart disease is the top killer in the United States, causing more than 26 percent of all deaths. Cancer comes in second, with 22.8 percent of deaths, then stroke (5.9 percent), chronic lower respiratory diseases (5.3 percent), unintentional injuries (4.8 percent), diabetes (3.1 percent), Alzheimer's disease (2.9 percent), and so on (CDC 2007b).

Before the 1990s, heart disease affected primarily men, but today almost as many women as men are dying of heart disease. One reason women are catching up may be the increase in the number of women who smoke cigarettes. Smoking was mostly a man's habit until the 1960s, but since then more women have taken it up. Women working outside of the home may be a contributing factor as well. In past decades it was more common for women to work in the home, and they had fewer workplace stresses. Working outside the home may also lead to eating more fast food with higher calories, fat, and cholesterol, which all contribute to heart disease (CDC 2007b).

Although it's the most serious, death isn't the only consequence of a chronic disease. More than 90 million Americans live with chronic illness, and chronic illness can progress into disability with time, lack of treatment, or an aggressive form of the illness (CDC 2007b). The life expectancy is higher for women with chronic illnesses, but women over the age of 70 are more likely to be disabled than men. Statistically, women live longer than men; however, those men who do live past the age of 70 have fewer illnesses. It may be that the men who live past the age of 70 are healthier and that is why they live longer than other men. Figure 8.2 illustrates the leading causes of disability in the United States.

Chronic disabling conditions severely limit daily activities for more than 1 out of every 10 Americans, or 25 million people (CDC 2007b). Arthritis, for example, can limit mobility, which makes it hard for people to bathe, dress, and feed themselves. Heart problems limit some people's activities because their heart condition is not controlled. Stroke patients often lose movement on one side of the body and lose memory. The lack of oxygen that comes with respiratory diseases causes severe fatigue, making it hard for a person even to walk from the bathroom to the living room. Diabetes can block the veins and arteries with plaque that builds up because of the stickiness of the blood. The blockage happens frequently in the lower extremities and results in toes and feet dying, which could require amputation. Diabetes patients with an amputated limb lose mobility until they can get a prosthetic limb to replace it (CDC 2007b).

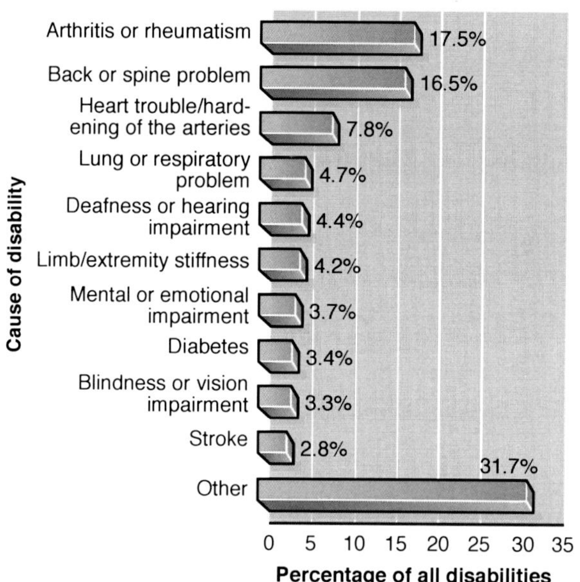

Figure 8.2 Leading causes of disability among people aged 15 and older from 1991 to 1998.

The economic burden of chronic disease is extremely high, contributing 75 percent of the $2 trillion of medical care costs incurred in the United States. For instance, direct and indirect costs of diabetes are $132 billion a year, arthritis results in medical care costs of more than $22 billion, smoking costs exceed $75 billion annually, $300 billion was spent on all cardiovascular disease in 2001, and physical inactivity costs were $76.6 billion in 2000 (CDC 2008a).

Tobacco is the number one cause of all diseases, including chronic disease. However, researchers expect that poor diet and exercise habits will surpass tobacco as the leading cause of disease in the next 10 years. In the 30 years between 1976 and 2006, obesity among adults aged 20 to 74 years increased from 15 percent to 33 percent. The picture is similar for younger people. The prevalence of overweight increased from 5 percent to 14 percent for children aged 2 to 5, from 7 percent to 19 percent for those aged 6 to 11, and from 5 percent to 17 percent for those aged 12 to 19 (National Association of Chronic Disease Directors [NAOCDD] 2007).

A newly coined term for some of these diseases is *lifestyle diseases*, meaning that the onset and disability of these diseases can be controlled by improving the lifestyle of a person or group. People may have a genetic predisposition toward a specific disease, but lifestyle may either reduce or increase the risk of that disease. As you may have guessed, exercising daily, eating a healthy diet, not smoking, and maintaining your weight at a normal level can reduce your risk for disease. Not only can a healthy lifestyle keep you from getting a disease, it can also reduce your chances for complications from a present disease and even stop the symptoms and progression of some diseases.

Lifestyle choices such as smoking and poor diet and exercise habits aren't the only causes of chronic disease, though. Microbial agents (germs) also cause many chronic diseases. For example, peptic ulcer disease has been linked with *Helicobacter pylori*, and cervical cancer has been linked with human papillomavirus (HPV). These discoveries will open the door to vaccines to prevent some chronic illnesses. The HPV vaccine, sold under the brand name of Gardasil, is one of the first.

We know what to do to prevent chronic disease, but we do not put the funds behind that knowledge to put preventive measures in place. Only 3 percent of health care dollars are spent on prevention programs in the United States. Only through the actions of policy makers will chronic disease be reduced and life spans increased through prevention efforts (NAOCDD 2007).

Although there are many chronic diseases, this chapter will cover the most prevalent. You might have friends or relatives who have chronic diseases not covered in this chapter, such as HIV or Lyme disease, but you probably know at least one person who has one of the chronic diseases discussed.

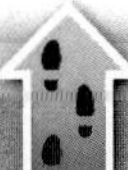

STEPS FOR BEHAVIORAL CHANGE

Increase Your Chances for a Long, Healthy Life

Lifestyle contributes more than genetics to developing chronic disease. That fact means you can change your lifestyle and reduce your chances of getting a chronic disease. One of the most important aspects of lifestyle is staying at a healthy weight.

If your lifestyle has caused you to gain weight, the first thing that you need to do is to acknowledge that you need to lose weight. That's not an easy thing to do!

The next step is to find a support group while you diet and exercise. Everyone wants a miracle pill that will melt the weight off effortlessly, but the key to weight loss is burning more calories than you eat. People in support groups such as Weight Watchers tend to lose more weight than people who go it alone.

The next step is to find an exercise that you enjoy, one that isn't boring or too extreme. Exercise 30 to 60 minutes a day to lose weight. Do activities that are fun, such as biking with friends or playing any game that gets your heart rate up for at least 30 minutes, such as basketball, tennis, or soccer. Exercise does not need to be painful to be effective, and you're more likely to continue an exercise program if you don't get so sore that you can't move.

You should eat between 1,200 and 2,000 calories a day, depending on your age, activity level, and gender. Men are able to eat more calories because they generally have more muscle mass than women, which means they burn more calories at rest. Take a look at the food pyramid (at www.mypyramid.gov) and use it to build balanced meals with low amounts of fat and sugar. Eat plenty of fruits and vegetables for adequate vitamins and minerals.

With this simple diet and exercise plan, you could lose up to 2 pounds (1 kilogram) per week. That may sound slow, but people who take off the weight slowly are more likely to keep the weight off.

CARDIOVASCULAR DISEASE

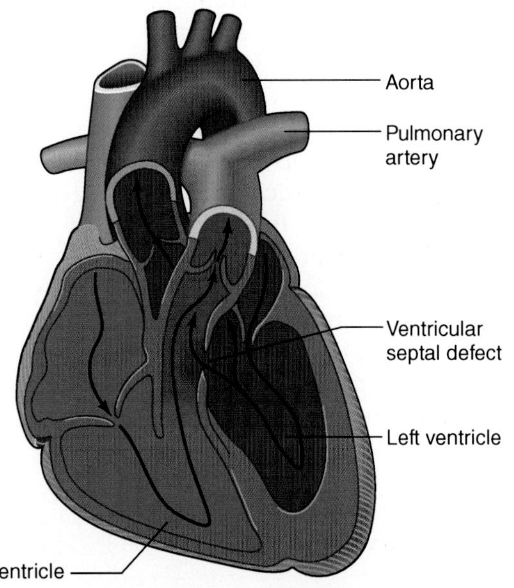

Figure 8.3 A ventricular septal defect allows oxygenated and unoxygenated blood to mix, forcing the heart to work harder than a healthy heart.

Cardiovascular disease (CVD) is an umbrella term that includes several diseases that affect the heart or blood vessels. CVD can develop even before a baby is born. **Congenital heart disease** is another broad term that covers a wide range of diseases and conditions that develop before birth and that can affect the formation of the heart muscle or its chambers or valves. These congenital conditions include narrowing of a section of the aorta (coarctation) or holes in the heart (atrial or ventricular septal defect; see figure 8.3). Some congenital heart defects may be apparent at birth, whereas others may not be detected until later in life (Mayo Clinic 2006). Nine out of every 1,000 babies born in the United States have a defect that originated as the heart was developing during pregnancy. Congenital heart defects are the most common birth defects (Lucile Packard Children's Hospital 2007).

When people typically think of heart disease, though, they're thinking about those that develop over time, including high blood pressure, coronary artery disease, peripheral artery disease, cardiomyopathy, aneurysm, valvular heart disease, pericardial disease, heart failure, arrhythmia, and stroke (Mayo Clinic 2006). In these forms, CVD causes more deaths for men and women than all forms of cancer combined.

High Blood Pressure

High blood pressure, or **hypertension**, is when blood pumps through blood vessels with excessive force against the walls. The heart has to work harder to pump the blood. Hypertension is one of the most common forms of CVD in the United States, affecting about one in three Americans. It is a precursor to many forms of coronary heart disease (CHD). Although hypertension is potentially life threatening, it's one of the most preventable and treatable types of CVD.

What Do You Do?

Go to a pharmacy or clinic and get your blood pressure checked. Which range described in this section is your blood pressure in?

Blood pressure measurements provide the information that leads to a diagnosis of hypertension. Blood pressure readings have two numbers and are usually reported as one number over another number (for example, 120 over 80 mmHg). The top number describes the systolic pressure, and the bottom number describes the diastolic pressure. (Systolic arterial pressure is the peak pressure in the arteries, which occurs near the beginning of the cardiac cycle. Diastolic arterial pressure is the lowest pressure, at the resting phase of the cardiac cycle.) When diastolic pressure is high, it is usually the result of stress. The arteries are restricted during the resting stage, indicating that stress hormones are tightening the arteries. Following are the stages of hypertension (D.W. Stein 2006):

- Normal blood pressure: Less than 120 over 80
- Prehypertension: 120 to 139 over 80 to 89
- Stage 1 hypertension: 140 to 159 over 90 to 99
- Stage 2 hypertension: More than 160 over 100

Most doctors do not diagnose hypertension in just one visit. Often people have elevated blood pressure when they are ill, are nervous about visiting the doctor, or hurried to the doctor's office. Repeated readings above the normal level under various circumstances will result in a diagnosis of hypertension. However, if the blood pressure reading is over 160, the doctor will most likely require patients to return in a short time to reread their blood pressure to see if it was a fluke or to prescribe them medication to control their blood pressure if a high reading occurs again.

Coronary Artery Disease

Coronary artery disease, in the forms of **arteriosclerosis** and **atherosclerosis**, is a common form of CVD. Arteriosclerosis is when the arteries lose some of their elasticity and harden, usually as a result of aging. Atherosclerosis, on the other hand, is when a fatty material called **plaque** builds up in the arteries around the heart (see figure 8.4). Coronary artery disease is the buildup of plaque in the arteries that supply the heart with blood. An unhealthy diet (lots of saturated fats), lack of exercise, being overweight, and smoking are major risk factors for developing atherosclerosis (Mayo Clinic 2006). Both arteriosclerosis and atherosclerosis can result in a lack of blood flow to the heart, which in turn can lead to chest pain (angina) and heart attacks.

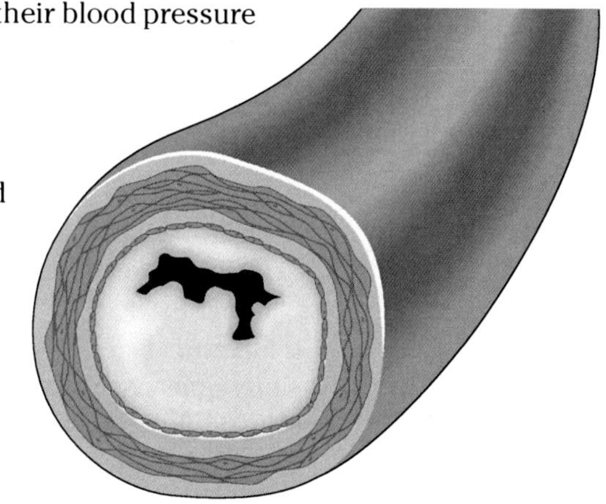

Figure 8.4 Plaque buildup in coronary artery disease.

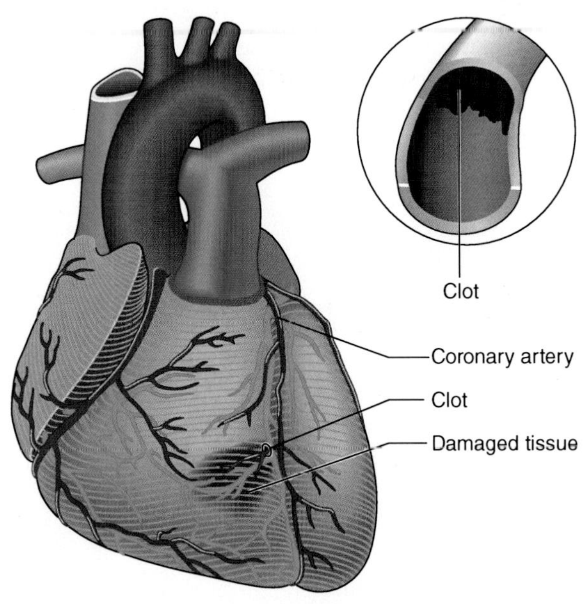

Figure 8.5 A blood clot can cause a heart attack, or myocardial infarction, by preventing the heart from getting enough oxygenated blood.

A heart attack is an injury to the heart muscle caused by a lack of oxygen. The medical term for a heart attack is **myocardial infarction (MI)**. Figure 8.5 illustrates how a small blood clot or piece of plaque can break loose from an artery and block oxygenated blood from reaching the heart. The lack of oxygen causes part of the heart muscle around the blocked area to die.

Peripheral Artery Disease

Peripheral artery disease occurs when plaque builds up on the inside walls of the arteries that carry blood from the heart to the head, internal organs, and limbs. It is also known as *atherosclerotic peripheral arterial disease*.

Here are some signs and symptoms of peripheral artery disease:

- Pain, numbness, aching, and heaviness in the muscles
- Cramping in the legs, thighs, calves, and feet
- Weak or absent pulse in the legs or feet
- Sores or wounds on toes, feet, or legs that heal slowly, poorly, or not at all
- Color changes in skin, paleness, or blueness (cyanosis)
- Decreased temperature in one leg compared with the other leg
- Poor nail growth and decreased hair growth on toes and legs
- Erectile dysfunction, especially among men with diabetes

Cardiomyopathy

Cardiomyopathy refers to diseases of the heart muscle. Some types of cardiomyopathy are genetic, and others have causes that are less well understood. Here are some types of cardiomyopathy.

- Ischemic—Caused by loss of heart muscle from reduced coronary blood flow, sometimes as a result of anemia (low iron levels in the blood) or sleep apnea (snoring and waking up many times during the night).
- Intrinsic cardiomyopathy—Not due to any known external causes; doctors must rule out the possibility of CHD. Can be caused by alcohol, drugs, hepatitis, or viruses.
- Dilated—Heart chambers are enlarged.
- Hypertrophic—Heart muscle is thickened.
- Restrictive cardiomyopathy—Uncommon cardiomyopathy in which the walls of the ventricles are stiff, but may not be thickened, and resist the normal filling of the heart with blood.
- Idiopathic dilated cardiomyopathy—Enlarged heart without a known cause (*idiopathic* simply means "unknown cause"); one of the most common types of cardiomyopathy (Mayo Clinic 2006).

Aneurysm

An **aneurysm** is a bulge or weakness in the wall of an artery or vein. Aneurysms usually get bigger over time. Because of that, they have the potential to rupture and cause life-threatening bleeding. Aneurysms can occur in arteries anywhere in the body. The most common sites include the abdominal aorta and the arteries at the base of the brain (Mayo Clinic 2006).

Valvular Heart Disease

Four valves in the heart keep blood flowing in the right direction. When any is damaged, a person has a **valvular heart disease**. Valves may be damaged by a variety of conditions, including narrowing (stenosis) or leaking (regurgitation or insufficiency). Another result of valve damage is improper closing (prolapse). A person could be born with valvular disease, or the valves could be damaged by such conditions as rheumatic fever, infections (infectious endocarditis), connective tissue disorders, and certain medications or radiation treatments for cancer (Mayo Clinic 2006).

Pericardial Diseases

Pericardial diseases are diseases of the sac that encases the heart (pericardium). They include inflammation (pericarditis), fluid accumulation (pericardial effusion), and stiffness (constrictive pericarditis). These conditions can occur alone or together. The causes of pericardial disease vary, as do the problems that the disease may lead to. For instance, pericarditis can occur after a heart attack and lead to pericardial effusion, or chest pain. Chest pain from blocked arteries is called *angina;* however, pain from fluid buildup around the heart is called *chest pain* and can be distinguished only through blood tests, electrocardiograms, or X rays.

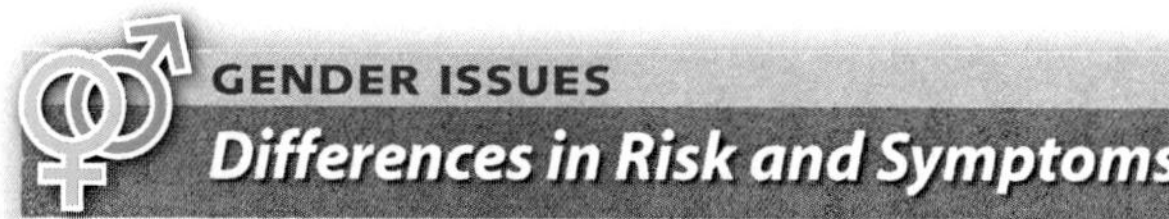

GENDER ISSUES

Differences in Risk and Symptoms

In a study of 2,794 people over 29 years, researchers found that women had a 1 in 6 chance of developing Alzheimer's disease (AD) and men had only a 1 in 10 chance of developing the disease. The overall risk of stroke or dementia in both sexes was about 1 in 3—higher than the risk of coronary heart disease (CHD) in women (Boston University 2008)

Women at risk for CHD may manifest their symptoms in different ways than men. Women can have CHD that does not show in traditional tests used on men. They may show smooth interior arteries in tests but may still have a high risk of disease. Some women manifest their disease with pain in their shoulders and jaw rather than the traditional sweating, heaviness in the chest, and pain. These women may incur a heart attack when experiencing stressful events or stressful exercise due to spasms in the arteries. Traditional medications are less effective with this population, and medications that reduce inflammation are more beneficial in reducing their risk of heart attack (R. Stein 2006).

Because of these findings, it is important for women and their doctors to become aware of the differences in symptoms, diagnosis, and treatment.

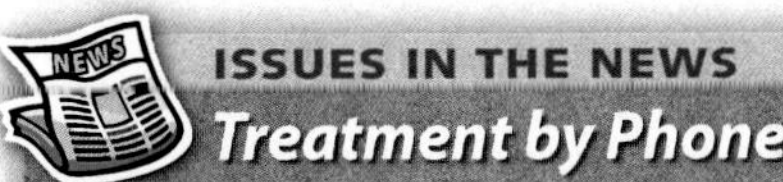

People with chronic diseases can now be monitored over the phone rather than having to go to the doctor. A health care provider can set up a monitoring station in a patient's home where the patient can test blood pressure, monitor weight, test blood sugar, or check heart rate. Monitoring chronic diseases over the phone improves the quality of life for the patient and saves money because regular checking in results in fewer hospital visits.

One such station was put into the home of an 82-year-old man with chronic heart failure. A weight gain of a single pound could signal that the patient was drowning in his own fluid. He used his monitoring station to check his blood pressure and weigh himself each day. The results were sent over the phone line to the doctor. If there was a problem, the doctor called to adjust the medication or have him come into the office for tests.

Researchers are conducting many studies in which they monitor patients with other types of electronic devices such as a bracelet that can monitor blood pressure, glucose levels, heart rate, and medication levels. After the information is taken, it is sent to the doctor's computer. If there is a problem with the patient, the doctor can call the patient, dispense more medication, or send an ambulance if the situation is severe.

Heart Failure

Heart failure is a condition in which the heart can't pump blood effectively enough to meet the needs of the body's organs and tissues. The term *congestive heart failure* (CHF) is technically reserved for situations in which heart failure has led to fluid buildup in the body. Not all heart failure is congestive, but the terms are often used interchangeably. Heart failure may develop suddenly or over many years. It may occur as a result of other cardiovascular conditions that have damaged or weakened the heart, such as coronary artery disease or cardiomyopathy (Mayo Clinic 2006).

The symptoms of heart failure are a direct result of the fluid buildup around the heart. Some of the symptoms include swelling of the feet, legs, and abdomen because of fluid retention. The fluid can cause chronic fatigue, confusion, difficulty breathing, and coughing with frothy sputum (mucus). A person who is experiencing any combination of these symptoms should see a doctor immediately. There are medications and treatments to control these symptoms.

Arrhythmia

An **arrhythmia** (also referred to as *dysrhythmia*) is an abnormal rhythm of the heart, which can cause the heart to pump less effectively. Arrhythmias can cause problems with contractions of the heart chambers in two ways: by not allowing the chambers to fill with an adequate amount of blood because the electrical signal is causing the heart to pump too fast, and by not allowing a sufficient amount of blood to be pumped to the body because the electrical signal is causing the heart to pump too slowly or too irregularly (Mayo Clinic 2006). Symptoms of arrhythmia are weakness, fatigue, palpitations, low blood pressure, dizziness, and fainting.

Stroke

High blood pressure can lead to other serious problems, such as heart failure and stroke (Mayo Clinic 2006). There are two kinds of strokes: ischemic and hemorrhagic. An **ischemic**

stroke is similar to a heart attack, because a blockage in an artery of the brain causes the part of the brain without oxygen to die. The death of this brain tissue can cause memory loss and paralysis of one side of the body. A **hemorrhagic stroke** is caused by a blood vessel breaking because of high blood pressure or an aneurysm bursting in the brain. The blood on brain tissue damages that part of the brain. More than 80 percent of all strokes are ischemic (WebMD 2006).

If you or anyone you know experience any of the following symptoms, call emergency medical services (911) immediately, because it could signal that the person is having a stroke (WebMD 2006):

- Sudden numbness or weakness in the face, arm, or leg (especially on one side of the body)
- Sudden blurred vision or decreased vision in one or both eyes
- Sudden inability to move part of the body (paralysis)
- Sudden dizziness or headache with nausea and vomiting
- Difficulty speaking or understanding words or simple sentences
- Difficulty swallowing
- Dizziness, loss of balance, or poor coordination
- Brief loss of consciousness
- Sudden confusion

Up to 50 percent of all strokes are preventable. Many risk factors can be controlled before they cause problems. These are some of the controllable risk factors:

- High blood pressure (greater than 140 over 90)
- Atrial fibrillation (heart condition)
- Uncontrolled diabetes
- High total cholesterol (greater than 200)
- Smoking
- Drinking alcohol (more than one drink per day)
- Being overweight
- Existing carotid or coronary artery disease

ARTHRITIS

According to the CDC, "Arthritis comprises over 100 different diseases and conditions. The most common are osteoarthritis, gout, rheumatoid arthritis, and fibromyalgia. Common symptoms include pain, aching, stiffness, and swelling in or around the joints. Some forms of arthritis, such as rheumatoid arthritis and lupus, can affect multiple organs and cause widespread symptoms" (CDC 2008b).

Arthritis is the leading cause of disability in the United States. Nearly 19 million American adults reported activity limitations due to arthritis each year from 2003 to 2005. Work limitations attributable to arthritis affect more than 5 percent of the general U.S. population and nearly 30 percent of people with arthritis. Each year, arthritis results in 750,000 hospitalizations and 36 million outpatient visits. Direct medical costs for arthritis were $81 billion in 2003. Arthritis is not just an old person's disease—nearly two-thirds of people with arthritis are younger than 65. Although arthritis affects children and people of all racial and ethnic groups, it is more common among women and older adults (CDC 2008b).

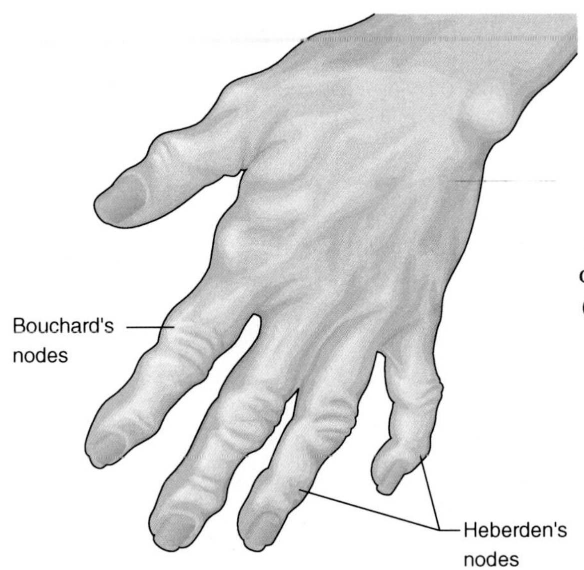

Figure 8.6 Late-stage osteoarthritis of joints in the hand.

Osteoarthritis

Osteoarthritis is a disease characterized by degeneration of cartilage and its underlying bone within a joint, as well as bony overgrowth. Joints most commonly affected are the knees, hips, and those in the hands and spine. In the hands, knobby deformities at the smallest joints near the ends of the fingers are called Heberden's nodes, and knobby deformities in the middle joints are called Bouchard's nodes (see figure 8.6).

The specific causes of osteoarthritis are unknown but are believed to be a result of both mechanical and molecular events in the affected joint. The disease comes on gradually, usually after age 40. There isn't a cure for osteoarthritis. A combination of patient education, physical therapy, weight control, and medicine helps relieve symptoms and improve function (CDC 2008b).

Gout

Gout is a rheumatic disease that develops when the body produces too much or doesn't excrete enough uric acid and deposits uric acid crystals (monosodium urate) in body tissues and fluids (see figure 8.7). Alcohol, certain foods, and common medications contribute to the development of gout. Alcohol can increase the levels of uric acid in the body due to its diuretic properties. Foods high in purine such as hearts, herring, mussels, yeast, smelt, sardines, and sweetbreads contribute to the onset of gout. Any medications that have diuretic properties can contribute to the onset of the disease.

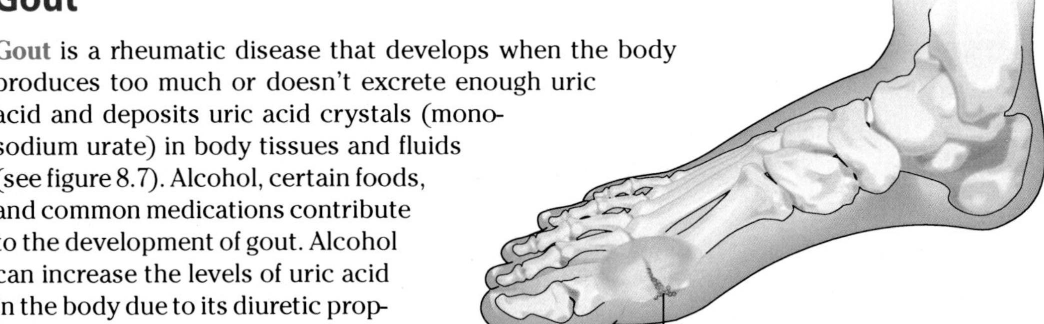

Figure 8.7 Gout causes uric acid crystals to be deposited in tissues and fluids.

Acute gout will typically manifest itself as a red, hot, and swollen joint with excruciating pain. These acute gouty flare-ups respond well to treatment with oral anti-inflammatory medicines, and they can be prevented with medication and diet changes. Recurrent bouts of acute gout can lead to a degenerative form of arthritis called *gouty arthritis* (CDC 2008b). Gouty arthritis is more common in men, striking after puberty and continuing until about age 75; women usually do not get gouty arthritis until after menopause.

Prevention of gout consists of adequate fluid intake to keep uric acid levels down. Also, alcoholic beverage intake should be restricted because alcohol acts as a diuretic, reducing fluid levels. The other important factor is severe weight gain. Controlling weight can help prevent attacks of gout. There are also medications that reduce the amount of uric acid in the body.

Rheumatoid Arthritis

According to the CDC, "Rheumatoid arthritis is a systemic inflammatory disease which manifests itself in multiple joints of the body. The inflammatory process primarily affects the lining of the joints (synovial membrane), but can also affect other organs. The inflamed synovium leads to erosions of the cartilage and bone and sometimes joint deformity" (CDC 2008b). Pain, swelling, and redness at the affected joints are common (see figure 8.8). People with **rheumatoid arthritis** can suffer from multiple joint pain or pain in just a few joints. Some patients have flares in different joints at different times, but most primarily have pain in the hands and feet. Medical experts believe that rheumatoid arthritis is the result of a faulty immune system. It can begin at any age, and it often causes fatigue and prolonged stiffness after rest. There is no cure for rheumatoid arthritis, but new drugs that specifically stop the immune response (such as Humira and Enbrel) are increasingly available. In addition to medications and surgery (to help restore joint mobility and repair damaged joints), good self-management, including exercise, is known to reduce pain and disability (CDC 2008b).

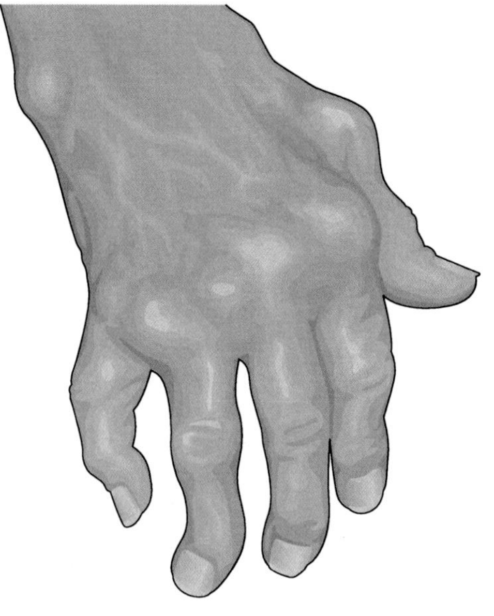

Figure 8.8 Late-stage rheumatoid arthritis of joints in the hand.

Fibromyalgia

Fibromyalgia is a syndrome predominately characterized by widespread muscular pain and fatigue. Researchers haven't found the cause of fibromyalgia, but they hypothesize that genetics and physical and emotional stressors might be contributing factors to development of the illness. It's hard for doctors to diagnose fibromyalgia, because its symptoms are similar to symptoms of other illnesses and there are no definitive diagnostic tests. One way doctors identify fibromyalgia is by locating certain tender points on the patient's body (see figure 8.9). Patient education, pharmacologic agents, and various nonpharmacologic therapies are used to treat fibromyalgia. Exercise can also improve outcomes for people with fibromyalgia.

Fibromyalgia is more common in women than in men. Generally it begins in middle to late adulthood, but it also can occur in children and older adults. There is no cure for fibromyalgia, and it is not progressive. However, because of the constant pain and lack of sleep, patients often become depressed and need help adjusting and creating healthier lifestyles to keep the pain under control.

There has been much controversy regarding the legitimacy of fibromyalgia as a true disease because there is no exact method of diagnosis. For many years people with fibromyalgia were considered constant complainers. However, rheumatologists, insurers, and now pharmacological companies believe that fibromyalgia is a true disease that causes pain and loss of work and leisure time. In 2007, Pfizer, one of the world's largest pharmaceutical companies, received approval from the U.S. Food and Drug Administration (FDA) for a new drug for people suffering from fibromyalgia. Patients with fibromyalgia cannot reduce their pain with drugs such as aspirin, ibuprofen, or naproxen sodium that work with other forms of arthritis. The new medication, Lyrica, does not block pain in the same way that those other pain relievers work; instead it affects the brain's perception of pain (Berenson 2008).

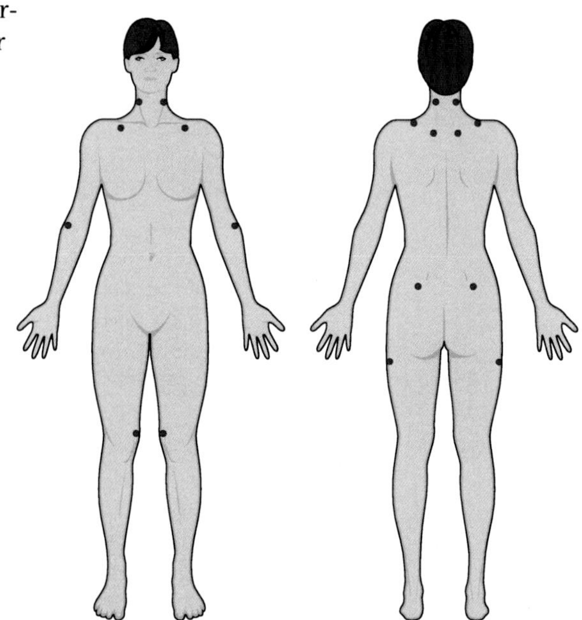

Figure 8.9 Tender points are used to help diagnose fibromyalgia.

Systemic Lupus Erythematosus

Systemic lupus erythematosus (SLE) is an autoimmune disease in which the immune system produces antibodies, or proteins used by the immune system to identify and neutralize foreign objects, such as bacteria and viruses. In SLE, however, the antibodies attack healthy tissue in the body, including internal organs, which leads to widespread inflammation and tissue damage. Medical experts don't know what causes SLE. They believe the disease is linked to genetic, environmental, and hormonal factors. People with SLE often experience cycles of illness and remission. SLE can affect the joints, skin, brain, lungs, kidneys, and blood vessels. People with SLE may experience fatigue, pain or swelling in joints, skin rashes, and fevers. A team approach to treating lupus is often warranted because of the number of organ systems involved (CDC 2007b).

SLE is more common in women than men and can start at any age, but it is more common in young adult women. The long-term outcome for patients with SLE is improving as more medications that suppress the immune system become available. Some patients have mild flares that cause pain in joints, and others have severe flares that affect major organs, including the brain. Patients with the more severe form of SLE are more likely to have serious complications.

LUNG DISEASE

Chronic obstructive pulmonary disease (COPD) refers to a group of diseases that cause airflow blockage and breathing-related problems, such as chronic bronchitis, emphysema, and asthma. Most people with COPD have both chronic bronchitis and emphysema. COPD is the fourth leading cause of death in the United States. It causes serious, long-term disability. Tobacco use is a key factor in the development and worsening of COPD. Asthma, exposure to air pollutants in the home and workplace, genetic factors, and respiratory infections also play a role in the progression of the disease.

In 2006, almost 9 million people were diagnosed with chronic bronchitis in the United States. Almost 4 million were diagnosed with emphysema, and 13,913 deaths were caused by that disease. Doctors diagnosed 15.7 million cases of asthma, and 3,816 people died from asthma (CDC 2008a).

Having a cough that doesn't go away and coughing up a lot of mucus are common signs of COPD. Those signs often occur years before the airflow into and out of the lungs is reduced. However, not everyone who coughs a lot and produces sputum goes on to develop COPD, and not everyone with COPD has a cough (CDC n.d.). Most cases of COPD develop after a person repeatedly breathes in fumes and other irritants that damage the lungs and airways. Cigarette smoke is the most common irritant that causes COPD. Pipe, cigar, and other types of tobacco smoke can also cause COPD, especially if the smoke is inhaled. In addition, breathing in other fumes and dust over a long amount of time may cause COPD. The lungs and airways are highly sensitive to these irritants, and the irritants destroy the elastic fibers that allow the lung to stretch and then return to its resting shape. The resulting inflammation and narrowing makes breathing air in and out of the lungs more difficult (National Heart, Lung, and Blood Institute [NHLBI] 2007).

Chronic Bronchitis

In **chronic bronchitis**, the airways become inflamed and thickened, and there is an increase in the number and size of mucus-producing cells (see figure 8.10). This results in excessive mucus production, which in turn contributes to coughing and difficulty getting air into and out of the lungs. Chronic bronchitis may last for several weeks or months or may recur frequently throughout the year. It is much different from getting bronchitis once a year in that it lasts longer and occurs more frequently. People who smoke are at a significantly higher risk for chronic bronchitis. In order to be diagnosed with chronic bronchitis, a person must

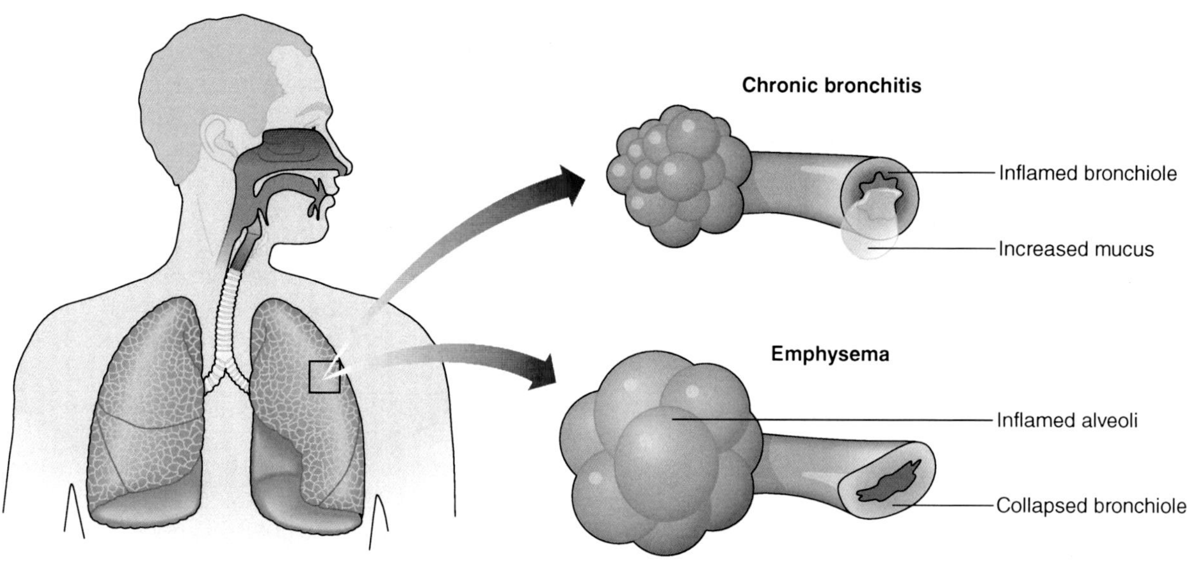

Figure 8.10 In chronic bronchitis, the airways become inflamed and filled with mucus. In emphysema, the airways collapse and damaged air sacs enlarge, causing shortness of breath and wheezing.

have bronchitis for 3 months or more in at least 2 consecutive years. Chronic bronchitis attacks can be brought on by exposure to allergens, viruses, or bacteria. There is no cure for chronic bronchitis, and people who are diagnosed should stop smoking, get medical treatment, and improve their lifestyles with moderate exercise, breathing exercises, and patient education. Sometimes lung transplants are suggested to increase the life span of patients.

Emphysema

In **emphysema**, the walls between many of the air sacs in the lungs are destroyed, leading to a few large air sacs instead of many tiny ones (see figure 8.10). Consequently, the lung looks like a sponge with large bubbles or holes instead of a sponge with tiny holes. The large air sacs have less surface area for the exchange of oxygen and carbon dioxide than healthy air sacs have. Poor exchange of oxygen and carbon dioxide causes shortness of breath. Signs and symptoms include the following:

- Coughing
- Sputum production
- Shortness of breath, especially with exercise
- Wheezing (whistling or squeaky sound with breathing)
- Chest tightness

Symptoms of emphysema are similar to the general category of COPD; however, they do not include the symptoms of chronic bronchitis, which include coughing and swelling of the feet and ankles due to fluid retention. Emphysema can also occur in people who have been exposed to powdered chemicals in the work environment. Many people who are farmers and factory workers are exposed to chemicals and metals in an aerosol form. For instance, farmers who spray pesticides and nutrients on their land often experience emphysema later in life. Factory workers in chemical plants and metalworking plants are often exposed and develop emphysema (CDC 2008a).

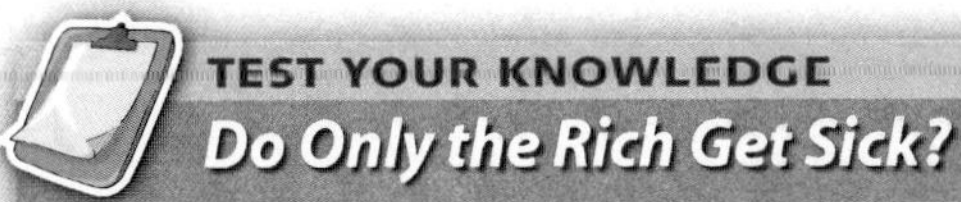

Do Only the Rich Get Sick?

Many people throughout the world believe that chronic diseases affect only rich people. That perception could be the result of the fact that poorer people do not seek medical care for regular checkups but visit only in times of illness (World Health Organization [WHO] 2005). Poorer people therefore may go undiagnosed. Also, it is possible that poorer people wait to see the doctor until the chronic condition is life threatening and live only a short time after diagnosis.

Asthma

More than 20 million people have been diagnosed with asthma, and 9 million of them are children. Asthma occurs when the body responds to cold, allergens, or chemicals and metals in an aerosol form. When the body reacts to inhaling these agents, the bronchial tubes become irritated and respond by swelling, which narrows the opening. When the bronchial tubes are narrowed, the air is restricted from entering the lungs, which causes shortness of breath and wheezing. Asthma attacks occur usually in the morning or at night. Some asthma attacks are so severe that they restrict oxygen from getting to vital organs and can result in death.

There is no cure for asthma, but there are treatments that reduce the chances of a severe attack. The first course of action is to go to the doctor to get a diagnosis and begin treatment. The first line of defense is to stay away from agents that irritate. The second is to carry an inhaler, usually Albuterol, to reduce the inflammation during an attack. If the patient uses this kind of inhaler more frequently than once or twice a month, then additional medication is prescribed to reduce the body's immune response.

Patients suffering from severe asthma attacks should go immediately to the emergency room. Indications of severe attacks include the following (CDC 2008a):

- Extreme difficulty breathing
- Bluish color in the lips and face
- Severe anxiety due to shortness of breath
- Rapid pulse
- Sweating
- Decreased alertness, such as severe drowsiness or confusion

CANCER

Many people have lost a loved one due to cancer. Survival rates for cancer have been increasing every year, however, resulting in cancer becoming a chronic disease rather than an acute disease that results in death.

Cancer is the unchecked growth of cells that form a tumor. Malignant tumors aggressively grow and invade surrounding tissue. Eventually, the tumors can spread through the bloodstream and affect other parts of the body in a process called *metastasizing.* Nonspecific symptoms of many cancers include weight loss and fatigue with depression and mood changes (Stoppler 2007).

Treatment for all cancers is generally surgical removal of the tumor and chemotherapy. Sometimes **radiation therapy** is used for smaller tumors. Radiation therapy uses high-energy X rays to kill dividing cancer cells. It only shrinks the tumor or limits its growth; however, in 10 to 15 percent of people, it leads to long-term remission (Stoppler 2007).

Chemotherapy uses drugs that target the rapidly growing cancer cells and destroy them. However, other cells in the body that grow quickly are also destroyed, such as hair cells, bone marrow cells, stomach and intestinal cells, and cells in the skin and mouth. The destruction of healthy cells results in many side effects. Damaged hair cells result in hair loss, damaged bone marrow cells result in fatigue, damaged stomach and intestinal cells result in diarrhea and vomiting, and damaged skin and mouth cells result in dry mouth and skin.

Chemotherapy can be used alone or in conjunction with radiation therapy or surgery. When used in conjunction with other treatments, it can extend a patient's life by three to four times longer than any other treatment alone would. Oncologists (cancer specialists) administer chemotherapy through pills, intravenously, or a combination of the two. Patients receive chemotherapy in cycles, where the drugs are given 2 to 3 months at a time followed by a time of recovery. Side effects of chemotherapy include increased susceptibility to infections, fatigue, weight loss, hair loss, nausea, vomiting, diarrhea, and mouth sores. The side effects disappear during the recovery (Stoppler 2007).

Prostate Cancer

The **prostate** is a walnut-shaped gland in men located in front of the rectum and under the bladder (see figure 8.11). It provides some of the fluid that protects and nourishes sperm cells in semen. When men have the proper level of testosterone, the prostate remains the same size after adulthood. Prostate cancer affects 70 to 90 percent of men over the age of 80, but not all of them have symptoms, so even their doctors may not be aware of the cancer.

Men may develop disorders of the prostate that aren't cancer. For example, older men may develop a noncancerous condition called **benign prostatic hyperplasia (BPH)** in which the inner part of the prostate continues to grow. BPH can cause the prostate to press on the urethra, resulting in frequent urges to urinate (American Cancer Society [ACS] 2007). Two other conditions—prostatic intraepithelial neoplasia (PIN) and atypical small acinar proliferation (ASAP)—aren't cancer but can be signals that prostate cancer may develop. PIN is a precancerous condition that affects nearly half of all men after age 50. Precancerous cells are in place, but they haven't invaded other parts of the prostate. After PIN is discovered, doctors may recommend that the patient have regular biopsies to monitor the health of the prostate. ASAP cells look similar to cancer under the microscope. If ASAP is found, there is a 40 to 50 percent chance that cancer is also present (ACS 2007).

Surgery sometimes provides the greatest chance for curing prostate cancer. Several types of surgical treatment are available for prostate cancer, including preventive, diagnostic, and curative. Preventive surgical treatment aims to prevent prostate cancer by removing ASAP cells that could become cancerous. Diagnostic surgery usually involves taking a tissue sample to be examined under a microscope. Doctors use a fine needle biopsy, a core needle biopsy,

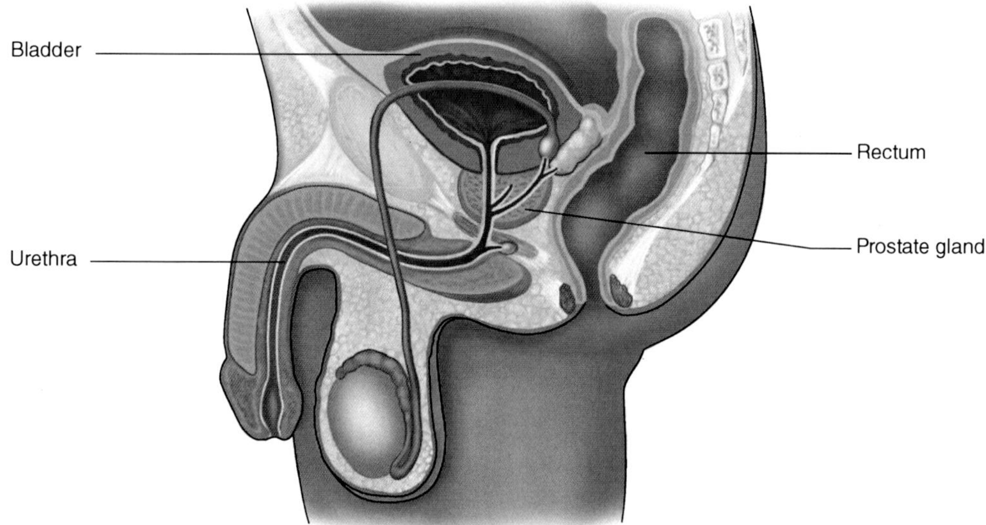

Figure 8.11 A doctor can check a man's prostate by inserting a gloved, lubricated finger in the rectum to feel the gland.

an incisional biopsy, or endoscopy to get the sample. The type of diagnostic surgery depends on the surgeon and the type of cancer that is suspected. Each type of surgery has drawbacks and advantages (ACS 2007).

Curative surgery is done when the cancer appears to be confined to one area. It may be combined with radiation therapy or chemotherapy. Sometimes doctors use radiation therapy during surgery. There are many new alternatives, such as laparoscopic, thorascopic, and laser surgery, and each can be just as effective as surgery using a scalpel (ACS 2007).

The ACS estimated that 218,890 new cases of prostate cancer would be diagnosed in the United States during 2007 but only 1 man in 35 would die from it. Even so, prostate cancer is the second leading cause of cancer deaths in men, behind lung cancer. Nine out of 10 cases of prostate cancers are found when the cancer is still within the prostate. The 5-year survival rate when prostate cancer is caught at this stage is almost 100 percent, the 10-year survival rate is 93 percent, and the 15-year survival rate is 77 percent. However, the 5-year survival rate for men whose cancer is diagnosed when it has metastasized to another part of the body drops dramatically, to 35 percent. Early diagnosis is done through a physical exam and blood work to identify an abnormal-sized prostate gland. Men over the age of 50 should have a yearly exam unless family history recommends earlier exams. Some symptoms are frequent urination, hesitation in urination, painful urination, painful ejaculation, lower back pain, and sometimes blood in urine. Prostate cancer is screened for by a PSA (prostate-specific agents) test, which is a simple blood test that measures the levels of PSA.

Lung Cancer

Although **lung cancer** is a lung disease, it's not a form of COPD. Many people with lung cancer are smokers or former smokers, but approximately 10 percent of lung cancer cases are diagnosed in nonsmokers. In 2005, 107,416 men and 89,271 women in the United States were diagnosed with lung cancer, and 90,139 men and 69,078 women died from the disease (CDC 2009).

Lung cancer is caught during a routine checkup in up to 25 percent of people diagnosed with the disease, because many people have no symptoms. Early symptoms of lung cancer include a cough that won't go away, constant chest pain, fatigue, shortness of breath, wheezing, chest pain, or coughing up blood. Sometimes lung cancer can paralyze the vocal cords and cause hoarseness. If the cancer invades the esophagus, a person may have difficulty swallowing.

Lung cancer is aggressive and spreads early to other parts of the body, especially to the adrenal glands, liver, bone, and brain. Because the heart pumps blood through the lungs to exchange carbon dioxide for oxygen, it's easy for lung cancer to spread from the lungs. The lungs are often the last place where other cancers metastasize. However, when cancer spreads to the lungs from another part of the body, it is not considered lung cancer; the cells retain the characteristics of their origin. For instance, when prostate cancer metastasizes to the lungs, it is prostate cancer in the lungs, not lung cancer (Stoppler 2007).

The overall prognosis for surviving lung cancer is poor compared with other cancers. The 5-year survival rate for lung cancer can be up to 16 percent, compared with 65 percent for colon cancer, 89 percent for breast cancer, and more than 99 percent for prostate cancer (Stoppler 2007). Early detection is always the best weapon against cancer.

Breast Cancer

In 2005, an estimated 188,231 cases of invasive breast cancer were diagnosed in the United States, and more than 41,000 women died from the disease. Breast cancer is also diagnosed in men; however, less than 1 percent of the diagnoses are in men, or approximately 1,764 cases in 2005 (CDC 2007a). Breast cancer is diagnosed most often in Caucasian women. African American women are more likely than Caucasian women to die as a result of breast cancer, though, because they're less likely to get early diagnoses from mammograms. A **mammogram** is a painless test that uses X rays to diagnose breast disease in women.

Known and probable risk factors for getting breast cancer include these (Susan G. Komen for the Cure 2007):

- Being a woman
- Getting older
- Genetics (having a mutation in the BRCA1 or BRCA2 breast cancer genes)
- Having a previous biopsy showing hyperplasia (abnormal cell growth) or carcinoma in situ (usually not a tumor, but a flat growth that can be a precursor of cancer)
- Having a family history of breast cancer or ovarian cancer
- Having high breast density on a mammogram
- Having a personal history of breast or ovarian cancer
- Starting menopause after age 55
- Never having children
- Having the first child after age 35
- Being overweight after menopause or gaining weight as an adult
- Having more than one drink of alcohol per day
- Currently or recently using combined estrogen and progestin hormone replacement therapy
- Having first menstruation before age 12

Warning signs of breast cancer shouldn't be ignored, including a change in the look of one breast, a change in breast size or shape, a lump or thickening, a warm sensation, a nipple turned inward or appearing sunken, an irregularly shaped nipple, a rash on the nipple, tenderness, nipple discharge, and breast pain (see figure 8.12). People with any of these signs should go to the doctor right away. The sooner the cancer is diagnosed, the better the chances of survival.

The available statistics sum up survival rates by breast cancer stage. The stages shown below are based on studies of a 5-year survival rate (CDC 2008a).

- Stage 0—No cancer. *Survival rate*: 100%.
- Stage I—Tumor is smaller than 2 cm and no lymph nodes are involved. *Survival rate*: 100%.
- Stage IIA—Tumor is smaller than 5 cm and there may be cancer cells in the lymph nodes under the arm that are not stuck together. *Survival rate*: 92%.
- Stage IIB—Tumor is bigger than 5 cm and the cancer has not spread. *Survival rate*: 81%.
- Stage IIIA—Tumor is bigger than 5 cm and the lymph nodes in the armpit contain cancer cells that may be stuck together, but there is no further spread. *Survival rate*: 67%.
- Stage IIIB—Tumor is fixed to the skin or chest wall and the lymph nodes may or may not contain cancer cells, but there is no further spread. *Survival rate*: 54%.
- Stage IV—Tumor can be any size, the lymph nodes may or may not contain cancer cells, and the cancer has spread to other parts of the body such as the lungs, liver, or bones. *Survival rate*: 20%.

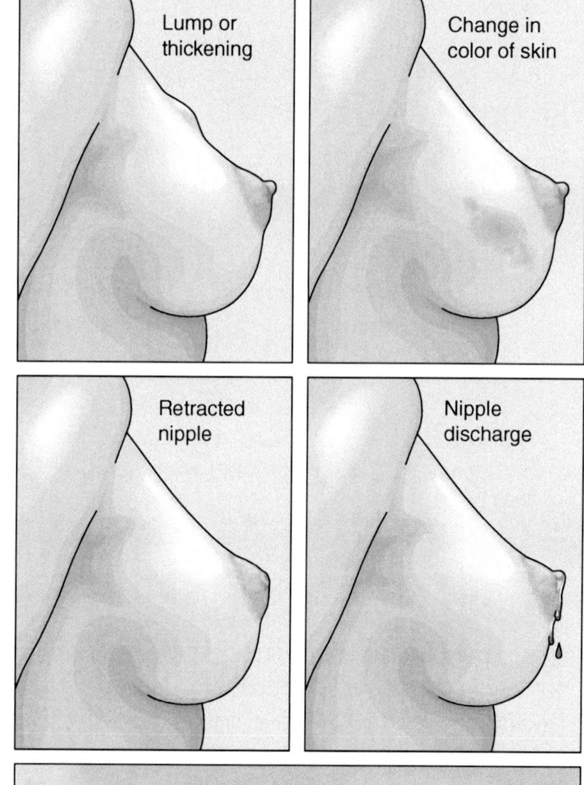

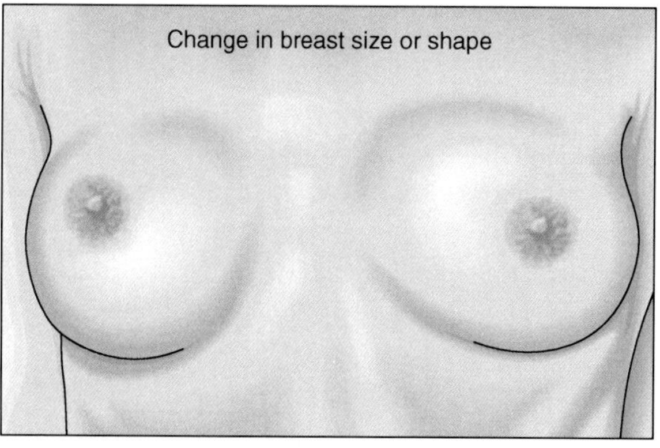

Figure 8.12 Warning signs of breast cancer.

The best way to detect breast cancer early is through monthly breast self-exams. Doing a self-exam requires a woman to lie down or stand with one hand raised and to examine the breast on the side of the raised hand (see figure 8.13). To determine if there is a lump or thickness in the breast,

- squeeze the area around the nipple with your thumb and index finger;
- move three flat middle fingers in a circular motion over the breast, starting in the middle and moving outward in bigger and bigger circles; and
- move three flat middle fingers up and down over the breast.

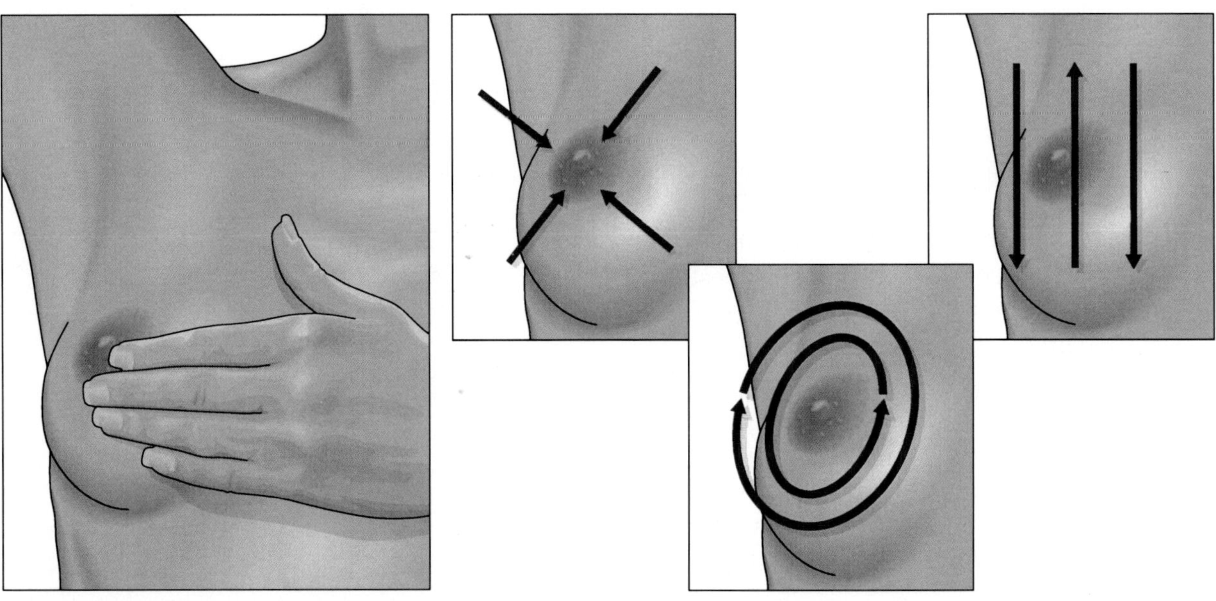

Figure 8.13 During a breast self-exam, squeeze the area around the nipple, and check the breast with circular motions and up and down motions using three flat middle fingers.

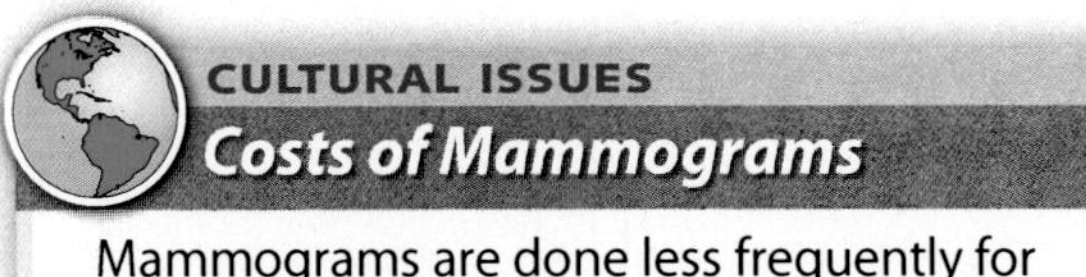

Mammograms are done less frequently for women from lower socioeconomic groups, including African American women, because of lack of insurance and time off from work for preventative procedures (Susan G. Komen for the Cure 2007). However, many social programs are available to help women who cannot afford mammograms. There are many mobile units that offer mammograms in low-income neighborhoods, women's clinics that provide mammograms with a sliding scale according to income, and other programs supported through nonprofit foundations such as the Susan G. Komen Breast Cancer Foundation and others.

Doctors detect breast cancer through a clinical exam or an MRI, digital mammography, and mammography (Susan G. Komen for the Cure 2007). Mammograms take X rays of the breast in several positions. Doctors then read the X rays to look for dark spots on the film. Digital mammograms are similar to regular mammograms, except the breast tissue can be viewed during the mammogram rather than waiting to review film. A technician can move the patient around and take several pictures of suspected areas. An MRI (magnetic resonance imaging) uses magnetic fields to create an image of the breast. They're being used more frequently because they can detect smaller tumors than traditional X rays. MRIs are more invasive because a radioactive dye is injected intravenously for contrast. If doctors suspect that there's a cancerous area, they may recommend surgery such as the kind described in the prostate cancer section, including needle biopsy, core needle biopsy, incisional biopsy, or large-needle aspiration. The tissue extracted from the biopsy is then sent to a lab for examination under a microscope (Susan G. Komen for the Cure 2007).

Treatment options for breast cancer are the same as for other cancers: surgery, radiation, chemotherapy, hormone therapy, and targeted therapies. Some women opt for a double mastectomy, which involves removing all the breast tissue from both breasts. Some women choose to have a double mastectomy even if cancer cells are only in one breast. Usually a combination of therapies is used. Recovery from surgery can be traumatic, especially if a large amount of breast tissue is removed. Support from family, friends, and other breast cancer survivors can be helpful (Susan G. Komen for the Cure 2007).

What Do You Think?

The breast cancer rate is lower among African American females than among other ethnic groups; however, the mortality rate is much higher. What do you think might contribute to the higher mortality rate? What steps should health educators or health professionals take to reduce the mortality rate of breast cancer in African American women?

DIABETES

As of 2007, the CDC estimates that 24 million people have diabetes in the United States, and almost 6 million of them aren't aware that they have diabetes (CDC 2008a). There are two types of diabetes: type 1 and type 2. Both types affect insulin, a chemical that helps the body use sugar or glucose. Diagnosis of **type 1 diabetes** is more common in young children than in adults. Type 1 diabetes develops when the body does not produce insulin. People with type 1 diabetes need insulin injections throughout their lives. **Type 2 diabetes** results from insulin resistance and is the most common type of diabetes in the United States. In **gestational diabetes**, a woman has uncontrolled glucose levels during pregnancy. Gestational diabetes is a form of prediabetes, which means that the glucose level is above 120 milligrams per deciliter (mg/dl), but it's not high enough to diagnose diabetes.

The risks for developing diabetes are being overweight, getting little or no regular exercise, having a family history of diabetes, or delivering a baby that weighs more than 9 pounds (4 kilograms). People who weigh in healthy ranges can develop type 2 diabetes because of problems with the pancreas or because they don't exercise and they have a poor diet.

Signs and symptoms of diabetes include:

- Being tired all the time
- Being hungry all the time (especially after eating)
- Craving extra liquids
- Frequent urination (especially during the night)
- Unexplained weight loss
- Numbness and tingling in your hands, legs, or feet
- Blurred vision
- Sexual dysfunction (difficulty with erection)

Type 2 diabetes is on the rise in the United States due to poor exercise and dietary habits. The primary risk factors for type 2 diabetes are family history of diabetes, lack of exercise, and obesity. With type 2 diabetes, the body either does not make enough insulin or the cells ignore the available insulin. Complications include kidney dysfunction, heart disease, and blindness. Diabetes has become an epidemic because of rising numbers of obese adults and young people. It is not uncommon for children as young as 10 to be diagnosed with type 2 diabetes, which was once considered an adult-onset disease.

What Do You Do?
The Web site of the American Diabetes Association offers an online calculator that can help determine your risk for having prediabetes or diabetes. Take the risk test at www.diabetes.org/risk-test.jsp.

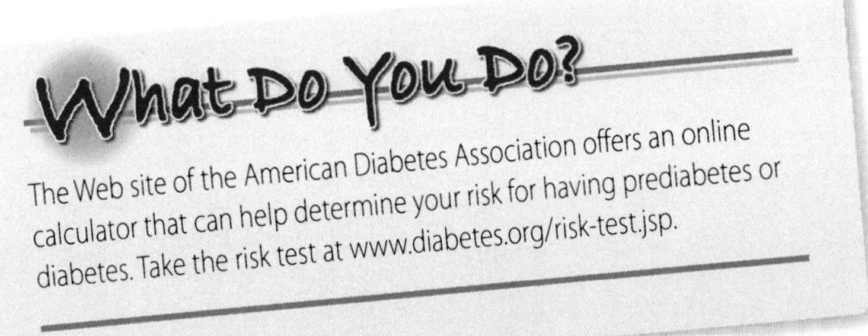

The best prevention for diabetes is exercising 30 to 40 minutes a day on 3 or 4 days a week, eating foods that are low in fat, eating fruits and vegetables high in fiber, and limiting carbohydrate intake. It's possible through weight loss and exercise to control some cases of diabetes without medication.

Treatment for diabetes may include adopting a healthy diet, exercising, and taking medicine to reduce glucose in the bloodstream. Early diagnosis can eliminate conditions that can result from uncontrolled diabetes. For example, diabetes increases the risk of heart disease and stroke because diabetes makes the blood sticky, which thickens the blood and helps attach cholesterol to the walls of veins and arteries.

Neuropathy is another possible health condition that comes from diabetes. Neuropathy affects the extremities by reducing blood flow, especially to the feet and lower limbs. Amputations are common among people with advanced diabetes. Reduced blood flow to the lower limbs makes it harder for the body to fight infection. Sometimes an infection occurs in the toes due to ingrown toenails or small cuts. The body can't send blood to the affected area, which can lead to an unchecked infection, which in turn can result in gangrene, or the death of the tissue. Amputation is the only way to stop the infection from spreading to the bloodstream after gangrene sets in.

ALZHEIMER'S DISEASE

Alzheimer's disease (AD) slowly hardens brain tissue, affecting the ability of the brain to function (see figure 8.14). AD is a degenerative disease that produces amyloid plaques and neurofibrillary tangles of proteins, or protein deposits that are surrounded by swollen neurons and dendrites making tangles on the surface of the brain (National Institute of Neurological Disorders and Stroke [NINDS] 2007). As many as 4.5 million Americans have AD. It usually begins around age 60, and the number of people diagnosed with AD doubles every 5 years as

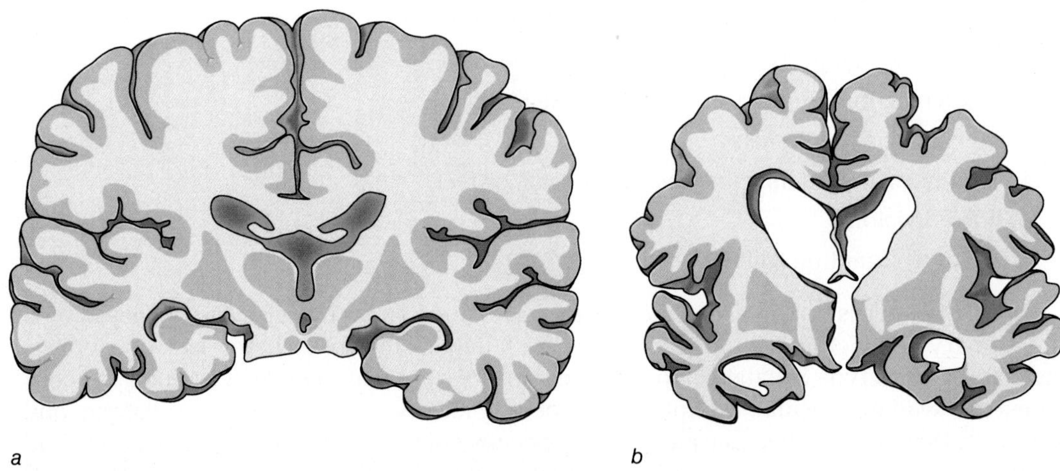

Figure 8.14 Compared to *(a)* a normal brain, *(b)* a brain with Alzheimer's disease is shriveled and reduced in size and has enlarged ventricles (cavities that contain cerebrospinal fluid).

CONSUMER ISSUES

Are Patients Medically Underserved?

A national survey (NCL News 2006) revealed that patients with chronic diseases are underserved and are not getting the treatment that they deserve. Survey respondents felt that patients with AD and Parkinson's disease are not getting the proper medication and treatment from their providers. The respondents also felt that the FDA was responsible for ensuring that the public has safe medications and treatments. However, the respondents felt that the FDA moves too slowly to provide new treatments for chronic diseases such as AD, Parkinson's disease, and multiple sclerosis. The message for the FDA and health educators is that people are not confident that enough is being done for those suffering from chronic ailments.

people pass the age of 65 (National Institute on Aging [NIA] 2007). Symptoms of AD include memory loss, language deterioration, impaired ability to mentally manipulate visual information, poor judgment, confusion, restlessness, and mood swings. Early stages of the disease are easily misdiagnosed because memory loss is a common complaint of older people. As the disease advances, usually over 5 to 20 years, people lose their ability to think and to function (NINDS 2007).

AD is named after Dr. Alois Alzheimer, who noticed changes in the brain of a woman who had died of a mental illness in 1906. He noticed the amyloid plaques and neurofibrillary tangles, which he had not seen before the death of this woman. There is no cure for AD, nor can it be slowed in its progression. There are drugs that assist with cognitive functioning, though, including donepezil, rivastigmine, and galantamine. Another drug recently approved by the FDA is memantine, which in combination with any of the previously mentioned drugs improves cognition better than any one drug alone (NINDS 2007).

The cause of AD is mostly unknown. Researchers have found that genetics plays a role in early-onset AD, which is rare and strikes people between the ages of 30 and 60. The presence of one gene, APOE, increases the possibility of getting AD in later life. APOE helps carry cholesterol in the blood, but only about 15 percent of the population has the form of APOE that indicates a risk for AD. Not everyone who has the gene gets AD. Researchers are now looking at possible environmental factors that may contribute to the disease.

CHRONIC DISEASES 101

Chronic diseases are long-term diseases such as cardiovascular disease, arthritis, lung disease, cancer, diabetes, and Alzheimer's disease. They account for 70 percent of all deaths in the United States, and they are costly for both the patients and society as a whole.

The degree to which you're able to prevent and control chronic diseases varies. Enjoying a healthy lifestyle can be the best prevention strategy for chronic disease. Eat well-balanced meals, control the intake of red meat and fats, and eat plenty of colored fruits and vegetables. Maintain a healthy weight and exercise on 3 or 4 days a week for at least 30 minutes each day. Remember, genetics plays only a small part in your risk factors for chronic diseases.

CHAPTER REVIEW

REVIEW QUESTIONS

1. What are some of the consequences of chronic diseases?
2. What are some factors of a healthy lifestyle that can reduce your risk for chronic disease?
3. Name and describe three types of cardiovascular disease.
4. Describe four symptoms of having a stroke, and describe four risk factors of stroke that can be controlled before they cause problems.
5. What is the leading cause of disability in the United States, and what are some of its symptoms?
6. What's the difference between chronic bronchitis, emphysema, and asthma?
7. Describe three general treatments for cancer.
8. List six known or probable risk factors for getting breast cancer.
9. What preventative measures that reduce the risks for diabetes would you recommend to a friend who is overweight?
10. What is the number one cause of all diseases, including chronic disease?

CRITICAL THINKING

1. Some women with a family history of breast cancer are choosing to undergo genetic testing to see if they have an altered gene (a mutation in the BRCA1 or BRCA2 breast cancer genes) that might make them more likely to develop the disease. Women who test positive for an altered gene can screen for cancer more thoroughly, take drugs to reduce their risk, or even have preventative double mastectomies, in which both breasts are removed surgically. However, the presence of an altered gene does not mean a woman definitely will develop breast cancer—only that her risk is higher—and some people consider the removal of healthy breasts to be dramatic and unnecessary. If you or a close friend or family member tested positive and were faced with a choice of treatments, how would you react? What factors would be important when making a decision?
2. As detailed in this chapter, direct and indirect costs for medical care for chronic disease are high. Currently, tobacco use is the number one cause of chronic disease, and the costs for treating tobacco-related disease exceed $75 billion annually. However, some people argue that those who choose to use tobacco should bear the costs of their resulting medical care. Do you think patients who smoked, ate poorly, or didn't exercise should be treated differently from patients who maintained a healthy lifestyle?

APPLICATION ACTIVITIES

1. Talk with family members about any chronic diseases in the family. Ask what they think caused the chronic disease. Find out who in the family has no chronic diseases and why they are healthy. Make a family tree and identify where chronic diseases are present on the family tree.
2. Visit a nursing home where patients with Alzheimer's disease live. Identify similarities and differences among the patients. Observe how the nursing home cares for and protects those clients, and see if you notice ways the facility could improve its care.

GLOSSARY

Alzheimer's disease (AD)—Degenerative disease that produces amyloid plaques and neurofibrillary tangles of proteins and affects brain function.

aneurysm—Bulge or weakness in a blood vessel wall.

arrhythmia—Abnormal rhythm of the heart, which can cause the heart to pump less effectively; also referred to as *dysrhythmia*.

arteriosclerosis—With age, the arteries become less flexible.

atherosclerosis—Progressive process in which fatty deposits form in arteries.

benign prostatic hyperplasia (BPH)—When the inner part of the prostate continues to grow, prostate may press on the urethra and cause frequent urges to urinate.

cancer—Unchecked growth of cells that form tumors and aggressively grow and invade surrounding tissue.

cardiomyopathy—Diseases of the heart muscle.

cardiovascular disease (CVD)—Range of diseases that affect the heart or blood vessels, including coronary artery disease, heart attack, heart failure, high blood pressure, and stroke.

chemotherapy—Drugs that target the rapidly growing cancer cells and destroy them. The destruction of healthy cells in addition to cancer cells results in many side effects.

chronic bronchitis—When the airways become inflamed and thickened, and there is an increase in the number and size of mucus-producing cells.

chronic diseases—Illnesses that persist over time.

chronic obstructive pulmonary disease (COPD)—Group of diseases that cause airflow blockage and breathing-related problems, including chronic bronchitis, emphysema, and asthma.

congenital heart disease—Form of heart disease that develops before birth.

coronary artery disease—Restriction of blood flow or blockage of arteries that lead to the heart.

emphysema—Lung disease that results from the walls between the air sacs being destroyed, leading to a few large air sacs instead of many tiny ones.

fibromyalgia—Syndrome characterized by widespread muscular pains and fatigue.

gestational diabetes—When a woman has uncontrolled glucose levels during pregnancy.

gout—Rheumatic disease resulting from deposits of uric acid crystals (monosodium urate) in tissues and fluids within the body.

heart failure—Condition in which the heart can't pump enough blood to meet the needs of the body's organs and tissues; often called *congestive heart failure* (CHF).

hemorrhagic stroke—Stroke caused by a blood vessel breaking because of high blood pressure or an aneurysm bursting in the brain.

hypertension—The excessive force of blood pumping through the blood vessels against the walls; commonly called *high blood pressure*.

ischemic stroke—Stroke caused by a blockage in an artery of the brain, which causes the part of the brain without oxygen to die.

lung cancer—The unchecked growth of cells that form a tumor in the lungs.

mammogram—X rays of the breast used to detect breast cancer. With digital mammograms, the breast tissue can be viewed during the mammogram rather than waiting to review film.

myocardial infarction (MI)—Heart muscle death due to loss of blood supply; also called *heart attack*.

osteoarthritis—Disease characterized by degeneration of cartilage and its underlying bone within a joint as well as bony overgrowth.

pericardial diseases—Diseases of the sac that encases the heart (pericardium).

peripheral artery disease—Occurs when plaque builds up on the inside walls of the arteries that carry blood from the heart to the head, internal organs, and limbs; also known as *atherosclerotic peripheral arterial disease*.

plaque—Fatty, cholesterol-rich, waxy substance that builds up in the coronary arteries.

prostate—Walnut-shaped gland in men located in front of the rectum and under the bladder.

radiation therapy—Cancer treatment using high-energy X rays to kill dividing cancer cells.

rheumatoid arthritis—Systemic inflammatory disease that manifests itself in multiple joints of the body. The inflammatory process primarily affects the lining of the joints (synovial membrane) but can also affect other organs. The inflamed synovium leads to erosions of the cartilage and bone and sometimes joint deformity.

systemic lupus erythematosus (SLE)—Disease in which the immune system produces antibodies that attack healthy tissue, leading to widespread inflammation and tissue damage to muscles surrounding joints and bodily organs.

type 1 diabetes—Develops when the body does not produce insulin. Type 1 diabetes is more common in young children than in adults, and people who have it need insulin injections throughout their lives.

type 2 diabetes—Results from insulin resistance and is the most common type of diabetes in the United States.

valvular heart disease—When the heart valves that keep blood flowing in the right direction are damaged.

REFERENCES AND RESOURCES

American Cancer Society (ACS). 2007. What is prostate cancer. www.cancer.org/docroot/CRI/content/CRI_2_2_1X_What_is_prostate_cancer_36.asp.

Berenson, A. 2008. Drug approved. Is disease real? *New York Times*, January 14.

Boston University. 2008. One in six women, one in ten men at risk for Alzheimer's disease in their lifetime. *Science Daily*. www.sciencedaily.com/releases/2008/03/080318114824.htm.

Centers for Disease Control and Prevention (CDC). 2007a. Breast cancer statistics. www.cdc.gov/cancer/breast/statistics/.

———. 2007b. Chronic disease prevention. www.cdc.gov/nccdphp/.

———. 2008a. Chronic disease overview. www.cdc.gov/nccdphp/overview.htm.

———. 2008b. Targeting arthritis: Improving quality of life for more than 46 million Americans. At a glance 2008. www.cdc.gov/nccdphp/publications/AAG/arthritis.htm.

———. 2009. Lung cancer fast facts. www.cdc.gov/cancer/lung/basic_info/fast_facts.htm.

———. n.d. Chronic obstructive pulmonary disease. www.cdc.gov/nccdphp/dach/.

Lucile Packard Children's Hospital. 2007. Congenital heart disease. www.lpch.org/DiseaseHealthInfo/HealthLibrary/hrnewborn/chd.html.

Mayo Clinic. 2006. Cardiovascular disease 101: Understanding heart and blood vessel conditions. www.mayoclinic.com/health/cardiovascular-disease/HB00032.

National Association of Chronic Disease Directors (NAOCDD). 2007. Public health advances through chronic disease prevention: 1986-2006. www.chronicdisease.org/files/public/Top10PublicHealthAchievements.pdf.

National Heart, Lung, and Blood Institute (NHLBI). 2007. What causes COPD? www.nhlbi.nih.gov/health/dci/Diseases/Copd/Copd_Causes.html.

National Institute of Neurological Disorders and Stroke (NINDS). 2007. NINDS Alzheimer's disease information page. www.ninds.nih.gov/disorders/alzheimersdisease/alzheimersdisease.htm.

National Institute on Aging (NIA). 2007. Alzheimer's disease fact sheet. www.nia.nih.gov/Alzheimers/Publications/adfact.htm.

NCL News. 2006. Survey: Consumers believe chronic disease patients to be medically underserved. www.nclnet.org/news/2006/Chronic_Disease_survey_02092006.htm.

Stein, D.W. 2006. High blood pressure causes. www.webmd.com/hypertension-high-blood-pressure/guide/blood-pressure-causes.

Stein, R. 2006. A gender difference in heart disease. *Washington Post*, February 1.

Stoppler, M.C. 2007. Lung cancer. www.medicinenet.com/lung_cancer/article.htm.

Susan G. Komen for the Cure. 2007. About breast cancer. http://ww5.komen.org/breastcancer/aboutbreastcancer.html.

WebMD. 2006. Stroke. WebMD and the Cleveland Clinic NeuroscienceCenter. www.webmd.com/stroke/default.htm.

World Health Organization (WHO). 2005. Preventing chronic diseases: A vital investment. www.who.int/chp/chronic_disease_report/full_report.pdf.

Other helpful resources include the following.

Beaglehole, R., J. Epping-Jordan, V. Patel, M. Chopra, S. Ebrahim, M. Kidd, and A. Haines. 2008. Improving the prevention and management of chronic disease in low-income and middle-income countries: A priority for primary health care. *The Lancet* 372 (9642): 940-949.

Center for Health Care Strategies, Inc. www.chcs.org. This nonprofit health policy resource center's mission statement is to improve health care quality for low-income children and adults, people with chronic illnesses and disabilities, frail elders, and racially and ethnically diverse populations experiencing disparities in care. Resources include sample educational materials for chronic disease management for providers and patients.

Disease Control Priorities Project. www.dcp2.org/pubs/GBD. This site includes background information and downloadable PDFs for a publication titled *Global Burden of Disease and Risk Factors*, which provides a multicultural and global perspective on the issue of diseases.

Indiana University. 2008. Chronic disease management: Does it improve health and save money? *ScienceDaily*, May 13. www.sciencedaily.com/releases/2008/05/080513054826.htm.

World Health Organization (WHO). www.who.int/topics/chronic_diseases/en/. This site provides general information, as well as links to fact sheets and publications.

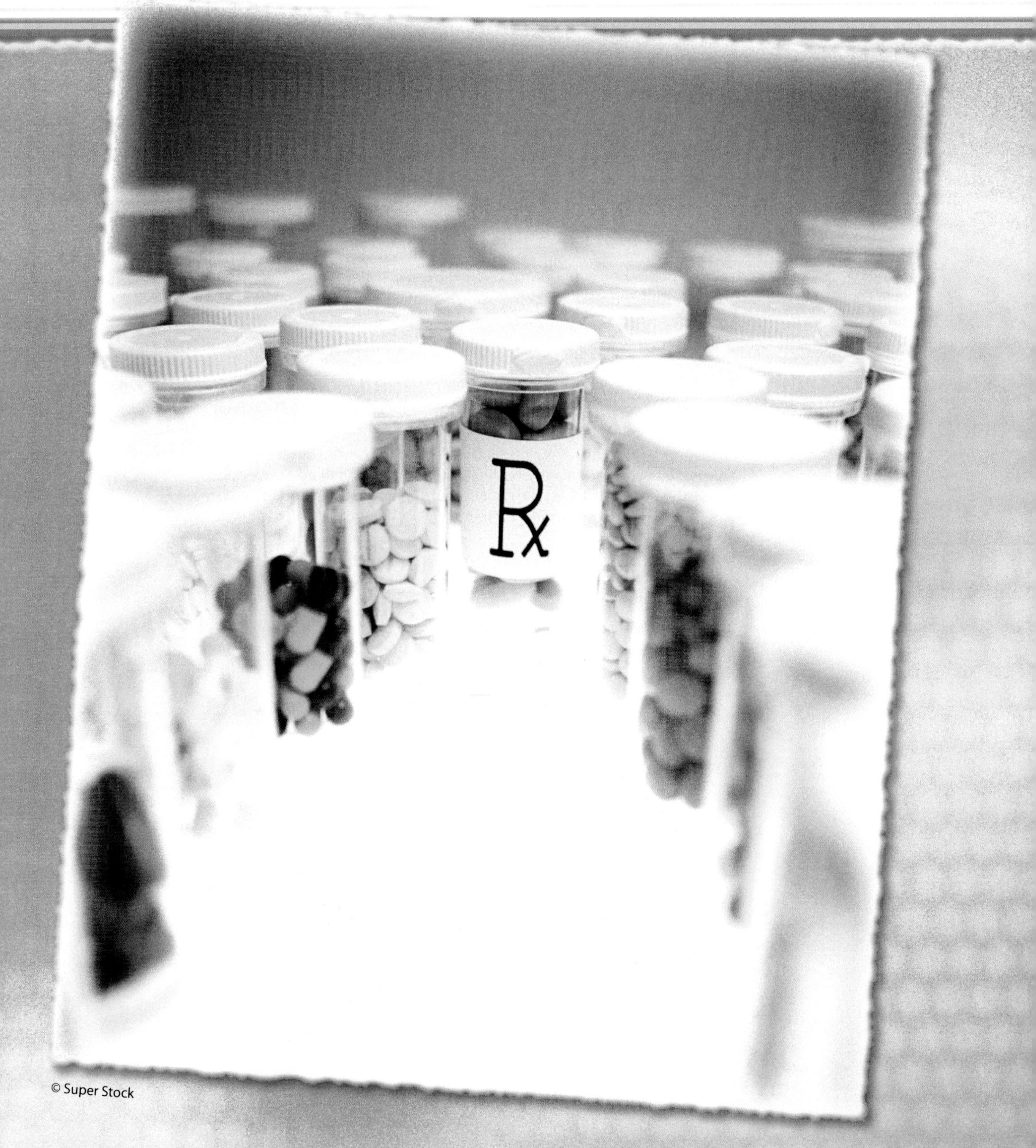

© Super Stock

CHAPTER 9

HEALTH CARE CONSUMERISM

PAMELA DOUGHTY, PHD, CHES
Institute for Obesity Research and Program Evaluation,
Texas A&M University

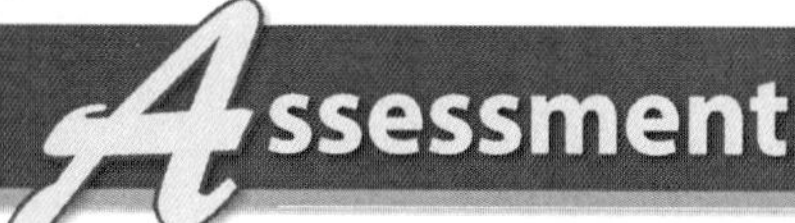

Assessment

- What's the difference between an HMO and a PPO?
- What type of health insurance is the *least* you should have?
- Do you know the best way to choose a doctor?
- How can you find reliable health insurance information online?
- Does acupuncture really work? How about herbal medicine?
- What are quacks, and how can you avoid them?

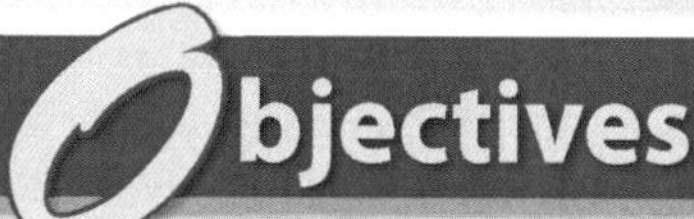

Objectives

- Define *consumer health*.
- Describe how to choose a provider, hospital, or treatment option.
- Define *alternative medicine* and *complementary alternative medicine*, and list the various treatment methods that they offer.
- Describe how to choose an affordable health plan.
- Describe how to talk with your doctor.
- Explain consumer-driven health care.
- List online resources for valid health care information.
- Describe how to assess online resources.
- Explain how to spot a health care scam.

If you're a college student, you might not have needed to think too much about your health care so far. Your parents may have chosen your physicians, covered your health insurance and health care costs, bought your medicine, and maybe even made most of your doctor appointments. Before long, though, those will be your responsibilities, and the decisions you'll have to make will be expensive ones. Figuring out which health plans meet your needs best and how you can afford them, choosing a qualified doctor whom you trust, and even knowing how to buy the right over-the-counter medicines are decisions that will cost you money. This chapter provides information you can use to make well-informed decisions about your health care.

Consumer health includes making decisions about health providers, hospitals, health plans, prescriptions, prevention strategies, quality of care, treatment choices, and reliable health information. Being an active health care consumer means that you take responsibility for your own health care. Not only do you adopt a healthy lifestyle, but you're also deliberate about choosing the right health care providers and treatment options for every aspect of your health—physical, mental, emotional, social, occupational, and spiritual.

Making informed decisions regarding your health also includes keeping the cost of health care within your budget as much as possible. The cost of health care has increased since the 1980s due to increased litigation, advancement in medical science that extends lives, and increased costs of insurance for doctors (National Center for Complementary and Alternative Medicine [NCCAM] 2007). Medical costs have increased dramatically in the past 10 years. In 2007, medical expenses increased to 16 percent of the U.S. gross national product, up from 14 percent in 2000 (Centers for Disease Control and Prevention [CDC] 2008). With the rising cost of health care, it is even more important to have health insurance.

Health insurance can be purchased as part of an employment package, where the employer pays part of the premium; it can be purchased directly from a health insurance company; and it can be provided at a low cost for children through state child insurance programs, Medicaid for low-income families, and Medicare for people over the age of 65 who have contributed to Social Security over the years. However, many people make too much money to get Medicaid and too little money to afford direct-pay medical insurance or employer-based health insurance.

In 2007, at least 20 percent of Americans were uninsured at least part of the time during the year (CDC 2008). As of 2007, less than 60 percent of Americans received health insurance as part of employment, less than 10 percent purchased their insurance themselves, less than 14 percent used Medicare, and less than 13 percent were on Medicaid. Table 9.1 shows that more than 60 percent of white and Asian males and females are insured, and less than 50 percent of black males and females and 40 percent of Hispanic males and females are insured. There is an inequity in those who are insured because many blacks and Hispanics have lower-paying jobs that do not include health insurance as a benefit or cannot afford insurance coverage.

What Do You Think?

Think insurance premiums are high? Check out the difference in the cost of a broken arm for an insured and uninsured patient (Anderson 2006):

- $8,094.21 is the total bill. This is what you would owe if you were uninsured.
- $1,755.15 is the bill after applying insurers' discounts.
- $309.57 is the amount that you would owe for your broken arm with health insurance.

FINDING THE RIGHT HEALTH INSURANCE PLAN

As a college student, you probably haven't had to be too involved in making decisions about your own health insurance coverage. You've probably been covered under a parent's or

TABLE 9.1 Participants in Health Insurance in 2007

Health insurance	Employment based	Direct purchase	Medicaid	Medicare
Total population covered	59.3%	8.9%	13.2%	13.8%
Males, all races	60.0%	8.5%	12.2%	12.2%
Females, all races	58.7%	9.4%	14.2%	15.4%
White, both sexes	61.2%	9.8%	11.4%	14.7%
White males	61.8%	9.2%	10.6%	12.9%
White females	60.5%	10.4%	12.1%	16.4%
Black, both sexes	49.1%	4.5%	24.2%	11.1%
Black males	49.5%	4.4%	22.5%	10.0%
Black females	48.9%	4.5%	25.7%	12.1%
Asian, both sexes	62.0%	8.4%	11.5%	8.6%
Asian males	61.6%	8.7%	11.2%	7.4%
Asian females	62.3%	8.1%	11.7%	9.7%
Hispanic, both sexes	40.3%	3.9%	22.5%	6.3%
Hispanic males	39.8%	4.0%	20.0%	5.3%
Hispanic females	40.8%	3.8%	24.5%	7.3%

Source: U.S. Census Bureau, Current Population Survey, 2000-2008 Annual Social and Economic Supplements.

guardian's plan, or you've been covered under insurance from your school. But sooner or later, finding good health insurance will be necessary, and you need to know how to find a plan that's affordable and gives you the coverage you need. Several types of health care plans are available to choose from, and you can purchase them as an individual or as part of a group plan.

Health Maintenance Organizations

A **health maintenance organization (HMO)** generally provides the cheapest health insurance plans. With an HMO, you choose your main physician from a list of physicians who have agreed to be part of the HMO plan. These physicians serve as gatekeepers for health care. As a patient, you have to see your primary care physician for routine visits. If you require special care, your primary care physician needs to refer you to a specialist and order X rays, sonograms, or other treatment outside of his practice. You usually pay a small fee, called a **copayment**, for your visit to the doctor. The copay is determined by the HMO contract. Copays usually range from as little as $10 to as much as $50, depending on the HMO and level of care.

The good thing about HMOs is that the cost is low and the copay covers all treatment that can be done in the doctor's office. Therefore, it's possible that a visit to the doctor for a broken finger that includes the doctor visit, X ray, blood work, splinting, and bandaging could cost only $10. Another positive aspect is there is a set fee for visits to specialists, emergency room visits, and hospital expenses.

There are some downsides to participating in an HMO, though. You have to choose your doctor from a list of providers in your area. Sometimes you might have to travel outside of your town to find an approved provider. If you've been with a certain doctor all your life and then you join an HMO, your doctor might not be on the list of approved providers, and either you'll have to pay extra to continue seeing your doctor or you'll need to choose a new one. In addition, it's possible that your primary care physician won't want to refer to you a specialist when you think you need to see one. Because your doctor is the gatekeeper for all your treatment options, she gets to decide whether you need to go to a specialist for your condition or whether she can treat you herself.

Furthermore, certain procedures aren't covered by HMOs. Organ transplants, in vitro fertilization (IVF), and other procedures are not routinely funded. Finally, doctors might need to book a lot of patients during a day to make up for the low cost per patient or because the doctor is on salary and the HMO determines the minimum number of patients seen in a day. That means you might feel rushed during your appointment, or the doctor might be running late to your scheduled appointment.

On the whole, HMOs are good options most of the time, because the cost is relatively low.

Preferred Provider Organizations

A **preferred provider organization (PPO)** isn't as restrictive as an HMO. PPOs allow you to choose your own doctor, but if he's not within the PPO network, your out-of-pocket cost is higher. The **premiums** for PPOs are significantly higher than for HMOs, and the **out-of-pocket expenses** are much higher, too. Even so, the freedom of choice attracts many people to this type of insurance. With PPOs, the doctor you've been with for years might be part of the network, or the PPO may allow you to see your established physician if you pay a little more. Some PPOs require a referral to specialists and others don't. PPOs are usually the first choice for people who can afford the higher premiums and higher out-of-pocket expenses. People in HMOs complain about the restrictiveness, and people in PPOs complain about the high costs.

Comparing Costs

The cost for medical insurance varies by the type of plan that is chosen and how much the employer contributes to the plan. Table 9.2 shows typical PPO and HMO costs for a family (the employee, a spouse, and children). Although PPOs have many advantages, it is easy to see that the costs are significantly lower for an HMO. Most of the cost for medical insurance is usually covered by the employer; it is only when adding a spouse or child that the costs increase. The advantage of purchasing health insurance from the employer is that the premiums are taken out before taxes are determined, called *pretax dollars*. This means that you only pay taxes on the amount left after removing the money used for the health insurance premium, resulting in lower taxes.

Government Plans

The U.S. government provides some insurance plans, such as Medicaid, state children's health insurance, and Medicare. **Medicaid** is state-administered health insurance for people whose

TABLE 9.2 Costs of Insurance Through an Employer

Type of insurance	Cost per month	Cost per year	Deductibles	Cost of $20,000 car accident
PPO	$850	$10,200	$500 deductible and 20% of balance	$4,400
HMO	$320	$3,840	$50 copay for emergency services	$50

income is below a certain level. Each state determines its own income level for eligibility. Medicaid pays the medical provider, not the person who receives the health care. The plan covers services from doctors and hospitals, diagnostic services, dental services, long-term care services, and other services as stated in the state's Medicaid law. The **State Children's Health Insurance Program (SCHIP)** is offered though the state. This insurance is offered to children whose parents do not qualify for Medicaid but have a low enough income that they cannot afford private insurance. It is easier for children to be eligible than adults for Medicaid. You can find information about each state's Medicaid program at www.cms.hhs.gov/MedicaidGenInfo/Downloads/MedicaidAtAGlance2005.pdf.

Medicare is available to all people in the United States who qualify for Social Security benefits.

- Part A pays a percentage for hospital visits, in-home health care, and inpatient skill nursing care and hospice, but it doesn't pay for visits to a physician. Most people do not pay a premium for Part A.
- Part B covers outpatient care, doctors' services, physical or occupational therapists, and additional home health care. Most people pay a premium for Part B.
- Part C is a combination of Part A and Part B.
- Part D is prescription drug coverage. It covers all medically necessary prescriptions and has a variety of plans to choose from. Part D coverage has a premium.

Dangers of Being Uninsured

Many people in the United States don't have health insurance coverage. People often are betweeners, making too much money to qualify for Medicaid but too little money to afford health insurance. In addition, people who are between jobs may not have insurance, and those

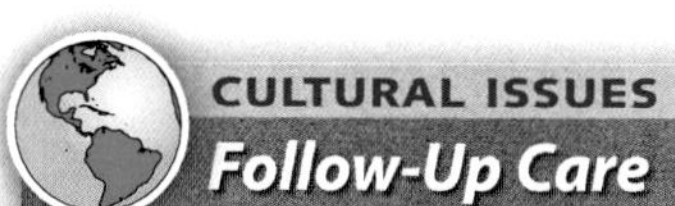

CULTURAL ISSUES

Follow-Up Care

A research study was designed to examine the influence of ethnicity and insurance coverage on health care access and healthy behaviors in adult survivors of childhood cancer in the United States. Twenty-five centers with 20,316 subjects diagnosed with cancer before age 21 participated. The observed subjects who remained in the study included 443 black, 503 Hispanic, and 7,821 non-Hispanic white subjects. Patients who qualified for public insurance such as Medicaid were more likely to report cancer-related follow-up care if they were Hispanic or non-Hispanic white than survivors with private insurance. Uninsured patients were less likely to report follow-up care in the years after treatment regardless of ethnicity (Casillas et al. 2005).

It would be expected that those without insurance would be less likely to follow up because the cost of follow-up care would be the survivor's responsibility. Survivors would most likely be young adults early in their careers and no longer covered under a parent's health insurance. As young professionals, they might not yet have insurance offered as part of their jobs. Perhaps those who did have jobs with private insurance didn't want to have cancer on their health record as they enrolled in their new health insurance plan because of fear that the policy would be canceled or that premiums would increase. Also, people with private insurance have copayments that people on public health insurance do not. Copayments for young adults might be too high. Missing work could be another factor that might inhibit the privately insured from getting follow-up care.

who've just started jobs may have to wait to become insured with their new employers. Often new employees have to wait 30 to 90 days to become eligible for their company-sponsored health insurance coverage to begin.

The **Consolidated Omnibus Budget Reconciliation Act (COBRA)** was passed into law in 1986. COBRA provides the opportunity for employees to buy group coverage for limited amounts of time and is available for terminated employees, those who lose coverage because of reduced work hours, or children who can no longer be on their parents' policy because of age. COBRA allows the person to continue with health insurance, prescription drug coverage, dental insurance, and vision care. It does not cover life insurance (Pension and Welfare Benefits Association [PWBA] 1994). COBRA can cost two to five times more than the health insurance provided by the employer, though, which makes it an expensive option.

Being uninsured can be a financial disaster for anybody who experiences a health care emergency. The cost of all the procedures, hospital stays, doctors, and prescriptions has to be paid by the uninsured person. Many people have declared bankruptcy because they experienced one health care emergency that put them into debt they could never repay. If an uninsured person has a health emergency, it can be helpful to speak with the hospital about the costs. Sometimes the hospital has resources available to patients who don't make enough money to pay their hospital bills. In addition, some practitioners will settle for less than the full cost billed to the uninsured. Don't be afraid to talk with everyone involved in providing care to find out options for repaying the cost of the care.

With the cost of medical care increasing every year, it is important that all people be able to pay for health care within their means. Any insurance is better than no insurance. Even if you can't afford much health insurance, you should try to purchase at least **catastrophic health insurance** coverage, which is much less expensive than most other health insurance. Catastrophic health insurance covers some of the medical bills from a health care emergency. It pays only a portion of the medical bills, sometimes 80 percent, but it protects against significant financial loss.

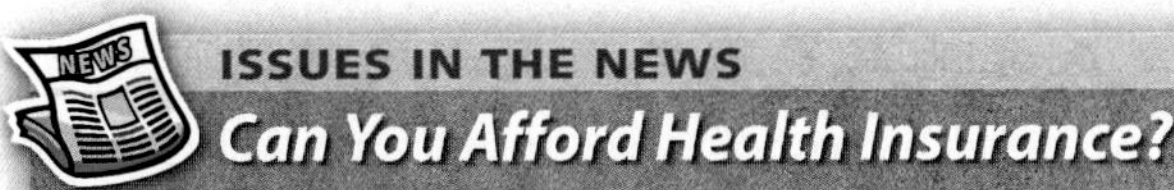

ISSUES IN THE NEWS

Can You Afford Health Insurance?

Health care has been in the news a lot lately as elected officials and interest groups discuss ways to lower costs and make insurance more accessible and affordable. For college students and others on their own, it's tempting to not purchase health insurance coverage because it can be expensive. Here's how you can figure out whether you can afford health insurance. (You'll need to do a little research to get these costs.) First, figure out the annual cost of the insurance premiums by multiplying the monthly premium by 12 months. Now, figure out the cost of your typical doctor visits annually. Include the cost of your annual checkup and blood work. Then add in the number of times you visit the doctor in a year for illnesses such as the flu, visits to the eye doctor, and so on. How do the costs compare?

Now add up 5 years' worth of premiums (forget about inflation for now). You're more likely to require an emergency room visit or hospitalization over that amount of time than over a single year. So, find out the cost of an emergency room visit for, say, a broken bone. Add in surgery to repair the bone and the cost of a day in the hospital. Subtract that amount from your 5-year premium cost.

Did you come out in the positive (you spent more money on health insurance than expenses), or did you come out in the negative (the actual cost was higher than the cost of insurance)?

CHOOSING A DOCTOR

Getting your insurance needs covered to the greatest extent possible is one important step in being a smart health care consumer. Choosing a doctor is another important step. You might have few choices because of the area you live in or the insurance coverage you have, but you probably have some choices in doctors. Just asking friends about the doctors they like might not be enough to find the right match for you, but if you ask several people and one doctor's name comes up repeatedly, that doctor might be a good choice. Ask around and listen to why others like or don't like a doctor.

Check the doctor's education and accreditation. Calling the doctor's office is a good way to check this out, and you can also do some research online. There are many Web sites that assist in finding a good doctor and hospital. The most important aspect of a good Web site is to determine if it is selling something. If it is not obvious whether or not the site has a bias, don't use it. For instance, WebMD (www.webmd.com) is an excellent Web site and doesn't promote specific doctors or sell information. The site runs advertising through banners, but the information provided doesn't back certain doctors or certain treatments, which makes it a reliable site. HealthGrades (www.healthgrades.com) is another reliable Web site.

Next, visit the doctor to find out her communication style. You may need to pay for that visit, but it's important to find a doctor who listens to you. During your visit, try to evaluate these things:

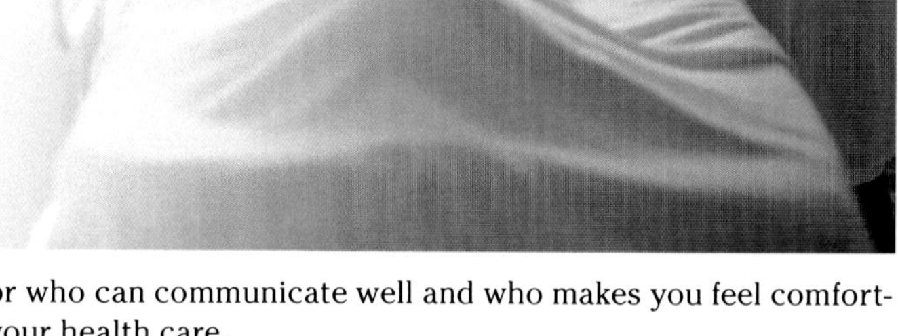

Find a doctor who can communicate well and who makes you feel comfortable about your health care.

© Photodisc

- Does the doctor talk with you about your concerns?
- Does the doctor take the time to listen to you?
- Does the doctor explain things in a way that you understand?
- Does the doctor use the information gained from listening to you to make diagnoses?

Communication can be the most important aspect of the doctor–patient relationship. You need to know you're heard and understood and that the doctor makes recommendations with your input in mind. Finding the right doctor you can trust may be one of the most important health care decisions you make.

Other considerations when choosing a doctor are culture, gender, and language. Health care disparity can be a result of cultural barriers. Finding a doctor who understands your cultural background can be a factor in determining your provider. Women who practice Islam, for example, require a woman doctor. Many women from all kinds of cultures prefer going to a female doctor, especially when they need to consult the doctor about gynecological concerns, because they think a female doctor will listen and understand them better than a male doctor will. Many men prefer a male doctor, especially when they experience health concerns such as erectile dysfunction or prostate problems. Being able to understand the doctor and have the doctor understand you is also important. People who are nonnative English speakers can feel reluctant to talk to the staff in the doctor's office because they're afraid that no one will understand them. When you're confident that the doctor and the staff can understand you, you're more likely to seek medical care.

You should also find out where your doctor has hospital privileges. Can your doctor see you and care for you if you're in the hospital? Most people want a doctor who has privileges at a nearby hospital. Some doctors don't have hospital privileges, which means if you need to go to the hospital, another doctor will need to see you.

Finding a doctor who's right for you may sound complicated, but you need to make the effort if you want to have good health care and a provider who will help you make good decisions in the future.

GENDER ISSUES

Doctor–Patient Relationships

Gender in medicine has been a topic of research in the United States since the women's movement began in the early 1970s. In the medical world, historically men were perceived as the norm for human beings and women were viewed as a deviation from the norm. Research in the 1970s showed that physicians associated a healthy adult with a healthy male, whereas a healthy female was described quite differently (Risberg, Johansson, Westman, and Hamberg 2003).

A 2003 study gave a questionnaire to faculty members of a medical college. The questionnaire asked about the importance of gender in doctor–patient relationships, faculty–medical student relationships, and faculty–faculty relationships. Results showed that women were significantly more aware of gender issues in all of the relationships, whereas men were unaware of the relationships or felt that they were not important (Risberg et al. 2003).

The study points out that gender differences influence behavior, expectations, and power inequities in doctors' relationships with patients and colleagues. When doctors ignore these gender differences, the result can be health disparity for women. It's good for doctors to be aware that female patients may feel powerless in a doctor–patient relationship and may not ask pertinent questions or refuse unnecessary treatment options. A female patient may have expectations that she will not be heard by her male physician, and as a result she might not adhere to prescribed treatments. Some patients may need to request same-gender physicians in order to have the best care.

IDENTIFYING RELIABLE INFORMATION

Sometimes you're not sure if you need to see a doctor. Or, your doctor might have diagnosed a condition that you want to find out more about. You need to know how to find reliable medical information, especially when there are so many resources to choose from. Seeing a doctor, visiting the hospital, and reading journal articles and resource books are the traditional means of finding good information about health care. The Internet has quickly replaced those sources as the primary source of information about any subject. Although the Internet has vast amounts of reliable information, it also has a wide variety of information that is misleading or wrong. Finding reliable information on the Internet can be easy if you follow the principles of evaluation provided by Health on the Net Foundation (HON 2007):

- Information must be authoritative.
- Information should support the doctor–patient relationship, not replace it.
- The site needs to respect the confidentiality of personal information.
- Information must be documented with references and dated.
- The site should include working links to additional external sources.

- Medical claims are supported by referenced research.
- The site provides a valid e-mail address to a webmaster.
- The site discloses its funding sources.
- The advertising policy of the site states a clear division between advertised content and editorial content.

Information that is authoritative means that the organizations or people publishing it know what they're talking about. Read about the authors of the Web site. What is their purpose? If it's to provide current, reliable information and they're from the medical or research community, then the information usually can be trusted. PhDs and MDs work for most of the authoritative organizations that publish health information Web sites. Those sites cite research and provide links to other research articles. Most of the time, the authors of the information on authoritative sites aren't selling products or information. Some health Web sites that give valid, reliable information do sell banner ads (advertisements on the Web site) to help support the site (HON 2007).

Reliable health care Web sites don't try to provide information that replaces medical care. In other words, the Web site always recommends that you see a physician if you have particular symptoms. The Web site does not offer health information for a fee, offer prescriptions without your seeing a doctor, or prescribe interventions without asking you to see a health care provider in person (HON 2007).

Your personal information remains personal on valid health information Web sites. The Web site should state that it won't sell your information to a third party. It won't ask for information that is not needed, such as your insurance information or other personal information. Some valid Web sites might request information about your age, gender, lifestyle habits, and so on, but they should never ask for birth dates, Social Security numbers, insurance information, or other personal information. A site that asks for personal information is selling something or stealing something from you (HON 2007).

A valid Web site has an administrator with a working e-mail address. Try to e-mail the webmaster. If the address is invalid, so is the Web site. On a valid Web site, all medical claims are referenced with articles and specific dates, so you can find and read the original articles. External resources with links to information for further reading and a statement that clearly defines advertising ethics are important in determining whether a Web site is reliable for health information (HON 2007).

What Do You Do?

Choose a health condition that you're interested in—one that you have or someone you know has. Do an Internet search to find at least three Web sites that provide information about the condition. Evaluate whether the three sites have reliable information using the criteria you learned about in this section.

BEING YOUR OWN HEALTH CARE ADVOCATE

Being a good consumer of health information and health care requires that you take responsibility for your own health care safety. Ask questions of your provider, keep a list of all your prescriptions, know the results of any test or procedure you have, learn which hospital best suits your needs, and understand the treatment options and their expected outcomes (Agency for Healthcare Research and Quality [AHRQ] 2004). Also remember that you can always get a second medical opinion. Many insurance companies encourage second opinions on expensive procedures or serious diagnosis. Tell your doctor that you would like a second opinion. She might give you the names of other doctors, or you might have to find another doctor on your own. Either way, you should always seek a second opinion for serious medical conditions or if you do not trust your doctor's expertise.

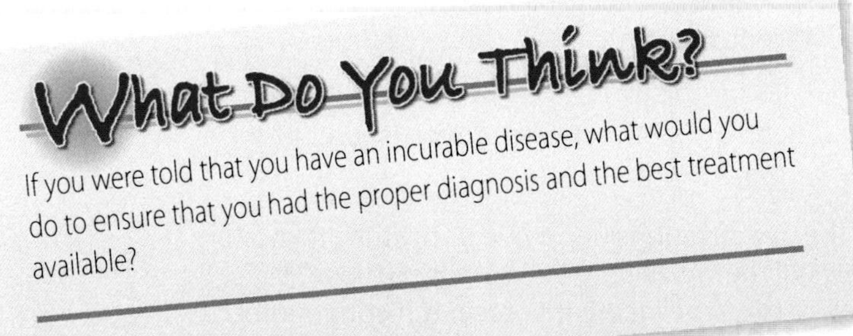

Doctors and their employees sometimes assume that a patient fully understands the results of tests and procedures. In those cases, your medical team might give you only the results, not necessarily the meaning behind those results. Or, they might give you only the meaning of the results, not the actual results of the tests and procedures. Here's an example: A nurse calls with news that your cholesterol is high and the doctor wants to put you on medication. But he doesn't give you the actual numbers, so you don't have the information you need in order to decide if diet and exercise might be a better initial approach than starting medication. In other cases, though, the doctor might give you only the cholesterol levels and assume that you understand the implications of those results. You need to ask your health care provider to give you the test result numbers, possible implications, suggestions for treatment, and expected outcome of the treatment. Then you need to use that information to make your own health care decisions.

It's your responsibility to request the information. If you don't understand what the numbers or results of tests and procedures mean, ask for clarification. Don't be reluctant to request additional information because you worry that the doctor will think you're stupid or that you don't trust him. Don't assume that the doctor knows best in every circumstance. Knowing test results will help make treatment decisions easier.

Decisions concerning treatment for any disease are based on the complications of the disease and the side effects of the treatment. The greater the long-term complications of the disease, the more side effects from the treatment are accepted. For instance, the side effects of chemotherapy are hair loss, vomiting, weight loss, lethargy, and so on. But, the long-term complication for cancer is a painful death, so the chemotherapy side effects are a more acceptable alternative.

READING MEDICINE LABELS

The next time you go to a pharmacy or drugstore, take a look around at the incredible number and variety of over-the-counter (OTC) medications, which are available without a prescription. Many people take OTC medicines without consulting a doctor first, so it's important to be able to read and understand the product label. In essence, the label explains what a medicine is supposed to do, who should or should not take it, and how it should be used. The U.S. Food and Drug Administration (FDA) requires that the labels of all OTC medicines present detailed usage and warning information in the same order and in a consistent style that is simple to understand (see figure 9.1).

Here is an explanation of the parts of the label (FDA 2006):

- **Active ingredient**. The amount of active ingredient (the therapeutic substance in the product) per unit.
- **Purpose**. The product action or category (such as antihistamine, antacid, or cough suppressant).
- **Uses**. Symptoms or diseases the product will treat or prevent.
- **Warnings**. When not to use the product; conditions that may require advice from a doctor before taking the product; possible interactions or side effects; when to stop taking the product and when to contact a doctor; warnings about consulting a health care professional if you are pregnant or breast-feeding, warnings to keep the product out of children's reach; and what to do in case of overdose.

Drug Facts

Active ingredient (in each tablet)	**Purpose**
Chlorpheniramine maleate 2 mg	Antihistamine

Uses Temporarily relieves these symptoms due to hay fever or other upper respiratory allergies:
■ sneezing ■ runny nose ■ itchy, watery eyes ■ itchy throat

Warnings

Ask a doctor before use if you have
■ glaucoma ■ a breathing problem such as emphysema or chronic bronchitis
■ trouble urinating due to an enlarged prostate gland

Ask a doctor or pharmacist before use if you are taking taking tranquilizers or sedatives

When using this product
■ You may get drowsy ■ avoid alcoholic drinks ■ alcohol, sedatives, and tranquilizers may increase drowsiness
■ be careful when driving a motor vehicle or operating machinery ■ excitability may occur, especially in children

If pregnant or breast-feeding, ask a health professional before use.
Keep out of reach of children. In case of overdose, get medical help or contact a Poison Control Center right away.

Directions

adults and children 12 years and over	take 2 tablets every 4 to 6 hours; not more than 12 tablets in 24 hours
children 6 years to under 12 years	take 1 tablet every 4 to 6 hours; not more than 6 tablets in 24 hours
children under 6 years	ask a doctor

Other information store at 20-25° C (68-77° F) ■ protect from excessive moisture

Inactive ingredients D & C yellow no. 10, lactose, magnesium stearate, microcrystalline cellulose, pregelatinized starch

Figure 9.1 Always read and follow the information presented in the labels on over-the-counter (OTC) medications. Do you know how to interpret the parts of an OTC label?

- **Directions**. Specific age categories, how much of the product to take, how to take it, how often to take it, and how long to take it.
- **Other information**. How to store the product properly and required information about certain ingredients (such as the amount of calcium, potassium, or sodium the product contains).
- **Inactive ingredients**. Substances such as colors or flavors.

The active ingredients on the label are the most important part of the label for consumers. Learn the generic terms for drugs that are commonly used and look for those terms on the label. When deciding between a brand-name medicine and a generic equivalent, compare the active ingredients and the amounts of those ingredients. If you are unsure of what the drug does, look it up on the Internet at WebMD.com or another reliable source of information. Learn what drugs work similarly and avoid taking those drugs together. For instance, NSAIDs are nonsteroidal anti-inflammatory drugs, such as aspirin or ibuprofen. You should not take ibuprofen and aspirin at the same time.

Learn to read labels by reading the active ingredients, learning what the active ingredients are used for, and learning how to prevent overdosing. If you're taking more than one over-the-counter medicine, stop and look at the active ingredients. Don't take two medicines with the same active ingredient at the same time unless instructed to do so by your doctor, pharmacist, or other health care professional.

CONSUMER ISSUES

Avoiding an Overdose of Acetaminophen

Acetaminophen is the active ingredient in Tylenol, Excedrin Migraine, many extra-strength headache medicines, and cold medicines (see the lists below). You should not take two or more products at the same time that contain acetaminophen because an overdose of acetaminophen can cause liver damage. Taking more than one dose every 4 to 6 hours is considered an overdose. Often people don't read the label on over-the-counter drugs and therefore don't realize that they're taking an overdose of acetaminophen, especially with cold medications.

Many cold medications have active ingredients that suppress coughs, relieve congestion, dry out nasal passages, and reduce fever. When people are sick with a cold and a fever, they often take both an all-purpose cold medication and acetaminophen, because they don't realize that the cold medication already contains acetaminophen. Reading the labels on over-the-counter medications can make the difference between relieving the symptoms of a cold and damaging your liver and shortening your life.

Common Prescription Drugs That Contain Acetaminophen

Darvocet	Hydrocodone bitartrate	Tapanol
Endocet	Lortab	Ultracet
Fioricet	Percocet	Vicodin
Hycotab	Phenaphen	Zydone
Hydrocet	Sedapap	

Common Over-the-Counter Drugs That Contain Acetaminophen

Actifed	DayQuil	Midol	TheraFlu
Anacin	Dimetapp	NyQuil	Triaminic
Benadryl	Dristan	Panadol	Tylenol products
Cepacol	Excedrin	Robitussin	Vanquish
Contac	Feverall	Sinutab	Vicks Formula 44
Coricidin HBP	Liquiprin	Sudafed	Zicam

COMPLEMENTARY ALTERNATIVE MEDICINE AND ALTERNATIVE MEDICINE

Traditional medical treatment for disease includes prescription drugs, over-the-counter drugs, surgery, radiation therapy, psychotherapy, physical therapy, and diet and exercise. What if those traditional medical treatments don't work? **Complementary alternative medicine (CAM)** and **alternative medicine** are other treatments you can consider. CAM adds alternative medical treatment methods to traditional medical care, and traditional methods aren't used at all in alternative medicine.

In this section of the chapter, we'll look at a few of the more common alternative medicine options, including acupuncture, chiropractic medicine, massage, and herbal medicine.

Acupuncture

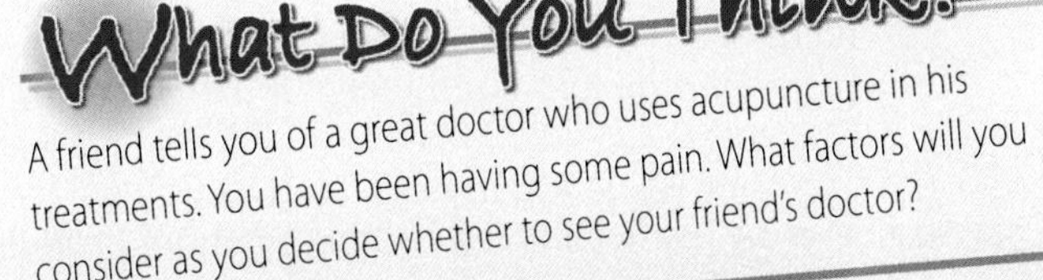

One of the oldest alternative medicine approaches is **acupuncture**, which comes from traditional Chinese medicine (TCM) and was written about in China more than 4,000 years ago. TCM is based on the belief that energy (chi) flows along meridians of the body. Chi is divided between the yin and yang and needs to be in balance for good health. Health problems result from blockages in the energy flow. Acupuncture, diet, exercise, herbal therapy, and meditation help to restore chi in the body.

Acupuncture helps to unblock the energy flow through acupoints. There are more than 2,000 acupoints on the body, and small needles—just larger than a strand of human hair—are inserted in some of these points. Proponents believe the acupuncture needles cause physical responses that initiate the production of proteins, hormones, and brain chemicals that control blood pressure, body temperature, and mood and that can boost the immune system and reduce pain (National Cancer Institute [NCI] 2007).

Research to determine the validity of acupuncture as a medical treatment began in 1976. Current research concerning acupuncture and pain has been inconclusive because of small sample sizes and inconsistent results. However, several studies have suggested that acupuncture prevents nausea in cancer patients undergoing chemotherapy, in pregnant women, and after surgery. Research continues to examine the effectiveness of acupuncture. If you're interested, you can keep up with new findings, which are published at www.pubmed.gov. The site includes a library of peer-reviewed articles on every aspect of health and medicine.

There are few complications from acupuncture unless the practitioner uses needles that aren't sterile. Finding a reliable practitioner is important to prevent minor infections, especially in cancer patients (NCI 2007).

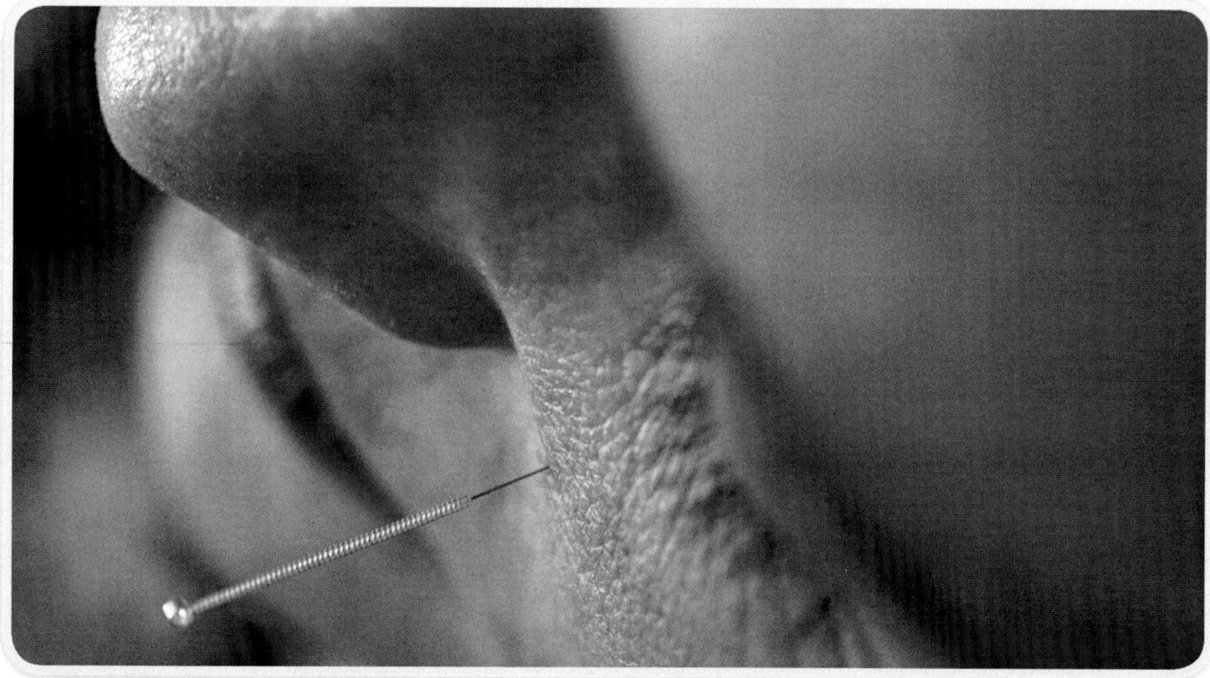

According to proponents of acupuncture, small needles inserted into acupoints on the body can provide various health benefits.

© Photodisc

Chiropractic Medicine

Chiropractic medicine is another alternative approach to traditional medicine. Chiropractic medicine treats neuromuscular problems by adjusting the spine into proper alignment. The term *chiropractic* combines the Greek words *cheir*, meaning "hand," and *praxis*, meaning "action" (NCCAM 2007).

Spinal realignment has a history going back to 2700 BCE in both China and Greece. In 1895, a doctor in Iowa named Daniel Palmer studied new developments in physiology and began treating patients using spinal manipulation. His son, P.J. Palmer, started the Palmer College of Chiropractic, which is still considered the top chiropractic school in the United States. In the 1970s, physicians and insurance companies began to recognize the benefits of chiropractic care, and it became more acceptable to the public and in the medical arena (NCCAM 2007).

Chiropractic doctors believe that the body is self-healing, and they don't advocate surgery or prescription medications. Chiropractors treat mostly neuromuscular problems such as headaches, joint pain, neck pain, and lower back pain. However, they also treat allergies, osteoarthritis, asthma, digestive disorders, carpal tunnel syndrome, tendinitis, sprains, and strains (NCCAM 2007).

Chiropractors earn degrees from college programs certified by the Council on Chiropractic Education (CCE). Chiropractors must pass an exam to get a license to practice. They must also take continuing education classes to maintain their licenses. Each state governs the scope of practice for chiropractors, including the selling of dietary supplements and the use of other CAM therapies such as acupuncture. Chiropractic care is covered by most insurance companies and by Medicare. Check with your insurance company before using chiropractic treatment to be sure (NCCAM 2007).

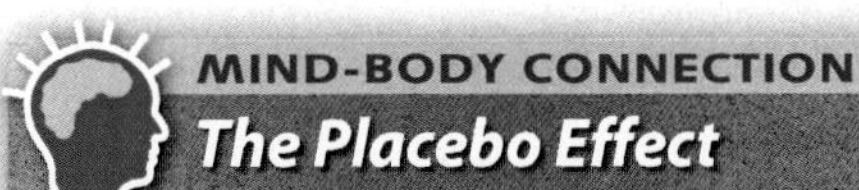

MIND-BODY CONNECTION

The Placebo Effect

The **placebo effect** can make even the most absurd treatment seem effective. A small percentage of adults will always believe strongly enough in a particular treatment that they'll get better. Researchers have been studying the placebo effect for decades. In 1955, researcher H.K. Beecher published his groundbreaking paper "The Powerful Placebo," in which he concluded that across the 26 studies he analyzed, an average of 32 percent of patients responded to placebos. In the 1960s, breakthrough studies showed the potential physiological effects of dummy pills. For instance, they tended to speed up pulse rate, increase blood pressure, and improve reaction speeds when participants were told they had taken a stimulant, and they had the opposite physiological effects when participants were told they had taken a sleep-inducing drug (Nordenberg 2000).

Dr. T.D. Wager from the University of Michigan used magnetic resonance imaging (MRI) to study the brains of volunteers who underwent a small amount of pain. Some received a placebo pain-reducing cream and others received no cream. The results showed that those who received the placebo had more activity in the prefrontal cerebral cortex and less activity in the areas of the brain that respond to pain, such as the thalamus. The placebo did not interfere with the ability of the body to feel pain but rather how the body interpreted the pain (Graham 2004).

If placebos can change the way the body reacts to painful stimuli, then any alternative treatment will help some people. The placebo effect could be one reason why people continue treatments that have no research to back up their effectiveness. For instance, many people wear copper bracelets to reduce arthritis pain. The effects of such bracelets have never been proven conclusively, but it would be difficult to convince the wearers that the bracelets don't work.

Research evidence is inconclusive regarding chiropractic care. There is no evidence to support that the manipulation of the spinal column reduces pain or illness. However, the relationship between patient and chiropractor may be the biggest benefit of chiropractic care. Patients believe that the chiropractor is helping, and that belief may in itself reduce the pain. Similarly, the understanding the chiropractor shows for the patient's life situations can bring relief.

Massage

Other forms of body manipulation include massage therapy, reflexology, Rolfing, and many others. **Massage therapy** is a therapeutic manipulation of the soft tissues of the body designed to promote relaxation and reduce stress. **Reflexology** is a therapeutic method of relieving pain by stimulating predefined pressure points on the feet and hands. **Rolfing**, also called *Rolf therapy* or *structural integration*, is a holistic system of bodywork that uses deep manipulation of the soft tissue to realign and balance the body's myofascial structure—the system of muscles and connective tissue. Although there is training to teach practitioners in all of these types of therapy, no certification standard exists. That means that people with little or no training can hang out a sign and place advertisements claiming expertise in the field. Poor training could result in unnecessary pain for clients or injury during therapy. When done by a trained practitioner, these therapies are safe for adults, unless the client has osteoporosis, broken bones, burns, open wounds, or deep vein thrombosis.

Research on the effectiveness of massage therapies has shown mixed results because it is difficult to employ a control group and because techniques differ from practitioner to practitioner, making it difficult to have a valid experimental design. The only conclusion from research is that hormones and brain chemicals are released through the manipulation of the body during massage.

Herbal Medicine

Herbs have been around as long as humans have, and people have used herbs to treat many aliments and symptoms of disease. **Herbal medicines** are sold as powders, tablets, extracts, teas, and fresh and dried plants and are used for their flavor, scent, or therapeutic applications. Herbs can cause health problems and may interfere with medications, so be sure to tell your doctors of any herbal medicines and vitamins that you are taking. Taking herbal supplements safely means that you take them under the guidance of medical personnel, take only the dose recommended on the package, and are extremely cautious if you're pregnant or nursing. Because there are hundreds of herbal medicines, we'll look at only a few of the most recognized, including aloe vera, chamomile, ginseng, echinacea, ephedra, garlic, ginkgo, green tea, hoodia, St. John's wort, and soy (NCCAM 2007).

Aloe Vera

Aloe vera is a tropical plant grown in the southwestern United States, Mexico, and South and Central America. The leaves of the plant contain a gel that is used topically for burns and wounds. The outside of the plant is used in an oral supplement as a laxative. The FDA has taken all laxatives that contain aloe vera off the market because they did not include the proper safety data. The FDA approves aloe vera only for topical use (NCCAM 2007).

Aloe vera improves the healing of burns, but one study showed that topical use of aloe vera for serious surgical wounds inhibited healing. Aloe vera taken orally can cause diarrhea and prevent the absorption of medications. People with diabetes should take extreme care using oral aloe vera, because it can lower blood sugar. Always inform your health care provider if you take any herbal supplements (NCCAM 2007).

Chamomile

Chamomile has been used by children and adults for hundreds of years for sleeplessness, anxiety, and gastrointestinal problems such as gas, diarrhea, and upset stomach. Today it's also used to help treat mouth sores from cancer treatment. The flowering tops of the chamomile plant are used in teas, tablets, creams, ointments, and oral rinses.

Little research has been done on chamomile, so no claims have been proven or disproven. Side effects from using chamomile are rare allergic reactions. People who react to chamomile also have allergic reactions to plants from the daisy family, including the ragweed family. Remember to tell your doctor if you're taking chamomile.

Ginseng

Asian **ginseng** contains ginsenosides (or panaxosides), which are chemicals that supposedly have healing properties. Ginseng root is dried and made into powders, tablets, teas, creams, and other applications. Ginseng is used to help recover from illness, increase stamina, cure erectile dysfunction, lower blood sugar, and reduce blood pressure. Some studies have shown that ginseng lowers blood sugar, so people with diabetes who take medicine to lower their blood sugar need to be cautious when using ginseng. Ginseng also increases the immune response. Most research has been inconclusive, with small sample sizes or animal testing only (NCCAM 2007).

If you take ginseng longer than 3 months, it's likely you'll experience more side effects, including headaches and sleep and gastrointestinal disturbances. If you take ginseng, be sure to talk it over with your doctor (NCCAM 2007).

Echinacea

Echinacea is used to prevent colds, flu, and other infections and is believed to boost the immune system. It is less commonly used for skin infections such as acne and boils. All parts of the echinacea plant are either dried to make teas and tablets or squeezed to make extracts or preparations for external use. Studies have shown that echinacea does not prevent or shorten the course of colds or flu, although one study did show some improvement in upper respiratory infections (NCCAM 2007).

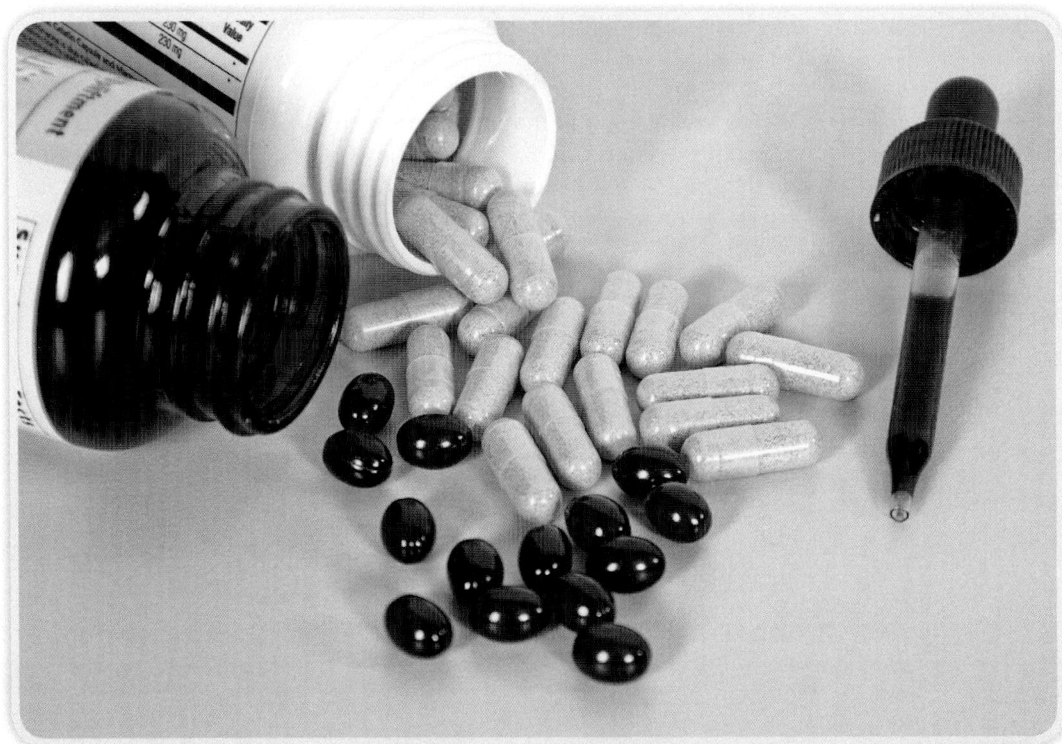

Some of the more widely used herbal supplements include St. John's wort (the dark brown capsules), echinacea (the light capsules), and ginkgo (the extract in the dropper).

Side effects are allergic reactions similar to those experienced by people who are allergic to ragweed or daisies. People who have asthma are more likely to have an allergic reaction to echinacea. Gastrointestinal problems have also been associated with echinacea. Tell your doctor if you're taking echinacea (NCCAM 2007).

Ephedra

Ephedra has been used for thousands of years in China and India to treat the symptoms of colds, flu, fever, headaches, and asthma. In the past, it has been used in over-the-counter supplements for weight loss. The main ingredient of ephedra is ephedrine, which is a strong stimulant of the nervous system and cardiovascular system (NCCAM 2007).

The side effects of ephedra are extremely serious. They include psychiatric problems, heart problems, high blood pressure, and stroke. In 2004, the FDA banned the sale of any supplement that contains ephedra, and it is no longer sold legally in the United States (NCCAM 2007).

Garlic

Garlic is a bulb plant that has been used for thousands of years as an herbal remedy and in cooking. Garlic can be eaten raw or cooked. It is also dried and made into powders and tablets. Raw garlic is made into liquid extracts. Garlic is used to improve the immune system and to reduce high blood pressure and cholesterol.

Studies have suggested that regular garlic use may slow the hardening of the arteries. There are mixed results showing that garlic in any form can reduce cholesterol, and no studies show positive results for reducing blood pressure. Some people believe that garlic can reduce the risk of stomach and colon cancers, but no studies support this belief. Side effects include breath and body odor, upset stomach, and occasional allergic reactions. These side effects are more common when garlic is eaten raw.

Precautions need to be taken when taking blood-thinning medication, because garlic can thin the blood. Tell your doctor if you use garlic as an herbal remedy (NCCAM 2007).

Ginkgo

Ginkgo has been used for thousands of years in China for asthma, bronchitis, fatigue, and tinnitus (ringing of the ear). Ginkgo seeds were eaten in China many years ago, but now leaf extracts are used to treat and prevent disease (NCCAM 2007). People have started using ginkgo to improve memory, to treat Alzheimer's disease and other dementias, and to treat tinnitus, multiple sclerosis, and sexual dysfunction.

Some small studies found that gingko improved dementia patients' memories, but a larger study of healthy adults over age 60 showed no memory improvement. Studies have found that tinnitus has shown improvement while taking ginkgo. Larger studies need to be done with positive results before recommendations can be made for using ginkgo (NCCAM 2007).

Green Tea

Another Asian herbal remedy that's been around for thousands of years is green tea. Since about 2002, it has gained popularity worldwide. **Green teas** have been used for cancers, including breast, stomach, and skin cancer, and they're currently used for improving mental alertness, lowering cholesterol, and protecting skin from sun damage (NCCAM 2007). Green tea is most often brewed for consumption, but it's sometimes made into capsules or skin ointments.

Research again shows mixed results. A small study suggests that green tea may slow the growth of certain cancers, but more research needs to be done. Another study shows that green tea improves alertness; however, that may be due only to the caffeine in the tea. Green tea is safe for most adults. It contains caffeine, which can cause sleeplessness, anxiety, and, in large dosages, seizures. It also contains small amounts of vitamin K that can make drugs such as warfarin (a blood thinner) less effective.

Hoodia

In 2006, **hoodia** became the rage for weight loss. Hoodia is a flowering cactus plant that grows in the Kalahari Desert in Africa. African bushmen have long used it to reduce their hunger and thirst during long hunts. The leaves and roots of the hoodia plant are dried and made into teas and extracts. Hoodia is often mixed with green teas. Currently, there is no published research regarding the effectiveness of hoodia, safe dosages, and its quality. However, there have been reports about products that claim to contain hoodia but really don't. Watch for new articles on hoodia at www.pubmed.gov.

St. John's Wort

St. John's wort has been used for years as a treatment for mental disorders, as a sedative, and as a malaria treatment. Today St. John's wort is used for depression, anxiety, and sleep disorders. The flowering portion of the plant is used for teas and extracts for tablets and capsules. Some studies have reported that St. John's wort is good for mild to severe depression. However, a large study showed that it worked the same as a placebo for people with moderate depression. St. John's wort has many side effects, including increased sensitivity to sunlight, anxiety, dry mouth, dizziness, gastrointestinal symptoms, fatigue, headache, and sexual dysfunction (NCCAM 2007). St. John's wort also interferes with birth control pills and with many medications used to treat cancer, human immunodeficiency virus (HIV), and heart problems.

Soy

Soy has been used as an extract, in tofu, in soymilk, in tablets, or in processed foods. Soy is believed to have many health benefits, including lowering cholesterol, relieving menopausal

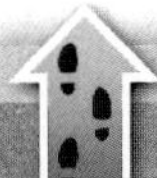

STEPS FOR BEHAVIORAL CHANGE

Alternative Treatments Go Mainstream

Some complementary treatments are now fairly mainstream, and you can use them in everyday life to reduce stress, increase mental alertness, and increase antioxidants. One of those treatments is for relaxation. Close your eyes and imagine yourself in your happy place—a place that you enjoy and feel relaxed in, such as lying on a beach under the warm sun. Close your eyes and take deep breaths as you settle into your place. Think about the surroundings and concentrate on feeling the wind or sun and hearing the birds, waves, or leaves around you. When you're fully relaxed, stay as long as you can. You might want to set a timer to prevent staying too long if you're working or have somewhere to be. Then slowly return in your mind to the chair or couch you're on and take another deep breath. You'll feel much more relaxed and less stressed. This is also a great technique to use when you have trouble falling asleep.

Another treatment that is fairly mainstream is drinking green and black teas. Research has shown that these drinks bring an elevated awareness (because of the caffeine) and might increase antioxidants that can reduce cell damage in the bloodstream. Preparing and drinking hot tea has a relaxing effect as well. Pouring hot water into a teapot with tea bags and waiting for the tea to steep can be a soothing and enjoyable process. Black tea or green tea consumed cold is just as good for mental alertness and antioxidant properties as hot tea, however.

Many people are now trying yoga and tai chi to improve their balance and muscle tone. Most cities have places that offer yoga and tai chi, and many universities offer classes that teach the basic moves.

Adding even one of these alternative medical treatments into your regular routine can reduce stress and improve your mood. Experiment with one or all of the techniques suggested here and see if you experience less stress and better moods and mental alertness.

symptoms such as hot flashes and osteoporosis, lowering high blood pressure, and helping treat some cancers. Research has shown that soy reduces some cholesterol and hot flashes, but those results came from small studies. No published research has shown soy to improve any other health conditions.

The use of soy is considered safe for most adults, with only rare stomach complaints as a side effect. However, there is some concern about the relationship between soy use and breast cancer. Therefore, if a person is at high risk for breast cancer, she should seek the advice of a doctor before using soy for long amounts of time.

AVOIDING QUACKS

Being a good health care consumer means taking responsibility for every aspect of your health care. It includes finding good, affordable health care; choosing a doctor; finding accurate information about disease and treatments; making decisions about alternative and complementary medicine; and knowing how to spot a **quack**, or a health provider who is more interested in making money than in providing good care.

Quacks don't show up only in complementary and alternative medicine. They exist in traditional medicine, too. Quacks are health care providers whose treatments don't work or, worse, are harmful. Quacks target people with chronic disease, those who are overweight, or the elderly. They promise quick solutions to complicated problems. You should be cautious when you encounter the following (Stoppler 2006):

- Products that claim to provide relief or cures for a number of conditions
- Special, ancient, or secret formulas, sometimes available from only one company
- Promises of quick and easy weight loss without diet or exercise
- Products that advertise prompt and painless cures
- Products that promise cures for diseases with no known cure
- Testimonials about miracles or breakthroughs that have not been documented in the medical literature
- Products that require advance payments or offer a free bonus or extra product with purchase, or suppliers who claim limited availability of their product
- Offers using terminology such as *scientific breakthrough*, *miracle cure*, and other superlatives or vague or scientific-sounding terms
- Money-back guarantees if success is not achieved

Legitimate treatment providers give plenty of time for decision making and explain the benefits and possible complications of the treatment. Every treatment option has pros and cons. Legitimate products acknowledge both the positive and the negative. Remember the old adage, "If it seems too good to be true, it probably is." If you have any questions about a medical product or treatment, ask your medical provider. To report a health product that you believe is being advertised falsely, contact the Federal Trade Commission (FTC):

- Call toll free at 877-FTC-HELP (877-382-4357); for TTY (for the hearing impaired), call toll free at 866-653-4261.
- Write to Federal Trade Commission Consumer Response Center, 600 Pennsylvania Avenue, NW, Washington, DC 20580.
- Go online at www.ftccomplaintassistant.gov.

You can also report quackery to your state attorney general's office, state department of health, or local consumer protection agency. These offices are listed in the blue pages of the telephone book (Stoppler 2006).

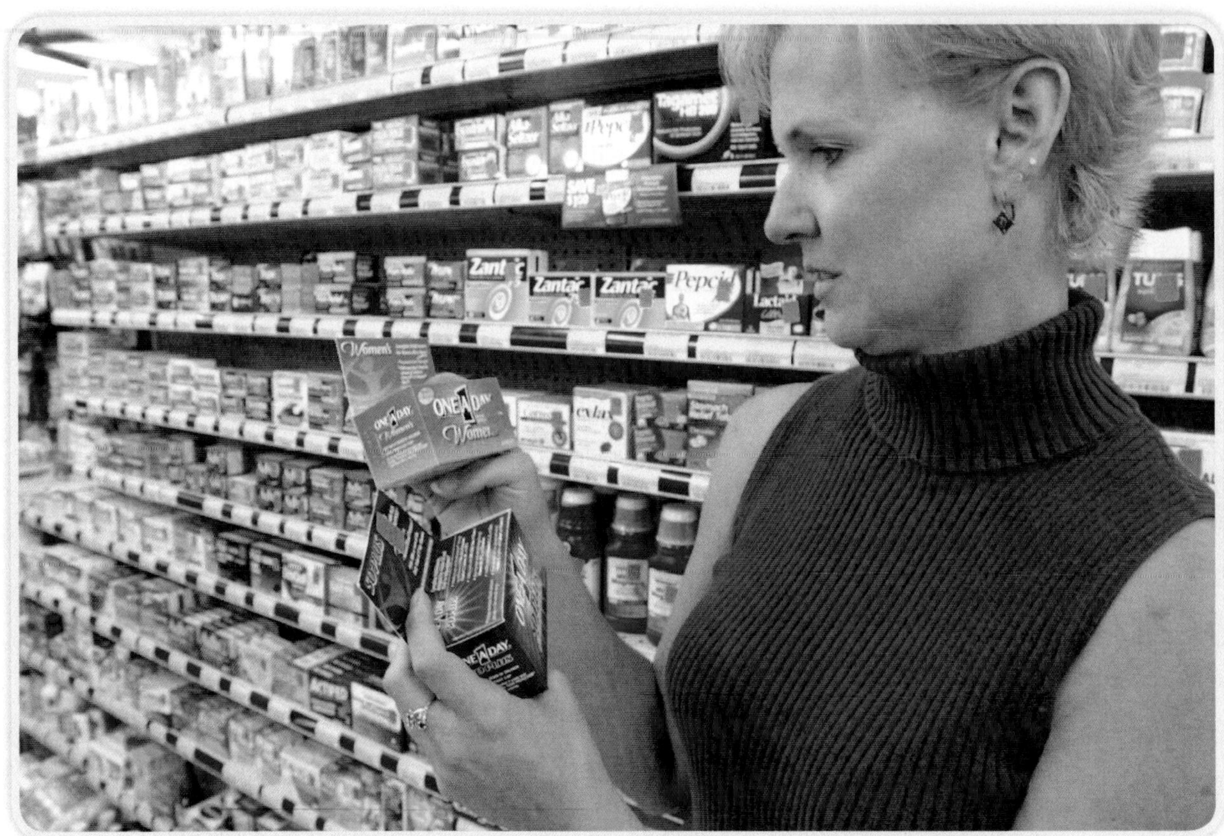

Good health care consumers check the labels on over-the-counter medicines and compare products to make sure they're getting what they need.

© Human Kinetics

HEALTH CARE CONSUMERISM 101

Becoming a good health care consumer has many steps. For one, you must know how to find a plan that's affordable and gives you the coverage you need. Several types of health care plans are available, including HMOs, PPOs, and government plans. You also need to know how to choose the right doctor for you and how to find accurate information from seeing a doctor, visiting the hospital, reading journal articles and resource books, and searching the Internet. Another important aspect of being a good health care consumer is taking responsibility for your health care by asking questions of your provider, knowing the results of any test or procedure you have, learning which hospital best suits your needs, and understanding the treatment options and their expected outcomes.

You may want to consider CAM and alternative medicine, which offer acupuncture, chiropractic medicine, massage, and herbal medicine. Be wary of quacks, though, who exist in both alternative medicine and traditional medicine. If it sounds too good to be true, it probably is, and it may even be dangerous.

Always ask questions of your doctor, and request information about all the available treatment options. Seek a second opinion if you get a diagnosis or treatment option you are unsure about. Know your rights as a health care consumer and research health care options. Being a good health care consumer can save you money, time, and, most of all, your good health.

REVIEW QUESTIONS

1. Name several ways that health insurance can be purchased.
2. Briefly explain one benefit and one drawback of an HMO, and one benefit and one drawback of a PPO.
3. Who is eligible for Medicare? Who is eligible for Medicaid?
4. What's the difference between SCHIP and COBRA?
5. When choosing a doctor, what is the most important aspect to consider?
6. Health on the Net Foundation provides several principles to help people evaluate information found online. List four of those principles.
7. For consumers of over-the-counter medications, what is the most important part of the product label?
8. Describe the placebo effect.
9. Name three common herbal medicines and describe how each is used to treat health problems.
10. What would you think about a health care product that offers a money-back guarantee if success is not achieved?

CRITICAL THINKING

1. You visit a doctor to explain a problem you're having. She listens to your concerns and a description of your symptoms, then hands you a prescription without saying much of anything. What should you do?
2. Your friend tells you about a new treatment for you to try. He says that there are no guarantees, but that you will get your money back if it doesn't work. How should you handle this situation?

APPLICATION ACTIVITIES

1. Find a doctor in your area who uses CAM. Interview the doctor about how he got started with CAM and what types of treatments he recommends to patients.
2. Find ads in the newspaper or magazines or on the Internet that describe a treatment from alternative medicine. Determine whether the claims are valid or are quackery based on the guidelines provided in the "Avoiding Quacks" section of the chapter.

GLOSSARY

acupuncture—Treatment using needles to unblock the energy flow through acupoints; based on the belief that energy flows along meridians of the body.

aloe vera—Tropical plant grown in the southwestern United States, Mexico, and South and Central America used topically for burns and wounds.

alternative medicine—Medicine that uses no traditional medical methods.

catastrophic health insurance—Covers some of the medical bills from a health care emergency.

chamomile—The flowering tops of the chamomile plant are used in teas, tablets, creams, ointments, and oral rinses for sleeplessness, anxiety, mouth sores from cancer, and gastrointestinal problems such as gas, diarrhea, and upset stomach.

CHAPTER REVIEW

chiropractic medicine—Treats neuromuscular problems by adjusting the spine into proper alignment.

complementary alternative medicine (CAM)—Adds alternative medical treatment methods to traditional medical care.

Consolidated Omnibus Budget Reconciliation Act (COBRA)—Terminated employees, those who lose coverage because of reduced work hours, or children who can no longer be on their parents' policy because of age may be able to buy group coverage for themselves and their families for limited amounts of time.

consumer health—Includes making decisions about health providers, hospitals, health plans, prescriptions, prevention strategies, quality of care, treatment choices, and reliable health information.

copayment—Amount of money the insured is responsible for paying for each visit or time of service.

echinacea—Herb used to prevent colds, flu, and other infections and believed to boost the immune system.

ephedra—Main ingredient is ephedrine, which is a strong stimulant of the nervous system and cardiovascular system. Ephedra is no longer sold legally in the United States.

garlic—Bulb plant that has been used for thousands of years in food and as an herbal remedy to improve the immune system and to reduce high blood pressure and cholesterol.

ginkgo—Used to treat and prevent disorders such as dementias, tinnitus, multiple sclerosis, and sexual dysfunction.

ginseng—Herb used to help recover from illness, increase stamina, cure erectile dysfunction, lower blood sugar, and reduce blood pressure.

green teas—Teas that have been used for cancers, including breast, stomach, and skin cancer, as well as for improving mental alertness, lowering cholesterol, and protecting skin from sun damage.

health maintenance organization (HMO)—Insurance provider with a main health care provider who is a gatekeeper for services. HMO insurance is usually provided through an employer.

herbal medicines—Herbal supplements used for their flavor, scent, or therapeutic applications.

hoodia—Flowering cactus plant that grows in the Kalahari Desert in Africa that is used for weight loss.

massage therapy—Therapeutic body tissue manipulation.

Medicaid—Insurance for people who meet financial need criteria and for people who are disabled.

Medicare—Insurance for everyone who has paid Social Security and is over the age of 65, as well as some disabled people.

out-of-pocket expenses—Costs that the consumer pays for medical expenses, including the copayment and deductible.

placebo effect—A small percentage of adults will always believe strongly enough in a particular treatment that they'll get better, regardless of whether the treatment is medically effective.

preferred provider organization (PPO)—Network of physicians who work with an insurance company with a negotiated rate for services.

premiums—Monthly cost for insurance.

quack—A health provider who is more interested in making money than in providing good care.

reflexology—Therapeutic method of relieving pain by stimulating predefined pressure points on the feet and hands.

Rolfing—Holistic system of body work that uses deep manipulation of the soft tissue to realign and balance the myofascial structure of the body; also called *Rolf therapy* or *structural integration*.

soy—Used as an extract, in tofu, in soymilk, in tablets, or in processed foods to lower cholesterol, relieve menopausal symptoms, lower high blood pressure, and help treat some cancers.

State Children's Health Insurance Program (SCHIP)—Insurance offered to children whose parents do not qualify for Medicaid but do not have health insurance.

St. John's wort—Flowering portion of the plant is used for depression, anxiety, and sleep disorders.

REFERENCES AND RESOURCES

Agency for Healthcare Research and Quality (AHRQ). 2004. Five steps to safer health care: Patient fact sheet. www.ahrq.gov/consumer/5steps.htm.

Anderson, G. 2006. Health care: The cost with and without insurance. *Washington Post,* April 7. www.washingtonpost.com/wp-dyn/content/graphic/2006/04/07/GR2006040700882.html.

Casillas, J.N., S.M. Castellino, M.M. Hudson, A.C. Mertens, J. Whitton, S.L. Brooks, L.K. Zeltzer, A. Abline, L.L. Robison, and K.C. Oeffinger. 2005. The effect of insurance and ethnicity on healthcare access and health behaviors: A childhood cancer survivor study. Paper presented at the 2005 ASCO Annual Meeting Proceedings.

Centers for Disease Control and Prevention (CDC). 2008. Health, United States, 2007. www.cdc.gov/nchs/data/hus/hus07.pdf.

Graham, S. 2004. Scientists see how placebo effect eases pain. *Scientific American.* www.sciam.com/article.cfm?id=scientists-see-how-placeb.

Health on the Net Foundation (HON). 2007. HON-accredited Web sites. www.hon.ch/providers.html.

National Cancer Institute (NCI). 2007. Questions and answers about acupuncture. www.cancer.gov/cancertopics/pdq/cam/acupuncture/patient/57.cdr.

National Center for Complementary and Alternative Medicine (NCCAM). 2007. Introduction to chiropractic. http://nccam.nih.gov/health/chiropractic/.

Nordenberg, T. 2000. The healing power of placebos. *FDA Consumer Magazine* 34: 14-17.

Pension and Welfare Benefits Association (PWBA). 1994. COBRA insurance summary. www.cobrahealth-insurance.com/Cobra_Health_Insurance_Summary.html.

Risberg, G., E.E. Johansson, G. Westman, and K. Hamberg. 2003. Gender in medicine: An issue for women only? A survey of physician teachers' gender attitudes. *International Journal for Equity in Health* 2: 10.

Stoppler, M. 2006. Watch out for health quacks. www.medicinenet.com/script/main/art.asp?articlekey=46696.

U.S. Census Bureau. 2008. Income, poverty, and health insurance coverage in the United States: 2007. www.census.gov/prod/2008pubs/p60-235.pdf.

U.S. Food and Drug Administration (FDA). 2006. The new over-the-counter medicine label: Take a look. www.fda.gov/buyonlineguide/OTClabel.htm.

Other helpful resources include the following.

Bachman, R.E. 2006. Healthcare consumerism: The basis of a 21st century intelligent health system. Available at www.healthtransformation.net.

Deloitte Center for Health Solutions. www.deloitte.com/dtt/section_node/0,1042,sid%253D80772,00.html. This site contains links to recent, relevant information regarding health care. Follow the Health Care Consumerism link to find the results from the 2008 and 2009 surveys of health care consumers.

National Center for Complementary and Alternative Medicine (NCCAM). http://nccam.nih.gov/health/decisions/. This site offers links to information designed to help people decide whether alternative treatment is right for them.

National Council Against Health Fraud (NCAHF). www.ncahf.org/index.html. NCAHF focuses on the threats of health misinformation, fraud, and quackery. As part of their mission statement, they advocate "(a) adequate disclosure in labeling and other warranties to enable consumers to make truly informed choices; (b) premarketing proof of safety and effectiveness for products and services claimed to prevent, alleviate, or cure any health problem; and (c) accountability for those who violate the law."

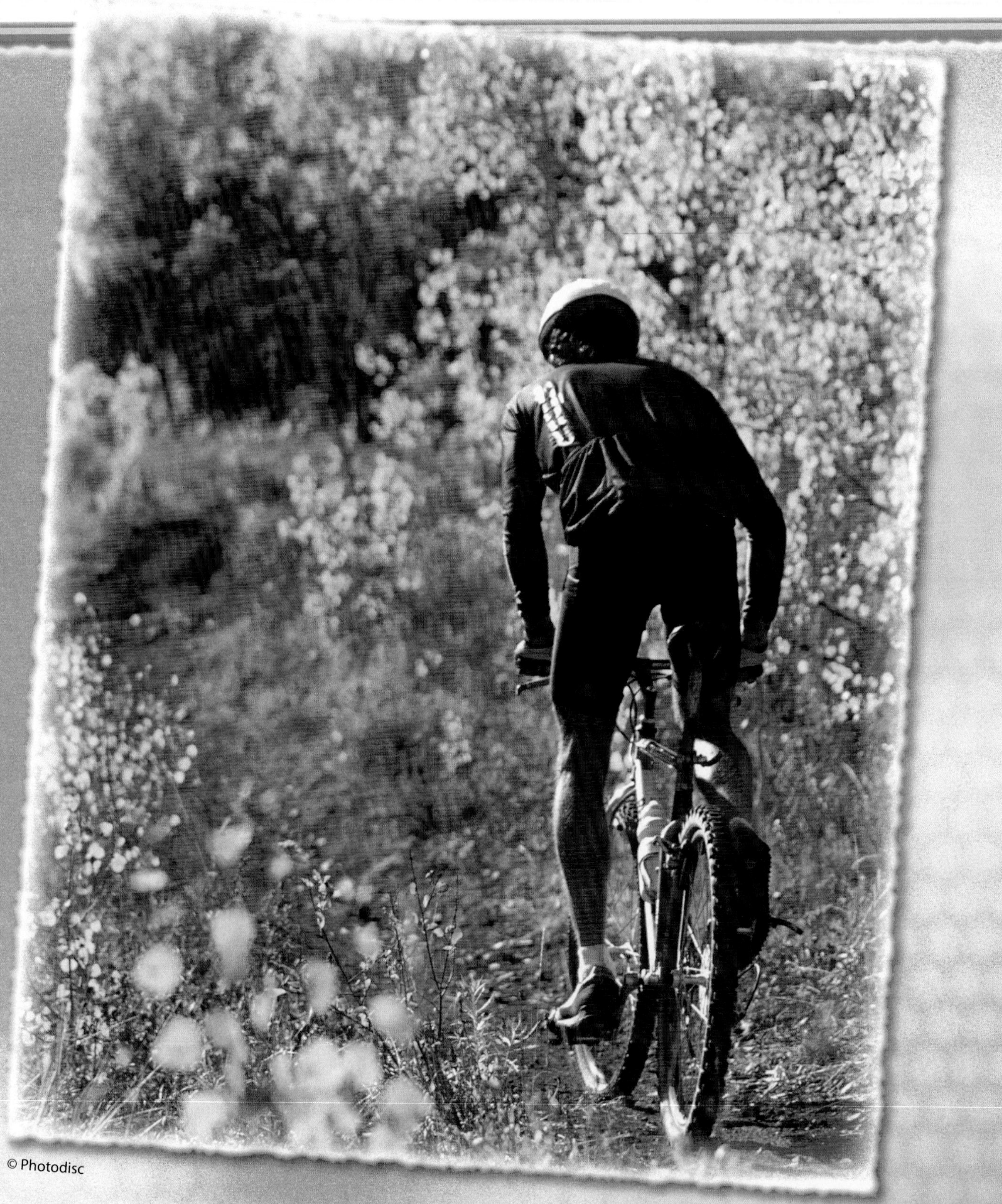

© Photodisc

CHAPTER 10

ENVIRONMENTAL HEALTH

PAMELA DOUGHTY, PHD, CHES
Institute for Obesity Research and Program Evaluation,
Texas A&M University

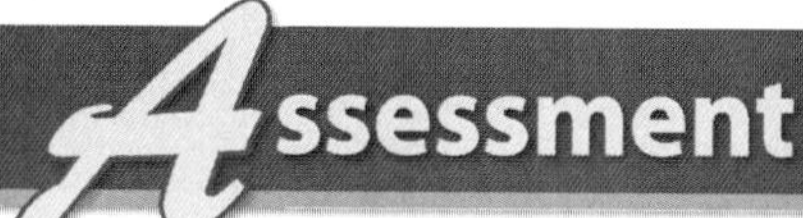

Assessment

- How much influence can a tree-lined street have on pollution?
- What do we mean by *global warming* or *climate change*?
- Do you think emissions of major air pollutants have increased or decreased since 1980?
- Would you pay more for food if farmers could reduce their use of chemicals?
- Are you being exposed to carcinogens in the environment? How often?

Objectives

- Define *environmental health*.
- List the various types of ecosystems.
- Define *urban ecosystem*.
- Explain how the agricultural ecosystem provides goods and services.
- Describe how trees affect the urban environment.
- Describe the relationship of the environment to human health.
- Explain how toxins get into the environment and how to prevent this from happening.

What's your fantasy vacation? Is it snorkeling in the turquoise water off the coast of a tropical island, with palm trees swaying on the white-sand beach? Is it a long road trip where you get to see the purple mountain majesties and amber waves of grain of "America the Beautiful" while driving under bright blue skies? Maybe it's camping in a pine forest next to a sparkling stream, or skiing on fresh powder. It could even be visiting a major city with great shopping, restaurants, and theater. The fantasy could be almost anything, but most likely the picture in your mind wouldn't include polluted water, smoggy air, or dead plants and animals. Polluted environments are unhealthy and depressing, and people have a responsibility to keep the environment healthy.

Environmental health is the science that studies how humans and nature interact to affect the health of humans. It addresses all the physical, chemical, and biological factors external to a person, including the assessment and control of those factors that can potentially affect health (World Health Organization [WHO] 2008). That definition suggests that if people don't manage it well, the environment will harm them. Hurricanes, tornados, volcanoes, earthquakes, tsunamis, animals, insects, bacteria, and viruses show how deadly the environment can be without the influence of people. However, many of the harmful things in the environment are attributable to humans, such as pollution, deforestation, and careless waste disposal.

A more comprehensive definition of environmental health is protection against environmental factors that may have an adverse effect on human health or the ecological balances essential to long-term human health and environmental quality (National Environmental Health Association 1996). This chapter will discuss environmental health using this definition and will present the factors that adversely affect human health, protection programs, and laws that influence the environment and ecological balances.

Ecological balance is a state of dynamic equilibrium, or balance, in which genetic, species, and ecosystem diversity remain relatively stable, though subject to gradual changes through natural succession (Ministry of Forests [MOF] 2008). An **ecosystem** is a place with unique physical features, including air, water, land, and habitats supporting plant and animal life (Environmental Protection Agency [EPA] 2008b). Each ecosystem has a similar food web. Figure 10.1 shows a soil food web, an ecosystem that has all the ingredients it needs to survive. Plants feed on organic matter; fungi, bacteria, and nematodes feed on the plants; nematodes feed on protozoa and fungi; arthropods feed on nematodes, fungi, and protozoa; and small animals and songbirds feed on arthropods. All of these plants and animals need sunlight and rain to survive. Too much or too little of any part of this food web will cause an imbalance in the system. For instance, too little rain will cause the organic matter to dry up, killing the plants, fungi, bacteria, protozoa, arthropods, birds, and animals and leaving little for humans to use as food.

ECOSYSTEMS

Humans need each of the six ecosystems described in this section for a good economy. The United States has all of these ecosystems and a few more, but not all continents have every ecosystem (Moyers 2001).

Forests

Forests have supplied the world with building materials since the beginning of time. Forests are defined as a canopy of overhead foliage from trees that covers a minimum of 10 percent of the ground area. Forests cover approximately 25 percent of the land area on earth. During the history of the United States, forests were depleted through logging. People began to notice that the forests were disappearing in the late 1800s, and it became popular to donate land for parks. Many laws were passed to protect the forests from being further destroyed and to plant trees to replace the lost forests (New York State Parks 2003). As the country expanded west, more forests were depleted and new laws passed to protect the forests. One example of a forest that was not replaced immediately after its loss was the forest around Carson City, Nevada. The hills surrounding Carson City are lacking trees, except for newly planted trees. Driving west just a few miles reveals the forests that were saved around Lake Tahoe.

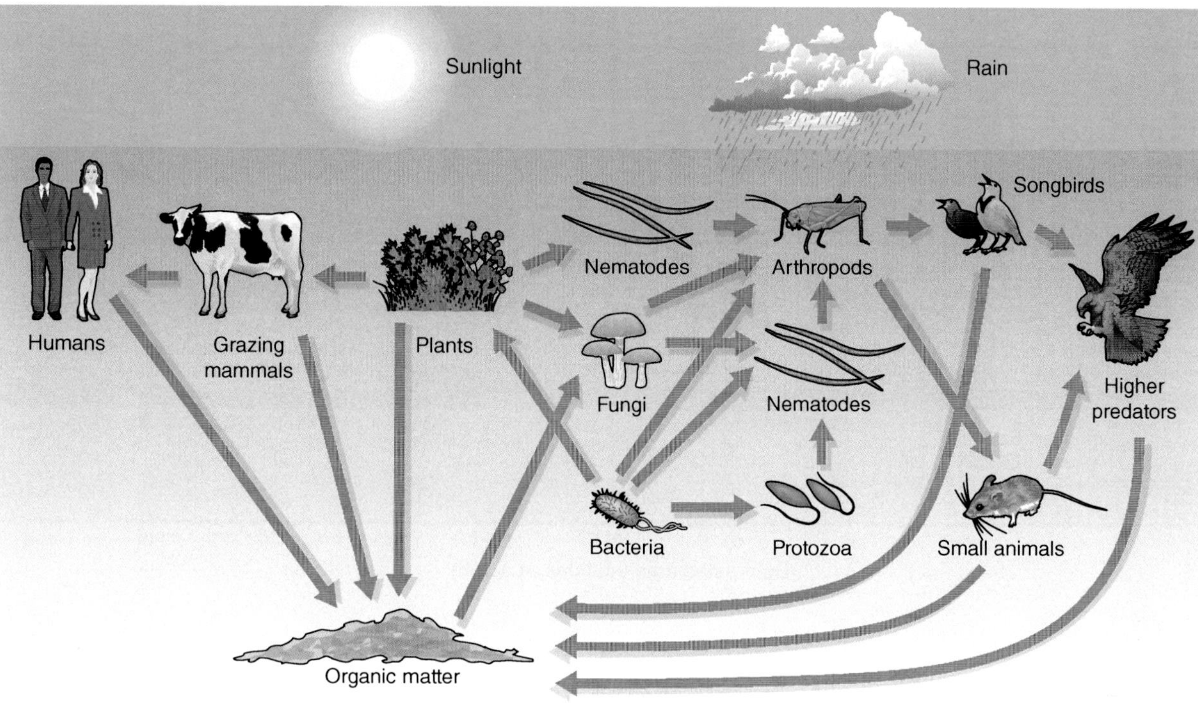

Figure 10.1 This soil food web shows the relationships between organisms in the ecosystem and how they contribute to the health of the soil that supports them all.

From Department of the Interior Bureau of Land Management.

Underdeveloped countries are beginning to see the economic advantages of supplying the world with wood because laws restrict logging in most developed countries. Figure 10.2 shows the 20 countries that cleared the most forest between 1990 and 2005. As the underdeveloped countries begin to overlog their forests, they will face the problems that the United States has spent years attempting to correct with its forests. The economic pull to cut down forests to sell the wood could endanger ecosystems in those countries. Many people live in the forests and depend on them for food (e.g., mushrooms, fruit, nuts, other edible plants, game), building and household materials (e.g., timber, vines, bamboo, leaves), and fodder to feed their livestock (Moyers 2001). The forests and their by-products are the economic basis for communities that live in and around the forests. Destruction of the forests will eventually destroy the communities' economies. As the economies decline, people will be forced out of the forest and into the urban populations. The challenge for these countries is to develop a plan that will keep the forests intact while still using timber as an economic support.

One community in Canada developed a plan with aboriginal Canadians, environmentalists, and loggers to cut only timber that would be destroyed naturally, such as trees fallen from weather. The plan keeps the aboriginal peoples employed by the logging companies, keeps the forests in place, and produces wood for the loggers to sell. Because of the difficulty finding and hauling trees from the interior of the forest, there are fewer trees to log and it is much more expensive. Hauling the trees is more expensive because it is necessary to move the trees through the existing forest, whereas traditional loggers cut a road through the forest to move the fallen trees. Overall, the cost of this lumber will go up. Will the builders who use the lumber pay the higher price if it means a better environment? If this plan works, it might spread to other areas of the world (Moyers 2001).

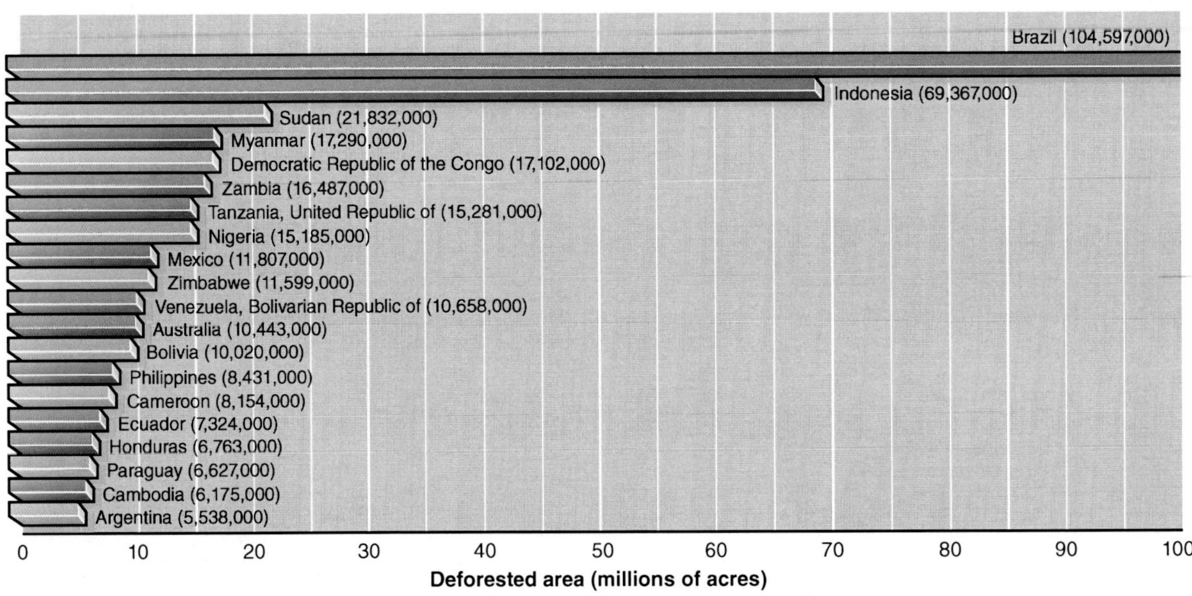

Figure 10.2 These countries cleared the most forest between 1990 and 2005 (based on data provided to the U.N. Foreign Agricultural Organization for the Global Forest Resources Assessment Report 2005). 1 acre = approximately 0.4 hectares.

Data from U.N. Foreign Agricultural Organization.

Freshwater Ecosystems

Freshwater ecosystems include lakes, groundwater, reservoirs, wetlands, ponds, rivers, and streams. All freshwater ecosystems are surrounded by land.

To determine the health of any body of freshwater, the U.S. EPA samples an area of water and examines the presence, condition, and types of fish, insects, algae, plants, and other aquatic life. If the samples are consistent over time, the EPA can get an accurate picture of the health of a body of water. Any changes in the balance of aquatic life could threaten the stability or balance of the water. For instance, if smaller fish start to die, the algae may get out of control because there are fewer fish to feed on the algae.

It is important for the aquatic life and humans to maintain **biological integrity**, or the maintenance of community structure and function that is characteristic of a particular area (EPA 2007b; Karr and Dudley 1981). Humans need to keep freshwater ecosystems healthy in order to preserve the water supply. Freshwater contains almost no salt, and all cultures use it for drinking, cleaning, cooking, and manufacturing. For instance, the paper industry needs clean freshwater because contaminants in water can change the color of the manufactured paper (Arrington 1998).

Forty percent of all fish species come from freshwater, and 18 percent of the freshwater fish are in danger of extinction. If even one species becomes extinct, it can affect other life in the freshwater ecosystem. Each species is dependent on another species for food or to control species growth. For instance, minnows are the food source for larger fish, and minnows help control the population of insects that land on the water surface (EPA 2007b).

Grasslands

Grassland ecosystems are biological communities and habitats with ground cover of grasses and other herbaceous plants. Examples include prairies, meadows, and savannas (U.S. Geological Survey n.d.).

Grasslands are considered the most threatened of all habitats (Mac, Opler, Puckett Haecker, and Doran 1998). The grasslands support many birds, lizards, small animals, and big game. Grasslands also supplied the original grasses that humans domesticated (wheat, corn, oats, barley, and rye). Many wild plants from grasslands are used now as alternative medicines, such as the extracts from the purple coneflower *(Echinacea purpurea)*, which is used to treat symptoms of the common cold. Another medicinal plant from the grasslands is goldenseal *(Hydrastis canadensis)*, which has been used as a tonic and as an astringent and yellow dye. Losing the grasslands could reduce medical discoveries from wild plants, as could happen with every ecosystem.

Human activities are threatening the grasslands. Some of those activities include farming, grazing, and killing off predators of livestock. As these changes take place, the greater sage grouse can't survive, and so the population of the sage grouse is used as an indicator of the health of the grassland ecosystem. State and federal agencies manage many grassland areas to protect them and the animals that live there.

Agroecosystems

Agroecosystems are the living communities of soil, plants, and animals that constitute farms, croplands, orchards, pastures, and rangelands where at least 30 percent of the land is used for cropland or pasture (Moyers 2001). Agricultural ecosystems are human-made systems from grasslands, forests, or arid areas to produce crops or livestock. They constitute 28 percent of the land area on earth, covering a total of 12.16 billion acres (4.92 billion hectares). Agroecosystems produce 90 percent of all crops and livestock worldwide.

Agricultural ecosystems are in danger from several elements. Runoff from herbicides, pesticides, and fertilizer sprayed on fields is polluting water. Many dryland farmers depend on irrigation systems to water the ground because of the lack of regular rain. Watering the soil artificially causes the salts in the soil to rise to the surface, which makes the soil become sterile. Soil erosion is causing farmers to fertilize more, which is causing the land to degrade, or lose necessary soil nutrients. Salts must be removed from the soil before the land can be replanted. The salts are removed by scraping the damaged soil. If the salts are not removed, the land cannot be replanted.

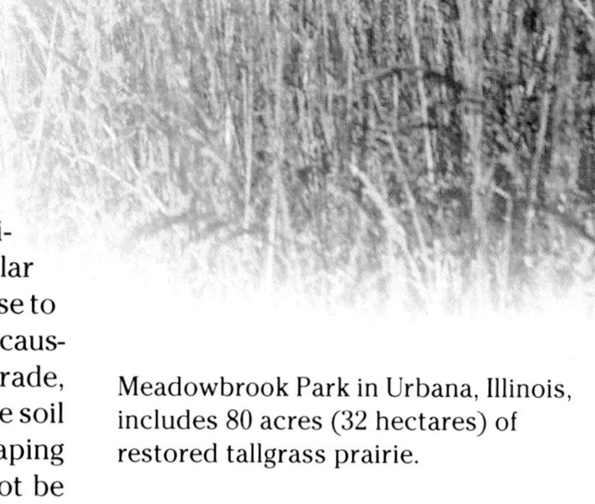

Meadowbrook Park in Urbana, Illinois, includes 80 acres (32 hectares) of restored tallgrass prairie.

If farmers don't restore the land, it will become a desert, but the cost of restoration can be high. A better alternative to investing in restoration is investing in prevention. Changing some farming practices could help preserve agroecosystems. For example, farmers could leave strips of ground unplanted and let natural grasses grow again on that land. The grasses help keep the soil from eroding, and they also bring some animals back to the land. That kind of farming can be more expensive for the consumer, though, because it might not yield as many crops.

Urban Ecosystems

An **urban ecosystem** refers to the plants, animals, and humans that inhabit an urban environment (Moyers 2001). Urban environments contain buildings, obviously, but they also contain street vegetation, lakes, ponds, yards, and parks.

Because much of the ground in urban areas is covered by parking lots, streets, and buildings, it can't absorb water. That makes it harder for the green areas to stay green during dry spells. Landscapers from urban areas try to develop green spaces; however, they usually bring in nonnative plants rather than restoring the indigenous plants that were removed to build streets and buildings. For example, a landscaper might replace plant life under trees with shade-tolerant grass. The lack of indigenous plants can damage soil because the natural ecosystem is disrupted.

Plants and animals in urban ecosystems face other dangers. Trees and shrubs are exposed to road salts in winter, physical barriers restrict the growth of plant roots, buildings restrict sunlight, and people and traffic pollute the air and water. Despite the tough environment of an urban ecosystem, many plants and animals live there. For example, a 1993 bird survey in Washington, DC, identified 115 bird species, and wild prairie grasses grow in Chicago (Moyers 2001).

Urban green spaces bring many benefits to the urban population. Trees shade streets and homes from sunlight, reducing temperatures. They also give off water vapor to help cool the atmosphere, they provide oxygen, and they're efficient air filters—they remove up to 70 percent of particulates on a tree-lined street (Moyers 2001). Urban forests in the area around Baltimore and Washington, DC, remove 17,000 tons (15,422 metric tons) of air pollution each year; without the trees, it would cost $88 million annually to do the same.

Urban green spaces also are home to deer, squirrels, muskrats, beavers, bats, opossums, raccoons, coyotes, foxes, minks, and weasels because those animals adapt well to environ-

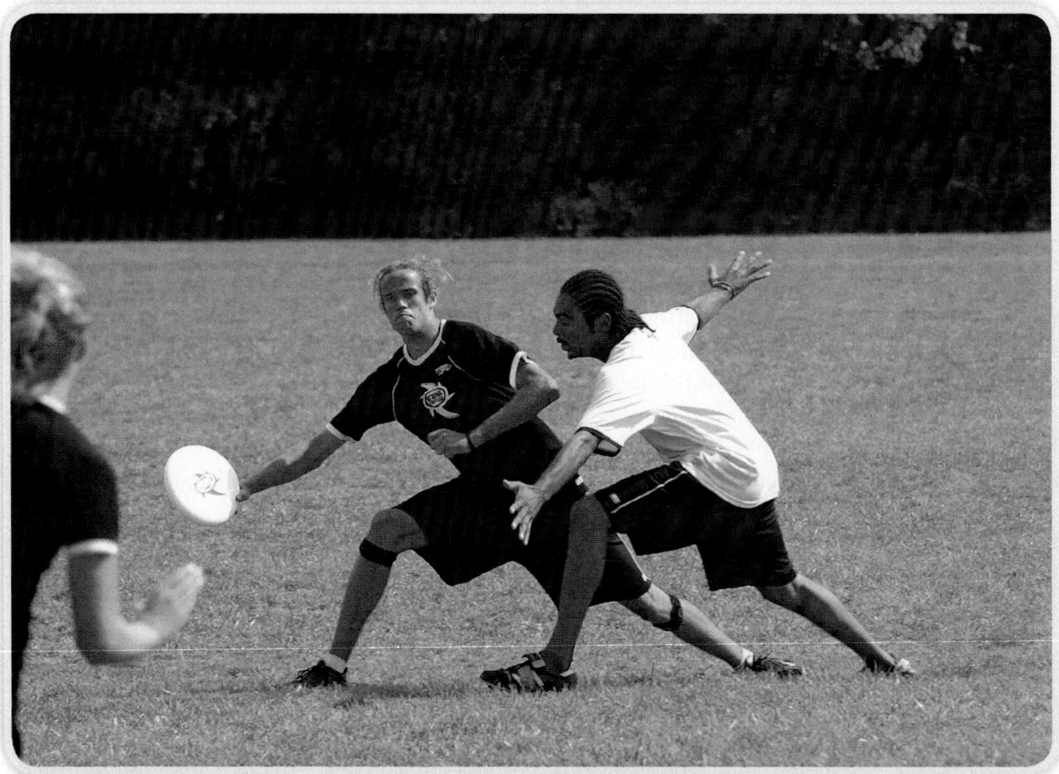

In urban ecosystems, green spaces such as parks provide homes for plants and wildlife and offer people opportunities for recreation.

© Human Kinetics

mental changes. People grow food in their backyards, enjoy the outdoors for recreation, and enjoy taking care of their own green spaces. Green spaces improve the environment for the people and animals that live in urban ecosystems. However, many places in the world need all the space they have to house humans and aren't able to include green spaces in their urban ecosystems (EPA 2007b).

Coastal Ecosystems

The United States includes four coastal ecosystems: the Great Lakes, the Chesapeake Bay, the Everglades, and the Gulf of Mexico. **Coastal ecosystems** are areas that are between the water and the land. They include estuaries, reefs, mangroves, islands, and salt marshes. Coastal ecosystems are home to many kinds of wildlife (Environmental Literacy Council 2007). Estuaries are semienclosed coastal bodies of water that have measurable salinity gradient from their freshwater drainage to the ocean entrance (National Oceanic and Atmospheric Administration [NOAA] 2008b). The status of estuaries has declined because of poor productivity of the plants and animals. The decline is attributed to the increase of land use, harmful algal blooms, and nutrient pollution. Studies are underway to understand the decline and to aid in the reduction of the harmful effects.

Coral reef ecosystems are experiencing similar stressors from natural and human-made sources. An increase in tourism reduces the coral reefs themselves. Hurricanes and other changes in weather and water temperature influence the coral through bleaching and a change in hard coral covers. Pollution causes disease outbreaks and a steady increase of algae (NOAA 2008a).

Mangroves have been studied for the last 2,000 years. Most of the older studies were about the use of the trees and shrubs and the wildlife in the area. About 12 families and more than 50 species are salt tolerant enough to live in mangroves. Mangroves have loose wet soil, salt, and periodic tides. They cover approximately 75 percent of tropical coastlines and prefer temperatures between 66 and 107 degrees Fahrenheit (19 to 42 degrees Celsius), so there are more mangroves near the equator. Mangroves also protect the land during hurricanes because they serve as a barrier to the wind and waves (U.S. Fish and Wildlife Service [FWS] 2008).

GENDER ISSUES

Women and Environmental Policy

Women have played an important role in the development of environmental health laws. The United Nations has had conferences for women and the environment since 1972. One group that was founded in 2002 is the Network of Women Ministers and the Environment, which believes that women offer new ideas and strategies for protecting people and the environment while practicing sustainable development (United Nations Environment Programme [UNEP] 2008). The network develops recommendations for practical solutions to environmental problems; builds network partnerships with civil society, nongovernmental, and intergovernmental agencies; exchanges best practices; and creates a critical mass of leadership to influence international and national policy (UNEP 2008).

This organization is just one example of women being involved in policy changes for environmental protection. Representation of women in policy-making groups has grown from zero to as many as 45 percent. Women's involvement in environmental policy gives lawmakers a new view, and women promote and practice conservation methods in their own countries. Change is happening in environmental protection around the world due to more women being involved in the grassroots efforts behind the policy and laws that are enacted.

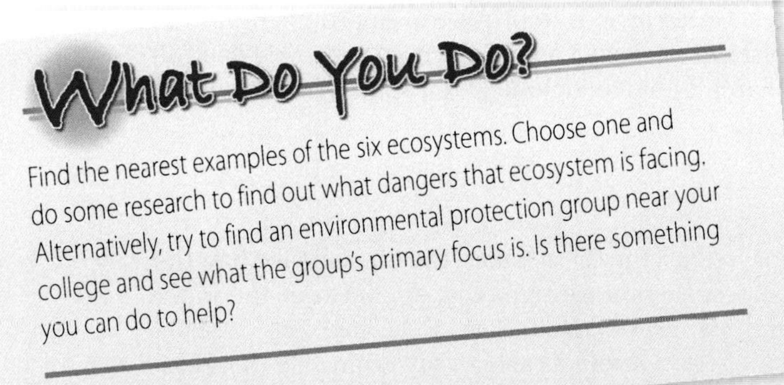

Salt marshes are not as plentiful as estuaries and are considered worthless by many people. Because society considers marshes to be unstable and unusable for building or for outdoor entertainment, they are often drained or dredged and filled. However, salt marshes have great value. They filter nutrients and pollutants from rivers before the water is emptied into the ocean. The plants in marshes have extensive root systems that provide stability during storm surges, and the protection of the vegetation provides nurseries for fish, shellfish, and crustaceans.

In Florida, salt marshes are decreasing due to major land developments. From 1944 to 1982, 51 percent of the salt marshes were lost in Palm Beach County. When there are fewer nurseries for commercial fish, the fish industry suffers as well as the public because prices increase for the few fish that can be caught in the area. In 1984, a law in Florida was passed to protect the remaining salt marshes (Florida Department of Environmental Protection 2008).

Natural disasters can have a devastating effect on the coastal ecosystems. Hurricanes can remove much of the existing land, plants, and animals, which are washed away during the high tides that move onto the shore. Salt marshes, mangroves, and estuaries are barriers that protect the land, but as these dwindle the land will be unprotected.

ENVIRONMENT AND PUBLIC HEALTH

Not only is the environment getting sick, but people are also getting sick from the damaged environment. Toxins and pollution, the way people manage waste, and the way they handle food can cause illness and disease. Humans have a symbiotic relationship with the environment, and this relationship requires using environmental products carefully, disposing of waste safely, and preserving resources for the next generation.

Global Warming

Although some find the topic controversial, in 2007 former U.S. vice president Al Gore won a Nobel Prize for his work in bringing **global warming** to the public's attention. Global warming is an increase in the temperature of the atmosphere that contributes to changes in global climate patterns (EPA 2008c). Scientists now prefer the term *climate change* because it suggests more than just the temperature changes, including wind and precipitation changes. Greenhouse effects are said to be the major contributor to the current climate changes. The greenhouse effect is a natural phenomenon that helps regulate temperature. Greenhouse gases (e.g., carbon dioxide, methane, nitrous oxide [NOx], chlorofluorocarbons) act as an insulating blanket, trapping solar energy that would otherwise escape into space. Without this natural greenhouse effect, temperatures would be about 60 degrees Fahrenheit (33 degrees Celsius) lower than they are now, and life as we know it today would not be possible (EPA 2008c).

The temperature increase is believed to have started during the industrial revolution and continued as humans have increased the burning of fossil fuels. The warmer temperatures could cause the melting of the glaciers and ice caps on both the north and south poles. If there is a complete melting of the ice caps and glaciers, it could cause the desalinization of the oceans. This desalinization, or decrease in the salt content of the water, could stop the flow of the atmosphere that warms the north and cools the south by stopping the conveyor belt of currents in the Atlantic Ocean. The warming of the planet will cause droughts in some areas and floods in others because of the change in weather patterns (EPA 2008c).

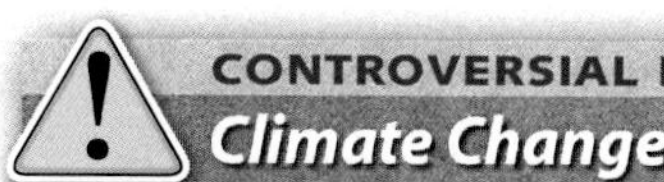

CONTROVERSIAL ISSUES

Climate Change Findings

Climate change has been a controversial issue for many years, but it came to a head after the documentary *An Inconvenient Truth* by Al Gore. The Intergovernmental Panel on Climate Change produced a summary of its findings to the United Nations in October 2007. The paper reported that warming of the climate system is unequivocal because the past 12 years have seen the warmest surface temperature since 1850. Seas have risen in response to the climate increase, but it is uncertain if this rise is a short-term or long-term trend.

The report says that the climate change is due to increased concentrations of carbon dioxide, methane, and NOx. These increases are from emissions released by industry and decomposing biological sources and agriculture. However, there is no mention of the increased number of people and decreased forests since 1750, which could cause an increase in carbon dioxide.

The paper gave several examples of effects associated with global average temperature change:

- Increased water availability in moist tropics and high latitudes
- Decreasing water availability and increasing drought in midlatitudes and semiarid low latitudes
- Hundreds of millions of people exposed to increased water stress
- Significant extinctions around the globe
- Increased coral bleaching
- Increasing species range shifts and wildfire risk
- Complex, localized negative impacts on small holders, subsistence farmers, and fishers
- Increased damage to coastal regions from floods and storms
- Increasing burden from malnutrition and diarrheal, cardiorespiratory, and infectious diseases
- Increased morbidity and mortality from heat waves, floods, and droughts

Some aspects to consider regarding global warming are that NASA (National Aeronautics and Space Administration) has been contracted to keep track of climate changes. NASA diversified in order to continue threatened funding for the department, and if it found no changes in the environment, the country might not continue to fund the project. Also, since Al Gore's movie there has been more public interest in the climate. With greater interest comes more research and more results that support the belief that global warming is caused by human interference rather than normal weather change patterns over time. Watch *An Inconvenient Truth* by Al Gore, read the summary written for the United Nations, and then read the information refuting the conclusions made by these two groups. Then, decide for yourself.

There are many ways that the United States is trying to slow down the rise in temperature. Currently, emission standards on gasoline and diesel engines are limiting the release of carbon monoxide, and the country has some of the most efficient vehicles on the road. The problem is that there are more motor vehicles on the road than ever before, causing an increase in emissions. Laws are in place that will reduce emissions of carbon monoxide for both cars and manufacturing. You can assist in reducing climate changes by reducing your **carbon footprint**—the amount of greenhouse gases you emit directly and indirectly through your daily activities, measured in units of carbon dioxide. Tips for reducing your carbon footprint include the following:

- Walk or ride a bicycle for short trips instead of driving.
- In the winter, set your thermostat to a few degrees cooler. In the summer, set it to a few degrees warmer.

- Only run the washing machine or dishwasher when they're full.
- Take shorter showers, and don't leave the water running when brushing your teeth.
- Use energy-efficient light bulbs.
- Unplug electronics after you've turned them off.
- Recycle.

Many Web sites are available to help you reduce your carbon footprint (EPA 2008c). One Web site will even calculate your carbon footprint for you (www.conservation.org/act/live_green/carboncalc/Pages/default.aspx).

Toxins

The environment is full of **toxins** in various amounts, and people are exposed to them daily. Some common toxins are pesticides, asbestos, and radon.

Pesticides are dangerous, especially to children under the age of 5 because they might ingest them. Almost half of all households with children under age 5 (47 percent) had at least one pesticide stored in an unlocked cabinet that was less than 4 feet (1 meter) off the ground (i.e., within the reach of children). Approximately 75 percent of households without children have pesticides stored in unlocked cabinets, which might explain why 13 percent of all pesticide poisonings of children happen outside the child's home (EPA 2007d).

Asbestos is a mineral fiber that was once used in homes and buildings for insulation and as a fire retardant. Asbestos is found in older homes in furnace insulation, shingles, floor tiles, and paint. When asbestos isn't disturbed, it isn't known to cause health hazards. However, many older buildings that have asbestos are deteriorating and are being renovated. When the asbestos in those buildings gets disturbed, it can cause lung cancer, cancer of the lining of the chest cavity, and scarring of the lungs with fibrous tissue. Illnesses caused by asbestos can be prevented by not disturbing asbestos materials and by using trained contractors to remove asbestos during renovation.

Radon is a cancer-causing natural radioactive gas that you can't see, smell, or taste (EPA 2007d). It is the leading cause of lung cancer among nonsmokers and is the second leading cause of lung cancer overall. Radon claims 20,000 lives each year. All homes should be checked for radon, no matter how old they are or where they're located. The gas comes from the degradation of natural radioactive substances such as uranium. As the radioactive substance breaks down, it gives off radon gas. The gas gets trapped between rock formations and can be found anywhere in the world. Any gas seeks to escape, and radon gas seeps through the soil and is released into the atmosphere. If a home is built on land where radon is seeping into the atmosphere, it will seep into the interior of the home.

The EPA regulates the release of most toxins and maintains standards for air and water purity. The government has set standards regarding what toxins and how much of them are allowed to be released into the atmosphere by any manufacturer. These standards are becoming stricter as new laws are passed to protect the environment.

What Do You Do?

Explore Tox Town on the Internet at http://toxtown.nlm.nih.gov. Describe what harmful environmental toxins are in your home, city, or town and what you can do to prevent your friends or family from exposure.

Air Pollution

The six major air pollutants are ozone, particulate matter, carbon monoxide, nitrogen oxides, sulfur dioxide, and lead.

Ozone is a gas that's created by a chemical reaction between oxides of nitrogen and volatile organic compounds in the presence of sunlight. Ozone is labeled as good or bad, depending on its position in the atmosphere. Bad ozone is near the earth and is caused by emissions from motor vehicles and industry. It's the main ingredient in smog. Good ozone, on the other hand, occurs naturally about 10 to 30 miles (16 to 48 kilometers) above the earth. Good ozone protects the earth from harmful ultraviolet rays (EPA 2007d).

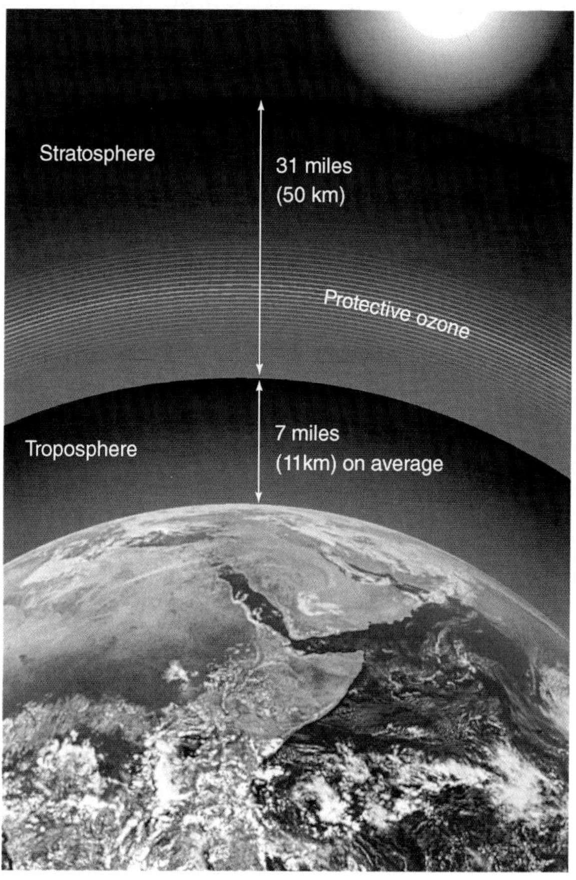

Figure 10.3 Bad ozone lies close to the earth's surface, but a layer of good ozone above the planet protects us from ultraviolet rays.

Figure 10.3 shows the troposphere and the stratosphere, the two atmospheric layers closest to the surface, along with the layer of protective ozone. The ozone layer protects the earth by reflecting light back to the sun, allowing only small amounts of sunlight into the atmosphere. Chemical reactions involving chlorine and bromine have created a "hole" in the ozone layer over the southern polar region (which you can monitor at http://ozonewatch.gsfc.nasa.gov/). If the hole gets too big or if the ozone layer in general gets too thin, more sunlight will penetrate the atmosphere and begin to heat up the earth. As the earth heats up, it is possible that the hole in the ozone layer will get larger and eventually burn off the ozone layer altogether. If this were to happen, the earth would be scorched and no longer would be able to support plant life or animal life. It is crucial to protect the ozone layer above the earth to ensure protection from the sunlight. The ozone layer near the earth is air pollution that can cause cardiovascular and respiratory problems.

In 1928, Freon, a hydrochorfluorocarbon, was invented and allowed for the proliferation of refrigerators. **Hydrochlorofluorocarbons (HCFCs)** are chemicals that pollute the air. HCFCs were used in refrigerants and air conditioners in both homes and cars, but the U.S. government has gradually phased out the use of HCFCs as coolants because they deplete the ozone layer. The reduced use of Freon as an air-conditioning coolant began several years ago, before laws were passed that required the reduced use of HCFCs.

Particulate matter is made up of small particles and liquid droplets, including acids, organic chemicals, metals, and soil or dust. The EPA is concerned about particles that are 10 micrometers or less in diameter (about the diameter of a human hair), because those can be inhaled by humans. Particles that small can enter the lungs and enter the bloodstream, which can cause serious health problems. Humans are not built to inhale particulates. Our noses and mouths are made to screen particulate matter as we breathe. However, we cannot screen particulate matter that is smaller than 10 micrometers in diameter. When particulate matter is prevalent in the atmosphere, there are higher incidences of cardiovascular events such as angina and heart attacks, as well as asthma-related deaths.

Carbon monoxide (CO) can have serious health effects for humans. It aggravates cardiovascular disease. Low levels can cause serious chest pain and reduce the ability to exercise, and prolonged exposure could result in other serious cardiovascular events. Carbon monoxide also is a major contributor to smog. National averages for carbon monoxide have decreased steadily over the last 26 years and are below the EPA standards for air pollution. Carbon monoxide is released during combustion of fossil fuels, and the majority of carbon monoxide comes from the manufacturing of electricity when using coal. Automobiles also release carbon monoxide from gas-burning engines. Diesel motors release more carbon monoxide than automobiles and account for the majority of carbon monoxide released by vehicles.

Nitrogen oxides (NOx) are a group of highly reactive gases that contain nitrogen and oxygen in varying amounts (EPA 2007d). These gases form when fuel is burned at a high temperature; primary human sources are motor vehicles, electric utilities, and industrial and commercial sources. They are also formed naturally in small amounts. Exposure to low levels of NOx can irritate the eyes and nose as well as the lungs, which results in fluid buildup. High levels of exposure to NOx can cause the lungs to become burned with an excess of fluid buildup, resulting in death (Environmental Defense Fund [EDF] 2002).

Sulfur dioxide (SO_2) is a gas that dissolves easily in water and creates an acid. Most emissions come from electric plants that burn coal. Sulfur dioxide contributes to respiratory illness and aggravates heart and lung diseases. It also contributes to acid rain, which damages trees, crops, historic buildings, and monuments and makes soil, lakes, and streams acidic. Sulfur dioxide doesn't just stay in the area around the plants that produce it but travels long distances through the air.

Emissions from motor vehicles used to contribute the most **lead** in air pollution. Lead was originally added to gasoline by oil companies to decrease the amount of gasoline in a gallon and thus increase profits. That's changed, though, since leaded gasoline was outlawed in 1986 to allow catalytic converters to reduce the amount of pollution released. Now most lead emissions come from metals processing. The highest levels of lead emissions are found near lead smelters, waste incinerators, utilities, and lead-acid battery manufacturers. Lead is a poison that affects brain functions in humans. It can cause learning disorders, brain dysfunction, slowed body growth, hearing problems, and kidney damage (Medline 2008).

Figure 10.4 shows how emissions for the six major air pollutants have declined between 1980 and 2007. The pollutants are measured using different scales, so the figure is split into three parts. The first section, measured up to 35 million tons, shows the emissions for nitrogen oxides (NOx), ozone (VOC, or volatile organic compounds, which form ozone), sulfur dioxide (SO_2), particulate matter that is smaller than 10 micrometers in diameter (PM_{10}), and particulate matter that is smaller than 2.5 micrometers in diameter ($PM_{2.5}$). The second section, measured up to 200 million tons, shows the emissions for carbon monoxide (CO). The third section, measured up to 80 thousand tons, shows the emissions for lead.

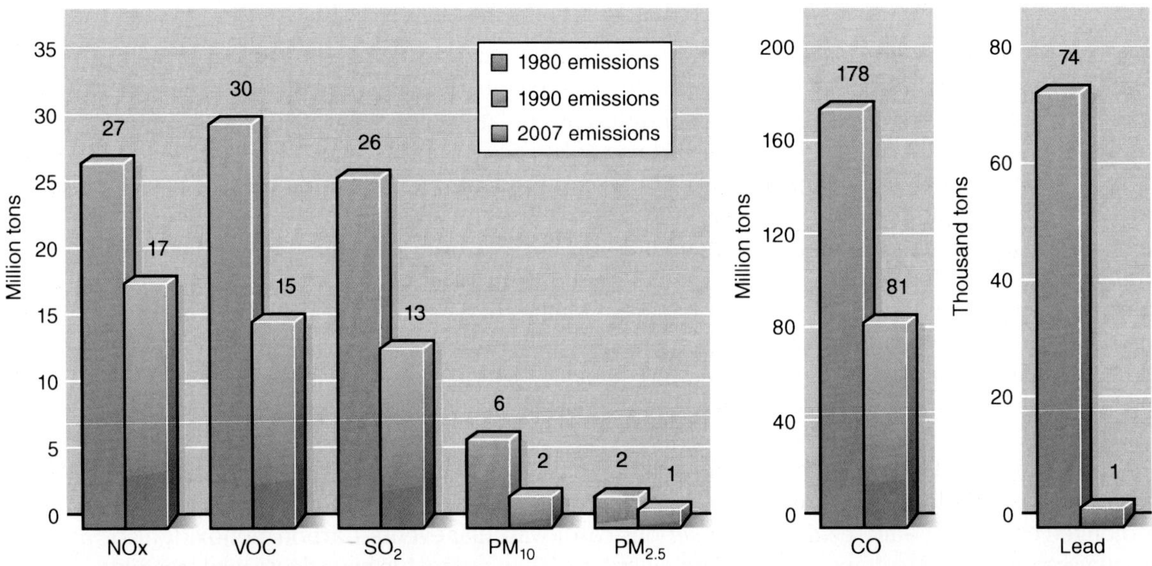

Figure 10.4 Emissions for major air pollutants have declined over the last few decades. This figure tracks the change in emissions from 1980 to 2007, except for $PM_{2.5}$, for which there's no estimated data until 1990.

Adapted from the EPA.

Water Pollution

The major water pollutants are arsenic, benzene, disinfection by-products, contaminated sediment and dredged material, lead, and microbial pathogens.

Arsenic is an odorless and colorless semimetal element found naturally in the soil. Arsenic can enter the water supply through natural deposits in the earth or through agricultural or industrial processes. An increase in the demand for drinking water can lower the levels of supply in natural reservoirs, causing arsenic to be released from rock formations. High levels of arsenic are found in some agricultural fertilizers and livestock feeds. Run-off from fields and feedlot can cause water contamination (EPA 2007a).

Benzene is an ingredient in plastics, rubber, resins, and synthetic fabrics such as nylon and polyester. It's also a solvent in printing, paints, and dry-cleaning chemicals. Short-term exposure can cause people to experience nervous system disorders, immune system depression, and anemia. With long-term exposure (such as years in an environment with a high benzene level), they're in danger of chromosome damage and cancer. Benzene will either evaporate very quickly or leach to groundwater if released to soil. It can be broken down by some soil microbes and may also be degraded in some ground waters. If benzene is released to surface water, most of it should evaporate within a few hours or be degraded by microbes. It's not likely to accumulate in aquatic organisms (EPA 2006b).

Disinfection by-products are the chemical outcomes of the treatment water goes through to become drinkable. These by-products are bromate, chlorite, haloacetic acids, and total trihalomethanes. Possible health effects of drinking water contaminated by disinfection by-products include anemia, increased risk of cancer, and liver, kidney, or central nervous system problems (EPA 2008a).

Sediments are loose particles of substances that settle at the bottom of bodies of water. They can become contaminated by various pollutants, including chemicals and pesticides. Dredged material is sediment that's dredged from waterways, ports, and harbors to maintain nations' navigation systems for commercial, national defense, and recreational purposes. The EPA and the U.S. Army Corps of Engineers share the responsibility for regulating the disposal of dredged material in United States waters and in ocean waters (EPA 2007c).

The toxic metal lead, which is found in small amounts in the earth's crust, has been used in a variety of consumer products. People who live in older homes can be exposed to lead-based paint, but lead can also enter tap water as a result of corrosion of plumbing materials. Homes constructed before 1986 are more likely to have lead pipes, solder, and fixtures, but even newer homes are at risk because "lead-free" plumbing can contain up to 8 percent lead. It can seep into water (especially hot water) from faucets and fixtures that are made of brass or chrome-plated brass. Lead can cause a variety of adverse health effects when people are exposed to it, even for relatively short periods of time. These effects may include interference with red blood cell chemistry; delays in normal physical and mental development in babies and young children; slight deficits in the attention span, hearing, and learning abilities of children; and slight increases in the blood pressure of some adults. Long-term effects of exposure can include stroke, kidney disease, and cancer (EPA 2007e).

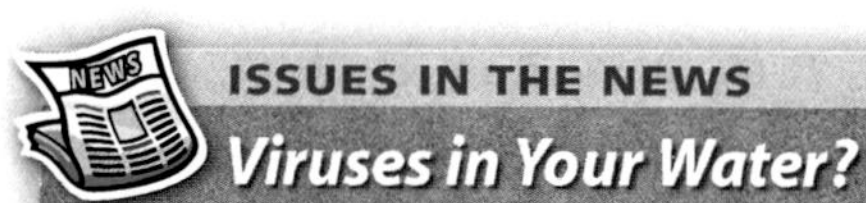

ISSUES IN THE NEWS

Viruses in Your Water?

Testing in a Wisconsin deep aquifer showed that human viruses migrated to the deepest portion of the water in about 40 years. It has always been assumed that deep water aquifers are pristine and contain no bacteria or viruses. With this new finding, it may be necessary to filter this water before drinking it.

Deep aquifers are layered under aquitards, which are impermeable, and it was assumed that bacteria and viruses could not penetrate the aquitard as water passed through. However, this new research showed that a virus might be small enough to pass through the aquitards or that it simply passed through cracks or thinned areas of the aquitards (Borchardt et al. 2007).

Whatever the reason for the presence of the viruses, scientists will have to develop new technologies to reduce the viruses in well water and municipal water sources. More information can be read about this and other environmental issues at www.environmentalhealthnews.org.

Microbial pathogens are microorganisms that can contaminate ground water, surface water, water used as food sources, and finished drinking water. These pathogens include *Giardia*, *Aeromonas*, *Legionella*, and *Cryptosporidium*.

- *Giardia* are protozoan parasites that are excreted in the feces of an infected host and can be ingested by others, spreading the infection. The infection can be acquired without producing any symptoms, but the most common symptoms are acute diarrhea, abdominal cramps, bloating, flatulence, weight loss, and occasional vomiting. Symptoms can last from 3 to 4 days up to several months or years, depending on severity (EPA 2000a).
- *Aeromonas* is found in water environments throughout the world as well as in foods such as dairy products and raw meat. Infections typically occur following trauma in an aquatic environment. Symptoms include diarrhea, wound infections, septicemia, meningitis, ophthalmitis, endocarditis, aspiration pneumonia, and biliary tract infections (EPA 2006a).
- Over 40 species of the *Legionella* bacteria are known to exist. *Legionella pneumophila* is responsible for the majority of human infections. The pathogen can cause Pontiac fever, which has flulike symptoms (fever, chills, headache, and muscle pain), or the more serious Legionnaires' disease, which has symptoms similar to those of pneumonia and can be fatal (EPA 2000b).
- *Cryptosporidium* is excreted in the waste of an infected host as oocysts (egglike structures) that are ingested by a new host. Symptoms include profuse diarrhea that lasts for approximately 48 hours, abdominal cramps, vomiting, lethargy, and general malaise. More severe cases can include renal failure and liver disease (EPA 2001).

The EPA is responsible for controlling water pollutants in municipal drinking water, but it doesn't control well water. People who have wells have to hire someone to come out and test their well water for them.

Waste Management

How people collect, move, dispose of, and recycle waste affects the environment and public health. Figure 10.5 illustrates the order in which strategies for **waste management** benefit the environment. The most effective technique is to design and manufacture products that turn into clean garbage rather than toxic waste in landfills. Other waste management strategies are to reduce, reuse, and recycle to minimize waste. It's also possible to recover energy from waste treatment, such as by burning waste to produce heat or gas that can be converted into electricity. The waste management strategy that's most harmful to the environment is disposing of waste in local dump sites (EPA 2007d; Waste Management [WM] 2007). Thirty-two percent of waste in the United States is recovered and recycled or composted, 14 percent is burned at combustion facilities, and the remaining 54 percent is dumped in landfills (EPA 2007d).

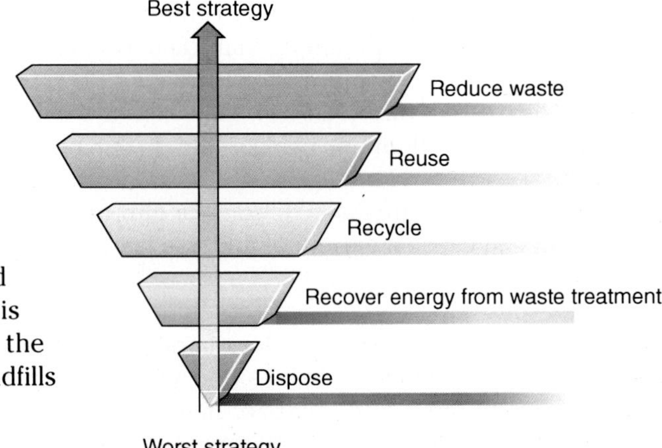

Figure 10.5 The waste management hierarchy ranks strategies from the best (reducing the amount of waste you produce) to the worst (disposing of waste).

CULTURAL ISSUES
Weighing Costs and Benefits

Environmental action is at the mercy of the cost to fix the problem and the harmfulness of the problem. It all comes down to a cost–benefit analysis. A simple example would be a home air filter. If home air filters reduced particulates in the home and decreased how often we got sick, we would all want to purchase one for our homes, right? But what if the cost of that filter was $5,000—would you still want to buy one? Most of us only miss a day or two of work per year because of illness and the cost of going to a doctor is much less expensive than $5,000, so most of us would not purchase the filter. However, if you had an autoimmune disease and easily spent that much in doctor's offices and hospitals while missing work, you might buy it.

Developing countries are in a similar situation. They produce great quantities of pollution and have poor equipment to reduce that pollution. We may think that they are being unfair to their population, which will be hurt from the harmful effects of pollution. However, the countries are poor and the populations even poorer. The population depends on the work provided by the factories. If factories were to pay for the pollution-reducing equipment, they would have to reduce the number of workers or increase the cost of their goods and services. The country as a whole would suffer from the loss of employment and the reduced sales of its goods and services. Is it ethical for these countries to pollute the environment and subject their citizens to the illnesses that result? The United States endured the same pollution in the early to mid-1900s. It is only recently that laws have begun to reduce pollution from factories.

The world still struggles with this ethical dilemma. It is important to reduce pollution, but in doing so it is also important that people do not suffer major economic consequences of pollution controls. A cost–benefit analysis will always be required when it comes to environmental safety.

Dump sites aren't healthy for the environment. They were worse in the past, when sites created leachate, a product of rainwater and decomposing materials that can pollute the water supply; methane gas and carbon dioxide from the decomposing material; and homes for vermin. Today, landfills try to protect groundwater by containing leachate with clay or a plastic lining material. Landfills also have gas-extracting systems that use perforated pipes to move the gas from inside the landfill to a gas engine, where the methane is burned off, generating electricity in the process (WM 2007). Trash is also compacted. The density of the compacted material stabilizes the land, and when it's covered vermin can't find a home.

Hazardous waste is dangerous to human health and the environment. It can come in many forms, including liquids, solids, contained gases, and sludges (semisolid materials). Hazardous waste can be the by-product of manufacturing processes or simply discarded commercial products, such as cleaning fluids or pesticides.

The EPA strictly regulates the disposal of hazardous waste. It follows the waste through its entire life cycle. Most EPA rules are specific to the kind of waste that needs to be disposed. For instance, a company with a certain type of hazardous waste may be required to transport it in sealed containers that travel no more than 10 days to the storage facility.

DISEASES AND DISORDERS

Researchers have discovered that the environment affects people's health in many ways. A lot of people are exposed to the same environmental dangers; some get sick and others don't.

The difference between the people who are affected and those who are not is **susceptibility**. When a person is sensitive to or can't resist something, such as a disease or drug, that person is susceptible. Your genetic makeup, the degree to which you've been exposed to something harmful, and the length of time you were exposed influences your susceptibility to disease. Just because you're exposed to pathogens, environmental particles, or disease doesn't mean you'll show symptoms. Exposure coupled with susceptibility is the key to whether or not you get sick.

In 2005, two government agencies, the Centers for Disease Control and Prevention (CDC) and the EPA, began to track diseases where the environment caused or contributed to the development of a disease. Those organizations track hospitalizations for asthma, myocardial infarction, birth defects, cancer, lead poisoning, and carbon monoxide poisoning (CDC 2006).

Asthma is a condition in which the airways constrict and breathing is difficult. Some people have asthma attacks when they're exposed to particulates in the environment. Children as young as 5 have been diagnosed with asthma, and doctors diagnose the condition in adults, too. The condition can develop at any time. People with asthma take medicine to reduce their reactions to triggers and to expand the airways during asthma episodes. Severe asthma episodes require emergency medical treatment. Asthma can be controlled but is never cured.

Research suggests that exposure to environmental factors such as air pollution can cause **myocardial infarction (MI)**, or heart attacks (Rückerl et al. 2007). Susceptibility is an issue with all environmental factors, but only since 2007 has research suggested that exposure to environmental factors could trigger a heart attack. More investigation is needed to understand the full scope of this relationship.

Scientists continue to study how exposure to various chemicals relates to birth defects. More than 60 percent of birth-defect causes are unknown (American Pregnancy Association [APA] 2007). Some studies suggest that autism may be caused by genetics combined with exposure to heavy metals such as mercury (Schettler 2004).

Cancer is the unchecked growth of cells that form tumors, which aggressively grow and invade surrounding tissue. Abuses of chemicals such as alcohol, tobacco, or marijuana is known to cause cancer in susceptible people. Many environmental substances called *carcinogens* are known to cause cancer, though a person's risk of developing cancer depends on the type and extent of exposure, genetics, and other factors. Known carcinogens include arsenic, asbestos, benzene, beryllium, cadmium, chromium, formaldehyde, lead, and nickel. The American Cancer Society lists the following exposure circumstances for known carcinogens (American Cancer Society 2008):

- Aluminum production
- Arsenic in drinking water
- Boot and shoe manufacture and repair
- Chimney sweeping
- Coal gasification
- Coal-tar distillation
- Furniture and cabinet making
- Hematite mining (underground) with exposure to radon
- Involuntary smoking (exposure to secondhand tobacco smoke)
- Iron and steel founding
- Isopropyl alcohol manufacture (strong-acid process)
- Painting (occupational exposure)
- Paving and roofing with coal-tar pitch
- Tobacco smoking and tobacco smoke

STEPS FOR BEHAVIORAL CHANGE

Reduce Your Waste

What can you do to make a difference in the environment? After all, you're just one person. One step to making a difference is reducing your own waste. How do you purchase your food? Do you use plastic bags or paper? Do you recycle? Do you purchase products wrapped in plastic?

Each of us has a responsibility to reduce the amount of waste we produce. There are many things that we can do to reduce our waste production. For instance, the number of plastic bags that are collected from grocery stores, department stores, and discount stores could be reduced by reusing sacks from home or by carrying canvas bags that can be used each time we visit a store.

Another way to reduce waste taken to the landfill is to recycle. Many cities and towns provide containers to separate waste into paper, plastic, glass, and aluminum. If your town provides these containers, it is easy to separate your garbage before you place it out on the curb for recycling pickup. Other towns do not provide this service, which requires a little more work.

Aluminum cans are great to recycle because there are many places in every city that will give money for collected aluminum. The price of aluminum has risen over the years and buyers can offer a reasonable amount of money for collected cans. Just place a container near your trash can to collect cans before recycling them.

Many grocery stores offer plastic bags for fruits and vegetables to make it easy for checkers to weigh the produce. However, it is possible to separate produce in the cart for weighing once you get to the checkout area. Although some checkers don't like unbagged produce, as long as the produce is together they don't mind too much. Not using plastic produce bags can reduce the amount of plastic that you take home.

Many products are housed in plastic, some for protection and some for security. Plastic used for protecting food is very thin and is necessary to keep food from spoiling. However, meats and vegetables can be purchased without plastic at the meat counter and in bins. Although you may pay a slightly higher price, you reduce the amount of plastic placed in the trash.

These are just a few ideas to reduce your trash; you might have many more. Discuss the possibilities with family, friends, and any organizations you belong to in order to come up with ways to save money and reduce the production of waste.

In the 1960s, health professionals discovered that children who ingested lead-based paint chips developed learning disabilities and behavioral problems, and some who ingested high levels of lead had seizures, went into a coma, and died (CDC 2007). Lead poisoning has been an environmental concern since that discovery. Approximately 310,000 children aged 1 to 5 have levels of lead in their blood higher than the CDC recommends. Lead paint can be found on toys, dishes that were manufactured before 1978 in the United States, and paint used in older homes. In 2007, there was a massive recall of toys made in China because lead was found in the paint and plastics of the toys (CDC 2007). Fortunately, the toys were recalled before children became poisoned from the lead.

Carbon monoxide is an odorless, colorless, tasteless gas. Each year, more than 500 Americans die from unintentional carbon monoxide poisoning, and more than 2,000 commit suicide by intentionally poisoning themselves (CDC 2008). Carbon monoxide is found in combustion fumes of small gasoline engines, stoves, lanterns, and burning charcoal and wood. In carbon monoxide poisoning, red blood cells latch on to carbon monoxide more quickly than oxygen cells, and they block oxygen from being absorbed. The lack of oxygen results in tissue damage and even death. The most common symptoms of carbon monoxide poisoning are headache, dizziness, chest pain, and confusion. The best way to prevent carbon monoxide poisoning is to make sure that all gas appliances are properly vented to the outside, avoid using portable gas heaters inside, and install a battery-operated carbon monoxide detector.

Carbon monoxide poisoning can happen outdoors, too. Never run a vehicle inside a garage with the door shut. If you ride with your trunk open or tailgate down, roll the windows down to keep the exhaust from entering the car or truck. If you're boating, don't ride with the bow too high or the smoke from the engine will draft over the back half of the boat. Traveling at slow speeds or idling can cause the carbon monoxide to build up in the cabin of the boat. Boats with generators can build up carbon monoxide at the rear, creating a potential hazard to boaters who are in the lower cabin or who are swimming at the rear of the boat.

GOING GREEN

You can help the environment by going green, a method of reducing your negative impact on the environment. Some ways to go green are reducing the amount of trash that is sent to landfills, reducing the amount of water that is used by households, using recycled products, and using energy efficiently.

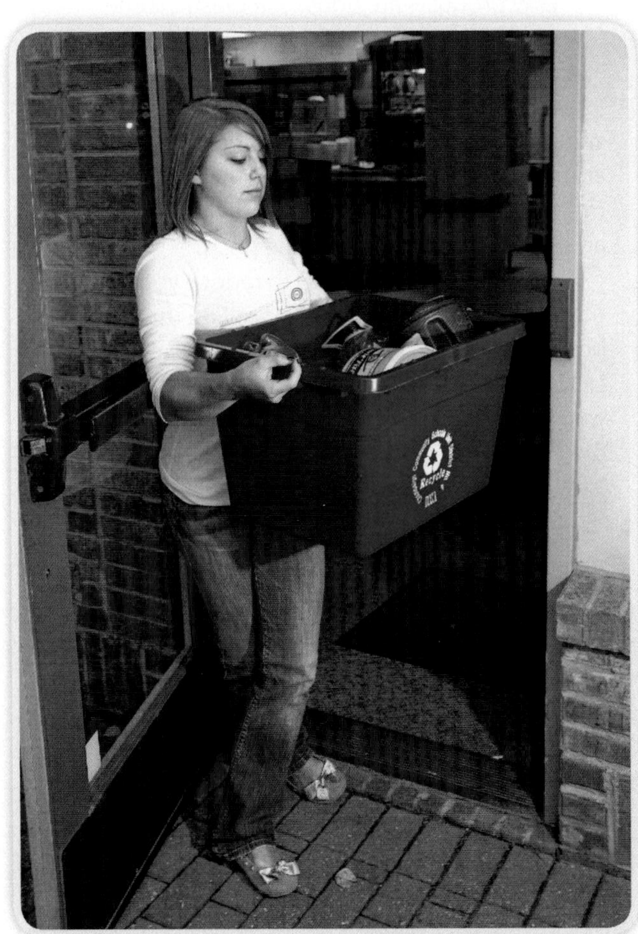

Standards for recycling plastic containers vary by community, so check into the practices followed in your area.

To reduce the amount of trash you produce, you can use a reusable bag for your groceries, buy products with less packaging, and recycle bottles, plastic, newspapers, and aluminum cans. Fast food is one example of overpackaging—it's wrapped and bagged. Donate toys instead of throwing them away. Create a compost pile of decaying organic matter, such as leaves and scraps of food, to provide nutrients and improve soil structure while throwing away food wastes.

You can also go green by changing your energy and water use. Change your lightbulbs to fluorescent bulbs, which use less energy. Don't leave your refrigerator door open too long, because every second adds up to more electricity usage. Ride a bike instead of taking the car to work or school. Turn the water off while brushing your teeth. Run the dishwasher only when it is full. Stop leaks as soon as they are noticed.

Improve your environment by planting a tree, growing a garden, and having indoor plants. Plants provide oxygen to the environment and use carbon dioxide in the process, which cleans up the air.

For even more suggestions on going green, visit the Environmental Health section of the textbook's online student resource.

TEST YOUR KNOWLEDGE
Myth Busters: Energy and Oil Demands

Take a look at these common misconceptions about energy and oil.

Myth: Most of the energy used in the United States comes from oil.

Busted: The United States gets approximately 60 percent of its energy from energy used to create electricity, which includes coal, nuclear power, natural gas, and renewable energy sources. Only 40 percent of energy use is from oil (Energy Information Administration 2008c).

Myth: Most of the U.S. oil supply comes from Saudi Arabia.

Busted: In 2007, about 58 percent of the petroleum (including crude oil and refined petroleum products like gasoline) consumed by the United States was imported from foreign countries. The top five sources of those imports were Canada (18 percent), Saudi Arabia (11 percent), Venezuela (11 percent), Mexico (10 percent), and Nigeria (8 percent) (Energy Information Administration 2008b).

Myth: Most of the domestic oil in the United States comes from Texas.

Busted: In 2006, the top crude oil-producing states were Texas (21 percent of the total U.S. domestic production), Alaska (15 percent), California (12 percent), Louisiana (4 percent), Oklahoma (3 percent), and New Mexico (3 percent). However, offshore production in the Gulf of Mexico accounted for about 25 percent of the total U.S. domestic production (Energy Information Administration 2008a).

Myth: Saudi Arabia produces more oil than any country in the world.

Busted: In 2006, the top five oil-producing countries were Russia (9.25 million barrels per day), Saudi Arabia (9.15 million barrels per day), the United States (5.1 million barrels per day), Iran (4.03 million barrels per day), and China (3.69 million barrels per day). Together, these five countries accounted for about 43 percent of the total world production (Energy Information Administration 2008a).

Myth: The United States produces more crude oil today than ever before.

Busted: In 1970, U.S. domestic production of crude oil average 9.64 million barrels per day. In 2006, that average had fallen to 5.1 million barrels per day—a decrease of about 47 percent (Energy Information Administration 2008a).

ENVIRONMENTAL HEALTH 101

When we talk about environmental health, we're referring to protection against factors in the environment that could be harmful to human health now or to the ecological balances that are necessary for our long-term health. We rely on ecosystems such as forests, freshwater bodies, grasslands, agricultural systems, urban areas, and coastal areas. Humans have a symbiotic relationship with the environment, so we must strive to ensure its health along with our own. People who are exposed to environmental hazards and who are susceptible can develop asthma or cancer, suffer from carbon monoxide poisoning or lead poisoning, and experience other diseases and disorders.

We must try to keep toxins, air pollutants, and water pollutants from contaminating the environment. It's also important to reduce the effects of global warming or climate change by reducing your personal carbon footprint and to manage your waste by reusing or recycling it instead of simply disposing of it. That's part of a larger movement known as going green, a general term used to describe ways to reduce the harmful impact of humans on the environment.

REVIEW QUESTIONS

1. Explain the concept of ecological balance and how it affects ecosystems.
2. How does deforestation present a dilemma to underdeveloped countries?
3. What are agroecosystems, and what dangers do they face?
4. The United States includes four coastal ecosystems. What are they, and what benefits do they provide?
5. What are some potential effects of global climate change?
6. Name three major air pollutants, and explain how they are released into the environment.
7. Describe waste management strategies, from most effective to least effective.
8. Exposure to certain environmental factors can cause diseases or disorders in people who are susceptible. Name three such diseases or disorders and the environmental factors that cause them.
9. What are some ways that you, personally, can help the environment by going green and reducing waste?
10. How can lead enter tap water in people's homes?

CRITICAL THINKING

1. Urban ecosystems—the plants, animals, and humans that inhabit urban environments—vary from city to city. What advice would you give to a city planner to ensure the creation of urban ecosystems that promote leisure activities, wildlife preservation, and low pollution?
2. Scientific research supports the belief that global warming exists and is caused, at least in part, by human activities that change the composition of the atmosphere. However, some people maintain either that climate change is not occurring or that human activity plays no role in it. Why do you think they make this argument, and how do they support it?

APPLICATION ACTIVITIES

1. Find out what your college's waste management strategy is. Get in touch with campus housing to see if there are recycling programs for the residence halls, and contact the maintenance department to find out the policies for disposing of cleaning materials, printer ink, paint, and so on. If you find that the policies aren't as environmentally friendly as you think they should be, develop a plan to take to the student government association to improve the policies.
2. Review the Household Products Database at http://hpd.nlm.nih.gov. Then look under your sink and find the brand names of two chemical cleaning products. Check the database for information taken from the product label or the manufacturer's Material Safety Data Sheet (MSDS) for those brands. Describe the harmful effects of the chemicals and the emergency advice for exposure or ingestion of the chemicals.

GLOSSARY

agroecosystems—Living communities of soil, plants, and animals that constitute farms, croplands, orchards, pastures, and rangelands (Moyers 2007).

arsenic—Odorless and colorless semimetal element that is found naturally in the soil.

CHAPTER REVIEW

asbestos—Harmful mineral fiber that was once used in homes and buildings for insulation and as a fire retardant.

asthma—Condition in which the airways constrict and breathing is difficult.

benzene—Toxic chemical used as a building block for making plastics, rubber, resins, and synthetic fabrics such as nylon and polyester.

biological integrity—The ability to support and maintain a balanced, integrated, and adaptive community of organisms (Karr and Dudley 1981).

cancer—Unchecked growth of cells that form tumors and aggressively grow and invade surrounding tissue.

carbon footprint—Total amount of carbon dioxide attributable to the actions of a person over the course of a year.

carbon monoxide (CO)—Odorless, colorless, tasteless gas that is very toxic.

coastal ecosystems—Areas that are between the water and the land, including estuaries, reefs, mangroves, islands, and salt marshes.

ecological balance—State of dynamic equilibrium within a community of organisms in which genetic, species, and ecosystem diversity remain relatively stable (MOF 2008).

ecosystem—Community of organisms and their environment functioning as an ecological unit.

environmental health—The science of how humans and nature interact to affect the health of humans.

forests—Trees with a canopy that covers a minimum of 10 percent of the ground area (Moyers 2001).

freshwater ecosystems—Ecosystems that include lakes, groundwater, reservoirs, wetlands, ponds, rivers, and streams.

global warming—Increase in the temperature of the atmosphere that contributes to changes in global climate patterns.

grassland ecosystems—Biological communities and habitats with ground cover of grasses and other herbaceous plants, including prairies, meadows, and savannas.

hazardous waste—Waste with properties that make it dangerous to human health and the environment.

hydrochlorofluorocarbons (HCFCs)—Air pollutants that were used in refrigerants and air conditioners in both homes and cars.

lead—Toxic metal that's one of the leading sources of both air and water pollution.

myocardial infarction (MI)—Heart muscle death due to loss of blood supply; also called *heart attack*.

nitrogen oxides (NOx)—Group of highly reactive gases that contain nitrogen and oxygen in varying amounts.

ozone—Gas composed of three oxygen atoms created by a chemical reaction between oxides of nitrogen and volatile organic compounds in the presence of sunlight.

particulate matter—Small particles and liquid droplets including acids, organic chemicals, metals, and soil or dust.

radon—Cancer-causing radioactive gas that you can't see, smell, or taste.

sulfur dioxide (SO_2)—Gas that dissolves easily in water and creates an acid.

susceptibility—Being predisposed to something or lacking the ability to resist something (such as a pathogen, familial disease, or drug).

toxins—Poisonous substances created by organic structures that cause disease or illness upon absorption.

urban ecosystem—Community of plants, animals, and humans that inhabit the urban environment (Moyers 2001).

waste management—Includes collection, transfer, disposal, recycling, and renewable energy.

REFERENCES AND RESOURCES

American Cancer Society. 2008. Known and probable human carcinogens. www.cancer.org/docroot/PED/content/PED_1_3x_Known_and_Probable_Carcinogens.asp.

American Pregnancy Association (APA). 2007. Birth defects. www.americanpregnancy.org/birthdefects/.

Arrington, D. 1998. Case study: Jackson Paper Manufacturing Company. www.p2pays.org/ref/07/06120.pdf.

Borchardt, M.A., K.R. Bradbur, M.B. Gotkowitz, J.A. Cherry, and B.L. Parker. 2007. Human enteric viruses in groundwater from a confined bedrock aquifer. *Environmental Science & Technology* 41: 6606-6612.

Centers for Disease Control and Prevention (CDC). 2006. CDC's National Environmental Public Health Tracking Program: National Network Implementation Plan. www.cdc.gov/nceh/tracking/pdfs/nnip.pdf.

———. 2007. General lead information: Questions and answers. www.cdc.gov/nceh/lead/faq/about.htm.

———. 2008. Carbon monoxide poisoning. www.cdc.gov/co/faqs.htm.

Energy Information Administration. 2008a. Crude oil production. www.eia.doe.gov/neic/infosheets/crudeproduction.html.

———. 2008b. How dependent are we on foreign oil? http://tonto.eia.doe.gov/energy_in_brief/foreign_oil_dependence.cfm.

———. 2008c. Petroleum products: Consumption. www.eia.doe.gov/neic/infosheets/petroleumproductsconsumption.html.

Environmental Defense Fund (EDF). 2002. Nitrogen oxides: How NOx emissions affect human health and the environment. www.edf.org/documents/2551_FactSheet_NOx.pdf.

Environmental Literacy Council. 2007. Coastal areas. www.enviroliteracy.org/subcategory.php/9.html.

Environmental Protection Agency (EPA). 2000a. *Giardia*: Drinking water fact sheet. www.epa.gov/waterscience/criteria/humanhealth/microbial/giardiafs.pdf.

———. 2000b. *Legionella*: Drinking water fact sheet. www.epa.gov/waterscience/criteria/humanhealth/microbial/legionellafs.pdf.

———. 2001. *Cryptosporidium*: Drinking water health advisory. www.epa.gov/waterscience/criteria/humanhealth/microbial/cryptoha.pdf.

———. 2006a. *Aeromonas*: Human health criteria document. www.epa.gov/waterscience/criteria/humanhealth/microbial/aeromonas-200603.pdf.

———. 2006b. Consumer factsheet on benzene. www.epa.gov/safewater/contaminants/dw_contamfs/benzene.html.

———. 2007a. Arsenic in drinking water: Basic information. www.epa.gov/safewater/arsenic/basicinformation.html.

———. 2007b. Biological integrity. www.epa.gov/bioindicators/html/biointeg.html.

———. 2007c. Dredged material management. www.epa.gov/owow/oceans/regulatory/dumpdredged/dredgemgmt.html.

———. 2007d. Indoor air quality. www.epa.gov/iaq/index.html.

———. 2007e. Lead in drinking water. www.epa.gov/safewater/lead/index.html.

———. 2008a. Drinking water contaminants. www.epa.gov/safewater/contaminants/index.html.

———. 2008b. Ecosystems. www.epa.gov/ebtpages/ecosystems.html.

———. 2008c. Frequent questions. www.epa.gov/climatechange/fq/index.html.

Florida Department of Environmental Protection. 2008. Salt marshes. www.dep.state.fl.us/coastal/habitats/saltmarshes.htm.

Food and Agriculture Organization of the United Nations. 2005. Global forest resources assessment 2005: Progress towards sustainable forest management. www.fao.org/DOCREP/008/a0400e/a0400e00.htm.

Karr, J.R., and D.R. Dudley. 1981. Ecological perspective on water quality goals. *Environmental Management* 5: 55-68.

Mac, M.J., P.A. Opler, C.E. Puckett Haecker, and P.D. Doran. 1998. *Status and trends of the nation's biological resources*. 2 vols. U.S. Department of the Interior, U.S. Geological Survey, Reston, VA. http://biology.usgs.gov/pubs/execsumm/page2.htm.

Medline. 2008. Lead poisoning. www.nlm.nih.gov/medlineplus/leadpoisoning.html.

Ministry of Forests (MOF). 2008. Glossary of forest terms in British Columbia. www.for.gov.bc.ca/hfd/library/documents/glossary/Glossary.pdf.

Moyers, B. 2001. Ecosystems [Television]. In *Earth on the edge,* producer P.B. Network. Public Affairs Television.

National Environmental Health Association. 1996. Environmental health. www.neha.org/position_papers/def_env_health.html.

National Oceanic and Atmospheric Administration (NOAA). 2008a. Coral reef conservation. http://oceanservice.noaa.gov/topics/oceans/coralreefs/.

———. 2008b. What is an estuary? http://oceanservice.noaa.gov/education/kits/estuaries/estuaries01_whatis.html.

New York State Parks. 2003. More about the Adirondack Park. www.apa.state.ny.us/About_Park/more_park.html.

Rückerl, R., S. Greven, P. Ljungman, P. Aalto, C. Antoniades, T. Bellander, N. Berglind, C. Chrysohoou, F. Forastiere, B. Jacquemin, S. Von Klot, W. Koenig, H. Kuchenhoff, T. Lanki, J. Pekkanen, C.A. Perucci, A. Schneider, J. Sunyer, and A. Peters. 2007. Air pollution and inflammation (interleukin-6, C-reactive protein, fibrinogen) in myocardial infarction survivors. *Environmental Health Perspectives* 115 (7): 1072-1080.

Schettler, T. 2004. Autism: Do environmental factors play a role in causation? *Science and Environmental Health Network*. www.healthandenvironment.org/autism/peer_reviewed.

United Nations Environment Programme (UNEP). 2008. Gender and the environment: Inspiring examples. www.unep.org/gender_env/inspiring/.

U.S. Fish and Wildlife Service (FWS). 2008. John H. Chafee Coastal Barrier Resource System. www.fws.gov/habitatconservation/coastal_barrier.html.

U.S. Geological Survey. n.d. Science topics: Grassland ecosystems. www.usgs.gov/science/science.php?term=499.

Waste Management (WM). 2007. About Waste Management. www.thinkgreen.com.

World Health Organization (WHO). 2008. Environmental health. www.who.int/topics/environmental_health/en/.

Other helpful resources include the following.

Booker, J., B. Keogh, D. Chu, J. Conner, and I. Hooper. 1998. *Mangroves.* Florida Department of Education and Seacamp Association.

Holmes, J. 2008. The unequal distribution of water. British Broadcasting Network: Global Eye. www.globaleye.org.uk/secondary_spring01/focuson/index.html.

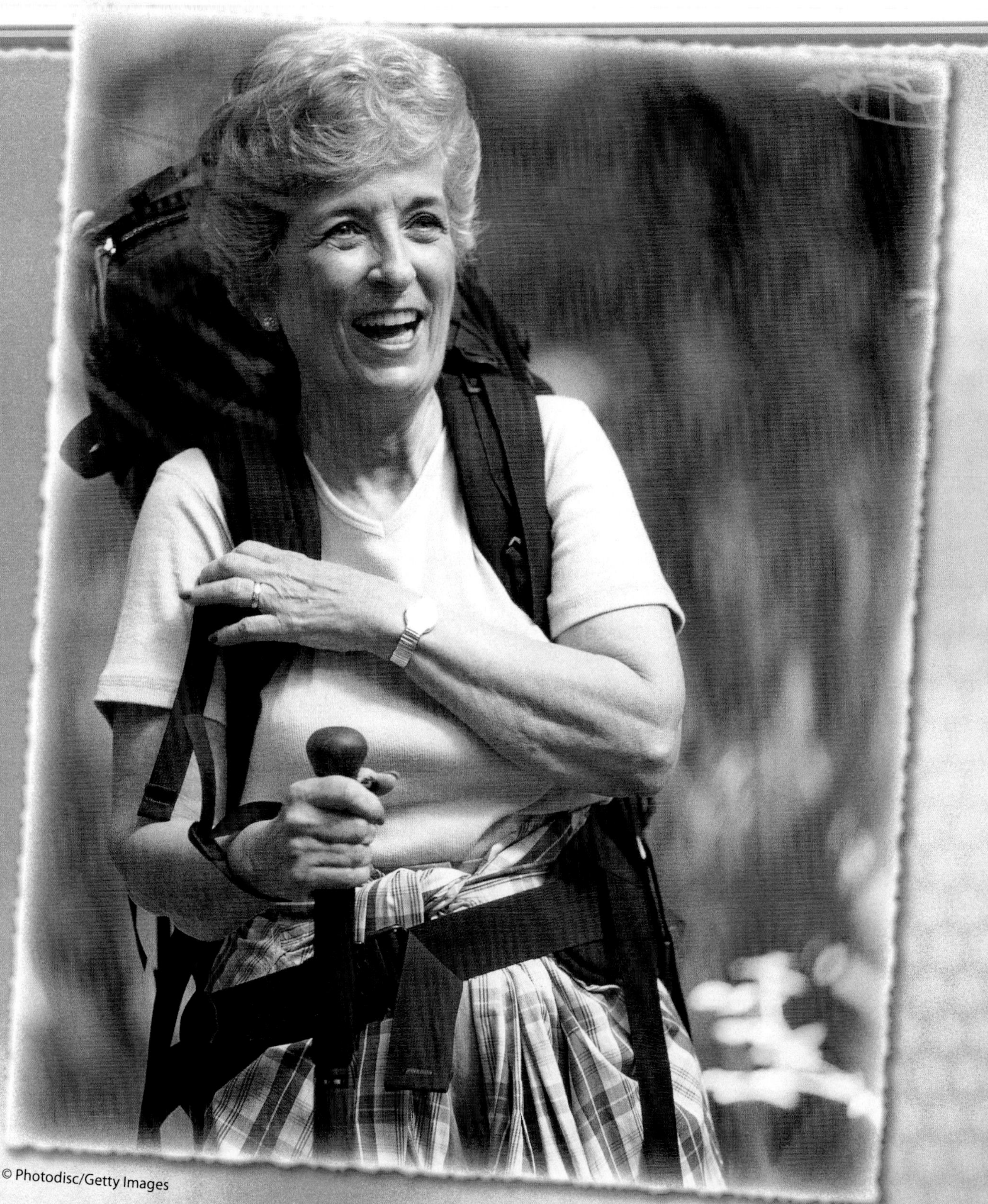

© Photodisc/Getty Images

CHAPTER 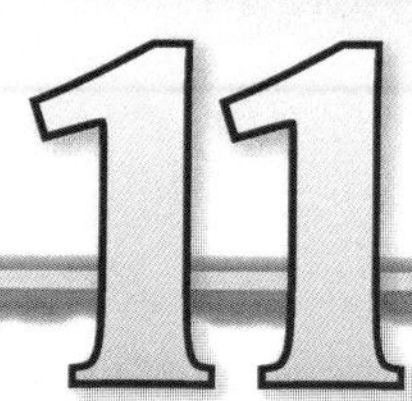

HEALTHY AGING

PAMELA DOUGHTY, PHD, CHES
Institute for Obesity Research and Program Evaluation,
Texas A&M University

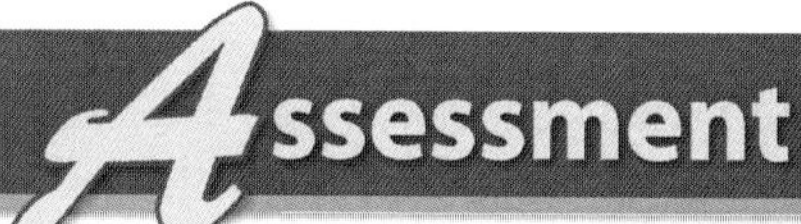

Assessment

- What age does someone have to be for you to consider that person "old"?
- Can smoking cause your skin to age?
- Do human bodies wear out from use?
- What is the number one killer of Hispanics, African Americans, Native Americans, and white non-Hispanics in the United States?
- Do you know anyone who has a brain disease such as Alzheimer's disease, Pick's disease, or Parkinson's disease?
- What is hospice care?

Objectives

- Identify how the aging process and onset of diseases relate to each other.
- Describe parts of the human body that undergo changes due to age.
- Describe what role genetics and lifestyle play in the way a person ages.
- Describe at least one theory of aging.
- Determine which theory of aging best explains how humans age.

If you were asked how old is *old*, what would you say? Chances are, you'd say people who are between 50 and 60 are old. Your parent or guardian, on the other hand, would have a different answer. And, if your grandparents are still living, they'd pick still a different age. One researcher found that no matter what age they are, people define *old* as 30 years older than they are presently. So, if you're 20 you think 50 is old, and 50-year-olds say 80 is old. The reason for this phenomenon is unclear. Maybe 30 years down the road is the farthest people can project themselves into the future. Defining age categories when speaking about older people is important because a simple number isn't enough. Scientists and researchers categorize age this way: *Older* is ages 65 to 75, *old* is 76 to 85, and *oldest old* is 86 and older. You might consider another age to be old, but those categories are the ones that will apply in this chapter.

You can't help getting older, but you can control *how* you age to some extent. Only 30 percent of how a person ages is due to genetics (Finch and Tanzi 1997). The remainder is due to **lifestyle**, including whether you smoke, how much you exercise, what you eat, whether you have friends, what your socioeconomic status is, and how much education you have. Many people in North America today will reach age 75, but whether they are healthy and to what extent they enjoy their remaining years will be influenced more by lifestyle than by genetic predisposition.

MORE PEOPLE ARE LIVING LONGER

In the mid-1930s, people in the United States died in their mid-50s, and 65-year-olds were usually old and frail. President Franklin Roosevelt signed the Social Security Act in 1935 to help frail, elderly people have an income. With the advent of better medical technology and sanitation, life expectancy has improved. Figure 11.1 illustrates how life spans have lengthened over time and projects trends for the future.

In the traditional pyramid of the U.S. population, children outnumbered all the other age groups in the population. Many children were being born, but few lived to old age. The population looked like a triangle, with most people in the lower age groups and few people in the older populations at the top of the pyramid. Beginning in the 1980s, the shape of the aging pyramid has become more rectangular, with projections estimating similar numbers of people in all age groups by 2020. The 85-plus age group is now the fastest growing population in the world. The change in the makeup of the U.S. population is similar in all populations of the world (Cheitlin 2003).

In 2007, 76 million Americans were between the ages of 43 and 62. Since their births, these baby boomers (people born between 1945 and 1964) have composed the largest segment of the population. They overburdened hospitals when they were born and schools as they grew up. It's hard to tell exactly what effect their aging will have on the population, but they're expected to overextend Social Security and Medicare, making both programs insolvent by 2020 (Office of Public Affairs 2005). Many boomers will live beyond 100. If they leave work at age 65, they'll spend 35 years in retirement, which means that one out of every five people in the United States in 2020 will be retired from work. Today's college students will benefit from what scientists learn about healthy aging as they watch the boomers age. What will current knowledge contribute to baby boomers aging well? How will this change over the next decades as young people age? Those questions will be answered throughout the chapter.

BODY SYSTEM CHANGES DURING AGING

Our organs and body systems age, including the integumentary (skin and hair), cardiovascular, renal, digestive, nervous, skeletal, and muscular systems. Research has shown that each system ages differently. However, when drawing conclusions from the research about how body systems age, it's important to differentiate the effects of aging from the effects of disease (Cheitlin 2003).

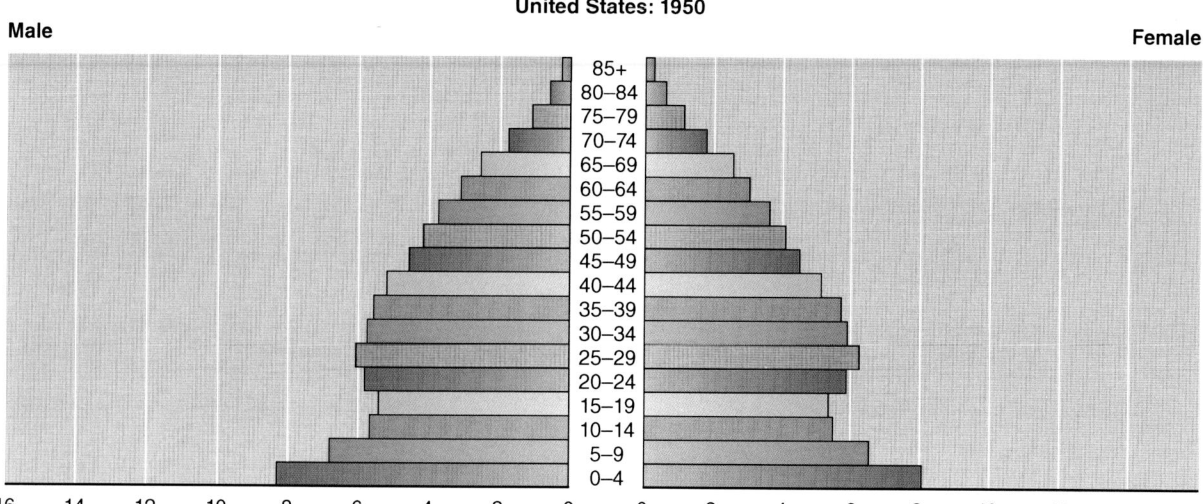

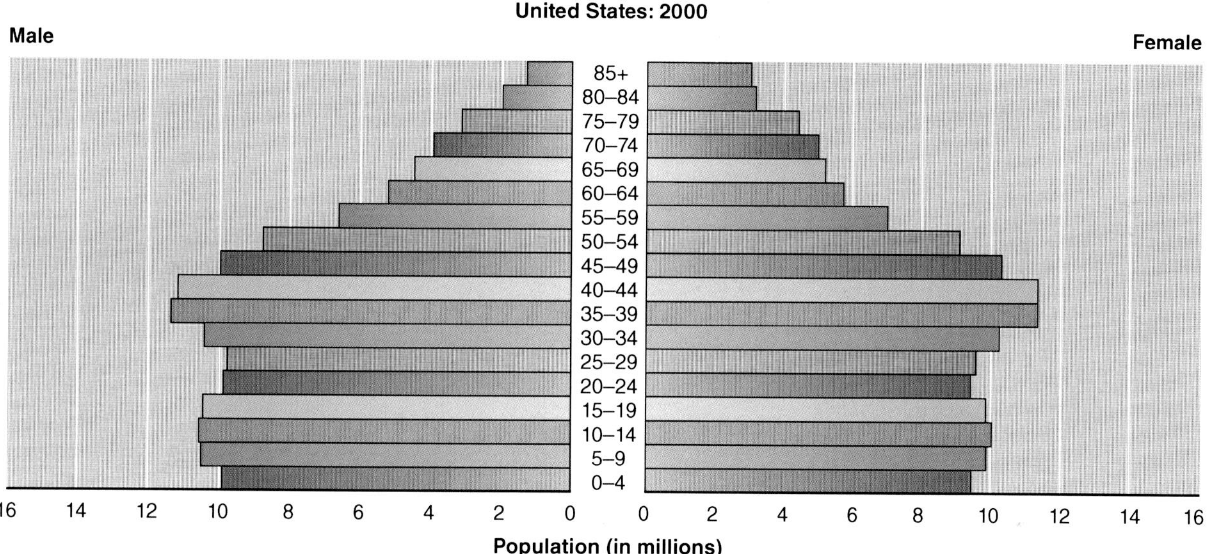

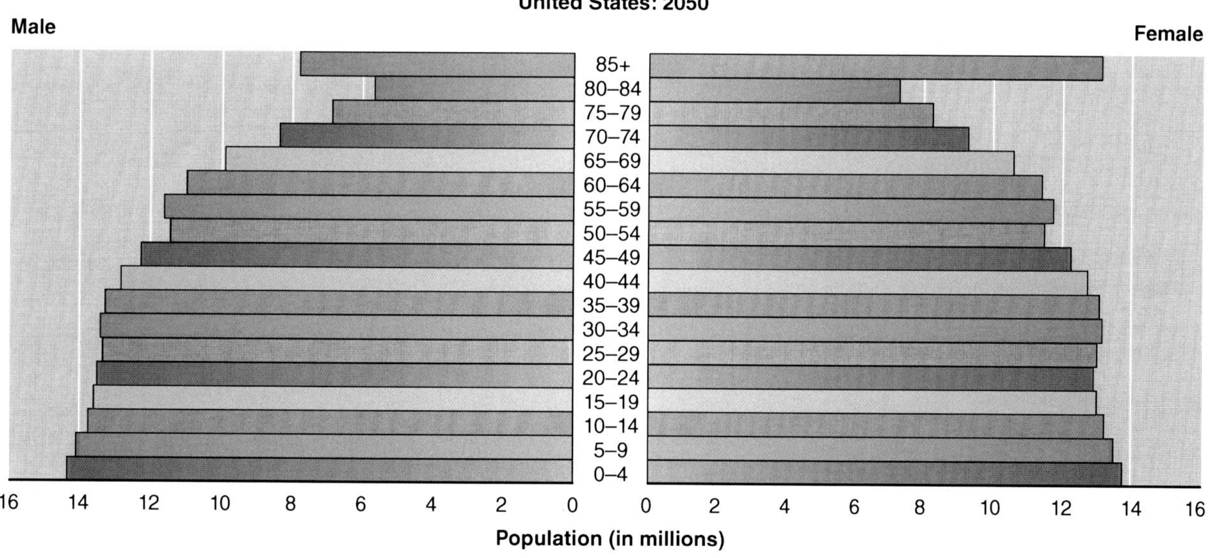

Figure 11.1 Traditionally, the U.S. population had most people in the lower age groups and few people in the older populations at the top of the pyramid. The aging pyramid has become more rectangular as people live longer.

Source: U.S. Census Bureau, International Database.

Skin and Hair

How old would you guess the men in figure 11.2 are? What did you think about as you made your guess? The condition of people's skin and hair influences how their age is judged. People with wrinkles and white hair (or no hair) are usually assumed to be older than those with few wrinkles and hair that's not gray or white.

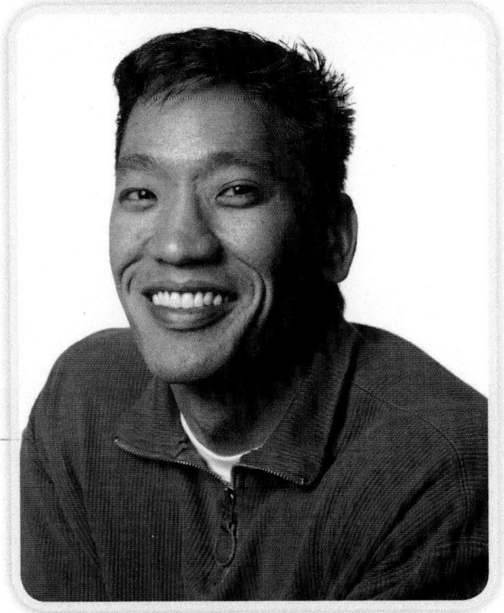

© Photodisc/Barbara Penoyar

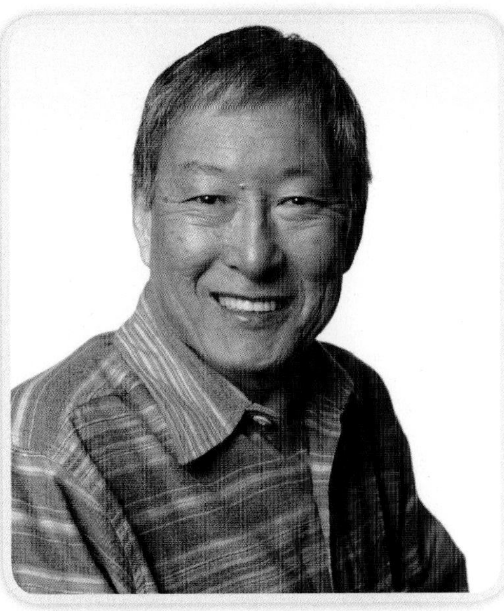

© Photodisc/Barbara Penoyar

Figure 11.2 Changes in skin and hair are obvious signs of aging.

After age 20, skin begins to show signs of aging. Here are some genetic signs that skin and hair are aging (AgingSkinNet 2005):

- Appearance of fine wrinkles
- Thinning skin
- Loss of underlying fat, leading to hollowed cheeks and eye sockets as well as noticeable loss of firmness on the hands and neck
- Bones shrinking away from the skin due to bone loss, which causes sagging skin
- Dry skin that may itch
- Inability to sweat sufficiently to cool the skin
- Graying hair that eventually turns white
- Hair loss
- Growth of unwanted hair, such as in the ears and nose
- Thinning nail plates where the half moons disappear and ridges develop

Those factors affect everyone as a normal part of the aging process. Other factors that aren't genetic, such as how much time you spend in the sun, whether you smoke, and how you sleep, may cause skin and hair to look prematurely old. You can control many of those effects.

What Do You Do?

Go to http://morph.cs.st-andrews.ac.uk/fof/. Upload a current photo of yourself and follow the directions on the Web site to see how you might look when you're 20 years, 30 years, or even 50 years older.

To prevent wrinkling from the sun, protect yourself with sunblock with an SPF over 30, wear protective clothing, and limit time in the sun between 10:00 a.m. and 2:00 p.m.

Smoking causes the skin to age due to the lack of oxygen to the skin and because the tobacco in cigarettes poisons the skin. Smoking narrows the blood vessels in the skin, which inhibits blood flow and thus reduces the amount of oxygen available to the skin cells. Smoking also damages the collagen and elastin in the skin, which reduces the flexibility of the skin and thus increases lines and wrinkles. Smiling and frowning a lot also causes wrinkles. Don't worry too much about trying to avoid repetitive facial expressions, though. You may avoid a few wrinkles, but you'd lose some personality in the process.

Sleeping positions can cause wrinkling, too. Sleeping on your front or side crumples the skin in the same way every night, causing wrinkles. Sleeping on your back can eliminate this cause of wrinkles (AgingSkinNet 2005).

Hair loss and hair gradually turning white or gray are genetic, and you can't do anything to change them. Products are available to regrow hair, but they must be applied every day because hair begins to fall out again when the applications stop. These products aren't always effective for male pattern baldness, but they can help men and women whose hair thins with age. Men and women also cover the signs of aging hair with hair coloring.

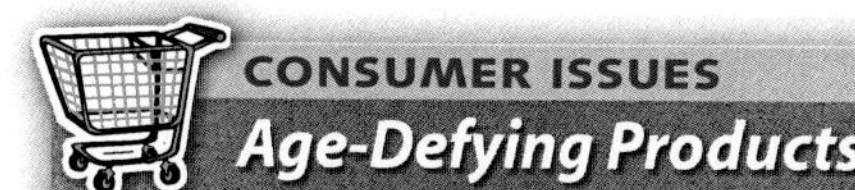

CONSUMER ISSUES

Age-Defying Products

Get the advertising circulars for a drugstore, such as Walgreens or CVS, from a Sunday newspaper. Count how many products are intended to reduce the signs of aging on the skin or hair. For example, treatments to rejuvenate the skin include creams, pills, microdermabrasion, peels, and home spa products, and treatments for younger-looking hair include color, thickeners, products to enhance shine, extensions, and more. After you've counted the products, consider which ones are most appealing or seem like they'd be the most effective, based on their ad alone.

Cardiovascular System

A study done in 2001 looked at the hearts of over 260 people who showed no symptoms of atherosclerosis, or hardening and narrowing of the arteries (WebMD n.d.). Nearly 52 percent of the subjects had some degree of atherosclerosis, including 17 percent of teenagers and 85 percent of people older than 50. In general, most people over 60 have some atherosclerosis, even if they don't notice any symptoms. The risk for coronary artery disease increases with age, as plaque builds up in arteries. In men, the risk increases after age 45; in women, after age 55 (National Heart, Lung, and Blood Institute n.d.). However, it can be hard to tell the difference between the changes in the heart that result from aging and those that result from disease.

Research has suggested that the heart ages when the number of myocardial cells in the heart is reduced, the fibrous valves harden, and the structure of the heart and its left ventricle hypertrophy. However, other research has shown that with consistent exercise, even seniors can grow new heart cells and improve the flexibility of the heart valves (Kemi et al. 2007). More research will need to be done before a distinction can be made between an inactive older adult and an active older adult and what part age plays in the decline of the cardiovascular system. The best defense against heart disease is controlling the factors that you can, which would include eating a healthy diet and getting adequate exercise to keep your heart as healthy as you can for as long as you can.

Renal System

The renal system includes the kidneys and the urine production system. As you age, the kidneys decrease from 250 to 270 grams at age 30 to 180 to 200 grams at age 70 (Beers 2007). The result is a less efficient kidney, because the volume of urine that it can accommodate is smaller, causing an older person to need to urinate more often than a younger person.

Digestive System

Few changes in the digestive system occur because of aging. Some minor changes do happen, but they don't have a big effect on how the digestive system functions. The stomach lining, for example, may become less resistant to disease due to the decline of the immune system and can make stomach ulcers more likely. Also, the contractions of the esophageal sphincter become weaker with age, but the weaker contractions don't restrict the passage of food. Compared with the other system of the body, the digestive system is relatively unaffected by the aging process (Beers 2007).

Brain

As the brain ages, it takes longer to retrieve information, but the store of information is greater and older people are better at problem solving than younger people (Blanchard-Fields 2007). Over time, brain mass declines, the outer surface thins, and white matter declines. The white matter (which contains the nerve fibers of the brain) is thought to shrink with age, particularly in the frontal lobe, which houses old memories, and in the hippocampus, where new memories are stored. Also, neurotransmitters such as serotonin and dopamine find fewer receptors to connect to, inhibiting information from being transferred from one nerve cell to the next. However, scientists are still discovering how amazing the brain is. One 2007 study discovered that even the oldest-old brain can still make neurons, repairing damaged connections and rerouting others. This process increases the availability of memories (Blanchard-Fields 2007).

Bones and Muscles

As the body ages, bones thin and begin to lose their strength and are also more prone to breaking. Older people lose height because the fluid-filled discs that separate the vertebrae in the spine tend to lose water and flatten and because the feet lose fat padding and grow flatter over the years. Joints become stiffer and lose cartilage. However, ankles change very little due to age. In women more often than in men, the fingers lose cartilage and the bones thicken; that may be hereditary. Muscles can lose their tone and become more rigid, and replacement of muscle fiber slows, even with exercise. These changes can affect the gait and can increase the chances of falling, which is one of the major concerns for the old and oldest old (Channel 2006).

Although aging does change the bones, muscles, and joints, exercise can help reduce those changes and keep the flexibility and strength needed for everyday activities and disease prevention. Exercise can also reduce the risk of osteoporosis, arthritis, and gait changes. Studies with master athletes, or people who train all of their lives, have shown that even though muscle mass decreases, strength and endurance do not decrease until later in life.

What Do You Think?

How many of the body system changes described in this chapter do you think are simply a result of genetics, and how many do you think can be controlled through lifestyle factors such as nutrition and exercise?

AGING THEORIES

You've just read about the changes that happen to the body as it ages. Scientists have long been studying what causes those changes to happen. Some theories have fallen out of favor whereas others have been widely accepted. There are somewhere around 300 theories, but this chapter discusses only the top 6. As you learn about these theories, consider which of them seems most reasonable to you.

Wear and Tear

The wear and tear theory of aging was one of the first to explain why people age. Scientists observed that older people lost muscle mass and had poor cardiovascular systems, joint problems, and chronic illnesses. They concluded that the body was wearing out. Now scientists are aware that although muscle mass declines with age, people can improve muscle tone and cardiovascular and mental health by exercising. The wear and tear theory is no longer considered valid.

Rate of Living

Another theory that has fallen out of favor is the rate of living theory. It suggested that a person's metabolic rate determines life span—the faster the body is used, the sooner it will burn out. In other words, people with a higher metabolic rate were thought to live fewer years than people with a lower metabolic rate.

It's easy to refute this theory—simply compare a bird with an animal of similar size. The metabolism of the bird is one-and-a-half to two times faster than any animal of comparable size, but the bird lives two to three times longer than the animal (Speakman 2005). Human bodies do not wear out from use, either; it's much more likely for a human to develop disease and mental decline because of disuse rather than overuse. Exercise improves the health of older and younger adults, increases metabolic rate, and does not wear out the body over time.

Evolutionary Programmed Senescence

Another theory about why we age is the evolutionary programmed senescence theory. Senescence is the process of aging whereby the capacity for cell division and growth and function are gradually lost (Beers 2007). The theory posits that within the genetic code is a switch that starts the aging, or senescence, process. Before the switch is turned on, certain genes are present to protect against disease. These protective features increase the chances that the organism will be healthy enough to reproduce in its younger years. After the possibility of reproduction ends, the aging switch is thrown. The body may have a protective feature that, for example, prevents younger people from getting cancer. When the reproductive years have passed, that feature would be turned off, allowing older adults to contract cancer. Evolutionary theory supports this hypothesis, because the key to the continuation of a species is reproduction. The continuation of protective features would be unnecessary after reproduction because the healthy parents produced healthy offspring.

Research was conducted with fruit flies that prevented them from mating until later in life (Arking 2005). The flies lived longer, healthier lives until after reproduction. However, the offspring of these flies were not as healthy when they were young as fruit flies born to younger parents, because the natural protective features were turned on later in life. The offspring without the protective features had a higher death rate at a younger age, keeping them from reproducing later in life. If these young adult fruit flies died before reproducing, eventually the species would no longer exist.

The results support the evolutionary aspect of programmed senescence occurring after reproduction, because human beings are the only animal that lives many years after the ability to reproduce ends. No information is available that tells us whether lifestyle can inhibit the start of these clocks.

Immune Theory

The immune theory could explain why we develop chronic illness late in life. It states that the immune system is compromised in some areas and overreacts in others as the body ages. With a poor immune system, the body can't fight off chronic diseases such as cancer, Alzheimer's disease, and Parkinson's disease or autoimmune diseases such as rheumatoid arthritis, lupus, and others. Autoimmune and other diseases cause a severe decline in function due to fatigue and joint pain, and they often eventually lead to death.

Free Radical Theory (Oxidative Damage)

The **free radical theory**, or oxidative damage theory, proposes that free radicals damage cells, including their DNA. Free radicals are released from the electron transport chain in the mitochondria during regular cell production, and cells leak hydrogen and oxygen molecules from the electron transport chain. The molecules are looking for the missing electrons for bonding, and they rip off hydrogen and oxygen molecules from cell walls.

This action damages the cells' outer membranes and can damage the DNA. Damage to the cells contributes to many age-related diseases, such as cancer, heart disease, diabetes, and Alzheimer's disease. Researchers are spending a lot of time studying free radical theory. One 2007 research project with sedentary mice showed that exercise increased the release of free radicals for the first few weeks. But when the mice continued to exercise, the number of free radicals released from the electron transfer chain was reduced. The cells had become more efficient with consistent exercise. In other words, it is thought that people who exercise consistently reduce the damage of free radicals by reducing the number of free radicals that can attack healthy cells. The results suggest that consistent exercise could reduce age-related diseases (Kwak, Song, and Lawler 2007).

Telomere Theory

Telomeres are the ends of the chromosome strands made from DNA, and their function is similar to that of the plastic ends of shoelaces. Just as those ends keep the shoelace from unraveling, telomeres keep chromosomes from unraveling ("UCSF's Elizabeth Blackburn receives Lasker Award" 2007). The **telomere theory** of aging states that as cells split, the telomeres shrink, getting smaller and smaller each time they divide. Eventually this causes the cell to die and increases the chance of getting a terminal disease.

UNHEALTHY AGING

No matter what causes body systems to age, the effects can be devastating for people who don't adopt behaviors that lead to healthy aging. Unhealthy older people often experience chronic diseases, dementia, and other health problems including stroke, heart attack, cancer, malignancies of the immune system, and pneumonia.

Chronic Diseases

Chronic diseases are diseases that affect a person's health over a long time. Some examples of chronic diseases are cardiovascular disease, osteoporosis, diabetes, and arthritis. For instance, cardiovascular disease occurs at rates of 52 per 100,000 in men between the ages of 35 and 44, but it occurs at rates of 3,239 per 100,000 in men aged 75 to 84. For women, the disease occurs at rates of 3 per 100,000 in women between the ages of 35 and 44, but it occurs at rates of 2,122 per 100,000 in women between the ages of 75 and 84 (Santoro 2007). In 2006 in the United States, 1.6 percent of Caucasian females younger than 45 years old had been diagnosed with type 2 diabetes, but 14.3 percent of Caucasian females over 75 years old had been diagnosed with the disease (Centers for Disease Control and Prevention [CDC] 2008).

What Do You Think?

You might notice that many of the chronic diseases covered in this section can be prevented or controlled with exercise and a healthy diet. Why, then, do you think so many people have those diseases as they get older?

Cardiovascular Disease

Cardiovascular disease (CVD) is the number one killer of Hispanics, African Americans, Native Americans, and white non-Hispanics in the United States. In 2005, cardiovascular disease caused nearly 27 percent of all deaths (Kung, Hoyert, Xu, and Murphy 2008). The risk factors for heart

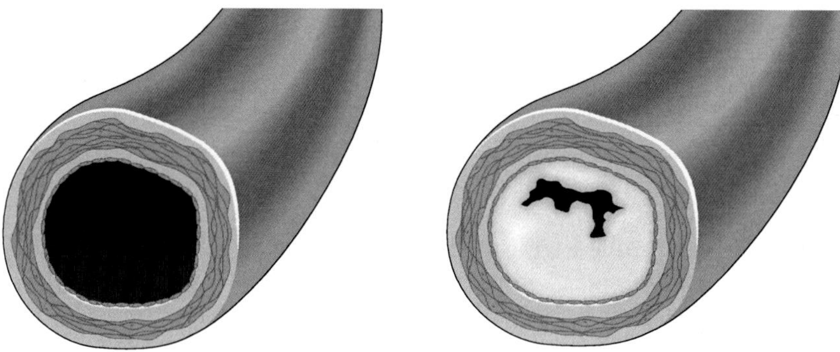

Figure 11.3 The risk for coronary artery disease, a form of cardiovascular disease, increases with age as a fatty material known as plaque builds up in the arteries around the heart.

disease are hypertension (high blood pressure), high cholesterol, diabetes, little no or physical activity, obesity, and smoking. CVD can result from atherosclerosis, which is caused when plaque gradually builds up in arteries due to poor exercise and eating habits (see figure 11.3). This buildup blocks the arteries to and within the heart. When the plaque breaks loose, the small particles block the blood to the heart and cause a heart attack. Depending where the particle breaks off, it can also go to the brain, causing a stroke and killing part of the brain.

CVD can be controlled by reducing cholesterol levels in the blood or by thinning the blood to allow blood to bypass the blockages. Both can be done with medication. However, exercising regularly, losing weight, and eating healthier can also help control CVD. Sometimes these methods can reduce or eliminate the need for medication.

Osteoporosis

Osteoporosis is a disease that occurs when bone density decreases due to a reduction of calcium and vitamin D. When this happens, the bones are gradually absorbed by the body as the calcium is used in the muscles. The people most at risk for osteoporosis are white non-Hispanic women and Asian women of slender build. Common signs of osteoporosis are hunched shoulders and a swayed back (see figure 11.4). However, early detection—the key to reducing the risk of fractures from reduced bone density—can be made with a bone density scan.

Spine fractures are the most common result of osteoporosis, with hip and limb fractures close behind. It takes a long time to recover from those fractures, and many older adults die within a year of the fracture. Load-bearing exercises and a diet rich in calcium and vitamin D can reduce the incidence of osteoporosis. Fosamax, a once-daily pill, can actually increase bone density, but a person must be able to sit or stand for 30 to 60 minutes after taking it, which prevents some frail older adults from using this remedy.

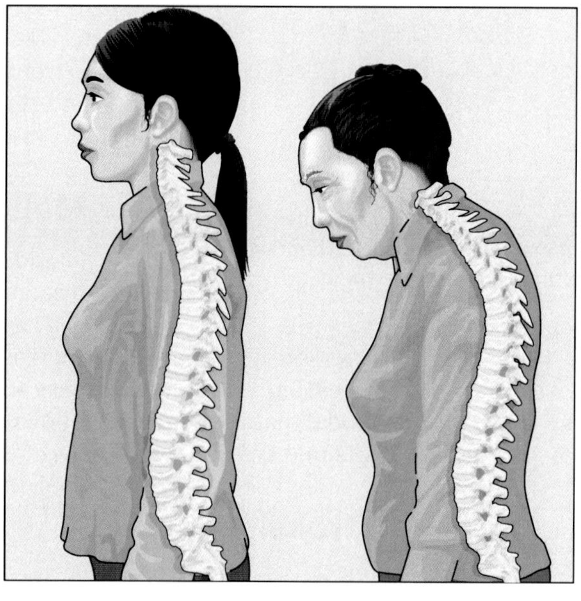

Figure 11.4 Hunched shoulders and a swayed back are signs of osteoporosis.

Diabetes

There are two types of **diabetes**: type 1 and type 2. Type 1 diabetes is genetic and usually starts in early childhood and sometimes early adulthood. In type 1 diabetes, the body does not produce insulin, which is the hormone that breaks down glucose. Without insulin, there is an overabundance of glucose in the blood, which causes damage to the heart, kidneys, liver, and eyes. When uncontrolled, type 1 diabetes causes blockages to the heart, lower extremities, and brain, leading to heart disease, stroke, and the need to amputate limbs. Type 1 diabetes is controlled through a combination of injections of insulin and diet, but there is no cure.

People develop type 2 diabetes when the body resists insulin. The pancreas produces insulin. In people with type 2 diabetes, the body stops using insulin because it does little to reduce the amount of glucose in the blood. As the body becomes more resistant to insulin, the pancreas reduces the amount of insulin it makes. Type 2 diabetes used to be called *adult-onset diabetes* because only adults contracted it. Now children as young as 10 have been diagnosed with the disease. Type 2 diabetes can be prevented by eating a healthy diet, exercising, and maintaining a healthy weight.

Type 2 diabetes is controlled with medication that increases insulin usage and insulin production. Good nutrition and exercise are also important in preventing and controlling type 2 diabetes. Most people with the disease should lose weight and reduce the amount of carbohydrate they eat. Thirty minutes of aerobic exercise a day increases the body's production and use of insulin.

Arthritis

Arthritis is inflammation of the joints, which causes pain, swelling, and limited movement (MedlinePlus 2008). Osteoarthritis is the most common type of arthritis and is caused by degeneration of the joints. It affects the hands, hips, and knees most often. Risk factors for osteoarthritis are being overweight, previously injuring the joint, and moving the joint in a repetitive motion (a baseball pitcher, for example, can develop osteoarthritis in the elbows and shoulders).

Rheumatoid arthritis is an autoimmune disease that usually develops in people between the ages of 25 and 55. Rheumatoid arthritis compromises the connective tissue in any of the joints, including the hands and feet. It causes swelling and can eventually deform the joints. Figure 11.5 shows the results of untreated late-stage rheumatoid arthritis of the hands. Medications now exist that can stop the progression of rheumatoid arthritis by keeping the immune system from damaging the joints; however, the side effects of the medication can bring an increase in bacterial infection and viruses because the immune system is compromised.

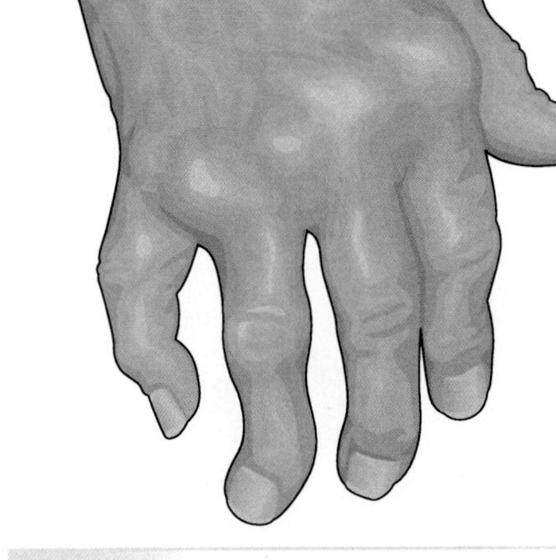

Figure 11.5 Late-stage rheumatoid arthritis of joints in the hand.

Malignancies of the Immune System

In addition to chronic diseases such as CVD, osteoporosis, diabetes, and arthritis, other health conditions become more prevalent with age. Because the immune system becomes compromised as a person ages, there is an increase in the incidence and severity of cancer in the old and the oldest old. The immune theory and evolutionary programmed senescence theory support the model that as people age, they become less resistant to diseases caused by a compromised immune system.

Stroke

When a person has a stroke, areas of the brain die due to broken blood vessels and the lack of blood in other parts of the brain. Symptoms of a stroke are tingling in the face or extremities, loss of bowel control, slurring speech, not comprehending written or spoken language, and loss of movement on one side of the body. People who experience any of these symptoms should seek immediate treatment. Early detection and treatment, including taking aspirin, can prevent some of the damage.

Dementia

Dementia is a general category for a group of symptoms caused by disorders that affect two or more functions of the brain. People with dementia may not be able to think properly, and it affects their ability to do routine activities such as eating or dressing. They may have difficulty controlling their emotions or making decisions. Some people with dementia see things that are not there and become agitated easily for no apparent reason. In the beginning of dementia, people are aware of the decline in memory and the change in personality. This awareness can result in depression, which should be treated with antianxiety or depression medication. Both the patient and the family need support as dementia progresses. Causes of dementia include Alzheimer's disease, Pick's disease, Parkinson's disease, and stroke (MedlinePlus 2007).

Alzheimer's Disease

Alzheimer's disease (AD) is a degenerative brain disease that affects memory, thinking, and behavior. Only 1 percent of people over age 65 have AD, but 25 percent of people over age 75 have the disease. A family history of AD increases the chances of having the disease in later life (MedlinePlus 2007).

AD prevents the neurons in the brain from sending messages by making tangles, or insoluble, twisted fibers that build up inside the nerve cell, and plaque, which is dense, mostly insoluble deposits of protein and cellular material outside and around the neurons (National Institute on Aging [NIA] 2006). Over time, the brain dies. AD progresses very gradually, and it might last 10 to 15 years from diagnosis to death. Figure 11.6 shows the physical effects of AD on a brain.

Early symptoms include memory decline and disrupted thinking, and the symptoms at this point may be subtle and are often attributed to natural aging. Symptoms are progressive and include the following:

- Repeating statements
- Misplacing items
- Having trouble finding names for familiar objects
- Getting lost on familiar routes
- Changing personality
- Losing interest in things previously enjoyed
- Having difficulty performing tasks that used to come easily, such as balancing a checkbook or learning new information or routines

In more advanced stages, symptoms are more obvious:

- Forgetting details about current events
- Forgetting events in one's own life history

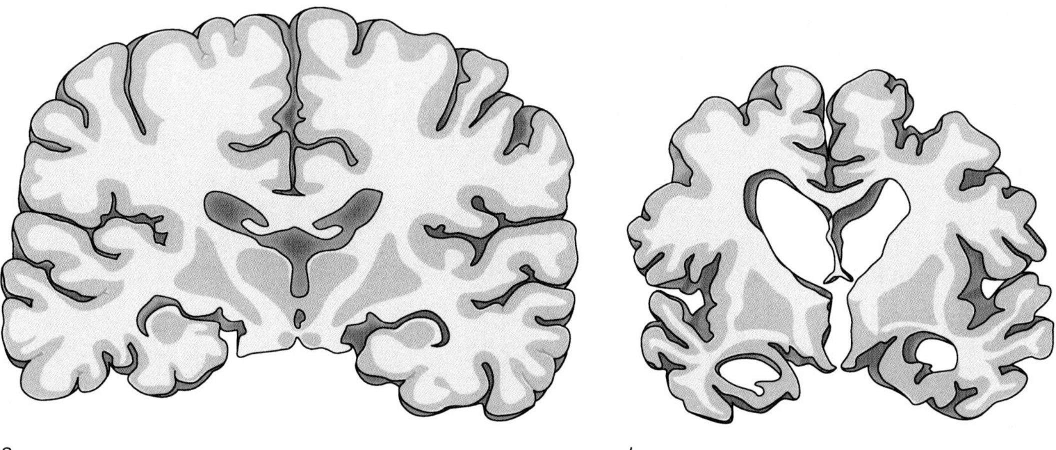

Figure 11.6 Compared to *(a)* a normal brain, *(b)* a brain with Alzheimer's disease is shriveled and reduced in size and has enlarged ventricles (cavities that contain cerebrospinal fluid).

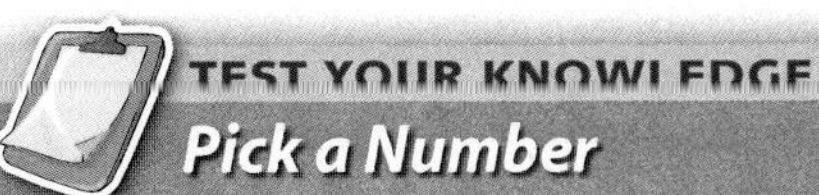

TEST YOUR KNOWLEDGE

Pick a Number

Try to supply the statistic to accurately complete the facts that follow. The answers are at the end of the list. Are you surprised at any of the facts? (All statistics apply to the United States only.)

1. People over age 65 do _____ percent of the volunteering in the United States.
2. People over age 65 are _______ (more, less, or equally) religious compared with the rest of the population.
3. Couples aged 75 and older engage in sexual intercourse _____ times per week, according to one survey.
4. The dating scene is fiercely competitive among older people, with only _____ single man to every _______ single women over age 75.
5. Approximately ____ percent of people over age 65 reside in long-term care facilities.
6. _________ percent of people over age 75 live on their own, with less than ______ percent living with relatives or in long-term care facilities.
7. The oldest old (over age 86) have many chronic and debilitating diseases, with _______ percent having some form of dementia and living in long-term care facilities.

Answers: 1) 95; 2) equally; 3) 1.5; 4) one, four; 5) 1; 6) 96, 5; 7) 20

- Choosing proper clothing with difficulty
- Hallucinating, arguing, striking out, and behaving violently
- Experiencing delusions, depression, or agitation
- Having difficulty performing basic tasks such as preparing meals and driving

At end stages of AD, people can no longer survive without assistance. Most people in this stage no longer understand language, recognize family members, or perform basic activities of daily living such as eating, dressing, and bathing (MedlinePlus 2007).

Pick's Disease

In the 1890s, Dr. Arnold Pick treated a man who had loss of speech and dementia. When the man died, Pick found that the man's brain had atrophied and had died in certain areas. This disease came to be known as **Pick's disease**, and it is a form of dementia that affects between 2 and 10 percent of dementia patients. Pick's disease affects the frontal and temporal lobes of the brain, which control speech, personality, and behavior. It can lead to changes in personality, loss of social skills, deteriorating intellectual function, and speech disturbances (MedlinePlus 2005). Similar to AD, Pick's disease cannot be diagnosed until an autopsy is performed, but some tests can rule out other diseases. The difference between AD and Pick's disease is that Pick's disease affects only one area of the brain, whereas AD can affect all of the brain.

Symptoms of Pick's disease include the following:

Behavioral Changes

- Inappropriate behavior
- Compulsive behaviors (e.g., overeating or only eating one type of food)
- Repetitive behavior
- Withdrawal from social interaction
- Inability to keep a job
- Problems with personal hygiene

Emotional Changes

- Abrupt mood changes
- No emotional warmth
- Indifference to events (apathy)
- Decreased interest in daily activities

Language Changes

- Echolalia (repeating spoken words)
- Aphasia (difficulty speaking or understanding speech)
- Difficulty finding a word
- Shrinking vocabulary
- Mute
- Decreased ability to read or write

Neurological Problems

- Rigidity of muscle tone
- Memory loss that continues to worsen
- Coordination problems

Parkinson's Disease

Parkinson's disease is a brain disease that can eventually result in dementia. In Parkinson's disease, the substantia nigra—the area in the brain stem that controls the production and release of dopamine, a neural transmitter—becomes damaged. The primary symptoms of Parkinson's disease are trembling in the hands, arms, legs, jaw, and face and impaired balance and coordination (U.S. Food and Drug Administration [FDA] 2006). At the end stages, people with Parkinson's disease can experience memory and personality changes. There is no cure for Parkinson's disease; however, there are some medications that can increase the production and use of dopamine, which reduces symptoms.

Multi-Infarct Dementia

Multi-infarct dementia (MID) is a common cause of memory loss in the elderly. MID is caused by multiple strokes in the brain. The strokes stop the blood flow to parts of the brain, resulting in cell death in that area of the brain. MID begins between the ages of 60 and 75. Memory loss begins suddenly and continues in a stair-step fashion, whereas AD, Pick's disease, and Parkinson's disease involve gradual losses.

Symptoms of MID include the following:

- Confusion
- Problems with short-term memory
- Wandering
- Getting lost in familiar places
- Walking with rapid, shuffling steps
- Losing bladder and bowel control
- Laughing or crying at inappropriate times
- Having problems following instructions, counting money, or making monetary transactions

There is no treatment for MID because parts of the brain are dead. Decline can be arrested if the cause of the strokes can be stopped or reduced. Blood-thinning drugs, cholesterol drugs such as statins, and other drugs can help keep strokes from occurring, which will stabilize the progression of dementia. Prevention is possible, however, with eating a healthy diet, exercising, not smoking, and maintaining a healthy weight.

Heart Attack

Most heart attacks are the direct result of heart disease. People often have minor heart attacks and don't pay attention to them. However, having a mild heart attack can often start people on a course of treatment, including weight loss and exercise, that can prevent a more serious heart attack in the future.

The National Heart Attack Alert Program notes three major symptoms of a heart attack. People who experience any of these symptoms should call emergency medical services (911) immediately:

- **Chest discomfort.** Most heart attacks involve discomfort in the center of the chest that lasts for more than a few minutes or goes away and comes back. The discomfort can be uncomfortable pressure, squeezing, fullness, or pain.
- **Discomfort in other areas of the upper body.** This can include pain or discomfort in the back, neck, jaw, stomach, or one or both arms.
- **Shortness of breath.** This often comes along with chest discomfort, but it also can occur before chest discomfort.

Other symptoms may include breaking out in a cold sweat or feeling nauseous or lightheaded.

Cancer

Lung cancer kills more people than any other cancer. It's most often caused by smoking, exposure to people who smoke, or other environmental exposures including asbestos and radon. Although smoking is the most prevalent cause of lung cancer, other causes exist.

Breast cancer is the second leading cause of cancer deaths in women. The risk factors for developing breast cancer are age, gender, family history of breast cancer, obesity, smoking, and sedentary lifestyle. Risk increases with age, and women are more likely than men to get breast cancer. As always, prevention is the best cure. Eating a diet of less than 30 percent fat, exercising 30 minutes or more a day, and getting a mammogram once before age 40 and yearly after turning 40 help prevent breast cancer or detect it early enough to treat it successfully.

A woman's chance of being diagnosed with breast cancer is as follows (National Cancer Institute 2006):

Ages 30 through 39	0.43 percent (1 in 233)
Ages 40 through 49	1.44 percent (1 in 69)
Ages 50 through 59	2.63 percent (1 in 38)
Ages 60 through 69	3.65 percent (1 in 27)

Prostate cancer is the second leading cause of cancer deaths in men. Some prostate cancers develop slowly and require no intervention, and others develop quickly and require surgery and chemotherapy. Sixty-five percent of all diagnoses occur in men over the age of 65. Here, too, lifestyle choices can reduce the chances of getting prostate cancer, such as reducing the amount of fat and red meat in the diet and getting a minimum of 30 minutes of exercise daily.

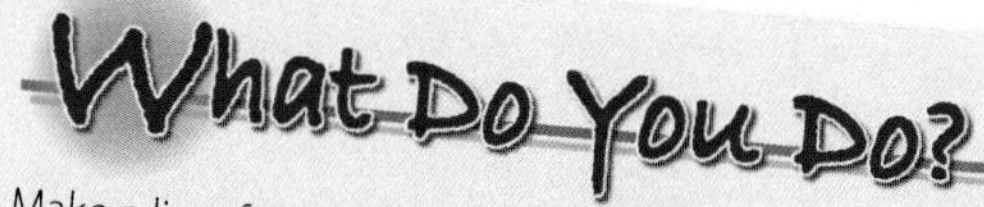

Make a list of people close to you who are older than 65. Ask them if they have received a pneumonia vaccine. If they haven't, contact the health department where they live and find out how they can receive the vaccine.

Pneumonia

Before the advent of penicillin in 1942, pneumonia was the number one killer of older adults. Now, a one-time vaccine is available to people over 65 or those with health problems, so no one should die from pneumonia anymore. However, not everyone gets the vaccine.

ISSUES IN THE NEWS

Report Card on Aging

The State of Aging and Health in America 2007 includes a national report card that looks at 15 indicators of older adult health (Centers for Disease Control and Prevention [CDC] and The Merck Company Foundation 2007). Those 15 indicators are grouped into four areas—health status, health behaviors, preventive care and screening, and injuries—and compared with targets set by the Healthy People 2010 initiative of the U.S. government. Healthy People 2010 establishes priorities to bring health to Americans and indicators of whether the public is healthy. The report card assigns a *met* or *not met* grade to indicators with specific Healthy People 2010 targets. Taken together, these indicators present a comprehensive picture of older adult health in the United States.

Of the 15 indicators in the report card, 10 are measured by Healthy People 2010. (The other 5 indicators were developed more recently and don't have corresponding targets.) The United States has met 4 of those targets several years ahead of schedule. (In the comparisons below, "people" refers to persons aged 65 and older.)

- In 2004, over 75 percent of people had a mammogram within the past two years, beating the Healthy People 2010 goal of 70 percent.
- In 2004, just over 9 percent of people were current smokers, beating the Healthy People 2010 goal of 12 percent.
- In 2004, over 63 percent of people aged 65 and older had colorectal cancer screenings, beating the Healthy People 2010 goal of 50 percent.
- In 2003, over 90 percent of people aged 65 and older had checked their cholesterol within the past 5 years, beating the Healthy People 2010 goal of 80 percent.

But there's room for improvement on the remaining targets. The following examples show results from 2004; again, "people" refers to persons aged 65 and older.

- Over 21 percent of people experienced complete tooth loss; the Healthy People 2010 goal is 20 percent.
- Almost 32 percent of people had no leisure-time physical activity in the past month; the Healthy People 2010 goal is 20 percent.
- Over 20 percent of people were obese; the Healthy People 2010 goal is 15 percent.
- Over 68 percent of people had a flu vaccine in the past year; the Healthy People 2010 goal is 90 percent.
- Over 64 percent of people reported ever having had a pneumonia vaccine; the Healthy People 2010 goal is 90 percent.

MANAGING THE CHANGES OF AGING

You've read about the changes in the body during aging and some theories about why those changes happen. You've also read about many of the diseases and other health conditions that become more prevalent with age. Many of those health conditions can be positively affected by lifestyle choices. This section will discuss some of the choices that can help you postpone many changes of aging.

Health is more than the absence of disease. It results from balance among the social, emotional, physical, and spiritual aspects of life. Healthy aging, then, is making lifestyle choices that have a positive influence on the 70 percent of aging that is not controlled by genetics (Finch and Tanzi 1997).

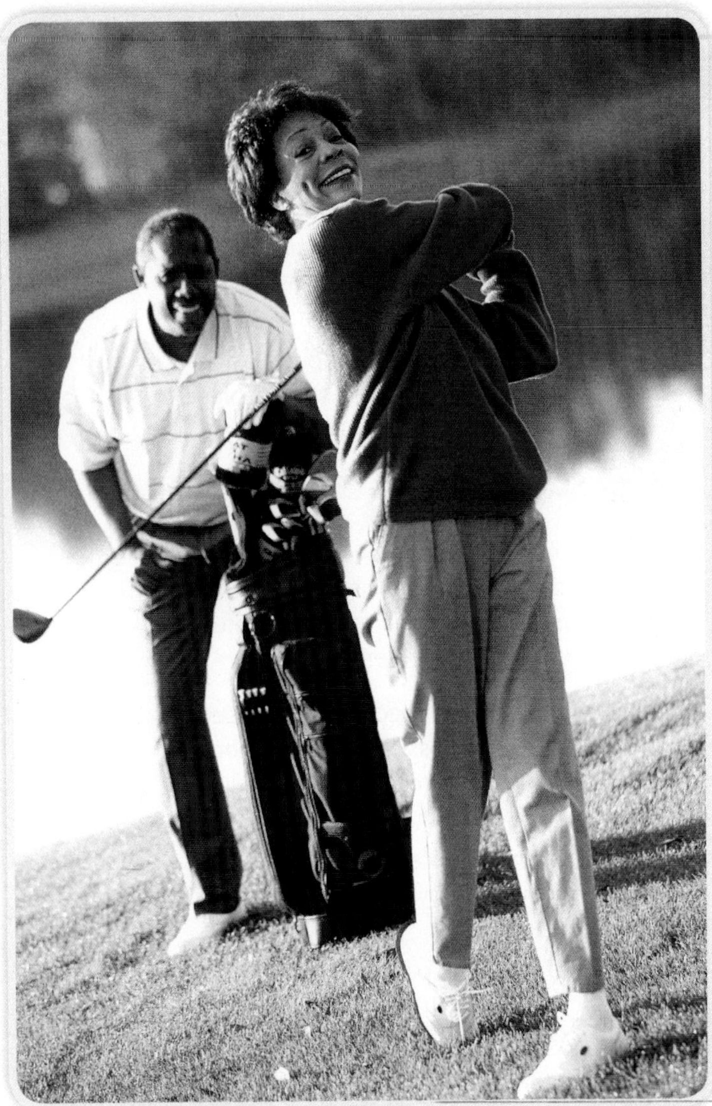

Although aerobic exercise provides the most health improvements, older adults also can benefit from less intense activities, such as golf.

© Photodisc/Getty Images

Physical Aspects

The lifestyle choices to exercise and eat well make up the physical aspects of healthy aging. Exercise makes improvements in the number of heart and brain cells at any age. To improve cardiorespiratory health, it is necessary to do a minimum of 30 minutes of **aerobic exercise** such as walking, jogging, jumping rope, bicycling, or swimming at least 5 days a week. Strength training, an **anaerobic exercise**, improves muscle tone, balance, and gait. Consistently doing both aerobic and anaerobic exercises can contribute to healthy aging. Aerobic exercise benefits the body more because it improves the cardiovascular system. Strength training is important for maintaining balance and strength, though.

Nutrition is another physical lifestyle factor that influences aging. Eating a balanced diet helps fight off free radicals and prevent disease. Using MyPyramid (see figure 11.7) can assist in choosing the correct balance. Protein and carbohydrate have 4 calories per gram, and each gram of fat has 9 calories. Keeping calories in mind when using the pyramid for food selection can help with maintaining, gaining, or losing weight. Food labels assume a 2,000-calorie diet when determining serving sizes for each food group.

Social Aspects

Studies have shown that membership in groups such as church and family lowers mortality risk (Christensen, Dornink, Ehlers, and Schultz 1999). People need other people to talk with and share their experiences for support. People who spend time with friends and family who support their activities are more likely to consistently maintain positive health behaviors. For instance, people with a support system tend to do better with medication and exercise compliance than those without supportive family and friends.

Spiritual Aspects

People who develop a spiritual connection with a power outside of themselves tend to live longer than people without that connection. Spirituality provides a sense of connection and can give people purpose and understanding beyond their circumstances. A meta-analysis of studies dealing with religiosity and spirituality suggests that most patients regard their spiritual health as equally important to their physical health. The study also found that 18 studies demonstrated that people involved with religion live longer. Religiosity or spirituality was defined as membership of a congregation or self-reported religiosity. The study concluded that most people have a spiritual life, they want that life to be addressed, and there is a direct relationship between religious involvement and spirituality and better health outcomes (Mueller, Plevak, and Rummans 2001).

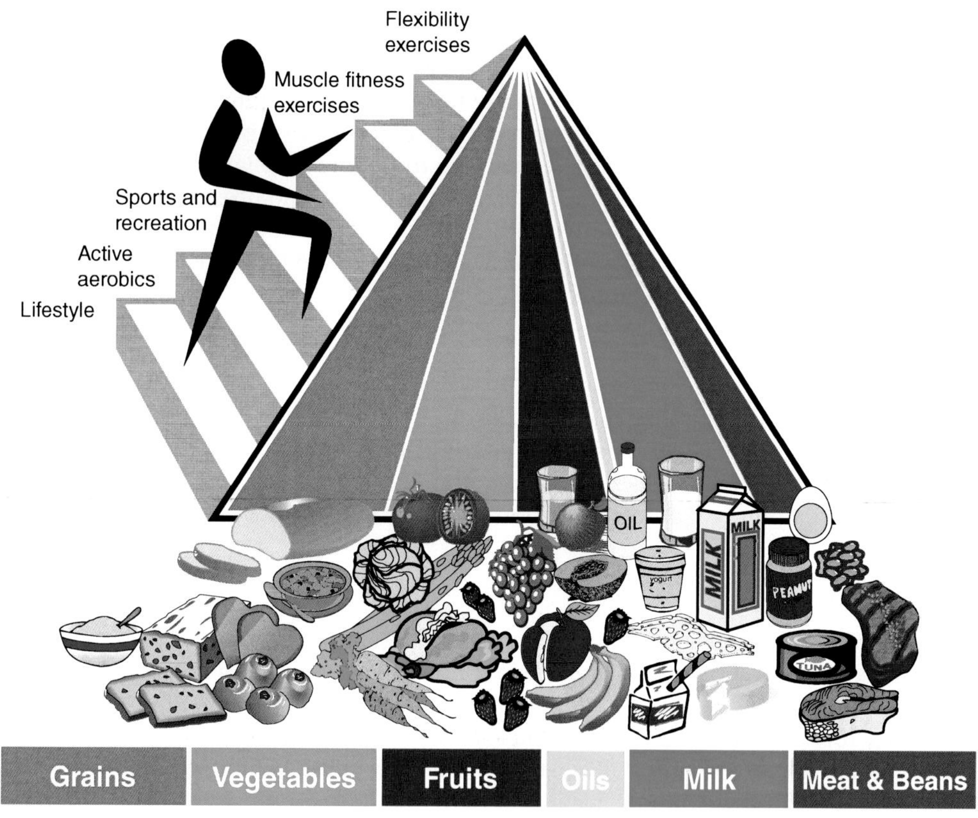

U.S. Department of Agriculture and the U.S. Department of Health and Human Services.

Figure 11.7 MyPyramid illustrates the dietary guidelines for Americans.

Lifestyle is defined by how you live and perceive life, and it determines how you will age. The lifestyle choices you make now will directly affect your health as you get older. If you perceive school as a stressor and you smoke to counter the stress, then the stress and results of smoking will likely shorten your life through disease. Exercising, eating nutritious meals, having a good social network of friends and family, and developing a spiritual component to your life will increase your chances of aging with health.

END-OF-LIFE ISSUES

Making healthy lifestyle choices can help prevent disease and delay many body changes as a result of aging. Medical advances have also prolonged life for many people. New drugs, more skilled surgical techniques, and machines that breathe and filter the blood extend the life of people who have a disease or who have been injured. However, at some point everyone will face the end of life, and in this section you'll read about options that are available for people at that stage.

Many times quality-of-life decisions can be made by the person affected by a health concern. Sometimes treatment for a disease can be difficult and painful and not extend life enough to make a person want to go through it. Other times treatment can extend a life for many years and the person may welcome that. Hospice, long-term care, and home-based care are three options that are available for people who are nearing the end of life.

STEPS FOR BEHAVIORAL CHANGE

Is Your Locus Internal or External?

Studies of centenarians (people over 100 years old) show that they share characteristics such as optimism, an internal locus of control, social support, and the ability to adapt well to change. An **internal locus of control** means that a person feels that he has power over his world; an **external locus of control** means he believes that things just happen to him. For instance, a person with an internal locus of control sees a poor test grade as a result of not studying enough rather than as a result of the instructor being unfair. She sees test grades as within her control.

Which lifestyle choices described in this section appear to be outside of your control? What could you do to change that?

Hospice

Hospice care is end-of-life care provided in the home by health professionals and volunteers. A doctor usually assigns a patient to hospice care. Dying at home often brings comfort to the patient and the family, and hospice provides a service to people who wish to die at home. Hospice offers visiting nurses, social workers, counseling services, and prescription services. Trained hospice workers act as liaisons between the patient and the doctor and often provide spiritual counseling. Patients can choose which services they would like to use. Families take part in the caregiving decisions and can take part in the caregiving itself.

Long-Term Care

Another option for people approaching the end of life is to enter a long-term care facility. Many long-term care facilities are similar to hospitals, offering nursing care and rehabilitation, but in an environment that's more homelike than a hospital. Some nontraditional long-term care facilities offer more community features and allow for more independent living.

Home-Based Care

People who can't afford the expense or don't like the environment of a long-term care facility often decide to take care of their family members at home. Caregiving can take many forms, such as taking meals to people each day at their home or staying with them full-time and having full responsibility for their care. Caregiving causes stress for caregivers and their families because most people do not stop their other responsibilities in the family. Many times adult children take care of both their parents and their own children. Support groups, adult day care, and other church and community groups can assist caregivers.

Adult day care facilities and some nursing homes offer an opportunity for release time for caregivers. Adult day care facilities provide a place to go for meals, entertainment, socializing, and medication management for adults who cannot take care of themselves during the day. This arrangement allows caregivers a chance to work or do daily chores. Some nursing homes and retirement facilities offer short-term care. This allows families to take a break from their caregiving duties, even if they just choose to stay home.

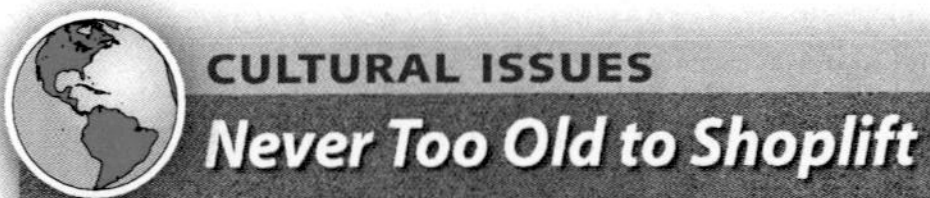

CULTURAL ISSUES

Never Too Old to Shoplift

When you think of shoplifters, do you picture kids and teenagers as the most likely culprits? That's not the case in Japan, where the crime rate among people 65 and older has increased fivefold in the past few decades (Harden 2008). Most of the offenses involve petty theft. A crime prevention task force in Hokkaido, one of Japan's largest islands, found that many elderly criminals break the law because they feel lonely, isolated, or out of touch with family and friends. Sometimes they crave simple human contact so much that they shoplift or engage in other petty criminal behavior to gain attention, even if that attention comes from the police. Another reason for an increase in shoplifting is the difficult financial situation experienced by many elderly in Japan. A government survey found that more than half of the elderly shoplifters questioned said they stole as a way of reducing their spending.

According to demographers, by the year 2040, Japan's elderly population will be nearly four times larger than its young population. It will be more important than ever to find ways to improve the social and financial problems that have led to increased criminal activity among that growing age group.

MIND-BODY CONNECTION

Attitudes About Aging

To what extent does looking old matter to you? Do any of the following statements describe your attitude at this point in your life?

- Wrinkles are natural, and I'm not going to worry about them. I'll consider my wrinkles a badge of honor when I'm older—as a sign that I've had a lot of life experiences.
- I want to keep my skin as healthy as I can naturally, so I'll control what I can now by being careful in the sun and not smoking.
- Old age is a long way off for me! I'm going to keep having fun, and I'll deal with how I look later, maybe with antiaging products or cosmetic surgery.

HEALTHY AGING 101

Growing old is not for the faint of heart! As we grow older, our organs and body systems age, including the integumentary (skin and hair), cardiovascular, renal, digestive, nervous, skeletal, and muscular systems. In addition, we become more susceptible to chronic diseases and other aspects of unhealthy aging. Regardless, at some point we all face the end of life, and there are many factors to consider during that stage, including quality of life and treatment and care options.

People can adjust their lifestyles and enjoy their retirement years by working, volunteering, or enjoying a hobby. Making sure that people have good quality of life during those years depends on their lifestyle during all the years before age 65. Exercising 30 minutes a day, eating a healthy diet, controlling weight, having good social relationships, continuing intellectual stimulation, being in a good environment, and enjoying life will help maintain a quality of life experienced at younger ages. Genetics plays a part in how people age and whether they are susceptible to disease, but lifestyle contributes to 70 percent of how people age. Most of the control over how people age is in their hands.

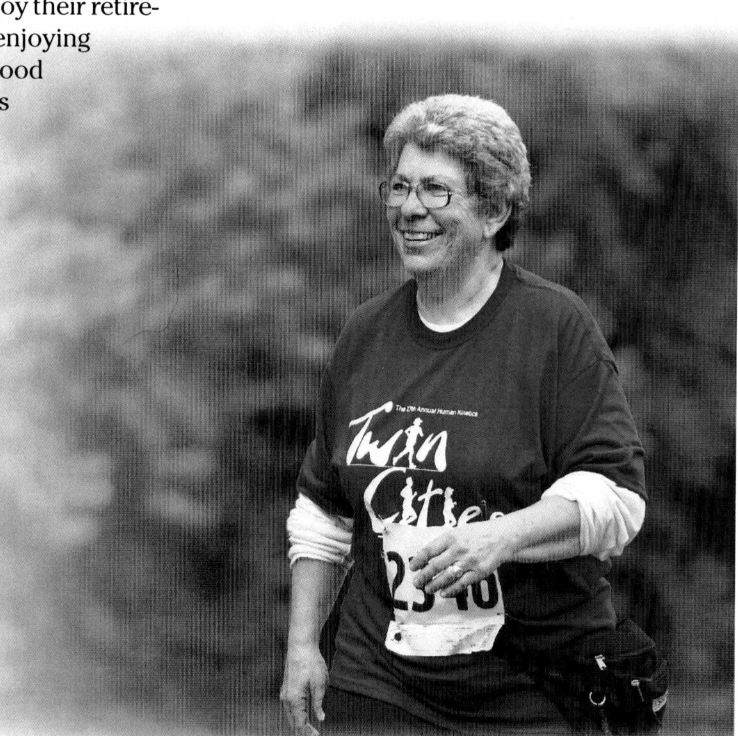

Getting the right amount of physical activity can improve your quality of life in your later years.

© Human Kinetics

REVIEW QUESTIONS

1. How has the traditional U.S. population pyramid changed, and what do the changes mean?
2. List at least six genetic signs of aging in skin or hair.
3. Describe how aging affects a person's bones and muscles and what can be done to help reduce those changes.
4. The chapter presented six aging theories. Compare and contrast three of them.
5. Hypertension, high cholesterol, and diabetes are risk factors for what kind of chronic disease?
6. Describe the general symptoms of dementia, and name two causes of dementia.
7. What is the second leading cause of cancer deaths in women? In men?
8. Explain several physical, social, and spiritual lifestyle choices that can help you postpone many changes of aging.
9. What is the difference between hospice care, long-term care, and home-based care?
10. Skin wrinkles as a normal part of the aging process. Name three causes of wrinkles that are not genetic and that you can control.

CRITICAL THINKING

1. In Texas, the government decided to put aging services under the umbrella of disability services. Do you agree or disagree with this decision, and why?
2. Genetics plays a small part in the aging process. If you were designing a media campaign on healthy aging, what lifestyle choices would you encourage and why?
3. What theory of aging best explains how people age? Describe the theory and defend your point of view.

APPLICATION ACTIVITIES

1. Besides being great problem solvers, the oldest old can certainly be creative. The Public Broadcasting Service (PBS) did a special on the aging brain and recorded the work of Stanley Kunitz, who was named poet laureate of the United States at the age of 95. Watch recordings of Mr. Kunitz reading three poems at www.pbs.org/wnet/brain/episode5/kunitz/index.html. Next, listen to a National Public Radio (NPR) report at www.npr.org/templates/story/story.php?storyId=1832793 about how poetry can help people with Alzheimer's disease. Finally, visit the Web site of the Alzheimer's Poetry Project at www.alzpoetry.com to learn more about the benefits that poetry can provide to Alzheimer's patients and their caregivers. Write an essay that summarizes your findings, and compare and contrast the information given by NPR and the Alzheimer's Poetry Project.
2. When people discuss the end of life, questions arise about quality of life. Each person should decide what quality of life means before making a decision for a loved one. Knowing what the minimum standards are for a life can assist in making that difficult decision about whether life support should continue. Talk with the older people in your life to learn their wishes so you can make the best decisions on their behalf about end-of-life issues.

CHAPTER REVIEW

GLOSSARY

aerobic exercise—Any physical activity in which increased oxygen uptake is needed.

Alzheimer's disease (AD)—Degenerative disease that produces amyloid plaques and neurofibrillary tangles of proteins and affects brain function.

anaerobic exercise—Any high-intensity activity in which oxygen is not needed.

arthritis—Disease characterized by inflammation of the joints.

cardiovascular disease (CVD)—Range of diseases that affect the heart or blood vessels, including coronary artery disease, heart attack, heart failure, high blood pressure, and stroke.

chronic diseases—Illnesses that persist over time.

dementia—Reduction of mental faculties, including memory loss, personality changes, or other signs of maladaptations.

diabetes—Disease where either the body cannot make insulin (type 1) or the body undermanufactures insulin and does not use insulin properly (type 2).

evolutionary programmed senescence theory—Theory of aging stating that there are genes that protect against disease before reproduction ends.

external locus of control—When people feel that events just happen to them and they have no control over their world.

free radical theory—Theory of aging proposing that free radicals, which are released during regular cell production from the electron transport chain, damage cells, including DNA; also known as *oxidative damage theory*.

immune theory—Theory of aging stating that with advancing age, the immune system is compromised in some areas and overreacts in other areas.

internal locus of control—When people feel they have power over their world.

lifestyle—The habits, attitudes, tastes, and so on that constitute mode of living.

osteoporosis—Condition in which the bones become less dense than they would during normal aging.

Parkinson's disease—Disease caused by a reduction of dopamine. Causes tremors and can result in memory and personality changes.

Pick's disease—Form of dementia that causes personality changes, loss of social skills, loss of intellectual function, and speech disturbances.

programmed senescence—Theory of aging stating that a switch within the genetic code starts the aging process.

rate of living theory—Disproved theory that a higher metabolism causes the body to burn out and age faster.

senescence—Process of becoming old.

telomere theory—Theory of aging stating that as cells split, the telomeres shrink, getting smaller and smaller each time they divide. Eventually this causes the cell to die and increases the chance of getting a terminal disease.

wear and tear theory—Disproved theory stating that the body wears out over time from overuse.

REFERENCES AND RESOURCES

AgingSkinNet. 2005. Causes of aging skin. www.skincarephysicians.com/agingskinnet/basicfacts.html.

Arking, R. 2005. Biology, fruit flies, and humans: Can extended longevity stretch from one to the other? *Gerontologist* 45 (3): 418-425.

Beers, M.H., ed. 2007. Merck Manual of Geriatrics. www.merck.com/mkgr/mmg/home.jsp.

Better Health Channel. 2006. Aging—muscles bones and joints. www.betterhealth.vic.gov.au/bhcv2/bhcarticles.nsf/pages/Ageing_muscles_bones_and_joints?OpenDocument.

Blanchard-Fields, F. 2007. Everyday problem solving and emotion: An adult developmental perspective. *Current Directions in Psychological Science* 16 (1): 26-31.

Centers for Disease Control and Prevention (CDC). 2008. Detailed data for prevalence of diabetes. www.cdc.gov/diabetes/statistics/prev/national/tprevwfage.htm.

Centers for Disease Control and Prevention (CDC) and The Merck Company Foundation. 2007. *The state of aging and health in America 2007*. Whitehouse Station, NJ: The Merck Company Foundation. Available at www.cdc.gov/aging and www.merck.com/cr.

Cheitlin, M.D. 2003. Cardiovascular physiology—changes with aging. *American Journal of Geriatric Cardiology* 12 (1): 9-13.

Christensen, A.J., R. Dornink, S. Ehlers, and S. Schultz. 1999. Social environment and longevity in schizophrenia. *Psychosomatic Medicine* 61: 141-145.

Finch, C.E., and R.E. Tanzi. 1997. Genetics of aging. *Science* 278 (5337): 407-411.

Harden, B. 2008. Silver-haired shoplifters on the rise in Japan. *Washington Post* (November 30): A15. Available at www.washingtonpost.com/wp-dyn/content/article/2008/11/29/AR2008112901913_pf.html.

Kemi, O., M. Høydal, P. Haram, A. Garnier, D. Fortin, R. Ventura-Clapier, and Ø. Ellingsen. 2007. Exercise training restores aerobic capacity and energy transfer systems in heart failure treated with losartan. *Cardiovascular Research* 76 (1): 91-99.

Kung, H.-C., D.L. Hoyert, J. Xu, and S.L. Murphy. 2008. Deaths: Final data for 2005. *National Vital Statistics Report* 56 (10). Available at www.cdc.gov/nchs/data/nvsr/nvsr56/nvsr56_10.pdf.

Kwak, H.B., W. Song, and J.M. Lawler. 2007. Exercise training ameliorates age-induced elevation in Bcl-2 family pro-apoptotic signaling in the aging rat heart. *FASEB Journal* 20: 791-793.

MedlinePlus. 2005. Pick's disease. www.nlm.nih.gov/medlineplus/ency/article/000744.htm.

———. 2007. Dementia. www.nlm.nih.gov/medlineplus/dementia.html.

———. 2008. Arthritis. www.nlm.nih.gov/medlineplus/arthritis.html.

Mueller, P.S., D.J. Plevak, and T.A. Rummans. 2001. Religious involvement, spirituality and medicine: Implications for clinical practice. *Mayo Clinic Proceedings* 76: 1225-1235.

National Cancer Institute. 2006. Probability of breast cancer in American women. www.cancer.gov/cancertopics/factsheet/detection/probability-breast-cancer/.

National Heart, Lung, and Blood Institute. n.d. Who is at risk for coronary artery disease? www.nhlbi.nih.gov/health/dci/Diseases/Cad/CAD_WhoIsAtRisk.html.

National Institutes on Aging (NIA). 2006. The hallmarks of AD. www.nia.nih.gov/Alzheimers/Publications/Unraveling/Part2/hallmarks.htm.

Office of Public Affairs. 2005. Treasury Secretary John W. Snow Statement on the 2005 Social Security and Medicare trust fund reports. www.ustreas.gov/press/releases/js2332.htm.

Santoro, N. 2007. Premenopausal protection against chronic diseases of aging. National Institutes of Health. www.nia.nih.gov/NR/rdonlyres/5A1CED8B-6BD5-4EA4-9197-58A6731D9614/2704/santoro.pdf.

Speakman, J.R. 2005. Body size, energy metabolism and life span. *Journal of Experimental Biology* 208: 1717-1730.

UCSF's Elizabeth Blackburn receives Lasker Award. 2007. University of California, San Francisco. http://pub.ucsf.edu/lasker/telomeres.php.

U.S. Food and Drug Administration (FDA). 2006. Coping with memory loss. www.fda.gov/consumer/features/memoryloss0507.html.

WebMD. n.d. What is atheroslerosis? www.webmd.com/heart-disease/what-is-atherosclerosis.

Other helpful resources include the following.

Burns, E.A., and E.A. Leventhal. 2000. Aging, immunity, and cancer. *Cancer Control* 7 (6): 513-522.

Cohen, S. 2006. Aging changes in the bones, muscles, and joints. www.nlm.nih.gov/medlineplus/ency/article/004015.htm.

MedlinePlus. 2007. Skin aging. www.nlm.nih.gov/medlineplus/skinaging.html.

Social Security and Medicare Boards of Trustees. 2008. A summary of the 2008 annual reports. www.ssa.gov/OACT/TRSUM/trsummary.html.

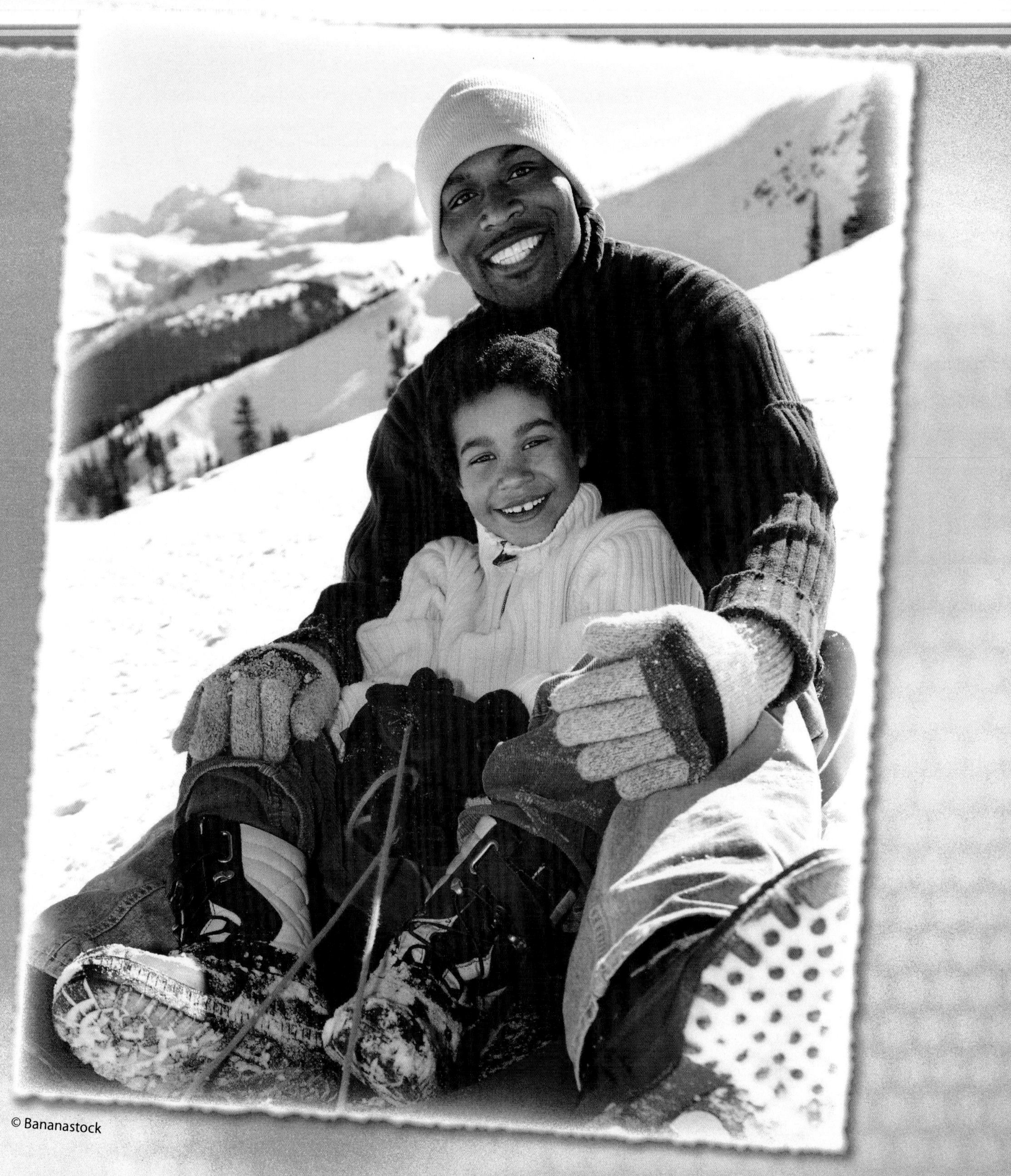

© Bananastock

CHAPTER 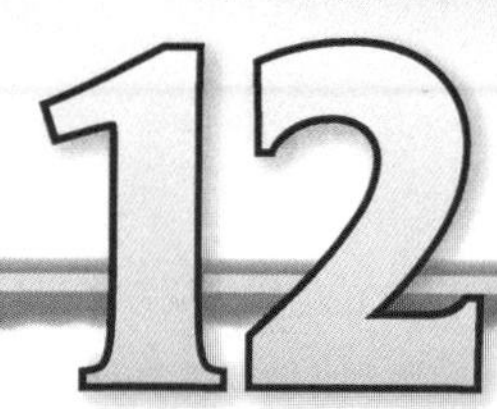

WELLNESS THROUGHOUT LIFE

BHIBHA DAS, MPH
University of Illinois

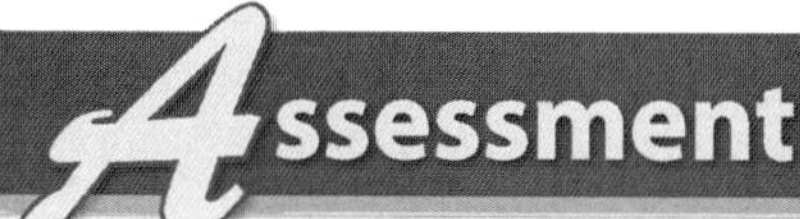

Assessment

- What would you say are some of the most important recent achievements in improving the health of the U.S. public?
- How can health insurance affect the type of health care people will receive?
- Other than physical wellness, what other kinds of wellness exist?
- What is one of the most important vaccinations that college students can get, and why?
- What five stages are described by the transtheoretical model of behavior change?

Objectives

- Understand the difference between health and wellness.
- Identify 10 significant public health achievements of the 20th century.
- Discuss challenges to wellness in the 21st century.
- Explain the six dimensions of wellness.
- Identify factors that influence your wellness.
- Understand behavior change models and why they work in creating wellness.
- Know how to set realistic goals.

Many people use the term *health*, and it probably means something different to each of them. Maybe it means they feel good, or they aren't sick, or that they live a healthy lifestyle. The World Health Organization (WHO) defines health as a state of complete physical, mental, and social well-being; in other words, it's not just the absence of disease and infirmity.

In recent years, there has been a shift in health-promotion circles away from the narrow concept of health and toward the more inclusive concept of wellness. In 1961, Halbert L. Dunn, a physician, introduced the concept of wellness (Oklahoma Cooperative Extension Services 2008). He defined it as a lifestyle approach for pursuing both physical and psychological well-being. Bill Hettler, cofounder and president of the board of directors of the National Wellness Institute, further described wellness as the overall quality of life, which encompasses an active, lifelong process with six interactive dimensions (National Wellness Institute 2007). These dimensions influence one another and help you achieve overall wellness.

The aim of this chapter is to help you realize that health and wellness aren't merely goals to achieve but the result of a lifelong process. To achieve wellness, you need to understand its dimensions, the factors that influence health and wellness, and how you can change your health behaviors if necessary.

CHANGES IN HEALTH AND WELLNESS OVER TIME

The 20th century saw significant progress in public health in the United States. From 1900 to 1999, continual changes in public health have added at least an extra 25 years to the life span of the average American. But that's not enough. The attention to public health is extending into the 21st century and beyond. The U.S. government continues to do research and establish national goals to help people improve their health and wellness in general.

Significant Public Health Achievements

The Centers for Disease Control and Prevention (CDC) selected the following as the top 10 significant public health achievements in the United States in the 20th century because of their influence on death, illness, and disability (CDC 1999).

1. **Vaccinations**. Vaccinations in the United States have eliminated smallpox and poliomyelitis and have controlled other infectious diseases such as measles, rubella, mumps, and diphtheria.
2. **Motor vehicle safety**. Vehicles and highways are safer, and personal behaviors such as using safety belts, car seats, and motorcycle helmets have improved. As a result, there has been a large decline of vehicle-related deaths.
3. **Safer workplaces**. Workplaces have become safer in the last century through advances in technology, stricter workplace regulations, and increased safety awareness. Occupational health problems, such as black lung disease among coal miners, are not nearly as prevalent now as they were in the earlier part of the 1900s. Mining, manufacturing, construction, and transportation injuries and fatalities have also seen a decline.

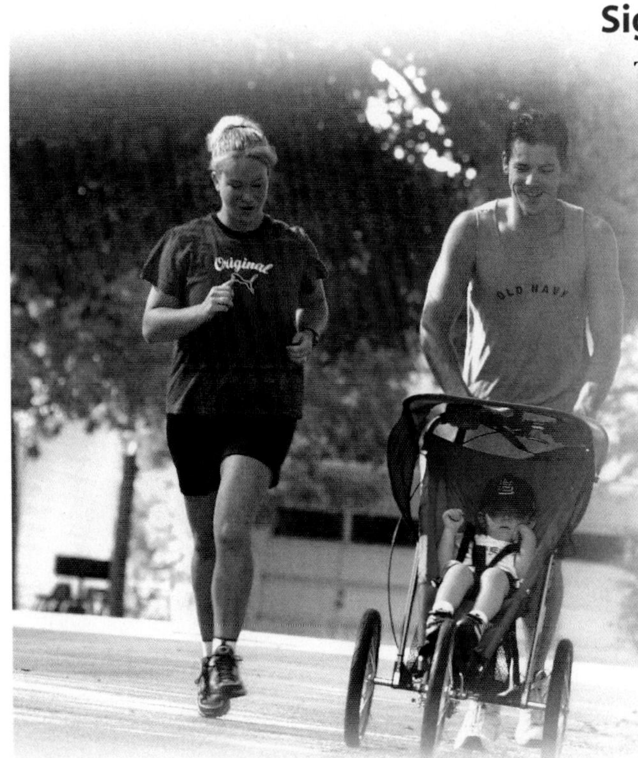

Families are healthier today because of numerous significant public health achievements of the 20th century.

© Human Kinetics

4. **Control of infectious disease**. These declines come from a combination of improved sanitation and clean drinking water. Improved sanitation has resulted in the decrease of diseases such as typhoid and cholera. Infectious diseases are also better controlled because of medical advancements such as antimicrobial therapy.
5. **Decline in deaths due to coronary heart disease and stroke**. This decline is a result of recognition of risk factors, such as tobacco use and high blood pressure, for cardiovascular disease (CVD). In addition, early detection and better treatment are available.
6. **Safer and healthier foods**. Safer and healthier foods are more readily available, and as a result, there have been decreases in microbial contaminations and increases in food-fortification programs. Nutritional deficiency diseases such as rickets are now rare in the United States.
7. **Healthier mothers and babies**. Mothers and babies have access to better hygiene and nutrition today than they did decades ago. They also have more access to timely and adequate maternal and neonatal health care, including access to antibiotics. Due to these factors, maternal mortality has declined 99 percent and infant mortality is down by 90 percent.
8. **Family planning**. Advances in family planning have helped create smaller families, longer intervals between children, fewer infant and maternal deaths, and contraceptives to prevent pregnancy and transmission of sexually transmitted infections (STIs).
9. **Fluoridation of drinking water**. Fluoridation of drinking water has been a cost-effective method of preventing tooth decay in both children and adults.
10. **Recognition of tobacco use as a health hazard**. After tobacco was recognized as a health hazard, smoking cessation programs and smoking prevention programs were introduced. In addition, exposure to secondhand tobacco smoke was reduced. As a result, fewer adults are smoking, which means smoking-related deaths have been prevented.

Challenges to Wellness

The field of wellness faces several challenges as the physical, geographical, and economic landscapes change. Obesity and overweight, infectious diseases, and access to health insurance are three of the biggest challenges to wellness.

Obesity and Overweight

In 2004, approximately 34 percent of U.S. adults over the age of 20 had a body mass index (BMI) of 30 or higher, which categorizes them as obese (CDC 2008a). More children are overweight today, too (CDC 2007g). Obesity and overweight are significant problems because they increase the risk of developing chronic diseases such as hypertension, CVD, and diabetes.

Infectious Diseases

Another new wellness challenge is the reemergence of infectious diseases. One of the top 10 public health achievements for the 20th century was control of infectious diseases, but they're becoming more prevalent (Mayo Clinic 2007). Bacteria that were once controlled with antibiotics are now resistant to even the most potent medications because antibiotics have been misused and overprescribed. These antibiotic-resistant superbugs cause deadlier versions of old diseases.

Another reason infectious diseases are on the rise is the popularity of global travel (Mayo Clinic 2007). As more and more people are traveling, they're carrying disease-causing pathogens with them or they're exposed to pathogens they don't have a natural immunity to. Animals and insects also spread disease globally. The West Nile virus came to New York City after an infected mosquito found its way onto an airplane coming from the Middle East.

Crowded living conditions are also contributing to the reemergence of infectious diseases (Mayo Clinic 2007). Cities and rural areas of developing nations are becoming more and more densely populated, which provides a prime opportunity for germs to spread not only from person to person but also from animals to people.

Access to Health Insurance

Access to health insurance is another challenge facing the field of wellness. These statistics from the Henry J. Kaiser Family Foundation point to this emerging problem:

- Nearly 46.5 million nonelderly Americans didn't have health insurance in 2006.
- People whose incomes are below 200 percent of the poverty level are at the highest risk of being uninsured.
- Sixty-one percent of people who are uninsured are over the age of 30.

Many Americans are uninsured for a variety of reasons. First, rising health care costs and insurance premiums have made getting job-based coverage difficult for many Americans. Since 2001, premiums for family coverage for health care have increased by 78 percent, but wages have increased only 19 percent (Henry J. Kaiser Family Foundation 2007). Fewer companies are opting to provide health care benefits to employees and their dependents.

Health insurance ultimately affects the type of health care people will receive. Many uninsured people don't have a primary care provider, and they often delay care or may not even receive medical care, which puts them at risk of developing more serious illnesses. Also, people without health care don't receive basic preventive care such as Pap smears, mammograms, annual physicals, or blood glucose screenings, and they are more likely to be hospitalized for medical conditions that could have been avoided if they'd received proper medical care from the beginning.

Healthy People 2010

Although wellness is largely a personal concern, the U.S. government has immense interest in the issue because people who aren't well have a tremendous cost to the nation. To help shape the nation's health, the United States started the Healthy People initiative with the goal of preventing disease and improving quality of life. As part of this initiative, the government publishes reports on the health status of the country every 10 years and sets national health goals for the following 10 years. The latest report, Healthy People 2010, sets the health goals to hopefully be accomplished by the year 2010 (Healthy People 2010 2000).

This report guides plans and goals for many parties, including state health departments, communities, professional organizations, and even individuals. The development of the goals was a time-consuming process that involved broad consultation, use of the best scientific knowledge at the time, and design of an evaluation process. The two overarching goals are to increase quality and years of healthy life and eliminate health disparities (Healthy People 2010 2000). In addition, the initiative focuses on 10 leading health indicators, including physical activity, tobacco use, environmental quality, and immunizations.

Using this national framework for health, groups and organizations can create comprehensive plans to improve and evaluate the health of communities. In addition, Congress has designated the Healthy People 2010 objectives as evaluation measures for the Indian Health Care Improvement Act, the Maternal and Child Health Block Grant, and the Preventive Health and Health Services Block Grant.

SIX DIMENSIONS OF WELLNESS

The six dimensions of wellness model (see figure 12.1) was developed by Dr. Bill Hettler, cofounder and president of the board of directors of the National Wellness Institute, which is an organization formed to provide health promotion and wellness resources to health professionals and individuals. The model demonstrates that all six types of wellness—physical, intellectual, emotional, social, spiritual, and occupational—must be present for a person to attain overall wellness (National Wellness Institute 2007). Efforts to attain wellness now will become a foundation for your life later.

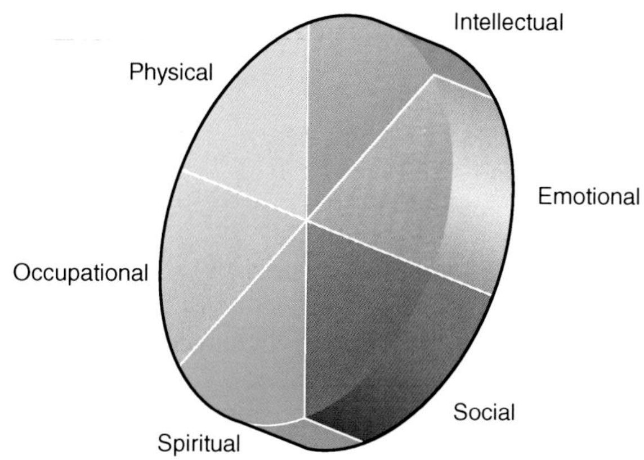

Figure 12.1 To attain overall wellness, you must have all six types of wellness.

Physical Wellness

Physical wellness—the wellness of the physical body—is important to overall health and wellness because when the body is sick or injured, it's harder to do physical and mental tasks well. You can't focus in class or complete homework assignments, for example. In the workforce, being physically ill may have a negative impact on your work productivity, ultimately affecting your career. Finally, if you continue being physically fit into your later years, you'll be able to maintain your independence and continue with your activities of daily life such as bathing, carrying groceries, and playing with your grandchildren.

You can do many things to maintain physical wellness, including getting regular physical activity. There are 1,440 minutes in a day; use at least 30 of them to do something active that you enjoy. Finding activities you enjoy will ensure that you continue participating in them. For instance, if you're a competitive person, you might want to join an intramural sport team.

Another important step you can take to being physically well is to have good eating habits. According to the U.S. Department of Agriculture (USDA), you should eat food from the grains, vegetables, fruits, milk, and meat and beans food groups (USDA 2008).

- At least half the grains you eat should be whole grains.
- Eat a variety of vegetables, especially dark green and orange veggies. Next time you're eating a salad, try to replace the iceberg lettuce with some spinach.
- Eat a variety of fruits. They can be fresh, frozen, canned, or dried. Beware, though: Fruit juices often add extra sugar, which adds calories.
- Dairy products should be low fat or fat free. If you're lactose intolerant, try eating lactose-free products and get your calcium from sources such as salmon, broccoli, or spinach.
- When choosing meat products, go lean. The best ways to prepare meat are to bake, broil, or grill it. Try to vary your choices in this food group. You can try fish and even nuts.
- The USDA food pyramid recommends eating sweets only in moderation. Every food fits, but in moderation.

Other things you can do to maintain physical fitness include not using tobacco products and illegal drugs such as marijuana or cocaine. Also, if you use alcohol, be sure to drink responsibly.

Remember these two tenets of physical wellness:

1. It is better to consume foods and beverages that enhance good health than those that impair it.
2. It is better to be physically fit than out of shape.

Intellectual Wellness

Intellectual wellness addresses creative and mental activities and your openness to new ideas (National Wellness Institute 2007). People who are intellectually well continually try to expand their knowledge and skills, and they're willing to share their knowledge and skills with others. You can achieve intellectual wellness by engaging in lifelong learning through both formal education and informal life experiences. If you're intellectually well, you'll welcome lifelong intellectual growth and stimulation and you'll look for interaction with the world around you. Intellectual wellness helps keep your mind sharp as you age.

Being enrolled in college is a step you're already taking to achieve intellectual wellness. As a college student, you are being exposed to a variety of ideas in both formal settings, such as the classroom, and informal settings, such as your dormitory or fraternity or sorority. Reading is another great way to stay well intellectually. If you don't like to read, you can watch or listen to programs with educational value. You can find a variety of educational television programming on the Discovery Channel, History Channel, Public Broadcasting Service (PBS), and so on. You can also learn new skills or pick up new hobbies throughout your life to help maintain intellectual wellness.

Remember these tenets of intellectual wellness:

1. It is better to stretch and challenge your mind with intellectual and creative pursuits than to become self-satisfied and unproductive.
2. It is better to identify potential problems and choose appropriate courses of action based on available information than to wait, worry, and contend with major concerns later.

Emotional Wellness

Emotional wellness gives you the ability to get through the rigors of life (National Wellness Institute 2007). Some aspects of emotional wellness include self-acceptance, self-confidence, self-control, and trust. Emotional wellness involves the ability to deal with stress, the ability to be flexible, and your attitude toward yourself and life in general. Emotional wellness will help you have a better outlook on life so that you enjoy it to its fullest.

You can do several things to help improve your emotional wellness. One of the most important is to develop a good social support network. In other words, make friends! Friends provide a sounding board, and their support helps you reduce stress and manage negative emotions.

MIND-BODY CONNECTION
De-Stress Your Life

College is hectic and fast paced. Classes, exams, papers, and research projects consume a lot of time, and the time that isn't spent on schoolwork is often spent on extracurricular activities, jobs, and the social scene. It's no wonder many college students feel stressed out!

Identify a stressful situation in your life. Develop a few creative solutions to help you de-stress the situation. Evaluate your list of solutions and decide which ones you are willing to try. Set a date for when you will implement these solutions, and then put them to work. Finally, analyze how well those solutions worked for de-stressing the situation and determine if revisions are necessary (Blair et al. 2001).

Even with a busy and sometimes chaotic schedule, make time to nurture relationships so you have a solid support system in times of need and in times of joy.

Another important step you can take to maintain emotional wellness is to build confidence. Each person has unique abilities and weaknesses. Accepting your strengths and weaknesses and doing the best with what you have can help build self-confidence.

Finding the optimal balance between work and personal life is another important step to maintaining emotional wellness. Try to schedule time to pursue activities that interest you, such as reading, exercising, or going to the movies. Finding a balance between schoolwork and the rest of your life will help you not only in school but as you enter the workforce and raise a family.

Remember these tenets of emotional wellness:

1. It is better to be aware of and accept your feelings than to deny them.
2. It is better to be optimistic in your approach to life than pessimistic.

Social Wellness

The emphasis behind the **social wellness** dimension is becoming a contributing member of society (National Wellness Institute 2007). A socially well person takes an active role in the community and encourages effective communication among community members.

Volunteering in the community provides a sense of satisfaction and purpose that paid work often can't give, so it's a good step toward social wellness. Another step is to expand your social support network. Your social support could be made up of people from work, school, professional organizations, and clubs. Being respectful of others will help you develop into a socially well person. You can also become socially well by joining a club or organization that is of interest to you. Most schools have a variety of clubs for virtually any interest. After college, you might want to join service organizations within your community. Joining clubs gives you a sense of community, which ultimately helps you achieve social wellness.

Remember these tenets of social wellness:

1. It is better to contribute to the common welfare of your community than to think only of yourself.
2. It is better to live in harmonywith others and your environment than to live in conflict with them.

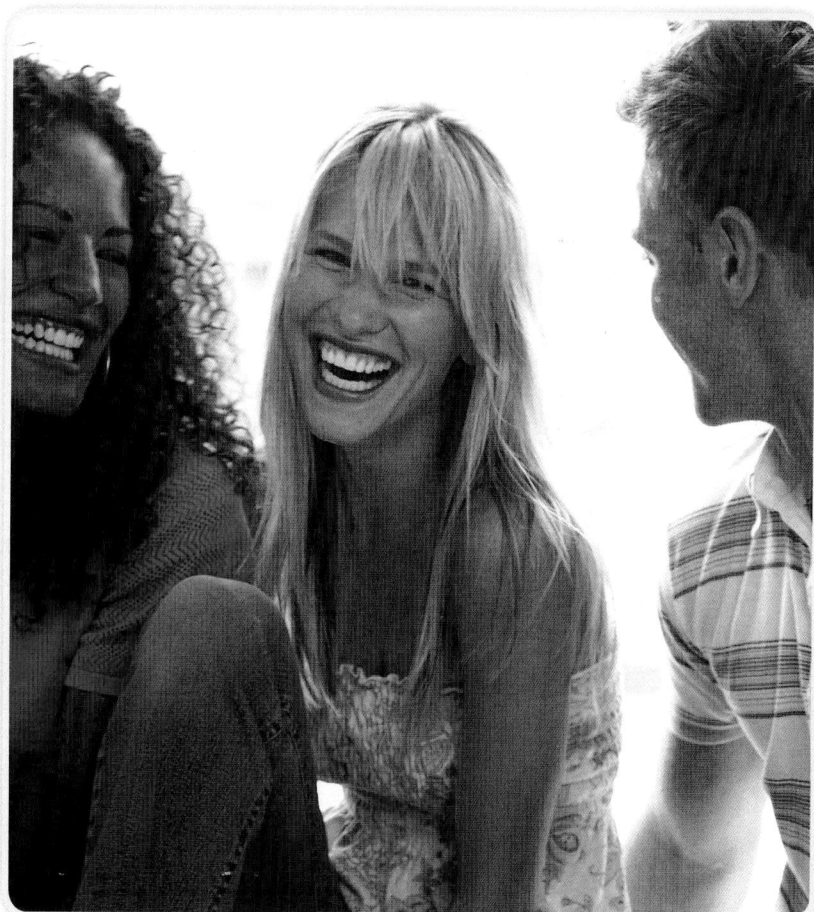

Having friends can help you deal with stress and improve your emotional wellness.

© Greg Hinsdale/Corbis

Spiritual Wellness

The dimension of **spiritual wellness** focuses on meaning and purpose in life (National Wellness Institute 2007). Aspects of spiritual wellness include the ability to forgive, to show compassion, and to love. Although traditional religious beliefs and practices are part of spiritual wellness, spiritual wellness can also encompass the broader range of relationships with other living things and your perception and appreciation of nature, the universe, and the meaning of life. The spiritual dimension also equips you with the ethics, values, and morals that help guide your decisions.

Developing spiritual wellness takes time, and there is no single approach that fits all. It's often hard to find time to develop spiritual wellness, but some simple things can help. Here are a few ideas that might get you started.

- Take a few minutes out of your day to pray or meditate. Taking just 5 minutes to clear your mind will help you become more focused.
- Use affirmations to change negative self-talk into positive self-talk—repeating positive ideas about yourself leads to positive feelings, which in turn increases spiritual wellness.
- Look for something inspirational to read every day, even if it's just a short quote.
- If you practice a religion, attending a church, synagogue, or temple will help with your spiritual wellness. Becoming involved in activities at your place of worship is another step you can take to becoming spiritually well.
- Practice breathing exercises—in a quiet place, breathe in slowly and deeply through your nose, and then let the breath out through your mouth.
- Spend time in nature, which can renew your sense of belonging to the world.
- Take care of yourself, including regular exercise and a balanced diet.
- Express yourself creatively through painting, drawing, singing, writing, and so on.

Remember these tenets of spiritual wellness:

1. It is better to ponder the meaning of life for yourself and to be tolerant of the beliefs of others than to close your mind and become intolerant.
2. It is better to live each day in a way that is consistent with your values and beliefs than to do otherwise and feel untrue to yourself.

Occupational Wellness

Occupational wellness applies to the personal satisfaction you get from your career (National Wellness Institute 2007). Satisfaction increases as you contribute your skills and talents to work that is meaningful and rewarding. Look for a job in a field you feel passionate about so work feels less like work and more like fun. Choose a career path compatible with your interests, talents, and personality.

Build strong working relationships with your coworkers. Creating strong relationships will help foster community in the workplace. Try to create a better work environment by avoiding gossip about your colleagues.

You can also achieve occupational wellness by working toward your career goals. Having a clear vision of your future will help you find ways to reach your career dreams. And, if you find that the current career path you are on is not fulfilling, be open to change and learn new skills.

Explore a variety of career options. During college, you can optimize your occupational wellness by visiting your campus career planning or placement office and using the resources there. Counselors can give you advice about a career path and give tips and suggestions for your résumé.

Remember these tenets of occupational wellness:

1. It is better to choose a career that is consistent with your personal values, interests, and beliefs than to select one that is unrewarding for you.
2. It is better to develop functional, transferable skills through structured involvement opportunities than to remain inactive and uninvolved.

FACTORS THAT INFLUENCE WELLNESS

Many factors influence wellness and overall health. This section covers several of these factors, including gender, race and ethnicity, income and education, genetics, location, health habits, environment, and access to health care and resources.

Gender

One of the most important factors that affects health is gender. For instance, although men are diagnosed with breast cancer, more women than men get the disease. In 2005, 186,467 women were diagnosed with breast cancer in the United States, but only 1,764 men were diagnosed with breast cancer (CDC 2007a). In addition, health care professionals diagnose and treat women differently than they treat men. Here's an example: Heart disease is the number one killer of women, but women often don't receive the proper medical care and attention to battle this disease. In addition, many medical studies have focused primarily on men. Conventional wisdom once held that women were just smaller versions of men because much of the male and female anatomy is similar. Because of the uniqueness of women, though, the National Institutes of Health (NIH) funded a 15-year, $625 million study, the Women's Health Initiative, beginning in 1991. The Women's Health Initiative focused on proving promising but unproven approaches to prevention, identifying predictors of disease, and studying community approaches to developing healthy behaviors (National Heart, Lung, and Blood Institute [NHLBI] 2007).

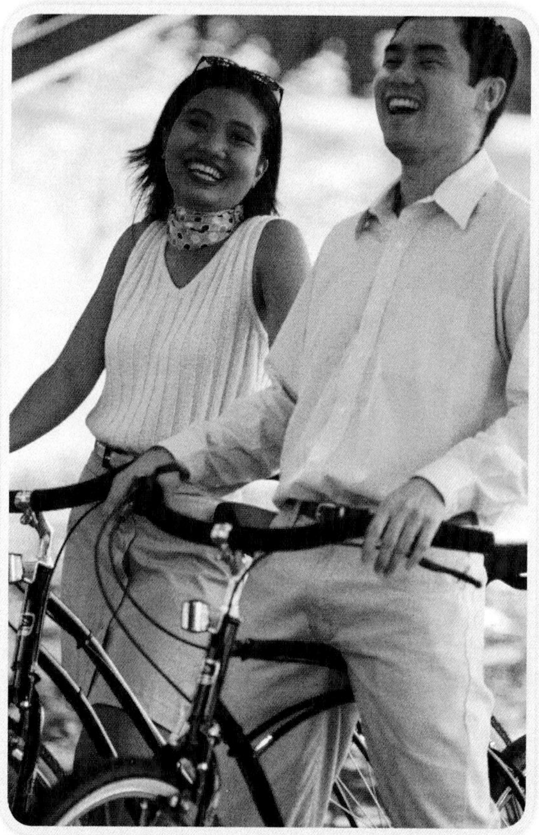

Gender and race are two factors that can affect your health and wellness.

© Eyewire

Race and Ethnicity

Other factors that can influence health are race and ethnicity. African Americans are more likely to have sickle cell anemia than any other race, for example. People who have ancestors from South or Central America, the Caribbean, the Mediterranean, India, and Saudi Arabia are also at a higher risk of developing sickle cell disease (CDC 2007h). People whose ancestors are from Northern Europe, on the other hand, are more likely to suffer from cystic fibrosis.

Each racial group has its health concerns. African Americans generally have the same leading causes of mortality as the rest of the U.S. population. However, there are higher infant mortality rates among this group. In 2000, infant mortality among African Americans reached 14.1 deaths per 1,000 live births, but the national average was only 6.9 deaths per 1,000 live births (CDC 2007c).

GENDER ISSUES

Heart Disease: Not Just a Man's Battle

Did you know that heart disease is the number one cause of death in American women? Of all American women who die each year, one in four die of heart disease. Although both men and women have heart attacks, women are more likely to die as a result. Also, while both men and women experience the common symptoms of a heart attack (including pain or uneasiness in the chest; pain in the arm, back, jaw, and neck; shortness of breath; and nausea), women are more likely to have other, less common symptoms, such as coughing, fatigue, loss of appetite, heartburn, and heart flutters.

The good news is that you can take steps to protect yourself from heart disease. First, know your numbers, especially your blood pressure, cholesterol level, and triglycerides level. High blood pressure can damage your arteries, and high levels of blood cholesterol can block your arteries; both problems prevent your heart from receiving the blood it needs. Triglycerides are fats that are found in your blood system. If you have high levels of triglycerides, you are at a higher risk of developing heart disease. Often, women who have high blood pressure, high cholesterol, or high triglyceride levels do not exhibit signs or symptoms, so it's important to have your numbers checked regularly by your health care provider.

Other important steps you can take to protect yourself from heart disease:

- Don't smoke. If you do, make your best possible attempt to quit. Various products and programs (such as nicotine patches and support groups) can help.
- Get tested for diabetes; being diabetic is a risk factor for getting heart disease.
- Maintain a healthy weight; being overweight or obese greatly increases your odds of getting heart disease. Engage in daily moderate-intensity physical activity and eat a healthy diet.
- Drink alcohol in moderation. Women should have no more than one 12-ounce (355 milliliters) beer, one 5-ounce (148 milliliters) glass of wine, or one 1.5-ounce (44 milliliters) shot of hard liquor a day.
- Learn to cope with stress, which is a factor in causing heart disease.

By being aware of the risk factors of heart disease and taking steps to protect yourself, you can avoid becoming another national statistic (Office on Women's Health 2008).

The African American population also tends to have higher rates of obesity, diabetes, high blood pressure, and stroke. For 2002, the death rate for African Americans was higher than Caucasians for CVD, including heart diseases, stroke, cancer, asthma, and diabetes. In 2004, African Americans were 1.4 times more likely to have high blood pressure compared with non-Hispanic whites (U.S. Department of Health and Human Services [USDHHS] 2006). Furthermore, African Americans were 10 percent less likely to have their blood pressure under control. Between 2001 and 2004, African American women were 70 percent more likely to be obese compared with non-Hispanic white women (USDHHS 2008). Finally, African American males are at a higher risk of developing prostate cancer, so earlier and frequent screenings are recommended for this group (CDC 2007d).

Hispanics also make up a large subsection of the non-Caucasian population in the United States. According to a 2006 estimate, approximately 44.3 million Hispanics live in the United States, and they make up approximately 15 percent of the population (USDHHS 2007b). Although Hispanics generally have lower rates of cancer, they have higher rates of obesity and diabetes than Caucasians have. The National Institute of Diabetes and Digestive and Kidney Diseases (NIDDK) reports that 73 percent of Mexican American women are overweight or obese, but only 57.6 percent of non-Hispanic white women are overweight or obese. Furthermore, in 2004, Hispanics were 1.5 times more likely to die from diabetes than their non-Hispanic counterparts (NIDDK 2007).

Asians generally have longer life expectancies than any other race in the United States. Asian American women have the longest life expectancy (85.8 years) of any group. Asian Americans usually have lower rates of CVD, and they are 50 percent less likely to die of CVD than their non-Hispanic white counterparts (USDHHS 2007a). However, Asian Americans have higher rates of osteoporosis because they generally have low bone mass and small body frames. They may experience bone fractures earlier and more frequently than other racial groups (USDHHS 2007c).

Income and Education

Socioeconomic status, which is often a reflection of income and education, is one of the main reasons for **health disparities** (inequalities in health care access and treatment) (Carter-Pokras and Baquet 2002). Socioeconomic status dictates where you live and where you obtain health services. Because income and education are closely related, people who live in poverty and have little education often suffer the most.

People with a low socioeconomic status are more likely to die prematurely and get chronic diseases. In addition, they usually have a poorer diet, don't engage in as much physical activity, and use more tobacco products than people with higher socioeconomic status (CDC 2007b, 2007e, 2007i). This population group often doesn't get adequate and timely health care for a variety of reasons. For example, women whose annual household income is less than $15,000 per year are less likely to receive mammogram screenings than their more affluent counterparts. Furthermore, women with less than a high school education are less likely to receive mammograms than women with college degrees (CDC 2005).

People with a low socioeconomic status might be uninsured or underinsured. As a result, they often must rely on hospital emergency rooms as the primary source of health care. Because they lack insurance benefits, they often put off seeing a physician until a condition has greatly worsened. This scenario then leads to missed work, and the vicious cycle continues.

Genetics

Although health habits influence wellness, genetics also play a large role in determining your health. Your genetics are determined by your parents, your grandparents, and their ancestors. Genetic makeup varies from person to person. Genes can also mutate within a person, and when they interact with other genes and other environmental factors, they can create susceptibility to a variety of illnesses such as diabetes, cancer, and stroke. For that reason, you should become aware of any chronic diseases that family members have.

What Do You Do?

Your family's health history is important to your own health. Even though health habits influence your health and wellness, genetics play a large role, too.

Talk to your parents about any chronic diseases they might have, and find out what chronic diseases your grandparents have. If your grandparents are deceased, find out the cause of death and age of death. It is also important to know of any chronic diseases that your biological aunts, uncles, and siblings may have. Knowing your family medical history is an important step to wellness. This information will also help your health care provider determine what screening tests you need to have and when.

Location

Geographic location also plays a role in overall wellness. People in the United States live mostly in rural, suburban, or urban areas. Those who live in rural areas are less likely to engage in physical activity and have less access to health care than people who live in either suburban or urban areas. In 2004, people living in rural areas reported fair or poor health, had more chronic conditions, and died from heart disease more frequently than their urban counterparts. Furthermore, rural residents reported fewer visits to health care providers and were less likely to receive recommended preventive services, such as annual mammograms or colonoscopies (USDHHS 2005). On the other hand, people in inner cities are more likely to engage in illicit drug use, unsafe sexual practice, and alcohol abuse than people who live in rural or suburban areas. They are also more likely to not get daily physical education in school and often don't have access to nutritious foods due to a condition known as a *food desert*—an urban area that provides little or no access to foods required to maintain a healthy diet.

Health Habits

Health habits influence wellness both now and in later years. Tobacco users are more likely to get emphysema, lung cancer, and CVD. Other health habits such as avoiding daily physical activity and eating a poorly balanced diet can have short-term and long-term health effects. In the short term, for example, if you don't get some activity every day and if you don't eat a balanced diet, you can compromise your immune system so that you get sick and fall behind on your work. Over the long term, if you keep getting too little daily physical activity and eating improperly, you can develop a lot of health problems. You might become overweight, for example, which can lead to other health problems such as joint pain, diabetes, and CVD. It is also vital to remember to practice safe sex, and if you use alcohol, use it in moderation.

CULTURAL ISSUES
How Does U.S. Public Health Policy Stack Up?

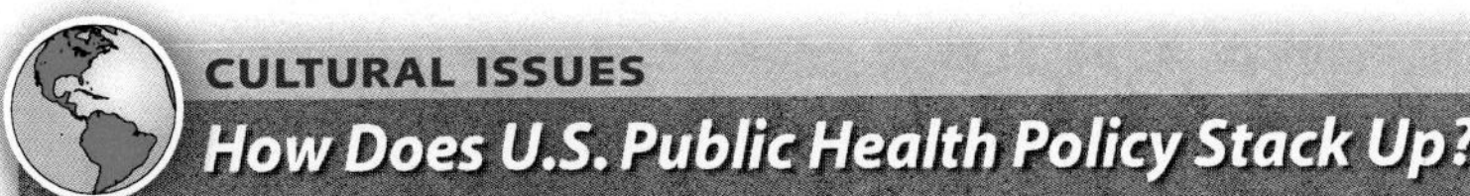

Although the United States has made considerable progress in the 20th century in the area of public health, much is left to work on. A research study published in the January and February 2008 issue of *Health Affairs* reveals that the United States is last among 19 other industrialized nations in preventable deaths (Nolte and McKee 2008). The three nations with the highest scores were France, Japan, and Australia. Preventable death is defined as death from certain causes before age 75 that could have been prevented with timely and effective health care. The idea of using preventable deaths as a way to measure health care progress came about in the 1970s. It is a way to assess the quality and performance of a health care system and track those changes over time.

What can you do to keep yourself healthy? The top three modifiable risk factors are physical inactivity, poor diet, and tobacco use. Get at least 30 minutes of moderate to vigorous physical activity on most days of the week. Also eat a well-balanced diet. If you don't know what food you should eat to be healthy and in what quantities, go to www.MyPyramid.gov, which is sponsored by the USDA and offers personalized eating plans so you can make smart food choices. Finally, if you are a tobacco user, the most important thing you can do for your health is quit! If you need help quitting, resources are available. You can receive free coaching, a free quit plan, free education materials, and referrals to local resources by calling 800-QUIT NOW.

Environment

Your environment also affects your wellness. It includes where you live, work, and play. It also reflects the quality of water you drink and the air you breathe. Where you choose to live, work, and play can greatly affect the quality of your life. If you choose to live in unsanitary conditions (such as among dirty dishes and piles of laundry), you can unknowingly affect your wellness and health. The unclean environment may cause stress and anxiety, and it could invite unwanted guests such as rodents and insects that could carry diseases. Living in an unsafe neighborhood also can affect your wellness. Constant worry about safety leads to stress and anxiety, which have an impact on wellness.

Access to Health Care and Resources

Access to health care and other health resources is a vital part of wellness. If you have adequate and timely access to proper health care, you will be treated for symptoms in a more effective and efficient manner. Preventive care is the first step to staying healthy. It helps you and your health care providers find health problems in the early stages so you can treat them more effectively.

Many services can be classified as preventive (see figure 12.2). One is obtaining a primary care physician who can help you make decisions that will help you stay healthy. You should also schedule annual physicals so that you can monitor your health over time and work with your doctor to watch for certain conditions. For example, if you know your family has a history of CVD, you will want to get a cholesterol screening at your annual physical.

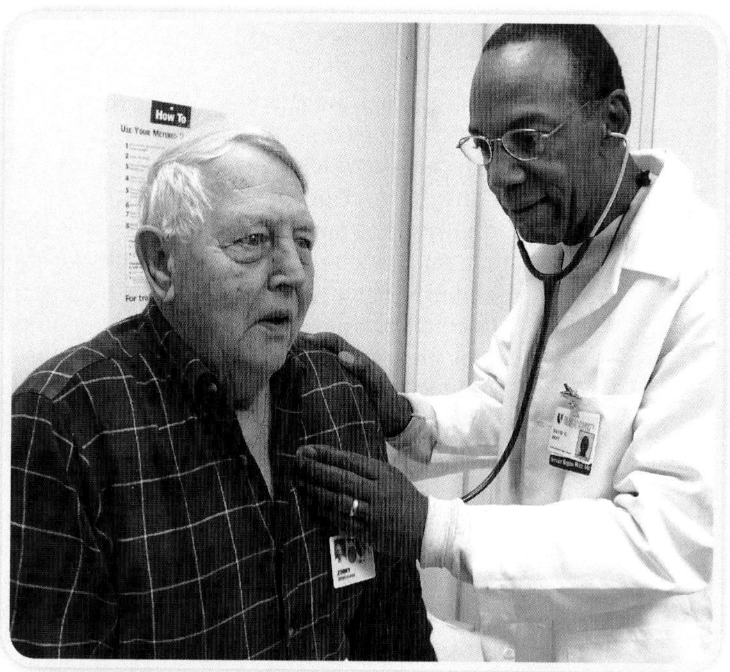

Choose a primary care physician, and visit him or her regularly to find and treat health problems efficiently.

© Human Kinetics

Males and Females

- Obtain a primary care physician
- Schedule annual physicals
- Have screenings: cholesterol, blood pressure, glucose, colonoscopy, vision
- Schedule dental exams twice a year
- Get required and recommended immunizations, especially the meningococcal vaccine

Females Only

- Schedule annual gynecological exams
- Get Pap smears (annually or less frequently)
- Have a mammogram
- Get the HPV vaccine

Figure 12.2 Follow these preventive care guidelines. The meningococcal vaccine is especially important for college students.

If you are a woman, it is crucial that you receive annual gynecological exams. The American College of Obstetricians and Gynecologists recommends women receive a Pap test within 3 years of being sexually active or starting at age 21, whichever comes first. A Pap smear is a test that helps detect cervical cancer in women by collecting cells from the cervix. Pap smears are a vital part of preventive care because detecting cervical cancer early increases the chances of successful treatment. Furthermore, regular Pap smears help detect any changes in cervical cells that could predict cancer development. Yearly Pap smears are recommended until age 30 (Mayo Clinic 2008). At that time, if a woman has at least three consecutive normal Pap smears, she can reduce the frequency of the test to once every 2 or 3 years, depending on her doctor's recommendation.

Other screenings are important to staying healthy. Typical screenings that you may have over the course of your life include cholesterol screenings, blood pressure screenings, glucose screenings for diabetes, colonoscopies to help detect colon cancer, mammograms to help detect breast cancer, and vision screenings to detect visual impairments such as cataracts or glaucoma. To determine when you should start these screenings, it is best to consult your health care provider. The age at which you should start receiving certain screenings depends not only on your personal medical history but on your family's medical history as well.

Another example of preventive care is twice-yearly dental exams. Routine dental exams and cleanings can help prevent dental problems such as gum disease, infection, and bone loss. Plus, regular dental exams can help you maintain good oral hygiene.

Receiving required and recommended immunizations is another preventive care measure. One of the most important vaccinations for college students is the meningococcal vaccine. Meningococcal meningitis is a bacterial disease that infects the fluids around the brain and spinal cord. Although anyone can get meningococcal meningitis, college students who live in dormitories and teenagers aged 15 to 19 are at an increased risk. The meningococcal meningitis vaccination protects approximately 90 percent of people who receive it (CDC 2008b).

Another important vaccination that college-aged females should receive is the human papillomavirus (HPV) vaccine. Genital human papillomavirus is the most commonly sexually transmitted virus in the United States, and more than 20 million people are infected. HPV is transmitted primarily through sexual contact. HPV detection and prevention is especially important because HPV has been linked to cervical cancer. The HPV vaccine protects against four major types of HPV, including two types that cause approximately 70 percent of cervical cancer cases and two types that cause about 90 percent of genital warts (CDC 2008b).

ISSUES IN THE NEWS

Is the HPV Vaccination for Me?

The HPV vaccine is recommended for girls aged 11 to 12. In some instances, it may be given to girls as young as 9. It is also recommended for girls and women between the ages of 13 and 26 who did not receive the vaccination when they were younger. Health care providers recommend that girls get the vaccine before their first sexual contact.

However, there are some instances where the HPV vaccination may not be right. Women who have had a serious allergic reaction to yeast, to any other part of the vaccination, or to a previous shot in the three-stage HPV vaccination should not receive the vaccination. The HPV vaccination also should not be given to pregnant women. Women who are moderately or severely ill when a new vaccination is scheduled should postpone the vaccination until they are healthy.

The HPV vaccination does have some possible side effects, including pain, redness, or swelling at the injection site; a mild to moderate fever; and itching at the injection site. Often, these symptoms do not last long and go away by themselves (CDC 2007f).

REACHING AND MAINTAINING WELLNESS

What Do You Do?

Get a copy of your immunization record and talk with your doctor about whether all of your immunizations are up to date. Plan to get any vaccinations that you may need.

To reach any sort of goal, including a wellness goal, you need to know your current status. It's also helpful to know some of the theories about why you develop specific behaviors and how you might change unhealthy ones. You can use both types of information to help set goals for developing lifelong health and wellness.

Determining Your Current Health Status

Before you can begin thinking about changing your habits to achieve wellness, you need to figure out your current behaviors and health status. Ask yourself what health habits you have now that have a positive influence on your overall wellness and then what health habits you have that have a negative influence.

People decide they want to change or adopt a health habit for a lot of reasons. For instance, serious illness may be a motivating factor for you to examine your current health habits. After you've assessed your current health status, pick one health habit you'd like to give up or one you'd like to adopt. Don't try to change all your health habits at once. Pick one habit to change, and after you've taken care of it, pick another one. You'll accomplish more by starting slowly and building on your success than if you try to focus all of your energy on changing everything at once.

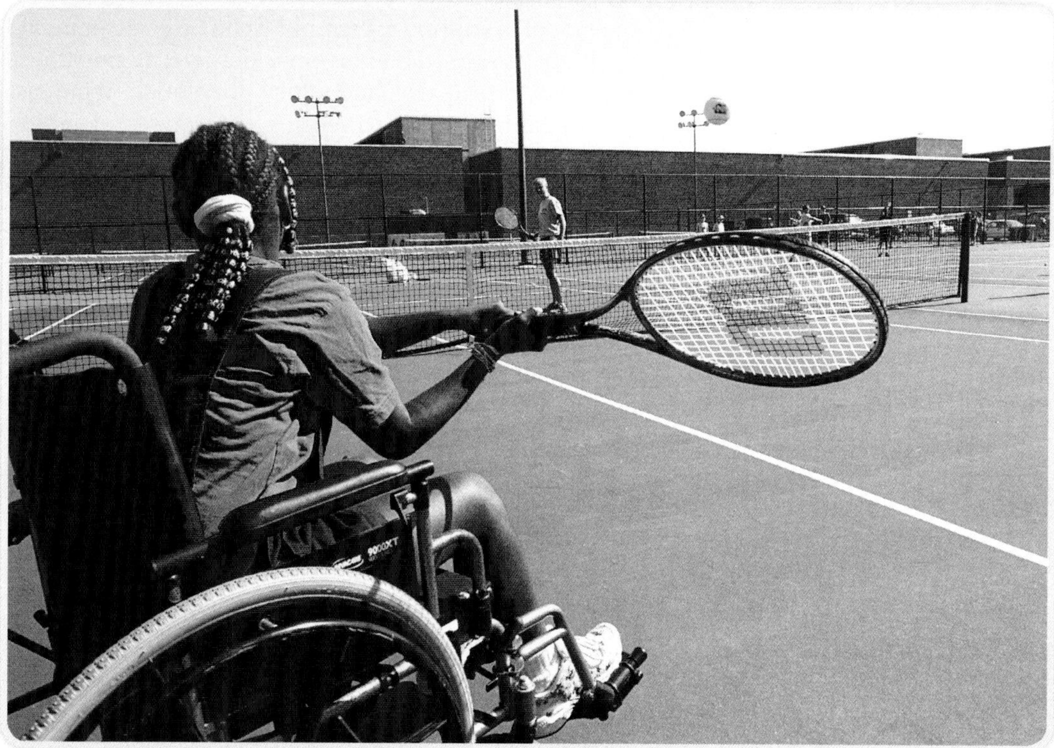

Playing active sports is a fun and healthy habit that can help improve your wellness.

© Human Kinetics

When you've decided what health behavior you're going to change, you need to find out more about it. Research the pros and cons of either adopting or eliminating a health behavior. You'll also need to figure out how to change your health behavior. That's easy for some health behaviors, but it's complicated for others. Quitting smoking is a clear-cut goal (though figuring out how to quit isn't quite so easy!). But a goal to eat a properly balanced diet is more difficult to pin down. For instance, you need to figure out if you're eating enough protein or whether you need to increase your fruit and vegetable intake. Because achieving proper nutrition is multifaceted, setting a specific goal and making a plan to achieve it might be complicated and require research.

As you work to change your health status, you might need to rely on outside resources for help. Most universities have campus health services with qualified health educators, nurses, physicians, and other health care practitioners who can help you in achieving your goal. They can provide reliable information and services. Many college campuses offer weight management programs and smoking cessation classes. In addition, you can visit your local health department to find information and to receive services.

Behavior Change Models

Determining your current health status is the first step in developing lifelong wellness. It's likely that the process revealed some health habits you'd like to change. Knowing what you want to change is the easy part; actually changing the behavior is hard. Many researchers have studied why it's so hard, and they've developed theories that provide some clues. Four of those theories are explained in this section. As you read, try to identify the theory that makes the most sense and applies most directly to you.

Transtheoretical Model

The **transtheoretical model** of behavior change was developed in the late 1970s by University of Rhode Island researchers James Prochaska and Carlo DiClemente (UCLA Center for Human Nutrition 2007). Prochaska and DiClemente initially used the model to study smokers, but it can be used for many health behaviors, including physical activity, nutrition, alcohol and drug use, and injury prevention. Whereas other health promotion theories focus on social or biological influences on behavior, this model focuses on the decision-making process. The core of the model is the **stages of change**, with the primary concept that behavior change is not a one-step process. Instead, people go through various stages on their way to adopting a healthy behavior (see figure 12.3). In addition, people progress through the stages of change at their own pace. Other concepts in the transtheoretical model include processes of change and decision balance (University of Rhode Island 2004; Kern 2008).

There are five stages of change in the transtheoretical model: precontemplation, contemplation, preparation, action, and maintenance. People need to move at their own pace through the stages if the change is to last for life. Going through the stages of change is an important part of creating and maintaining a healthy behavior (University of Rhode Island 2004).

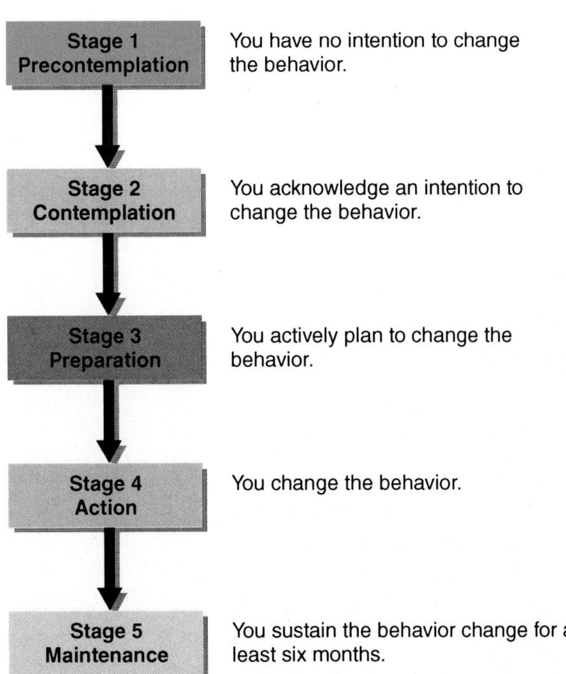

Figure 12.3 The stages of change are not necessarily linear; you can cycle through stages or jump back and forth between them.

Self-Efficacy and Social Cognitive Theory

Self-efficacy was defined by psychologist Albert Bandura as people's belief in their ability to succeed in specific situations. People with high self-efficacy believe they can master difficult tasks, and they don't avoid those kinds of challenges. Self-efficacy is a vital part of changing health behaviors because it helps determine your confidence in yourself and in your ability to change. The idea of self-efficacy is at the core of Bandura's **social cognitive theory**, which says that people behave in a certain way because of the interaction between personal factors, behavior, and the existing environment (York University 2006). It also offers these five principles:

1. People learn from watching others.
2. Learning is an internal process that may or may not change behavior.
3. Behaviors are targeted toward specific goals.
4. Behavior eventually becomes self-regulated.
5. Reinforcement and punishment have both direct and indirect effects.

Social cognitive theory is important to the field of health and wellness because it helps explain behavior change, it helps explain how people develop and maintain behavioral patterns, and it helps in designing interventions (Purdue University 2000).

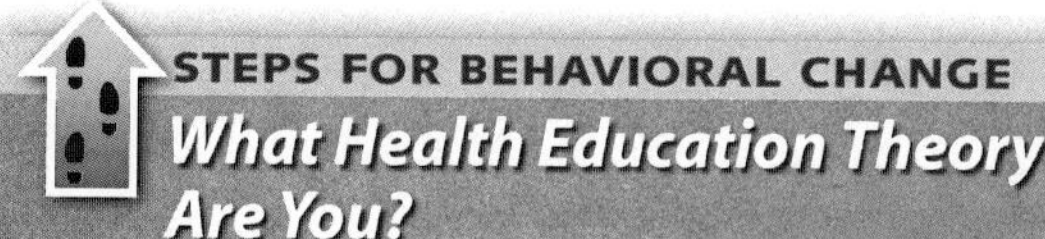

What Health Education Theory Are You?

Under "Behavior Change Models," you were asked to think about which behavior change theory was most applicable to you. Write down that theory and then make some notes about how that theory might help you change a specific health behavior. For example, say you want to get at least 7 hours of sleep each night. You've been blaming your roommate's late-night noise and the amount of homework you have for your lack of sleep. After reading about the locus of control theory, you might realize that you can take some control over the situation by asking your roommate to respect some quiet hours and by managing your time differently to get on top of your homework. Put your plans into action and evaluate your success after a week.

Health Belief Model

The **health belief model** was developed in the 1950s by social psychologists Godfrey Hochbaum, Irwin Rosenstock, and Stephen Kegels (University of Pittsburgh Graduate School of Public Health 2008). The model was developed in response to the failure of a free tuberculosis screening program. Since then, the model has been adapted for a variety of public health issues, ranging from drug use and abuse to physical activity and nutrition.

The health belief model incorporates four basic beliefs (University of Twente 2004). People will engage in a health-related action if

1. they have an interest in health matters (health motivation),
2. they think they are susceptible to a particular illness (perceived vulnerability),
3. they think the benefits of the treatment outweigh the barriers to it (perceived barriers and benefits), and
4. they think a particular illness could be severe (perceived seriousness).

We can use smoking as an example of how the health belief model might work. The first step is to identify health motivation. It could be something as simple as not taking up smoking. Then you need to figure out what your perceived vulnerability is. Are you a former smoker, for example? Third, assess what the perceived barriers and benefits to smoking would be. For instance, if you are friends with a lot of smokers, a barrier would be that your social network is made up of smokers. However, a benefit would be healthier lungs. You'd need to decide whether the benefits of not being a smoker outweigh the barriers. Finally, you need to understand the perceived seriousness of a particular disease. In our example, you'd need to decide how serious diseases such as emphysema or lung cancer are to you.

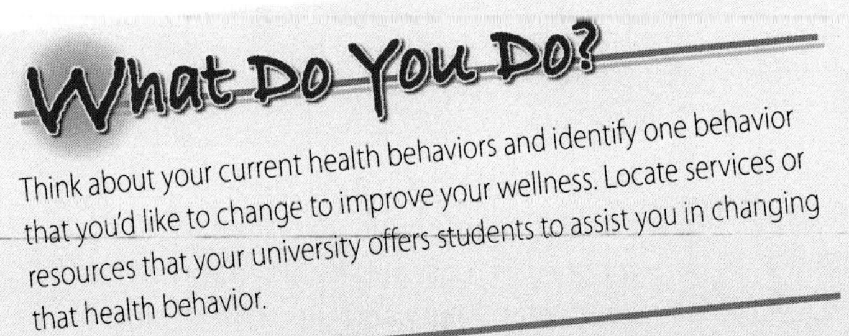

Locus of Control

Locus of control is an important aspect of personality. There are two loci of control: external and internal (Teague, Mackenzie, and Rosenthal 2006). The concept of locus of control was developed by psychologist Julian Rotter in the 1950s. Your locus of control depends on your view about the main causes of events in your life. If you have an external locus of control, you believe that outside circumstances, such as fate or destiny, guide your behaviors. People with an external locus of control often don't have the confidence in themselves to succeed in obtaining or overcoming certain health habits. But if you have an internal locus of control, you believe that your personal decisions affect your actions. As a result, you're more confident in your ability to change a behavior.

Setting SMART Goals

Now that you know how to determine your current health status and what behavior change models you can use to reach your goals, it's time to set effective goals. SMART goals have five characteristics, and each one builds on the one before it. SMART goals are **s**pecific, **m**easurable, **a**chievable, **r**ealistic, and **t**imely (adapted from Doran 1981).

Make your goals specific and measurable and develop a plan of attack to accomplish them. Write down when and where you'll try to change your behavior. For example, if your goal is to get 30 minutes of moderate physical activity a day, your plan of action can include walking to and from class each day instead of taking the bus. If your goal is to increase your fruit intake by one serving daily, you can plan to eat an extra banana every morning as part of your breakfast. A plan of action provides strategies and techniques to help you change your behavior.

If your goals are hard to achieve, you'll become frustrated easily and give up. Small goals make the overall goal seem manageable and easier to accomplish. If you've had a sedentary lifestyle, for example, a goal of doing a triathlon in the next 6 months is probably unrealistic. Instead, start small and build on small successes. You may not be able to do a triathlon in the next 6 months, but if you set and accomplish small goals, you may be able to do one eventually.

Set a date for when you will begin and when you hope to achieve your goals. Establishing a time restriction will help you plan a route to get there and measure your progress along the way.

Remember to reward yourself whenever you reach a goal. If your goal is to increase your physical activity, find a way to treat yourself each week that you get more exercise than the week before. And don't be afraid to look for support. Include the people close to you in your plan so that you'll have the support and encouragement to help you progress toward your goal.

WELLNESS THROUGHOUT LIFE 101

Achieving and maintaining wellness is an integral part of living a healthy, happy, and productive life. It is important to understand the difference between the concepts of health and wellness. It is also important to understand that health and wellness are not goals to achieve but rather the result of a lifelong process that takes time and dedication. By taking responsibility for your health and wellness, you will become a happier and more productive person.

In order to become and stay well, you need to understand the six dimensions of wellness, which are physical, intellectual, emotional, social, spiritual, and occupational wellness. As discussed, there are many ways to maintain wellness throughout your life.

Behavior change models help explain how to create wellness, including the transtheoretical model, self-efficacy and social cognitive theory, health belief model, and locus of control. The use of behavior change models is important to people who are trying to maintain a healthy lifestyle. Finally, setting SMART goals will help you in your journey to achieving and maintaining wellness.

CHAPTER REVIEW

REVIEW QUESTIONS

1. How does the World Health Organization define health?
2. Name 5 of the top 10 significant public health achievements in the United States in the 20th century.
3. Why are bacteria that were once controlled with antibiotics becoming resistant to even the most potent medications?
4. Name three ways to stay well intellectually.
5. Volunteering in the community can contribute to which dimension of wellness?
6. What is the number one cause of death in women in the United States?
7. Which racial group has higher rates of osteoporosis, and why?
8. Name two important vaccinations that college-aged females should receive.
9. What are the four basic beliefs of the health belief model?
10. What is the belief of someone who has an external locus of control? An internal locus of control?

CRITICAL THINKING

1. In your own words, describe wellness. What are some things you do on a daily basis that help improve your wellness?
2. Pick 3 of the top 10 greatest public health achievements of the 20th century. Discuss how these three achievements have had a direct impact on your wellness.

APPLICATION ACTIVITIES

1. Think about the six dimensions of wellness. Identify one thing you are currently doing to improve your wellness for each dimension. Identify one thing you can begin doing to improve your wellness for each dimension.
2. Visit your primary care facility or student health center. Talk with a physician, physician's assistant, or nurse practitioner about appropriate screening exams based on your gender, age, and family history. Get a list of these appropriate screening exams, and make sure you have them completed at the appropriate times.

GLOSSARY

emotional wellness—Ability to get through the rigors of life; aspects include self-acceptance, self-confidence, self-control, and trust.

health belief model—Behavior change theory that explains why people will participate in a health-related behavior.

health disparities—Inequalities in health care access and treatment.

intellectual wellness—Ability to engage in creative and mental activities and be open to new ideas and schools of thought.

locus of control—Behavior change theory that focuses on how people view the main causes of events in their lives. There are two loci of control: external and internal.

occupational wellness—Personal satisfaction from your career. As you strive for occupational wellness, you contribute your skills and talents to work that is meaningful and rewarding.

physical wellness—Wellness of the physical body; influenced by factors such as body weight, physical fitness, and ability to perform day-to-day functions.

self-efficacy—Your belief in your ability to succeed in specific situations.

social cognitive theory—Theory that people behave in a certain way because of interactions among personal factors, behavior, and the existing environment.

social wellness—Wellness that comes from being a contributing member of the community and society. Relates to the depth of interpersonal relationships and how you develop and maintain associations in a variety of settings.

spiritual wellness—Meaning and purpose in life; aspects include the ability to forgive, to show compassion, and to love. Traditional religious beliefs and practices are part of spiritual wellness, but it also encompasses relationships with other living things and perception and appreciation of nature, the universe, and the meaning of life.

stages of change—Core of the transtheoretical model; states that people go through five stages on their way to adopting a healthy behavior: precontemplation, contemplation, preparation, action, and maintenance.

transtheoretical model—Model of individual readiness to change a behavior that involves five stages of change: precontemplation, contemplation, preparation, action, and maintenance.

REFERENCES AND RESOURCES

Blair, S.N., A.L. Dunn, B.H. Marcus, R.A. Carpenter, and P. Jaret. 2001. *Active living every day.* Champaign, IL: Human Kinetics.

Carter-Pokras, O., and C. Baquet. 2002. What is a "health disparity"? www.publichealthreports.org/userfiles/117_5/117426.pdf.

Centers for Disease Control and Prevention (CDC). 1999. Ten great public health achievements—United States, 1900-1999. www.cdc.gov/mmwr/PDF/wk/mm4812.pdf.

———. 2005. Breast cancer screening and socioeconomic status. www.cdc.gov/mmwr/preview/mmwrhtml/mm5439a2.htm.

———. 2007a. Breast cancer statistics. www.cdc.gov/cancer/breast/statistics/.

———. 2007b. Cigarette smoking among adults. www.cdc.gov/mmwr/PDF/wk/mm5644.pdf.

———. 2007c. Eliminate disparities in infant mortality. www.cdc.gov/omhd/amh/factsheets/infant.htm.

———. 2007d. Eliminate health disparities in cancer screening and management. www.cdc.gov/omhd/amh/factsheets/cancer.htm.

———. 2007e. Fruit and vegetable consumption among adults. www.cdc.gov/mmwr/preview/mmwrhtml/mm5610a2.htm.

———. 2007f. HPV (human papillomavirus) vaccine: What you need to know. www.cdc.gov/vaccines/pubs/vis/downloads/vis-hpv.pdf.

———. 2007g. Prevalence of overweight among children and adolescents: United States, 2003-2004. www.cdc.gov/nchs/products/pubs/pubd/hestats/overweight/overwght_child_03.htm.

———. 2007h. Sickle cell disease. www.cdc.gov/ncbddd/sicklecell/faq_traits.htm.

———. 2007i. U.S. physical activity statistics. http://apps.nccd.cdc.gov/PASurveillance/DemoCompareResultV.asp?State=1&Cat=2&Year=2006&Go=G.

———. 2008a. New CDC study finds no increase in obesity in adults; but levels still high. www.cdc.gov/nchs/pressroom/07newsreleases/obesity.htm.

———. 2008b. Vaccine information statements. www.cdc.gov/vaccines/pubs/vis/default.htm.

Doran, G.T. 1981. There's a S.M.A.R.T. way to write management's goals and objectives. *AMA Forum* (November): 35-36.

Healthy People 2010. 2000. *Healthy People 2010.* www.healthypeople.gov.

Henry J. Kaiser Family Foundation. 2007. Uninsured and their access to health care. www.kff.org.

Kern, M.F. 2008. Stages of change model. www.addictioninfo.org/articles/11/1/Stages-of-Change-Model/Page1.html.

Mayo Clinic. 2007. Are infectious diseases on the rise? www.mayoclinic.com.

———. 2008. Pap smear. www.mayoclinic.com/health/pap-smear/MY00090.

National Heart, Lung, and Blood Institute (NHLBI). 2007. Women's Health Initiative. www.nhlbi.nih.gov/whi/background.htm.

National Institute of Diabetes and Digestive and Kidney Diseases (NIDDK). 2007. Prevalence statistics related to overweight and obesity. http://win.niddk.nih.gov/statistics/#preval.

National Wellness Institute. 2007. Six dimensional model of wellness. www.nationalwellness.org/index.php?id_tier=2&id_c=25.

Nolte, E., and C.M. McKee. 2008. Measuring the health of nations: Updating an earlier analysis. *Health Affairs* 27 (1): 58-71.

Office on Women's Health. 2008. Frequently asked questions: Heart disease. www.womenshealth.gov/faq/heart-disease.cfm.

Oklahoma Cooperative Extension Services. 2008. Wellness for older adults in daily life. http://pods.dasnr.okstate.edu/docushare/dsweb/Get/Document-4989/T-2237web.pdf.

Purdue University. 2000. Social cognitive theory. www.edst.purdue.edu/moon/EDPS235/lectures/00-01-19%20Social%20Cognitive%20Theory%20Outline.htm.

Teague, M.L., S.L.C. Mackenzie, and D.M. Rosenthal. 2006. *Your health today: Choices in a changing society.* New York: McGraw-Hill.

UCLA Center for Human Nutrition. 2007. Prochaska and DiClemente's stages of change model. www.cellinteractive.com/ucla/physcian_ed/stages_change.html.

University of Pittsburgh Graduate School of Public Health. 2008. Health belief model. www.publichealth.pitt.edu.

University of Rhode Island. 2004. Cancer Prevention Research Center transtheoretical model. www.uri.edu/research/cprc/transtheoretical.htm.

University of Twente. 2004. Health belief model. www.cw.utwente.nl/theorieenoverzicht/Theory%20clusters/Health%20Communication/Health_Belief_Model.doc/.

U.S. Department of Agriculture (USDA). 2008. MyPyramid. www.mypyramid.gov.

U.S. Department of Health and Human Services (USDHHS). 2005. Health care disparities in rural areas. www.ahrq.gov/research/ruraldisp/ruraldispar.htm.

———. 2006. Heart disease and African Americans. www.omhrc.gov/templates/content.aspx?ID=3018.

———. 2007a. Asian American/Pacific Islander profile. www.omhrc.gov/templates/browse.aspx?lvl=2&lvlID=53.

———. 2007b. Hispanic/Latino profile. www.omhrc.gov/templates/browse.aspx?lvl=2&lvlID=54.

———. 2007c. Osteoporosis. www.4woman.gov/minority/asianamerican/osteoporosis.cfm.

———. 2008. Obesity data/statistics. www.omhrc.gov/templates/browse.aspx?lvl=3&lvlid=537.

York University. 2006. Theories used in IS research: Social cognitive theory. www.istheory.yorku.ca/socialcognitivetheory.htm.

Other helpful resources include the following.

Donatelle, R.J., and P. Ketcham. 2007. *Access to health.* 10th ed. San Francisco: Benjamin Cummings.

Eastern Illinois University. 2007. Health belief model. www.ux1.eiu.edu/~jcdietz/HST%203700/The%20Health%20Belief%20Model.ppt.

Eastern Michigan University. 2007a. Six dimensions of wellness. www.emich.edu/uhs/sixdimensions.html.

———. 2007b. Wellness. www.emich.edu/wellness/.

Insel, P. 2005. *Core concepts in health.* 10th ed. New York: McGraw-Hill.

Payne, W.A. 2007. *Understanding your health.* 9th ed. New York: McGraw-Hill.

INDEX

B

F

N